A Concise Textbook
of Radiology

A Concise Textbook of Radiology

Edited by

Peter Armstrong MB, BS, FMed Sci, FRCP, FRCR
Professor of Radiology
St Bartholomew's Hospital
London, UK

Martin L. Wastie MB, BChir, FRCP, FRCR
Consultant Radiologist
University Hospital
Nottingham, UK

A member of the Hodder Headline Group
LONDON
Co-published in the USA by Oxford University Press, Inc., New York

First published in Great Britain in 2001 by
Arnold, a member of the Hodder Headline Group,
338 Euston Road, London NWI 3BH

http://www.arnoldpublishers.com

Co-published in the USA by
Oxford University Press, Inc.,
198 Madison Avenue, New York, NY 10016
Oxford is a registered trademark of Oxford University Press

Whilst the advice and information in this book is believed to be
true and accurate at the date of going to press, neither the
author[s] nor the publisher can accept any legal responsibility or
liability for any errors or omissions that may be made. In
particular (but without limiting the generality of the preceding
disclaimer) every effort has been made to check drug dosages;
however, it is still possible that errors have been missed.
Furthermore, dosage schedules are constantly being revised and
new side-effects recognized. For these reasons the reader is
strongly urged to consult the drug companies' printed instructions
before administering any of the drugs recommended in this book.

British Library Cataloguing in Publication Data
A catalogue record for this book is available from the British
Library

Library of Congress Cataloging-in-Publication Data
A catalog record for this book is available from the Library of
Congress

ISBN 0 340 75938 0

Publisher: Nick Dunton
Project Editor: Sarah de Souza
Production Editor: James Rabson
Production Controller: Martin Kerans
Project Manager: Anne Waddingham
Cover design: Terry Griffiths

Typeset in 10/12 pt Minion by
Scribe Design, Gillingham, Kent, UK
Colour separation by Tenon & Polert Colour Scanning Ltd,
Hong Kong, China
Printed and bound in Great Britain by The University Press,
Cambridge

What do you think about this book? Or any other Arnold title?
Please send your comments to feedback.arnold@hodder.co.uk

Contents

Contributors

Andreas N. Adam MB, BS, FRCP, FRCR, FRCS
King's College, London, UK

Peter Armstrong MB, BS, FMed Sci, FRCP, FRCR
St Bartholomew's Hospital, London, UK

Sarah Burnett MB, BS, MRCP, FRCR, MBA
St Mary's Hospital, London, UK

Iain R. Colquhoun MB, BS, FRCS, FRCR
Charing Cross Hospital, London, UK

Andrew J. Evans MB, ChB, MRCP, FRCR
City Hospital, Nottingham, UK

Richard Farrow BSc, MB, BS, MRCP, FRCR
Treliske Hospital, Truro, UK

Stuart Field MA, MB, BChir, DMRD, FRCR
Kent & Canterbury Hospital, Canterbury, UK

Roger H. S. Gregson BSc, MB, BS, FRCR
University Hospital, Nottingham, UK

Donald M. Hadley PhD, MB, ChB, FRCR, DMRD
Institute of Neurological Sciences, Glasgow, UK

Jane M. Hawnaur MB, ChB, MRCP, DMRD, FRCR
University of Manchester, Manchester, UK

Jeremiah C. Healy MB, BChir, MRCP, FRCR
Chelsea and Westminster Hospital, London, UK

Tim Jaspan BSc, MB, ChB, FRCP, FRCR
University Hospital, Nottingham, UK

James McIvor FDSRCS, FRCR
Late of Charing Cross Hospital and Eastman Dental
Institute, London, UK

Ivan Moseley MD, PhD, FRCP, FRCR
Moorfields Eye Hospital, London, UK

Rodney H. Reznek FRCP, FRCR
St Bartholomew's Hospital, London, UK

Asif Saifuddin BSc, MB, ChB, MRCP, FRCR
Royal National Orthopaedic Hospital, Stanmore, UK

Giles W. Stevenson FRCP, FRCR, FRCP(C)
McMaster University Medical Center, Hamilton, Ontario,
Canada

Peter Twining MB, BS, FRCR
University Hospital, Nottingham, UK

Martin L. Wastie MB, BChir, FRCP, FRCR
University Hospital, Nottingham, UK

Anthony F. Watkinson BSc, MSc, MB, BS, FRCS, FRCR
Royal Free Hospital, London, UK

Judith A. W. Webb BSc, MD, FRCP, FRCR
St Bartholomew's Hospital, London, UK

Simon C. Whitaker MB, BChir, MRCP, FRCR
University Hospital, Nottingham, UK

Brian K. Wignall MB, ChB, MRCP, FRCR
Charing Cross Hospital, London, UK

R. Peter H. Wilde BSc, BM, BCh, MRCP, FRCR
Bristol Royal Infirmary, Bristol, UK

A. Robin M. Wilson MB, ChB, FRCR, FRCP(E)
City Hospital, Nottingham, UK

Acknowledgements

Many individuals are involved in the production of a medical text book. Our heartfelt thanks go to the many contributors who revised their chapters from *Diagnostic and interventional radiology in surgical practice* to make the book suitable for a wider readership. Our special thanks go to the new contributors of the additional chapters. In spite of being hassled and cajoled, everyone has managed to keep to a strict timetable.

Our many thanks go to the secretaries who typed the manuscripts and revisions. In particular Tiina Wastie gave much assistance in the production of the book. Secretarial help was also provided by Linda Hopkinson, Julie Jessop and Veronica Nettleship.

We would like to thank Anne Waddingham for her part in creating such an excellent layout and Michèle Clarke for her copyediting and indexing skills. Sarah de Souza of Arnold has been a tower of strength during the whole production of the book. Our thanks go to her and the staff of Arnold.

Preface

The radiological literature abounds with elementary texts and specialized books on different body systems or imaging modalities. Various multivolume reference series exist, but what is lacking is a succinct single volume work covering the whole field of radiology that gives basic radiological knowledge to the trainee in the initial stages of training. The greater use of imaging by clinicians, the introduction of new imaging modalities and the wide acceptance of interventional radiology has greatly increased the scope and importance of radiology.

A version of this book was previously published as *Diagnostic imaging and interventional radiology in surgical practice*. It quickly became apparent that the book would be very suitable for radiologists, so the current version has been expanded to cover the whole of radiology by including 'medical' as well as 'surgical' conditions.

Each chapter describes the use of various imaging modalities and then gives an account of the radiological changes in disease enumerating the likely diagnosis and signs rather than producing encyclopaedic lists. The important role of interventional radiology is brought to the fore.

It is not possible in a book of this size to give details of the pathological aspects of the various conditions nor to discuss patient management. The aim is to give the radiology trainee and the interested clinician an introduction to the wide field of radiology. The most appropriate imaging modalities are suggested together with the indications for interventional procedures.

We hope this book will be of use to radiologists at the beginning of their specialist training.

PA
MLW
November 2000

Imaging techniques

PETER ARMSTRONG, JANE M. HAWNAUR, RODNEY H. REZNEK, MARTIN L. WASTIE,
SIMON C. WHITAKER

USE OF THE IMAGING DEPARTMENT

X-ray and imaging departments need to be efficiently used in order to minimize radiation hazard and be cost-effective. Good communication between clinician and radiologist is vital: the radiology staff need to know and understand the clinical problem in order to carry out appropriate tests and to interpret the results in a meaningful way; the clinicians need to understand the strengths and limitations of the investigations they request.

Sensible selection of investigations is most important. Laying down precise guidelines for requesting the various imaging examinations is difficult because patients are managed differently in different centres and the information required varies significantly. The Royal College of Radiologists has published a very useful booklet *Making the best use of a department of clinical radiology: guidelines for doctors* (4th edn, 1998, Royal College of Radiologists, London, UK). It gives the following advice:

> A useful investigation is one in which the result – positive or negative – will alter management or add confidence to the clinician's diagnosis. A significant number of radiological investigations do not fulfil these aims. Unnecessary investigations increase waiting times, waste limited resources, lower standards and may add unnecessarily to patient irradiation.

The chief causes of the wasteful use of radiology are:

1 Investigation when results are unlikely to affect patient management: because the anticipated 'positive' finding is usually irrelevant, e.g. degenerative spinal disease (as 'normal' as grey hairs from early middle age) or because a positive finding is so unlikely. DO I NEED IT?

2 Investigation too often: i.e. before the disease could have progressed or resolved or before the results influence treatment. DO I NEED IT NOW?

3 Repeating investigations which have already been done: e.g. at another hospital, in an Outpatient Department, or in Accident & Emergency. HAS IT BEEN DONE ALREADY?

4 Failing to provide appropriate clinical information and questions that the radiological investigation should answer: deficiencies here may lead to the wrong radiographs being obtained (e.g. the omission of an essential view). HAVE I EXPLAINED THE PROBLEM?

5 Doing the wrong investigation: imaging techniques are developing rapidly; it is often helpful to discuss an investigation with a radiologist before it is requested. IS THIS THE BEST INVESTIGATION?

X-RAY PRODUCTION

The production of X-rays is the same for both conventional radiography and computed tomography (CT).

X-rays are produced when a stream of electrons from a heated tungsten filament, the cathode, hits a target anode, usually made of tungsten. The electrons are accelerated by applying a high voltage in the range of 70–140 kV between the anode and cathode both of which are enclosed in a vacuum tube. Metal shielding around the X-ray tube absorbs unwanted X-rays and allows a beam of X-rays to emerge (Fig. 1.1). Less than 1% of the energy of the electrons is converted into X-rays; the rest is converted into heat and the dissipation of heat is an important factor in the design of X-ray tubes, especially those used for CT.

Figure 1.1 *X-ray tube.*

CONVENTIONAL RADIOGRAPHY

PHOTOGRAPHIC EFFECT

The formation of images in a conventional radiograph is dependent on the differential absorption of X-rays by calcified structures, soft tissues, fat and gas. The resulting unabsorbed X-rays passing through the body cause blackening of a photographic film that is then processed. The film, which is sensitive to both light and radiation, is enclosed in a light-proof cassette and the film is sandwiched between two intensifying screens. These screens convert the radiation to light that is detected by the film. It is mainly the light emitted from these intensifying screens that cause blackening of the developed film. The use of intensifying screens allows lower exposures and, therefore, a reduction in radiation dose to the patient.

GRIDS

Grids are employed to improve the image quality by removing scattered radiation which would otherwise cause blurring of the film. A grid consists of thin strips of lead separated by transparent material.

PROJECTION

By convention the projection assigned to a radiograph is determined by the direction of the X-ray beam through the body. Hence in a postero-anterior (PA) film, which is the normal projection for a chest X-ray, the patient has the sternum against the X-ray cassette and the X-ray beam traverses from the back to the front of the chest, whereas for an anteroposterior (AP) film the beam passes from front to back and the patient's back is against the film.

HORIZONTAL BEAM

For the detection of air–fluid levels or free abdominal gas, the film must be taken with a horizontal beam. The analogy can be made with a glass of water: the only way to see the fluid level is to look from the side in a horizontal direction. Another use of a horizontal beam is in a lateral decubitus film for which the patient lies on either the right or left side. The result is an AP projection, but with a horizontal beam.

PORTABLE FILMS

Films taken on the ward with the use of portable X-ray equipment should be avoided if possible. The films tend to be of inferior quality as positioning of the patient is difficult and longer exposures are needed, resulting in blurring from respiratory movement. Also, the radiation dose to patients and staff is higher than with films taken in the radiology department.

FLUOROSCOPY

X-rays striking a fluorescent screen cause it to emit a minute amount of light. By means of an image intensifier the image can be made sufficiently bright to be viewed on a television monitor and, if necessary, a permanent record may be made of the image. Fluoroscopy has had a profound impact on imaging as it allows interventional procedures (such as biopsy, catheterization and orthopaedic manoeuvres), to be performed under direct vision. All examinations of the gastrointestinal tract are performed with fluoroscopy, as peristalsis can be observed and the patient positioned for the optimum images to be recorded.

SUBTRACTION

This technique of removing unwanted images from a film is normally used in angiography to eliminate the bone and soft tissue images, so leaving the contrast-filled vessels clearly visible. Nowadays this is performed electronically and is widely used in the form of digital subtraction angiography (DSA).

RADIATION HAZARDS

Because of the energy they possess, X-rays cause ionization and so alter molecules in tissue leading to adverse biological effects. Most ionizing radiation comes from the sun and from the earth's core; medical radiation accounts for about 12 per cent of the total radiation received by humans. Other artificial sources, such as nuclear fallout, account for only 1 per cent of the total amount.

Some organs are more sensitive to radiation than others. The gonads are highly sensitive and are irradiated in X-rays of the lumbar spine and pelvis; they receive a particularly high dose from a barium enema and pelvic CT.

The major adverse effects of radiation are the induction of cancer and genetic effects. There is no dose threshold below which no harmful effect will occur; thus all ionizing radiation is potentially harmful.

Irradiating the fetus *in utero* is especially hazardous as rapidly dividing cells are particularly radiosensitive. The main risk if the induction of childhood cancer and leukaemia. The natural risk in childhood is 1:650 but a high radiation examination such as barium enema or pelvic CT during pregnancy doubles this risk. The natural frequency of genetic disease manifesting at birth is between 1 and 3 per cent. A high radiation examination in pregnancy increases this risk by only 0.1 per cent.

DOSE MEASUREMENT

The maximum radiation dose limit for the general public and occupationally exposed workers has been determined by the International Commission on Radiological Protection (ICRP). Hospital personnel can wear small dosemeters to measure the radiation that they receive. This may be a film badge, which will show blackening when exposed to radiation, or a thermoluminescence dosemeter (TLD), which stores the energy from the radiation. TLD monitors may be sufficiently small to enable the dose to the fingers to be measured.

DOSE LIMITATION

Because all ionizing radiation is harmful and there is no safe lower threshold of radiation, everyone must strive to keep the radiation dose to the patient as low as reasonably achievable. The radiology department must use a meticulous radiographic technique and up-to-date equipment. However, there is an onus on the referring clinician who should contribute by:

- avoiding unnecessary examinations or examination not of direct relevance, e.g. there is no indication for a routine preoperative chest X-ray;
- ensuring the examination has not already been performed, and waiting an appropriate time before requesting a repeat examination, e.g. a week should elapse before a follow-up film is requested in an uncomplicated pneumonia;
- using an alternative technique, such as ultrasound or MRI, which does not involve ionizing radiation;
- avoiding whenever possible the use of X-rays during pregnancy.

It has been calculated in the UK that if these radiation-reducing methods were implemented, including the elimination of unnecessary examinations, it would be possible to reduce the number of radiation-induced cancer fatalities by over 100 cases a year.

PICTURE ARCHIVING AND COMMUNICATION SYSTEMS (PACS)

Over the past three decades, digital recording has developed dramatically. CT, ultrasound, MRI, nuclear medicine, fluoroscopy and angiography are all now recorded in a digital format. Even conventional radiographs, which currently use analog film/screen combinations, can be based on digital information. For digital radiography, the radiograph is produced on a special phosphor screen and read by a laser, which then writes the image onto film, or the image can be displayed on a TV monitor. A TV image can be altered by adjusting the window level or width as described (see p. 12) in the section on CT.

One of the advantages of digital data is that it can be processed by a computer and allows electronic transmission between sites, buildings and even countries and, most importantly, allows computer storage. Another advantage of digital data is that computers can be used to manipulate the images, an ability most dramatically illustrated by three-dimensional or multiplanar reconstructions.

A fully digital department would obviate the need for X-ray films with a potential saving in film costs. Also, images with their report could be viewed in the wards and clinics on television monitors. Outlying hospitals could send images into a central radiology department. Lost films would become a thing of the past. The inability to lose images, the simultaneous display of different studies and the ability to enhance these images are all great advantages of a digital system, but further technical developments will be needed before filmless radiology departments become widespread and cost-effective.

INTRAVENOUS CONTRAST AGENTS FOR UROGRAPHY, ANGIOGRAPHY AND COMPUTED TOMOGRAPHY

The intravenous and angiographic contrast agents rely on iodine in solution to absorb X-rays. The same agents are used for urography, angiography and contrast enhancement at computed tomography (CT). Usually they are given in large doses, often with rapid rates of injection. Since their only purpose is to produce opacification, ideally they should be pharmacologically inert. This has not yet been totally achieved, though the introduction of low-osmolality agents, such as the non-ionic media, has been a great advance in reducing adverse effects. The advantage of the newer agents is that they have a lower osmolality than the ionic contrast media previously in general use and are therefore safer. The disadvantage of the newer agents is that they are considerably more expensive than their predecessors. The following discussion applies particularly to the older ionic agents: the same complications occur with the newer low-osmolality agents, but with lesser frequency.

Patients may experience a feeling of warmth spreading over the body as the contrast medium is injected; a few find this feeling objectionable. Sometimes, particularly with slow injections of the more concentrated solutions, pain occurs in the upper arm and shoulder due to stasis in the veins. When this occurs it is helpful to raise the patient's arm at the end of the injection.

Nausea, vomiting or light-headedness are experienced by a few patients and some will develop an urticarial rash. All these phenomena usually subside spontaneously. Contrast inadvertently injected outside the vein can be very painful and should be carefully guarded against.

Bronchospasm, laryngeal oedema or hypotension occasionally develop and may be so severe as to be life-threatening. It is, therefore, essential to be prepared for these dangerous reactions and to have available the equipment and drugs to cope with them. Approximately one in 160 000 patients dies as a consequence of ionic contrast agents, a risk which, although small, should not be ignored.

Patients with known allergic manifestations, particularly asthma, are more likely to have an adverse reaction. Similarly, patients who have had a previous reaction to contrast agents have a higher than average risk of problems during the examination. Such patients are usually premedicated with steroids, preferably for at least 18 hours prior to the examination. Antihistamine drugs may also be given shortly before the contrast injection.

High-risk groups are given low-osmolality agents to help minimize complications from contrast injections. Patients with a higher than average risk of complications from intravenous contrast injections include:

- **infants**, who are at risk from a rapid rise in plasma osmolality because of the high osmolality of the injected contrast agent; even with low-osmolality agents the injection rate in infants should, when possible, be slow;
- **elderly patients**, who often tolerate the injected contrast medium poorly;
- **those with known heart disease**; arrhythmias are a risk in these patients;
- **those with renal failure, myeloma or severe diabetes**; even the non-ionic agents have a temporary adverse effect on renal function. (Patients are more likely to show a deterioration of renal function owing to the contrast medium if they are deprived of fluids prior to the examination.)

RADIONUCLIDE IMAGING

Radionuclide imaging depends on the fact that radionuclides can be tagged to certain substances which concentrate selectively in different parts of the body. These substances are known as radiopharmaceuticals and are most often administered by intravenous injection (Fig. 1.2). For most diagnostic tests in nuclear medicine, radionuclides emitting gamma radiation are used. The gamma radiation can be detected and an image produced by means of a gamma camera. When a photon of gamma radiation strikes an activated sodium iodide crystal, the crystal scintillates emitting a small flash of light. A gamma camera consists of a large activated sodium iodide crystal with a large number of photomultiplier tubes facing the crystal. Nowadays, most gamma cameras are double headed, with each head having a separate sodium iodide crystal. Each photomultiplier tube generates a signal proportional to the amount of light it receives. The location of the scintillations can be determined and so an image can be produced which, if desired, may be recorded on X-ray film. Each detected photon is recorded as a count. Between 300 000 and 500 000 counts are needed to produce a satisfactory image, necessitating about 3–5 minutes to obtain the image.

EMISSION TOMOGRAPHY

In this technique the gamma camera moves around the patient. A computer can analyse the information and produce sectional images which, as in MRI, may be reconstructed in any plane. However, the spatial resolution of emission tomography is inferior to both CT and

Figure 1.2
Radionuclide bone scan. The patient has received an intravenous injection of a ⁹⁹ᵐTc-labelled complex organic phosphate. This agent is taken up by the bones in proportion to bone turnover and blood flow so that an image of the skeleton can be produced.

Figure 1.4 *FDG PET scan in a patient with lung cancer showing tumour in the mediastinum, and rib metastases.*

POSITRON EMISSION TOMOGRAPHY

Positron emission tomography (PET) uses short-lived positron emitting isotopes to study a variety of biochemical and metabolic processes. The positron travels less than 3 mm before being annihilated with an electron producing two gamma rays, which can be detected with a specialized gamma camera to produce cross-sectional images. Because of the short half-lives of these isotopes, they must be produced by a cyclotron immediately before use. Positron emitting isotopes in use are carbon-11, nitrogen-13 and oxygen-15, but the one most commonly employed is fluorine-18 as the pharmaceutical F-18 fluorodeoxyglucose (FDG). This is an analogue of glucose and is taken up into cells in proportion to glucose metabolism, which is increased in tumour cells. PET using FDG is used in the staging and follow-up of cancer (Fig. 1.4) and the differentiation of benign from malignant lung nodules. Additional uses are in cardiology to detect viable myocardium prior to surgical revascularization, and in neurology to evaluate patients with intractable epilepsy for possible surgery. With other pharmaceuticals, complex biochemical processes such as neurotransmitter binding and storage, and protein and DNA synthesis can be studied.

MRI. Since only one usable photon is emitted for each disintegration, the technique is also known as single photon emission computed tomography (SPECT). Conventional radionuclides such as technetium-99m or thallium-201 are used.

The main applications of SPECT are in the spine, especially in the detection of focal abnormalities such as spondylolysis (Fig. 1.3), in the heart for the diagnosis of myocardial ischaemia, and in the brain in conjunction with blood flow or tumour-localizing agents.

Figure 1.3 *SPECT bone scan through L5 showing increased uptake in a spondylolysis of the pars interarticularis of L5 (arrow). The increased uptake was much more clearly seen on SPECT than on planar views.*

DYNAMIC IMAGING

Another advantage of radionuclide imaging is that not only are anatomical images produced, dynamic scans

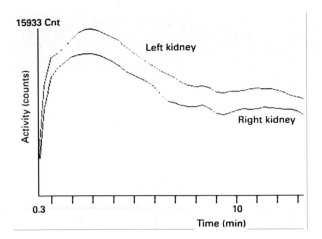

Figure 1.5 *Renogram. When rapid serial images are taken after an intravenous injection of ^{99m}Tc-DTPA, which is excreted by the kidneys, an activity–time curve is produced giving information on renal function.*

may also be performed so that function may be measured. With the use of a computer, rapid serial images may be taken and an activity/time curve produced. This technique is employed in renography to measure renal function (Fig. 1.5).

RADIOPHARMACEUTICALS

Radiopharmaceuticals must be regarded from both their biological and radiation standpoint. The radiopharmaceutical must localize safely in a certain organ or compartment within the body and stay there long enough to be imaged. Technetium-99m is the most commonly used radionuclide. It has a convenient half-life of 6 hours which is short enough to limit the radiation dose to the patient but sufficiently long to enable the imaging study to be completed. Technetium-99m emits only gamma radiation and this radiation is of a suitable energy for detection by the gamma camera. Moreover it is easily prepared at any time from a molybdenum-99 generator. Because of its chemical nature it can be incorporated into various radiopharmaceuticals in order to localize in different parts of the body.

Other radionuclides in common use include iodine-123, thallium-201, gallium-67, indium-111, and the gases krypton-81m and xenon-133.

Cell labelling, usually with technetium-99m, has become an important technique. Labelled leucocyte scanning is employed for the detection of inflammation and abscesses. Labelling of the red blood cells enables gastrointestinal blood loss to be detected and, because it provides blood pool imaging, it permits cardiac imaging to be performed. Monoclonal antibodies that are raised against tumours can be radiolabelled and thereby detect sites of tumour in the body.

SAFETY OF RADIONUCLIDE IMAGING

Although radionuclide imaging employs ionizing radiation, the patient dose in most examinations is quite low. Once the patient has received the radiopharmaceutical, no further radiation is incurred by repeated imaging, unlike in CT or conventional radiography.

ULTRASOUND

Ultrasound has become a readily available and much used examination in a wide variety of situations. Ultrasound imaging is based on the fact that if high frequency sound is directed into the body from a transducer placed on the skin, some of the sound is reflected by tissue interfaces in the body to produce echoes, which are picked up by the same transducer and converted into an image. All ultrasound examinations are now performed with real-time imaging, a system which produces images fast enough to allow motion to be followed. In any position of the transducer, the image obtained is that of a slice; thus to obtain information about the whole of an organ or region, the transducer must be moved and angled to produce a number of slices. Hence there are no fixed projections and the image acquisition and subsequent interpretation depends greatly on the skill of the operator.

Since air and bone absorb the ultrasound beam, gas-filled and bony structures are unable to be imaged. Ultrasound is unable to cross a tissue–gas or tissue–bone boundary; therefore deeper structures may be obscured. Bowel gas frequently limits visualization of abdominal structures, and ultrasound plays little part in the diagnosis of lung or bone pathology.

Ultrasound is produced by a transducer constructed of a piezoelectric crystal, which changes thickness when a voltage is applied across it. When electrically pulsed, the crystal resonates, producing high frequency sound depending on the thickness of the crystal. Not only is the transducer the transmitter, it also acts as the receiver producing a small electric signal when an ultrasound wave strikes it. Very short pulses of sound lasting about a millionth of a second are transmitted by the transducer about a thousand times a second.

For diagnostic use the frequency of the ultrasound ranges from 2.5 MHz to 13 MHz. The skin is smeared with a jelly-like substance in order to effect acoustic coupling between the skin and the transducer. The ultrasound beam travels through tissue at a near constant velocity of 1540 m/s. The time delay between the initiation of a pulse and the return of an echo is proportional to the distance the beam has travelled. This distance can be calculated from the velocity of sound in tissues. Distance is essential information needed to place the echoes in the correct position. It also allows accurate measurement to be made from ultrasound images.

Figure 1.6 *Acoustic enhancement. The area behind the cyst (C) in the upper pole of the right kidney shows brighter echoes as more sound traverses the cyst. No echoes are seen from the cyst itself. D = diaphragm.*

Figure 1.7 *Acoustic shadowing. The area behind the stone (S) in the gall bladder shows reduced echoes as sound does not pass through the stone.*

Reflection of sound is greatest when there is a large difference between the acoustic impedance of two structures, which explains why cysts and cystic structures, such as the gallbladder and the fetus in its sac of amniotic fluid, are so well demonstrated with ultrasound. Strong echoes are produced from the cyst walls but no echoes arise from the fluid within the cyst. As more sound traverses the cyst, more echoes are received from the area behind the cyst, a feature known as **acoustic enhancement** (Fig. 1.6). Conversely with a calcified structure, such as a stone, there is a reduction in the sound passing through, causing a band of reduced echoes beyond the stone, known as **acoustic shadowing** (Fig. 1.7).

As sound waves pass through the body the amount of reflection is determined by the difference in the acoustic impedance of the tissues. A liver metastasis may have a different acoustic impedance from the surrounding normal liver, so the sound is reflected differently to enable the metastasis to be visualized.

Small ultrasound probes have been developed that can be placed close to the region of interest, so producing highly detailed images but with only a small range of a few centimetres. Examples include rectal probes for examining the prostate, and anal canal and transvaginal probes for the examination of pelvic structures. Tiny ultrasound probes may be incorporated into the end of an endoscope. With an endoscope in the oesophagus, lesions of the heart and aorta may be detected and abnormalities of the pancreas may be demonstrated with an endoscope passed into the stomach and duodenum.

Harmonic imaging is a recently introduced modification designed to improve tissue visualization by reducing artefacts, particularly those that arise from superficial structures, by using harmonics of the transmitted ultrasound beam. When an ultrasound signal is transmitted, the sound is reflected off tissues at multiples or harmonics of the transmitted frequency. There is increased generation of these harmonic frequencies as the sound travels deeper through tissues. With the use of appropriate filters, the various frequencies can be selected for processing.

DOPPLER EFFECT

The Doppler effect is the shift in frequency of a wave when the source moves relative to the receiver. The rise in pitch of a train whistle as a train approaches is a familiar example. The assessment of blood flow is based

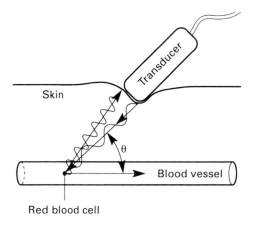

Figure 1.8 *Principle of Doppler ultrasound. With blood flowing towards the transducer the frequency of the received sound is increased. The difference in frequency between the transmitted and received sound is known as the Doppler shift. θ = angle between the vessel and the transmitted sound wave: an angle known as the Doppler angle.*

on the Doppler effect as sound is reflected from the blood cells flowing in the vessels. When blood flows towards the transducer, the received signal is of higher frequency than the transmitted frequency (Fig. 1.8), whilst the opposite occurs if blood is flowing away from the transducer. This frequency shift can be measured and blood flow velocity calculated from the formula:

$$\text{frequency shift} = \frac{2 \times Fi \times v \times \cos \theta}{C}$$

Where C equals the speed of sound in tissues, and Fi the incident frequency of the beam. As these are constant and if the Doppler angle θ is kept constant, the frequency shift depends on the blood flow velocity v.

The Doppler signals fall in the audible range so, when amplified, they give a characteristic sound for arterial and venous flow that may be altered if flow is disturbed. In addition the flow velocity wave form may be recorded by plotting the Doppler signal against time.

For imaging, pulsed Doppler is employed. The ultrasound transducer operates with repeated bursts of sound in between which it remains quiet for echo reception. This enables a Doppler trace to be available simultaneously with an ultrasound image, and the position of the Doppler gate from which the signal arises can be chosen at will. This combined system of Doppler and an ultrasound image is known as **duplex scanning**. A further development is **colour Doppler** which shows flow patterns over the whole ultrasound image. Direction of blood flow towards or away from the transducer can readily be determined and can be assigned a colour, usually red or blue (Plate 1, opposite p. 358).

Both duplex and colour Doppler ultrasound are affected by the angle of insonation and also limited by the pulse repetition frequency (PRF), the frequency with which the bursts of ultrasound are emitted. The maximum frequency shift that can be resolved is half the pulse repetition frequency – the **Nyquist limit**. Higher frequencies than this will 'wrap around' the frequency scale and appear as frequency shifts in the opposite direction – a situation known as **aliasing**. Increasing the PRF in order to display, or measure, high frequency shifts (such as might be encountered in a stenosis) will reduce the depth at which the probe can operate. Duplex ultrasound not only allows precise location of the Doppler sample site to a specific vessel but also enables calibration of the system for the angle of insonation so that measurements can then be given in terms of velocity rather than frequency shift.

The velocity/time graph, or spectral display, is a useful qualitative display of the flow pattern. Each vessel has its own characteristic appearance or 'signature', which is determined partly by the characteristics of vessels upstream from the measuring point but predominantly by characteristics of the vascular bed beyond. Arteries that supply low resistance vascular beds have persistent flow through diastole. Examples of this type are the internal carotid (Plate 1) and renal arteries. Conversely, arteries that supply structures with a high vascular resistance show absence or reversal of flow in diastole. An example of this pattern is found in the superficial femoral artery when the leg is at rest (Plate 2a, opposite p. 358). The shape of the velocity waveform in some vessels may change considerably with physiological or pathological changes in the arterial bed. For instance, the demands of the leg on its femoral artery supply vary considerably depending on its level of activity. During periods of exercise, the peripheral vessels dilate and the flow pattern alters to the low resistance pattern. Various parameters may be measured to quantify the velocity waveform. Commonly used indices are the peak systolic velocity, end diastolic velocity, resistive index, pulsatility index, acceleration time and acceleration index (Plate 2b).

At any instant, blood cells within a given sample volume will be moving with a range of different velocities. For laminar flow in the centre of the lumen the range of velocities and therefore the spectrum of measured frequency shifts will be narrow. The spectral display will then show a clean velocity waveform that approximates to a single line with clear space between it and the baseline (Plate 2a). When the flow is turbulent (e.g. downstream from a stenosis), blood cells within the sample volume will be moving with greatly varying velocities and directions. The spectrum of frequency shifts will be very wide in this situation, known as **spectral widening**.

Power Doppler

To overcome some of the limitations of conventional Doppler, such as artefacts and dependence on the angle of insonation (Doppler angle), **power Doppler** has been introduced. Power Doppler measures the energy of the moving red cells, which depends on the amplitude of the Doppler signal, the density of the red blood cells and the attenuation by intervening tissue. This energy is assigned a colour. Power Doppler has the advantage that it is less affected by artefacts, is not dependent on the angle of insonation and is more sensitive to low flow states than conventional Doppler, so allowing better demonstration of the calibre and course of a vessel. A limitation of power Doppler is that it gives no indication of direction of blood flow or information on blood flow velocity (Plate 3, opposite p. 358).

ULTRASOUND CONTRAST AGENTS

The action of ultrasound contrast agents depends on highly reflective gas-filled microbubbles that, when exposed to an ultrasound beam, return signals many times more reflective than blood. Carrier agents such as albumin or galactose in solution are used to stabilize the microbubbles which are 1–7 μm in size. When injected into the blood stream, these microbubbles traverse even the smallest capillaries, and contrast agents can be used to evaluate and detect tumours that otherwise may not be demonstrated if contrast is not used. Ultrasound contrast agents are also used in cardiac and Doppler studies and, when injected into the uterine cavity, can be used to demonstrate fallopian tube patency.

INTERVENTIONAL PROCEDURES

Percutaneous biopsies can conveniently be performed under ultrasound control because the course of the needle can be viewed as it passes to the target. Similarly, abscess aspiration and placement of drainage tubes can readily be performed using ultrasound. Intraoperative ultrasound can be valuable in certain situations, such as in localizing an endocrine tumour of the pancreas during surgery.

SAFETY OF ULTRASOUND

Although high power ultrasound can inflict damage to tissues, no harmful effects have been recorded at the intensities used for diagnostic purposes. Follow-up has failed to detect any abnormality resulting from ultrasound scans performed during pregnancy, despite the many millions of such scans over several decades that have been performed.

COMPUTED TOMOGRAPHY

Computed tomography (CT) overcomes some of the limitations of plain radiography by removing the problem of superimposition of structures and by enabling very small density difference between tissues to be shown.

The problem of superimposition of structures is achieved by collimation of the X-rays into a thin beam that only passes through the 'slice' of tissue being imaged. Having passed through the patient, the X-ray beam strikes very sensitive detectors which can distinguish and quantify subtle differences in tissue density.

Compared to conventional plain radiography, the range of densities recorded is increased from approximately 20 to 2000 or more. CT scanning is a digital imaging system based on three essential components:

- data acquisition
- data processing
- image display, manipulation, storage and recording.

DATA ACQUISITION

There are two methods of data acquisition, 'slice-by-slice' and 'volume-acquisition'. The X-ray detectors measure the radiation transmitted through the patient from all the different locations of the X-ray tube, in both the slice-by-slice and volume-acquisition techniques.

Relative transmission values (or penetration measurements) can then be calculated. The **relative transmission** depends almost entirely on the attenuation of the X-rays by the body, which in turn depends on the number of atoms in the path of the beam, and their atomic number.

In the conventional slice-by-slice method, data are collected by the X-ray tube rotating around the patient, thus giving information from a single slice. The tube comes to a stop and the patient is then moved into position so that the next slice can be scanned (Fig. 1.9). This process continues until all slices have been scanned.

In the newer method of volume acquisition, a special X-ray beam geometry, referred to as **spiral or helical CT**, is used to scan a volume of tissue rather than one slice at a time (Fig. 1.10).

The patient is transported continuously through the scanner. As the X-ray tube rotates continuously around the patient, the X-ray beam traces a spiral or helical path with respect to the moving patient while data are

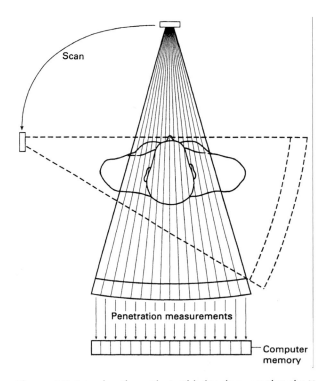

Figure 1.9 *Scanning the patient. This involves rotating the X-ray tube and detectors around the patient to collect transmission or penetration measurements; these are stored in the computer memory.*

(a)

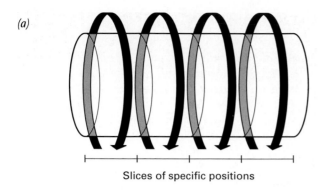

Slices of specific positions

(b)

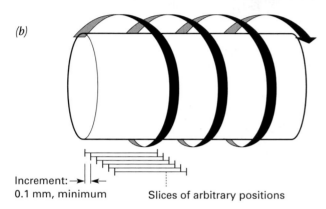

Increment: → ‖ ←
0.1 mm, minimum   Slices of arbitrary positions

Figure 1.10 *Two methods of data collection in CT (a) through conventional scanning and (b) through spiral scanning.*

Figure 1.11 *3D reconstruction of the facial bones.*

removed as there is no shifting of anatomical structures between the slices and lesions can be localized accurately.

• Slices can be reconstructed at any arbitrary position within the volume after the data have been acquired.

acquired continuously through each 360° rotation. This images a volume of tissue (rather than a slice) so the technique is also referred to as **volume scanning**.

A major requirement of spiral scanning is an increase in the capacity of the X-ray tube which has to deliver X-rays continuously during the time it takes to scan the volume of tissue. Usually patients are moved by 10 mm/s so that a typical 24-s scan covers 240 mm (24 cm). The maximum scanning time is usually in the order of 32 s. Slice thickness may range between 1 mm and 1 cm (Fig. 1.10).

THE ADVANTAGES OF SPIRAL (HELICAL) CT

Several advantages are associated with the use of spiral (helical) CT.

• The examination time is reduced by elimination of an interscan delay so that whole organs can be scanned on a single breath-hold.
• The potential for a gap between slices is removed because a volume of tissue is scanned rather than scans being obtained slice by slice.
• The effect of different depths of respiration is

Figure 1.12 *3D reconstruction of the pulmonary vasculature. The relationship of a small nodule to the adjacent vessels is clearly seen (arrow).*

(a)

(b)

Figure 1.13 *CT angiography. (a) Sagittal planar reconstruction of the CT data showing an aortic aneurysm, which is being planned for endovascular stent insertion. (b) The aneurysm shown on 3D surface reconstruction.*

- There is greater accuracy in multiplanar and 3D reconstruction; this has proved particularly valuable in studying the facial bones (Fig. 1.11), complex joints such as the elbow, in demonstrating the vascular system (Figs 1.12, 1.13) and for virtual endoscopy (Fig. 3.4, p. 50).

MULTISLICE CT

Very recently, the ability to acquire the data from more than one slice simultaneously has been developed using parallel banks of detectors. Scanners are now capable of acquiring four CT slices in one X-ray tube rotation; soon this will be increased to eight and even 16 slices. Numerous clinical advantages result from this multislice technology. With a four-slice system the data can be acquired four times faster than with a single-slice spiral scanner. This is particularly useful in studies where patient motion is a limiting factor, as in examinations in paediatric patients or in patients who have sustained trauma. The other main advantage of multislice systems is the possibility of acquiring a large number of thin slices quickly, improving spatial resolution and providing good quality 3D reconstruction for applications such as CT angiography and virtual endoscopy. Multislice systems can also provide CT 'fluoroscopy'; by simultaneous

imaging of a number of slices, real-time display is possible resulting in improved localization for interventional procedures.

DATA PROCESSING AND CT NUMBERS

The X-ray transmission values collected during scanning are stored as raw data in the computer and then converted into numbers – CT numbers (Hounsfield units [HU]) or attenuation values – by a mathematical process referred to as a **reconstruction technique** or **algorithm**. The computer prints images based on these CT numbers. Thus X-rays passing through bone/calcification (+1000) undergo the most attenuation and those passing through air (–1000) are least attenuated (Fig. 1.14). The final image is converted to a grey-scale image by relating the attenuation value of the tissues to that of water, the CT number of which is designated zero. The relationship of CT numbers to brightness level is shown in Fig. 1.15, in which the upper (+1000) and lower (–1000) limits of the scale represent white and black respectively.

IMAGE DISPLAY

The image so obtained consists of a matrix of picture elements (**pixels**), each representing the degree of

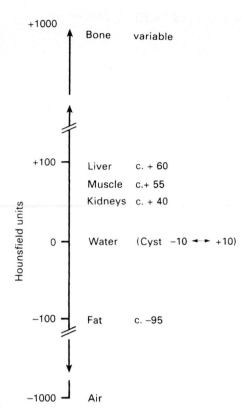

Figure 1.14 *Chart depicting the Hounsfield scale, showing the values for some normal structures.*

(a)

(b)

Figure 1.15 *Relationship between CT numbers and the brightness level (grey scale).*

Windowing

Since only a limited number of grey-scale steps can be appreciated by the human eye, only a limited range of values can be distinguished simultaneously. For this reason, the viewing console is provided with controls which enable the observer to select a range of values for display and recording appropriate to the tissue being examined. The centre of the range is known as the window level, and the range of density, the window width. The smaller the range of density values represented by each grey-scale step, the greater the contrast. For this reason, a narrow width is used when structures such as the liver or brain are being examined where

Figure 1.16 *An example of varying the window width and level by manipulating the data of one thoracic image. (a) At conventional soft tissue settings (width 400 HU, level 40 HU) the normal mediastinal soft tissue striations are shown but the lung detail is not seen. (b) At lung settings (width 1000 HU, level −700 HU), bone and soft tissue detail are now all lost as they all appear white. Lung detail is well seen.*

attenuation of X-rays at a particular point in the body. Since each image represents a certain thickness of tissue, the attenuation value recorded at a point represents the mean value obtained from a tiny volume of tissue (the **voxel**). This image is displayed on a television monitor. An important parameter of the grey-scale display monitor is resolution, which is related to the size of the pixel matrix (**matrix size**).

small differences in density can be important. Relatively wider widths are commonly used in body scanning when the shape and contours of structures are the main criteria for diagnosis (Fig. 1.16).

ARTEFACTS

Partial volume effect

When CT numbers are computed, the calculations are based on the measurement of attenuation for an entire voxel of tissue. If the voxel contains only one tissue type, then the calculations give the true attenuation of the tissue. On the other hand, if the voxel contains more than one tissue type, then the CT number for that voxel is based on an average of those tissues. This is known as **partial volume averaging** and may lead to inaccuracies when tissues are being characterized and their size estimated (Fig. 1.17). This potential artefact can be minimized by scanning thinner slices, so that the likelihood of different tissues being present in a given voxel is reduced.

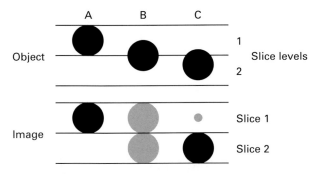

Figure 1.17 *Partial volume effect. Object A occupies the full height of the slice and so its diameter and density are accurately represented on the images. Object B lies half in slice 1 and half in slice 2 so the images will indicate its correct size but the density on each image slice will be half its true value. Object C lies partly in slice 1 but mainly in slice 2 and so the upper slice of the image will underestimate both its diameter and density.*

Streak artefacts

Movement, either voluntary or involuntary, such as peristalsis or cardiac motion, during scanning can result in the appearance of streak artefacts on the image which are tangential to the high density difference edges of the moving part. Very high density materials, including metals, barium, surgical clips and electrodes, can also give rise to streak artefacts on the image.

THE USE OF CONTRAST MEDIUM

Ooral contrast medium

The use of dilute oral contrast material to opacify the gastrointestinal tract is essential when the abdomen is scanned, so that homogeneous fluid-filled bowel loops are not confused with masses or abscesses. Proper opacification of the gastrointestinal tract is especially valuable in patients who are extremely thin and lack the usual amount of intra-abdominal fat necessary to outline structures. Gastrografin (an iodine-containing compound) diluted to 2% solution or dilute barium sulphate are the most commonly used contrast agents for abdominal and pelvic scans. If the examination is being performed primarily to study the stomach, the patient is given 300–500 ml contrast medium immediately before the study. If the examination extends to the remainder of the abdomen, then the small bowel is opacified by the patient being given contrast medium to drink 45 minutes to 1 hour before the examination. Rectal contrast medium may also be administered before pelvic examination.

Intravenous contrast agents

Intravenous contrast medium is most frequently used to increase the density difference between the normally enhancing parenchyma of an organ (such as the liver, pancreas or kidney) and a focal abnormality (such as a tumour or an abscess) which takes up the contrast medium to a lesser extent. This improves the sensitivity with which focal abnormalities are detected. Contrast is also useful for distinguishing between vessels and a mass, and for identifying the extent of vascular displacement or invasion. Intravenous contrast material may be used to opacify blood vessels to determine the relative vascularity of a mass. The contrast media are the same as those used for angiography and urography.

RADIATION DOSE FROM CT

When a CT examination is requested, consideration must be given to the radiation dose to the patient, particularly in view of the potential for high patient doses. Examinations on children require an even higher level of justification since children are at greater risk from radiation than are adults. When clinically appropriate, the alternative use of safer non-ionizing techniques (such as ultrasound and MRI) or of low dose X-ray techniques must always be considered. Currently, in the United Kingdom, by far the highest collective patient dose arises from the use of CT. The effective dose of a chest or abdomen CT (which includes a weighting for the relative risks of fatal malignancy) is

(a)   (b)

Figure 1.18 *MRI of brain. Axial sections through the lateral ventricles of a normal brain. (a) T1-weighted image. (b) T2-weighted image. The CSF is low signal on the T1-weighted image but high signal on the T2-weighted image. Note the different signal intensity of the grey and white matter on the two images.*

equivalent to 200 chest X-rays, approximately the same as the dose for a barium enema.

MAGNETIC RESONANCE IMAGING

Magnetic resonance imaging (MRI) depends on the magnetic properties of the nuclei of certain elements. The basic physical principles centre on the concept that the nuclei of hydrogen behave like small, spinning bar magnets and align with the magnetic field when placed in a strong magnetic field. Hydrogen nuclei (**protons**) are present in large numbers in water molecules and lipids. If a radiofrequency pulse at an appropriate frequency (**resonant frequency**) is beamed into the patient, a proportion of the protons change their alignment, flipping through a preset angle, and rotate in phase with one another. Following this radiofrequency pulse, the protons return to their original positions. As the protons realign (relax) they induce a radio signal which, though very weak, can be detected by coils placed around the patient. The site of origin of

this radio signal can be determined and an image representing the distribution of the hydrogen protons can be built up. The strength of the signal depends not only on proton density but also on two relaxation times, T1 and T2: T1 depends on the time the protons take to return to the axis of the magnetic field and T2 depends on the time the protons take to dephase. A T1-weighted image is one in which the contrast between tissues is due mainly to their T1 relaxation properties, while in a T2-weighted image the contrast is due to the T2-relaxation properties (Fig. 1.18). Some sequences produce mixed (often called 'balanced') images which approximate to proton density. Most pathological processes show increased T1 and T2 relaxation times which appear lower in signal (blacker) on a T1-weighted scan and higher in signal (whiter) on a T2-weighted scan than the surrounding normal soft tissues. The T1 and T2 weighting of an image can be selected by appropriately altering the timing and sequence of radiofrequency pulses. The types of sequences, such as spin-echo and gradient-echo, are also of great importance because they influence image contrast and affect speed of acquisition.

(a)

(b)

Figure 1.19 *MRI contrast enhancement of craniopharyngioma. Sagittal T1-weighted scans (a) precontrast and (b) postcontrast with gadolinium. There is contrast enhancement of the tumour (*). The rim of the cystic component of tumour also enhances (arrows).*

An MRI scanner consists of a large, strong magnet. Inside the magnet are the radiofrequency transmitter and receiver coils, as well as gradient coils to allow spatial localization of the MRI signal. Ancillary equipment converts the radio signal into a digital form which is then processed by a computer to form a final image. One advantage of MRI over CT is that the information can be directly reconstructed in any plane. Currently MRI requires longer scan times compared to CT, with the disadvantage that it is necessary to keep the patient still during the scanning procedure. Unavoidable movements owing to breathing, cardiac pulsation and peristalsis often degrade the image. Machines and sequences capable of shorter scan times and various electronic gating devices are being actively developed. **Cardiac gating** is already widely available.

In the same way that contrast media have been of great value in CT, magnetic contrast media are providing useful diagnostic information with MRI. These agents depend on magnetic and paramagnetic properties to produce contrast. The most widely used agent is gadolinium DTPA which dramatically decreases the T1 relaxation time (Fig. 1.19).

MRI is now widely used to scan the brain and spinal cord, where it has significant advantages over CT and few disadvantages. It is also an established technique for imaging the spine, bones, joints and pelvis.

The physical basis of non-contrast enhanced vascular MRI is complicated and beyond the scope of this book. With some sequences, fast-flowing blood produces no signal, whereas with others it produces a bright signal. This 'motion effect' can be exploited to image the vascular system; for example, large arteriovenous malformations can be readily demonstrated without contrast media; hilar vessels can be distinguished from masses, and even stenoses of blood vessels can be demonstrated. Special flow sequences have been developed which give images of vessels, resembling a conventional angiogram without the need for contrast media. More recently, a technique has been developed for contrast-enhanced **magnetic resonance angiography** (MRA) which uses intravenously injected gadolinium and very rapid acquisition of data using gradient-echo techniques. High field strength magnets plus rapidly switching large gradients are currently necessary for good contrast-enhanced MRA (Fig. 1.20).

Figure 1.20 *MR angiogram of the cerebral arteries. This flow sequence produces images of the arteries forming the circle of Willis at the base of the brain without the need for contrast media.*

Cardiac MRI uses electronic gating to obtain images during a specific proportion of the cardiac cycle. With this technique it is possible to limit the degradation of the image by cardiac motion and, therefore, demonstrate the cardiac chambers, valves and myocardium. Recently developed rapid scanning techniques allow the beating heart to be directly visualized as a cine image.

SAFETY OF MRI

One of the advantages of MRI is that it involves no ionizing radiation; also no adverse biological effects from diagnostic MRI have been demonstrated. It is, however, contraindicated in patients with metallic intraocular foreign bodies, certain types of aneurysm clips and cardiac pacemakers, because of the strong magnetic fields involved.

GENERAL PRINCIPLES OF ULTRASOUND, CT AND MR IMAGE INTERPRETATION

Familiarity with the appearance of component tissues in pathological processes on the various cross-sectional imaging modalities is vital to provide a useful differential diagnosis. In many situations, however, different diseases have similar appearances radiologically and a specific histological diagnosis cannot be given.

The ultrasound appearance is dictated by the pattern of transmission and reflection of a beam of high-frequency sound waves, determined by tissue interfaces and the acoustic impedance of tissues in the path of the beam. Structures containing watery fluid, such as the bladder or simple cysts, transmit ultrasound extremely well, appearing echo-free and allowing a high proportion of the beam to reach deeper structures, resulting in posterior acoustic enhancement. Tissues such as fat and bone, calcification and gas reflect a high proportion of the ultrasound beam, appearing echogenic, with reduced ultrasound transmission to deeper structures, i.e. acoustic shadowing. Complex cystic masses, solid organs and soft tissue masses produce a variable echo pattern.

On CT, the appearance of tissues depends on their electron density and atomic number: the higher the value of these parameters, the more X-rays are absorbed by the tissue and the whiter the tissue appears on the grey-scale image. The CT density, measured in Hounsfield units (HU), ranges from −1000 for air to +1000 for compact bone. Water has a value of 0 HU, but most fluids *in vivo* contain electrolytes and protein increasing the range up to about 20 HU. Most soft tissues are denser than water, in the range 20–50 HU, overlapping in density with proteinaceous or haemorrhagic fluid. Fat is an exception, having a density less than water. The presence of blood, calcium or administered contrast medium increases the density of tissues. Cortical bone has an extremely high density, measuring several hundred HUs.

On MRI, signal intensity of tissue can be made to reflect many variables but, for the purpose of clinical diagnosis, image interpretation is based on changes in proton density, T1 and T2 relaxation times. Many pathological processes are associated with an increased number of mobile protons which provides more signal, and prolongation of relaxation times which reduces signal intensity on T1-weighted sequences and increases signal on T2-weighted sequences. Muscle, including that in the walls of viscera such as the bladder and rectum, has a low signal on T2-weighted sequences, but increases in signal if inflamed or involved by tumour. Fat is characterized by a short T1 relaxation time, causing high signal intensity on T1-weighted sequences, a pattern also seen in certain components of haemorrhage. Signal voids occur in gas, bone and calcification (where hydrogen protons are absent or unable to generate signal), in flowing blood on certain sequences and when there is local distortion of the magnetic field caused by metal or haemosiderin.

FURTHER READING

Curry, T.S., Dowdey, J.E. and Murray, R.C. 1990: *Christensen's physics of diagnostic radiology* (4th edition). Baltimore: Lea and Febiger.

Dendy, P.P. 1999: *Physics for diagnostic radiology* (2nd edition). Bristol: Institute of Physics Publishing.

Dowd, S.B. and Tilson, E.R. 1999: *Practical radiation protection and applied biology* (2nd edition). Saint Louis: Saunders.

Farr, R.F. and Allisy-Roberts, P.J. 1998: *Physics for medical imaging*. Saint Louis: Saunders.

Hashemi, R.H. and Bradley, W.G. 1997: *MRI the basics*. Baltimore: Williams & Wilkins.

NRPB 1993: Board statement on diagnostic medical exposures to ionising radiation during pregnancy. London: National Radiological Protection Board, Stationery Office, **4**(4).

NRPB 1995: *Doses to patients from medical X-ray examinations in the UK*. London: National Radiological Protection Board, Stationery Office, Report 289.

Perkins, A. 1995: *Nuclear medicine, science and safety*. London: John Libbey.

Westbrook, C. and Kaut, C. 1998: *MRI in practice* (2nd edition). Oxford: Blackwell Science.

2

Plain abdomen

STUART FIELD

In patients presenting with acute abdominal pain, plain films remain one of the most valuable initial investigations. The main purpose of the plain radiograph is to try and establish a diagnosis so that the clinician can decide whether or not a patient with acute abdominal pain needs an operation and, if an operation is needed, whether it needs to be performed immediately or whether time can be spent resuscitating or performing other investigations to confirm the diagnosis.

NORMAL APPEARANCES

The formation of a radiographic image depends on the structure and size of the organs within the abdomen. Gas which absorbs least X-rays appears black or dark grey, fat is usually seen as dark grey lines, the soft tissues appear very light grey with large soft tissue masses appearing almost white and finally calcification, which absorbs most X-rays, appears white (Fig. 2.1).

Relatively large amounts of gas are normally present in the stomach and colon, but only a small amount of gas is usually seen in the small bowel. The duodenum often contains air and a fluid level is frequently seen in it on horizontal X-ray films. The presence of bowel gas

Figure 2.1 *Normal abdomen. A relatively gasless bowel and good fat lines outlining the psoas muscles, kidneys, liver, spleen and bladder can be seen.*

is important in assessing the diameter and position of the bowel and judging the amount of fluid within it.

When the stomach is empty it is usual to be able to identify the gastric rugae on a radiograph taken with the patient supine and to see a relatively long air–fluid level in the fundus of the stomach when the patient is erect. Because the antrum and body are normally contracted, small amounts of fluid and air result in a relatively long fluid level in the fundus on the erect film. There is rarely sufficient gas present in the small bowel to outline more than a short length and although the mucosal pattern may be seen, the thin bands of the valvulae conniventes, which extend across the full width of the jejunum, are seldom identified in a normal patient. However, air and fluid are normal contents of the small bowel and short fluid levels are not abnormal. The significance of air fluid levels is often overstated. Fluid levels may occur in the colon in normal people. Three to five fluid levels less than 2.5 cm in length may be seen, particularly in the right lower quadrant without any evidence of intestinal obstruction or paralytic ileus. However, more than two fluid levels in dilated small bowel (calibre > 2.5 cm) is abnormal and usually indicates paralytic ileus or intestinal obstruction but may also be seen in normal radiographs. Most of the gas seen within the bowel has been swallowed and it normally reaches the colon within 30 minutes. However, when severe pain is present anywhere in the body or when respiration is laboured, such as in pneumonia or asthma, more air is swallowed producing a dramatic plain abdominal radiograph showing gas-filled, slightly dilated loops of bowel throughout the abdomen. The term 'meteorism' is sometimes given to this appearance (Fig. 2.2). It is sometimes difficult to differentiate air swallowing, produced for example by renal colic, from intestinal obstruction. The clinical history and examination frequently enable the radiological findings to be correctly interpreted.

The amount of gas present in a normal colon is extremely variable from almost none to what may appear to be pathological gaseous distension. Sufficient gas is usually present for colonic haustra, which form thick incomplete bands extending across most of the large bowel, to be readily identified. Numerous colonic fluid levels, some several centimetres in length, may be a common finding and up to 20 per cent of normal people may have a fluid level in the caecum.

Large bowel calibre is very variable with considerable overlap between the normal and abnormal: a reliable measurement for the upper limit of normal diameter of the large bowel cannot be given. However, a transverse colonic diameter of 5.5 cm has been suggested as the upper limit of normal in patients with colitis and, if the diameter of the transverse colon is greater, then megacolon should be suggested. The caecum is readily distensible, particularly in large bowel obstruction, and it has been suggested that a diameter of 9–10 cm is a

Figure 2.2 *Normal abdomen. The entire alimentary tract is gas-filled owing to air swallowing. The stomach, duodenal cap, varying lengths of small bowel and entire left half of colon are filled with gas but not unduly distended.*

critical level beyond which there is a great risk of perforation.

The outlines of the kidneys, psoas muscles, bladder and the posterior borders of the liver and spleen can often be identified by the fat which surrounds them (Fig. 2.1). These fat lines can be displaced by enlargement of these organs or effaced by inflammation or fluid. It is, however, important to realize that in a number of normal people these fat lines may be blurred or even absent. The outline of the spleen cannot be identified in around 40 per cent of normal individuals and the right psoas is blurred in nearly 20 per cent. In children, owing to the small amount of body fat, loss of the psoas outlines may occur in up to 50 per cent of normal individuals and the proprcritoneal fat lines may not be visible in almost 20 per cent of normal children. These factors must be considered carefully before undue emphasis is placed on fat-line changes.

ABDOMINAL CALCIFICATION

Although the history and clinical examination may contribute important clues, the finding of calcification on a plain abdominal radiograph is often unexpected and it may not be possible to elucidate the exact cause.

The commonest types of abdominal calcification are non-visceral and often unrelated to the presenting clinical problem:

- **Common**
  - atherosclerosis
  - mesenteric lymph nodes
  - phleboliths
  - aneurysm
  - rib cartilage (normal)
  - injections in the buttocks
- **Uncommon**
  - infestations
    - ▶ *Armillifer armillatus*
    - ▶ cysticercosis
    - ▶ guinea worm
    - ▶ hydatid
  - tumours
    - ▶ lipoma
    - ▶ haemangioma
    - ▶ neuroblastoma
    - ▶ osteo/chondrosarcoma
    - ▶ retroperitoneal sarcoma
    - ▶ peritoneal metastases
    - ▶ phaeochromocytoma
  - tuberculosis
    - ▶ peritonitis
    - ▶ psoas abscess
  - meconium peritonitis
  - pseudomyxoma peritonei
  - dermoid cyst
  - mesenteric cyst
  - pancreatitis with saponification
  - lithopaedion
  - appendices epiploicae
  - ligaments
  - foreign bodies
  - post-traumatic buttock cysts.

Abdominal calcification associated with an acute abdomen is relatively uncommon. The associations are summarized below:

- **Gallstones**
  - cholecystitis
  - pancreatitis
  - biliary colic (stone may be close to spine)
  - empyema of gallbladder
  - gallstone ileus (stone in abnormal location)
- **Calcified gallbladder wall**
  - cholecystitis
- **Limey bile**
  - cholecystitis
- **Appendix calculus**
  - appendicitis
- **Calculus**

- Meckel's diverticulum ⎫
- jejunal diverticulum ⎬ Showing acute inflammation or perforation
- colonic diverticulum ⎭
- **Pancreatic calculi**
  - pancreatitis – chronic and acute (rare)
- **Ureteric calculus**
  - renal colic
- **Calcified aneurysms** (aortic, splenic, hepatic)
  - rupture
- **Teeth/bone in ovarian dermoid**
  - torsion.

THE ACUTE ABDOMEN

Patients with acute abdominal pain form one of the largest groups presenting as an emergency to the general surgeon. Plain radiographs have become established as an essential investigation in these patients. Interpretation of the radiographs may present a formidable challenge. While in many cases a specific diagnosis can be made, plain radiographs are often non-specific or occasionally even misleading, and further investigations with contrast agents, ultrasound, radionuclides or computed tomography may be necessary. When the radiological diagnosis is specific or supports the clinical diagnosis, surgery is often indicated. If immediate surgery is indicated on clinical grounds, negative or equivocal radiological findings should be ignored.

RADIOGRAPHIC TECHNIQUE

A supine abdomen and erect chest can be regarded as the basic standard radiographs. The bladder should be emptied before the supine radiograph is taken and the film should include the area from the diaphragm to the hernial orifices.

A horizontal ray abdominal radiograph, either erect or left lateral decubitus (right side raised), is frequently taken to add information and to demonstrate fluid levels. The clinical condition of the patient will determine whether erect radiographs are taken with the patient standing or sitting. In a patient who is too ill even to sit, it may only be possible to obtain a lateral decubitus or supine radiograph with a horizontal ray. Ideally the patient should always remain in position for 10 minutes prior to the horizontal ray radiograph to allow time for any free gas to rise to the highest point.

A chest radiograph is essential because the following chest diseases may mimic an acute abdomen:

- pleurisy
- pneumonia
- pulmonary infarction
- myocardial infarction

- leaking or dissecting thoracic aneurysm
- congestive cardiac failure
- pericarditis
- pneumothorax.

Furthermore the erect chest radiograph is superior to the erect abdominal view for the demonstration of free intra-abdominal gas under the diaphragm and, therefore, it is essential that the chest film includes the diaphragmatic area. Up to one third of patients presenting with acute abdominal pain may have an abnormal chest X-ray: either pleural effusions or evidence of pneumonia and occasionally the chest condition may actually simulate an acute abdomen. It is also helpful to have a chest radiograph as a baseline because chest complications and subphrenic abscess are frequent postoperative complications in patients presenting with acute abdominal pain and who proceed to emergency surgery.

Further abdominal views may be needed to obtain additional information when the standard radiographs have been viewed or a specific diagnosis is suspected. A left lateral decubitus radiograph (one taken with the patient lying on their left side and with the use of a horizontal ray) may be taken to confirm equivocal free gas suspected on an erect chest radiograph. A left lateral decubitus film may also demonstrate a dilated gas-filled duodenum in acute pancreatitis. However, the supine abdominal radiograph is the most useful single view and, in many conditions, it is the only plain film of the abdomen that is required. Although in some centres as many as six different plain film views have been suggested, this is time-consuming and expensive if done on every patient with abdominal pain! There is a body of opinion which believes that an erect chest and supine abdomen should be taken and viewed, and additional films taken only if the clinical story warrants it or abnormalities are identified which require further elucidation. A management change as a result of information gleaned from radiographs of the chest and abdomen can be expected in 10–15 per cent of patients presenting with an acute abdomen.

DILATATION OF BOWEL

Dilatation of bowel occurs in mechanical intestinal obstruction, pseudo-obstruction, paralytic ileus and air-swallowing. However, in some individuals, particularly those who are institutionalized or intellectually impaired, the diameter of the colon may be enormous without any evidence of obstruction. Differentiation of the causes of dilated bowel will depend on the clinical history and examination together with the determination of the size and distribution of the various loops of bowel.

GASTRIC DILATATION

An enlarged stomach can be caused by any of the following conditions.

- **Mechanical gastric outlet obstruction**
  - duodenal or pyloric canal ulceration
  - carcinoma of pyloric antrum
  - extrinsic compression, e.g. annular pancreas
- **Paralytic ileus**
  - postoperative
  - trauma
  - peritonitis
  - pancreatitis
  - cholecystitis
  - diabetes
  - hepatic coma
  - drugs
- **Gastric volvulus**
- **Intubation**
- **Air swallowing**
- **Intestinal obstruction**.

Mechanical gastric outlet obstruction caused by peptic ulceration or a carcinoma of the pyloric antrum usually leads to a huge fluid-filled stomach or a stomach which contains inspissated food (Fig. 2.3). The dilated stomach may occupy most of the upper abdomen and may be identified as a soft-tissue mass containing bubbles of air with little or no bowel gas in the remainder of the bowel. Usually, however, a little gas is present in the stomach which allows the organ to be identified, particularly if a long fluid level is visible in the fundus on the erect chest radiograph. **Paralytic ileus** (often referred to as acute gastric dilatation) may predominantly affect the stomach, particularly in old people (Fig. 2.4). Acute gastric dilatation is associated with considerable fluid and electrolyte disturbance and carries a high mortality.

A **gastric volvulus** is relatively rare and may result from the stomach twisting around the longitudinal, transverse or mesenteric axis. The dilated stomach owing to a gastric volvulus is frequently spherical and may contain a long fluid level. The stomach is displaced upwards and is often associated with elevation of the left hemidiaphragm. The small bowel is usually collapsed and it is unusual to see any gas shadows beyond the stomach. If oral contrast medium is given, there may be complete obstruction at the lower end of the oesophagus or, if contrast does enter the stomach, it may not pass beyond the obstructed pylorus.

Gastric dilatation sometimes occurs simply due to **air swallowing**. After the patient has been resuscitated and intubated, large amounts of gas frequently enter the stomach, often leading to massive dilatation. On the supine radiograph a gas-filled stomach can usually be identified with the wall of the greater curvature appear-

Figure 2.3 *Gastric outlet obstruction, supine abdomen position. The gas- and fluid-filled stomach gives rise to an upper abdominal soft-tissue mass which is indenting the gas-filled transverse colon. The patient had chronic duodenal ulceration.*

Figure 2.4 *Acute gastric dilatation. Air swallowing has produced a hugely distended gas-filled stomach in a patient with acute cholecystitis. (Source: S. Field, in D.J. Nolan (ed.), A radiological atlas of gastrointestinal disease; published by John Wiley, Chichester, 1983.)*

ing convex caudally and the pyloric antrum pointing cranially.

It is important to differentiate a distended stomach from a caecal volvulus which may also be positioned beneath an elevated left hemidiaphragm. In both small or large bowel obstruction gastric dilatation may be prominent in addition to the dilated bowel.

SMALL AND LARGE BOWEL DILATATION

When a radiograph shows dilated bowel it is important to try and determine whether the small or large bowel or both are dilated. Useful differentiating features depend on the size, distribution and markings of the loops, features summarized in Table 2.1. The presence of solid faeces is the only reliable differentiating sign, the others being sometimes misleading. Dilated lower ileum may be difficult to distinguish from the sigmoid colon because both may be smooth in outline and occupy a similar position low in the central abdomen. Although haustra usually form thick incomplete bands across the colonic gas shadow they sometimes form complete transverse bands. However, these can usually be differentiated from valvulae conniventes because haustra are thicker and further apart than the small bowel folds. Haustra may be absent from the descending and sigmoid

colon but can usually still be identified in other parts of the colon even when it is massively distended.

The small bowel folds or valvulae conniventes form thin complete bands across the bowel gas shadow, prominent in the jejunum but becoming less marked as the ileum is reached. The valvulae conniventes are much closer together than colonic haustra and become thinner when stretched but still remain relatively close together even when the small bowel calibre increases. However, if the small bowel blood supply is compromised and the bowel becomes oedematous or gangrenous, the valvulae conniventes may become thickened and then be difficult to differentiate from colonic haustra.

Table 2.1 *The distinction between small bowel and large bowel dilatation*

	Small bowel	Large bowel
Haustra	Absent	Present
Valvulae conniventes	Present in jejunum	Absent
Number of loops	Many	Few
Distribution of loops	Central	Peripheral
Radius of curvature of loop	Small	Large
Diameter of loop	30–50 mm	50 mm +
Solid faeces	Absent	May be present

(a)

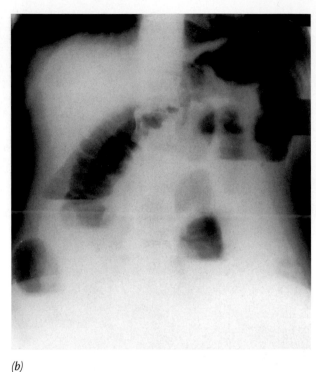

(b)

Figure 2.5 *Small bowel obstruction seen on (a) supine abdomen and (b) erect abdomen. The gas-filled loops of small bowel clearly identified by the valvulae conniventes can be seen filling the central part of the abdomen. There is no gas in the colon. Multiple fluid levels are present on the erect film.*

Although the bowel calibre is extremely variable, it is unusual in small bowel obstruction for the small bowel diameter to exceed much more than 5 cm. In large bowel obstruction it is unusual for the large bowel calibre to be less than 5 cm, indeed, it usually greatly exceeds this value.

SMALL BOWEL OBSTRUCTION

Mechanical obstruction of the small bowel normally causes small bowel dilatation with an accumulation of both gas and fluid and a reduction of the calibre of the large bowel (Fig. 2.5).

The amount of gas present in the large bowel depends on the duration and the completeness of the small bowel obstruction. Valvulae conniventes are more prominent in the jejunum, and the knowledge of this, together with an assessment of the number and position of the dilated loops, allows an estimate to be made as to the site of the obstruction. Plain film changes may appear after 3–5 hours with complete small bowel obstruction, and changes are usually very marked after 12 hours. However, with incomplete obstruction, the plain radiographic changes may take hours or days to appear and even then may be undramatic. Barium studies or ultrasound may be required to establish the

diagnosis. The dilated, gas-filled loops of small bowel are readily identified on the supine radiograph with multiple fluid levels present on the erect or lateral decubitus radiographs. In most cases there is little difficulty in diagnosing small bowel obstruction (Fig. 2.6); there are, however, many causes of small bowel fluid levels:

- normal (always < 25 mm in length)
- small bowel obstruction
- large bowel obstruction
- paralytic ileus
- gastroenteritis
- hypokalaemia
- uraemia
- jejunal diverticulosis
- mesenteric thrombosis
- saline cathartics
- peritoneal metastases (usually < 25 mm in length)
- cleansing enemas.

In some cases of small bowel obstruction relatively little air is swallowed and the small bowel is predominantly filled with fluid. Dilated fluid-filled loops of small bowel may then be identified as sausage-shaped, oval, or round soft-tissue densities that change position in different views. The **string of beads sign**, which is due to bubbles of gas trapped between valvulae

(a)

(b)

Figure 2.6 *Small bowel obstruction seen on (a) supine abdomen and (b) left lateral decubitus abdomen. In patients who are unfit to sit or stand for an erect film, the left lateral decubitus is a valuable alternative horizontal ray film to an erect abdomen.*

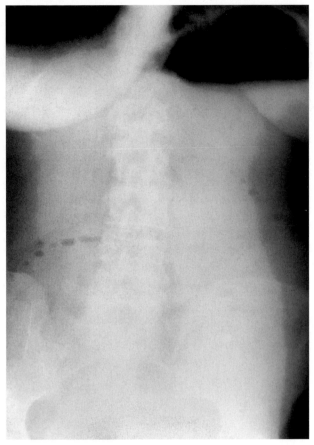

Figure 2.7 *'String of beads' sign. This is a valuable sign indicating a predominantly fluid-filled small bowel obstruction. Tiny bubbles of gas trapped between the valvulae conniventes are identified on this erect film. (Source: S. Field, in D.J. Nolan (ed.),* A radiological atlas of gastrointestinal disease; *published by John Wiley, Chichester, 1983.)*

conniventes, occurs when very dilated small bowel is almost completely filled with fluid, and this appearance is virtually diagnostic of small bowel obstruction (Fig. 2.7). Normal or equivocal initial radiographs that may result in delayed diagnosis are found in a proportion of patients with small bowel obstruction, particularly those with high obstruction (Fig. 2.8). There may be no gas fluid visible in the small bowel of patients with high

jejunal obstruction who have substantial vomiting. As a result the small bowel diameter cannot be assessed and the diagnosis from the plain film is difficult or impossible to make. If there are suggestive clinical findings, repeat plain films after a few hours, ultrasound or barium studies should be performed (Fig. 2.9).

In the developed world about 80 per cent of individuals with mechanical small bowel obstruction will have **adhesions** due to previous surgery. The obstruction will be caused by a strangulated hernia in less than 10 per cent of cases. However, in developing parts of the world nearly three quarters of cases of small bowel obstruction are caused by a **strangulated hernia** (Fig. 2.10). It is important to look for a hernia on the radiograph which may be identified as a small gas-filled viscus below the level of the inguinal ligament. However, visualization of a hernia does not always mean it is the cause of the small bowel obstruction. If, however, a dilated small bowel loop can be identified, which points directly to the inguinal region and which also contains

(a)

(a)

(b)

Figure 2.8 *Small bowel obstruction seen on (a) supine abdomen and (b) CT scan. The abdominal radiograph is within normal limits. The CT scan, however, clearly demonstrates a grossly dilated loop of small bowel with bubbles of gas trapped beneath the valvulae conniventes, the CT equivalent of the 'string of beads' sign.*

(b)

an abnormally located gas shadow, a confident diagnosis of obstruction due to the hernia can be made.

Although hernias other than inguinal or femoral hernias may cause intestinal obstruction, it is extremely uncommon for these hernias to be identified on plain abdominal radiographs. Rarely, a hernia through the foramen of Winslow, an umbilical or incisional hernia can be identified on the abdominal radiograph.

Figure 2.9 *Small bowel obstruction seen on (a) supine abdomen and (b) barium small bowel examination. The abdominal radiograph demonstrates borderline dilatation of one or two loops of bowel in the left upper quadrant. The barium study clearly demonstrates markedly dilated small bowel which is obstructed proximally owing to small bowel lymphoma. (Source: S. Field, in D. Sutton (ed.), Textbook of radiology and imaging, published by Churchill Livingstone, Edinburgh, 1992.)*

Figure 2.11 *Isolated strangulated loop of small bowel seen on supine abdomen. An isolated loop of small bowel can be identified in the right upper quadrant. Closed loop obstruction was secondary to band adhesions.*

Figure 2.10 *Strangulated left femoral hernia seen on supine abdomen. Markedly dilated loops of small bowel can clearly be identified passing into the left femoral region in child aged 4 months with persistent vomiting.*

Causes of small bowel obstruction that may be identified on a plain abdominal radiograph include:

- hernia
- volvulus
- gallstone ileus
- intussusception
- constipation
- tumour
- mesenteric infarction
- foreign body
- malrotation.

STRANGULATING OBSTRUCTION

Strangulating obstruction occurs when a loop of obstructed small bowel becomes incarcerated by a band or by the neck of a hernial sac in such a way as to compromise the blood supply by compression of the mesenteric vessels (Fig. 2.11). The closed loop thus formed may fill with fluid, be palpable and be visible on a radiograph as a soft tissue mass or 'pseudo-tumour'.

The strangulated loop may contain gas and the arms of the loop, separated only by thickened intestinal walls, may resemble a large coffee bean. If gangrene occurs, mucosal nodularity, small bubbles and linear gas shadows may be seen in the wall of the bowel (Fig. 2.12). However, the appearances in strangulating obstruction, with all its lethal potential, may be indistinguishable from simple small bowel obstruction. A raised white cell count is a pointer that strangulation may have occurred.

VOLVULUS OF THE SMALL INTESTINE

Volvulus of the small bowel may occur as an isolated abnormality or in combination with obstruction owing to adhesive bands. It may be associated with anomalies of the mesentery and there is often associated malrotation of the bowel. In children incomplete rotation, malrotation or non-rotation of the gut may be associated with a massive small bowel volvulus that may occur in the neonatal period or sometimes months or even years after birth. Impairment of the blood supply frequently occurs in small bowel volvulus so that intramural gas or nodular thickening of the bowel wall may be seen. It is not usually possible to differentiate between strangulating obstruction, small bowel volvulus or simple small bowel obstruction from plain radiographs alone.

Figure 2.12 *Gangrene of small bowel in obstruction secondary to adhesions. Linear gas can be identified within the wall of the small bowel (arrows). (Source: S. Field, in Clinics in Gastroenterology 1984; **13**: 1.)*

Figure 2.13 *Gallstone ileus seen on supine abdomen. Small bowel obstruction is present. Gas can be identified within the bile ducts in the right upper quadrant (arrows). (Source: S. Field, in D.J. Nolan (ed.), A radiological atlas of gastrointestinal disease; published by John Wiley, Chichester, 1983.)*

GALLSTONE ILEUS

Gallstone ileus is the term given to mechanical intestinal obstruction caused when one or more gallstones impact in the intestine. This usually occurs in the distal ileum at its narrowest point just proximal to the ileocaecal valve but may also rarely occur in the duodenum or colon. Following an attack of cholecystitis, a gallstone may pass through the inflamed gallbladder wall and into the duodenum. The patient, who is most commonly a middle-aged or elderly woman, will frequently have had recurrent episodes of right hypochondrial pain characteristic of cholecystitis. However, the most recent attack will usually have been more severe and associated with prolonged vomiting. Gallstone ileus accounts for around 2 per cent of patients presenting with small bowel obstruction. The diagnosis is frequently delayed or missed even though the characteristic radiological features of gallstone ileus are present in nearly 40 per cent of cases. Over half of the patients will have evidence of intestinal obstruction and about one third will have gas present in the biliary tree (Fig. 2.13). The radiological features of gallstone ileus include:

Figure 2.14 *Gallstone ileus seen on supine abdomen. Oedematous dilated loops of small bowel can be identified in the lower abdomen. The calcified ring shadow of the obstructing gallstone can be identified, with difficulty, overlying the sacrum (arrow).*

(a) (b)

Figure 2.15 *Ileocolic intussusception seen on (a) supine abdomen and (b) barium enema. A soft-tissue mass can be clealry identified within the transverse colon on the plain abdominal radiograph with a crescent of gas outlining the head of the intussusception in a child aged 2 years. These findings are confirmed on the barium study.*

- incomplete or complete small bowel obstruction;
- gas within the gallbladder and/or bile ducts;
- abnormal location of a gallstone;
- change in position of a gallstone;
- relatively large fluid-to-gas ratio in distended bowel.

Gas in the biliary tree can be recognized by its branching pattern with the gas being more prominent centrally. Gas in the biliary tree has to be differentiated from gas in the portal vein, which tends to be more peripherally located in small veins around the edge of the liver. The gallstone that is causing obstruction usually lies in the loops of ileum overlying the caecum and, therefore, is often difficult to identify (Fig. 2.14). However, the gallstone can be seen in around one third of patients either on plain radiographs or on subsequent barium examinations. Although the obstructing gallstone is usually larger than 2.5 cm in size it may be difficult to identify on plain films because it is frequently composed almost entirely of cholesterol and may possess only a thin rim of calcification. The changing position of a previously observed gallstone is a rare sign. Gas in the biliary tree may also be seen in a number of other conditions:

- fistula between gallbladder and bowel from passage of a gallstone;

- following biliary surgery or endoscopic sphinctero-tomy;
- following percutaneous or endoscopic cholangiography;
- malignant fistula;
- perforated peptic ulcer (into bile duct);
- emphysematous cholangitis (gallbladder usually enlarged);
- physiological – owing to lax sphincter.

Small bowel obstruction may develop following biliary surgery and the radiological appearances may mimic gallstone ileus.

INTUSSUSCEPTION

Two groups of patients develop small bowel intussusception. It is most frequently seen in children under the age of 2 years when the most usual form of intussusception is the ileum invaginating into the colon. Inflammation of the lymphoid tissues in the ileum causes enlarged lymphatic patches to project into the lumen of the bowel and peristaltic movement then pushes one part of the lumen into another (Fig. 2.15). In adults intussusception is almost invariably associated with a tumour arising either in the small bowel or colon.

Figure 2.16 *Small bowel pseudo-obstruction seen on supine abdomen. Numerous loops of small bowel and gas-filled, but not unduly dilated, ascending colon can be identified in a patient aged 82. History of abdominal pain and vomiting for 3 weeks accompanied by marked abdominal tenderness. No obstructing lesion was found at laparotomy.*

Figure 2.17 *Mesenteric embolus with small bowel infarction seen on supine abdomen. Multiple small bubbles of gas and linear intramural gas lie within infarcted small bowel in the right side of the abdomen. This caused functional obstruction; gas-filled loops of distended proximal small bowel can also be seen. The patient was aged 79 years and reported sudden onset of right hypochondrial pain. (Source: S. Field, in Patrick C. Freeney and Giles W. Stevenson (eds), Margulis and Burhenne's alimentary tract radiology, published by Mosby, St Louis, 1994.)*

Intussusception is usually recognized clinically by pain, vomiting, blood in the stool and a palpable abdominal mass, although the diagnosis is sometimes difficult to make.

Plain film radiographs in infants often show evidence of small bowel obstruction. The intussusception itself may be identified as a soft-tissue mass, frequently situated in the right hypochondrium. This mass may sometimes be surrounded by a crescent of gas giving rise to the 'crescent' sign, whereas the 'target' sign consists of two concentric circles of fat density. Although visualization of a mass is the most common sign of intussusception, the crescent and target signs are more specific. The target sign is seen almost twice as frequently as the crescent sign. Depending on local practice, ultrasound or a barium or gas enema are frequently performed to confirm the diagnosis of intussusception. The gas, barium or a saline enema may be used in an attempt to reduce the intussusception under ultrasound or fluoroscopic control.

Intussusception in adults develops either as a result of surgery, e.g. following gastroenterostomy, or more commonly secondary to a tumour in the bowel. Plain film diagnosis depends on identifying the soft-tissue mass which may be either spherical or oval, the crescent-shaped gas shadow at the apex of the mass or gas within the intussuscepting bowel resembling a 'coiled spring'.

SMALL BOWEL PSEUDO-OBSTRUCTION

Although pseudo-obstruction most commonly affects both the large and small bowel, it may occur in small bowel alone and simulate small bowel obstruction (Fig. 2.16).

MESENTERIC THROMBOSIS – SMALL BOWEL INFARCTION

Infarction of the small bowel is a most serious abdominal condition caused by thrombosis or embolism of the

(a)

(b)

Figure 2.18 *Large bowel obstruction seen on (a) supine abdomen and (b) prone abdomen. In the supine position gas rises to the most superior part of the bowel which is the transverse colon, fluid fills the ascending and descending colon. In the prone radiograph fluid fills the transverse colon. This cannot be visualized but gas has filled the ascending and descending colon. It is important to recognize how different positions affect the distribution of gas.*

superior mesenteric artery. The clinical diagnosis is often uncertain until laparotomy but the sudden onset of severe abdominal pain, sometimes associated with bloody diarrhoea, in an elderly person who may have other stigma of atherosclerosis, is very suggestive of small bowel infarction (Fig. 2.17). Gas-filled, slightly dilated loops of small bowel with multiple fluid levels, or fluid-filled loops of small bowel, are the most common plain film findings. However, the walls of the small bowel loops may become thickened and nodular, secondary to submucosal haemorrhage and oedema. Bubbles of gas and linear gas streaks may be identified within the bowel wall if gangrene develops, and free gas may be present if perforation has occurred. Frequently there is also a generalized peritonitis, which may also cause colonic distension. In advanced cases intraluminal gas in the mesenteric or portal veins may be identified, which indicates a very grave prognosis.

MECHANICAL LARGE BOWEL OBSTRUCTION

Although adhesive bands are the commonest cause of small bowel obstruction, only very rarely do they cause obstruction in the colon. Common causes of colonic

obstruction include tumour, particularly carcinoma of the sigmoid colon, abscesses secondary to perforated diverticular disease, large bowel volvulus and, more rarely, extrinsic compression from a pelvic tumour (Fig. 2.18). In the developed world over 80 per cent of mechanical large bowel obstructions, are caused by a carcinoma and most of these are situated in the sigmoid colon. Diverticulitis, commonly associated with a small pericolic abscess, is the next most common cause. In the developed world volvulus accounts for only around 10 per cent of cases of colonic obstruction, but in Iran and Africa volvulus may comprise more than 80 per cent of cases of large bowel obstruction.

Obstruction to the left side of the colon is more common than to the right. The plain film findings depend on the site of obstruction and whether or not the ileocaecal valve is competent. If the ileocaecal valve remains competent, marked distension of the caecum will occur. The competent ileocaecal valve may also result in small bowel distension. Consequently in large bowel obstruction both small and large bowel dilatation may be seen. However, if the ileocaecal valve is incompetent, the caecum and ascending colon do not become distended but there is marked small bowel distension. When the ileocaecal valve is competent, massive caecal distension may occur and the caecum is then 'at risk' of

Figure 2.19 *Large bowel obstruction causing impending perforation of the caecum. The ileocaecal valve is competent and the caecum and small bowel are distended. There is gaseous distension of both small and large bowel. The transverse caecal diameter measures 11 cm and the wall of the caecum is oedematous and thickened auguring impending perforation. An ischaemic caecum was confirmed at surgery for carcinoma of the sigmoid colon. (Source: S. Field, in Clinics in Gastroenterology 1984; **13**: 1.)*

Figure 2.20 *Large bowel obstruction with a large fluid-filled caecum. A carcinoma of transverse colon was found at laparotomy. The hepatic flexure is gas-filled but the caecum, although markedly distended, is filled with fluid. There is obvious gas-filled small bowel distension. This radiograph could be misinterpreted as small bowel obstruction.*

perforation secondary to ischaemia (Fig. 2.19). It has been suggested that a caecal diameter of > 10 cm renders the caecum increasingly liable to perforation.

The obstructed colon almost invariably contains large amounts of gas and can usually be identified by the presence of haustra and by its position in the periphery of the abdomen. When both small and large bowel dilatation are present, the radiographic appearances may be indistinguishable from paralytic ileus. The variation in colonic diameter in normal individuals is very considerable and some people with large bowel obstruction may have colonic diameters that are less than those observed in some normal individuals.

There are numerous causes of colonic distension without obstruction, and all causes of paralytic ileus may also lead to massive colonic distension. In many centres a single contrast barium enema or water-soluble contrast enema is performed as an emergency investigation to differentiate between mechanical obstruction and pseudo-obstruction or colonic ileus. A barium study increases both the sensitivity and specificity of the plain film findings in large bowel obstruction. Although obstructed large bowel usually contains varying

amounts of gas, a fluid-filled caecum can simulate small bowel obstruction (Fig. 2.20) and a completely fluid-filled large bowel can simulate ascites (Fig. 2.21).

LARGE BOWEL VOLVULUS

Volvulus of the large bowel is relatively common in developing countries but is less frequent in the developed world where it comprises about 10 per cent of all cases of large bowel obstruction. Volvulus of the colon can only occur where there is a long freely mobile mesentery. The sigmoid colon and caecum are, therefore, the most commonly affected sites, and torsion of other parts, such as the flexures or transverse colon, is rare. A compound volvulus involving the intertwining of two loops of bowel, such as an ileosigmoid knot, is very rare in developed countries but is not uncommon in Africa, Iran and parts of Russia.

CAECAL VOLVULUS

Caecal or right colonic volvulus can only occur when there is a degree of malrotation and the caecum and

Figure 2.21 *Fluid-filled large bowel obstruction seen on supine abdomen. The walls of the distended fluid-filled descending colon are outlined by fat in this patient with carcinoma of the sigmoid. (From Field S. in: Patrick C. Freeney and Giles W. Stevenson (eds.)* Margulis and Burhenne's alimentary tract radiology, *published by Mosby, St. Louis, 1994.)*

(a)

(b)

ascending colon are on a mesentery. Compared with sigmoid volvulus it occurs in a relatively young age group, 30–60 years being most common. In around half the cases, the caecum twists and inverts so that the pole of the caecum and the appendix occupy the left upper quadrant (Fig. 2.22). In the other half of cases, the twist occurs in an axial manner without inversion and the caecum still occupies the right half of the abdomen, usually the right lower quadrant. Even though there is considerable distension of the rotated caecum in a caecal volvulus, one or two haustral markings can usually be identified. The distended caecum can usually be identified as a very large gas- and fluid-filled viscus that may be situated almost anywhere in the abdomen. Identification of the attached gas-filled appendix confirms the diagnosis. Marked gaseous or fluid distension of small bowel is often present and may sometimes obstruct the caecum itself. The left side of the colon is usually collapsed.

SIGMOID VOLVULUS

Sigmoid volvulus is the classic large-bowel volvulus normally occurring in old age. The usual mechanism is twisting of the sigmoid loop around the mesenteric axis;

Figure 2.22 *Caecal volvulus seen on (a) supine abdomen and (b) erect abdomen. A dilated gas-filled caecum can be identified in the left upper quadrant; there is also evidence of small bowel obstruction. (From S. Field in:* Clinics in Gastroenterology *1984;* **13**: *1.)*

Figure 2.23 *Sigmoid volvulus seen on supine abdomen. A huge mainly ahaustral loop of sigmoid can be identified rising out of the pelvis. The ahaustral margin can be seen overlapping the liver (liver overlap sign) and overlapping the haustrated descending colon (left flank overlap sign).*

(a)

only rarely does one limb twist in axial torsion. Sigmoid volvulus is usually chronic with intermittent acute attacks although a true acute torsion may occur. Although plain film diagnosis may be easy, up to one third of cases are difficult to diagnose radiologically and further investigations may be needed. Signs of a sigmoid volvulus include:

- ahaustral margin
- left flank overlap sign
- liver overlap sign
- apex under left hemidiaphragm
- apex above 10th thoracic vertebra
- inferior convergence on left
- pelvis overlap sign.

When a sigmoid volvulus occurs, the inverted 'U'-shaped loop is usually massively distended and commonly devoid of haustra – an important diagnostic feature (Fig. 2.23). The margin of this ahaustral loop can often be identified overlapping:

- the haustrated dilated descending colon – **the left flank overlap sign**;
- the lower border of the liver shadow – **the liver overlap sign**;
- the left iliac bone – **the pelvis overlap sign**.

(b)

Figure 2.24 *Sigmoid volvulus seen on (a) supine abdomen and (b) following passage of a flatus tube. The massively distended ahaustral sigmoid loop can clearly be identified on the plain film. Following the passage of a rectal tube, there has been dramatic deflation of the volvulus with gas remaining in a relatively undistended descending colon.*

(a)   *(b)*

Figure 2.25 *Sigmoid volvulus seen on (a) supine abdomen and (b) emergency barium enema. There is marked distension of large bowel which contains faeces and air. The diagnosis cannot be made from the plain films alone. The barium enema demonstrated tapering of the sigmoid at the point of twist where the 'cork-screw' appearance of the mucosal folds is also seen (arrow). (Source: S. Field in Patrick C. Freeney and Giles W. Stevenson (eds),* Margulis and Burhenne's alimentary tract radiology, *published by Mosby, St Louis, 1994.)*

The superior aspect of the sigmoid volvulus usually lies very high in the abdomen, above the level of D10 with its apex lying on the left side beneath the left hemidiaphragm. Sometimes the gas in the sigmoid loop may simulate free intraperitoneal gas.

Inferiorly, where the two limbs of the volved loop converge, three white lines meet representing the two outer walls and the contiguous inner walls of the twisted loop. This point is called the **inferior convergence** – it is usually on the left side of the pelvis at the level of the upper sacral segments. It is usual for a large amount of air to be present in the volvulus. A recent evaluation of the radiological signs suggested that apex of the loop under the left hemidiaphragm, inferior convergence on the left and the left flank overlap signs were highly specific as well as being very sensitive.

The initial management of a sigmoid volvulus frequently involves the insertion of a rectal tube (Fig. 2.24). If this fails and there is still doubt about the diagnosis on plain radiographs, a barium enema should be performed. Features seen at the point of torsion include smooth curved tapering like a hooked beak (**bird of prey sign**) and the mucosal folds often showing a 'screw' pattern at the point of torsion (Fig. 2.25).

VOLVULUS OF TRANSVERSE COLON AND COLONIC FLEXURES

These types of volvulae are rare but careful evaluation of the plain film findings can often suggest the diagnosis.

COMPOUND VOLVULUS – ILEOSIGMOID KNOT

A compound volvulus – specifically an ileosigmoid knot – is well recognized in developing countries but is rare elsewhere. An abnormally mobile loop of small bowel passes around the base of the pelvic colon below the attachment of the pelvic mesocolon and forms a knot. The clinical onset is abrupt with a fulminating course and intense pain in the abdomen and back. The key radiological features are a dilated loop of pelvic colon and evidence of small bowel obstruction with retained faeces in an undistended proximal colon.

ISCHAEMIC COLITIS

Ischaemic colitis is characterized clinically by the sudden onset of abdominal pain followed by bloody

Figure 2.26 *Ischaemic colitis seen on supine abdomen. There is extensive mucosal abnormality with irregular outline and wall thickening ('thumb printing') involving the entire transverse colon and proximal descending colon. (Source: S. Field in Patrick C. Freeney and Giles W. Stevenson (eds), Margulis and Burhenne's alimentary tract radiology, published by Mosby, St Louis, 1994.)*

diarrhoea. The splenic flexure and proximal descending colon are most frequently involved although other areas may be affected (Fig. 2.26). The wall and mucosa of the colon are thickened owing to haemorrhage and oedema; this can sometimes be detected on plain radiographs but in most cases a barium enema is necessary. The term **thumb printing**, showing crescentic margins, has been used to describe the appearance of the submucosal haemorrhage. The part of colon, normally on the left side, involved by the ischaemia acts as an area of functional obstruction, so that the right side of the colon is frequently distended, although the bowel wall and mucosa usually appear normal.

PARALYTIC ILEUS

Paralytic ileus occurs when intestinal peristalsis ceases and there is an accumulation of fluid and gas in the bowel. It is very common, occurring most frequently in the postoperative period and in peritonitis (Fig. 2.27). However, numerous conditions, many of which are not intra-abdominal, can cause bowel paralysis:

- peritonitis
- postoperative

(a)

(b)

Figure 2.27 *Paralytic ileus seen on (a) supine abdomen and (b) erect abdomen. Multiple loops of distended small and large bowel are present in this patient aged 57, who had profuse vomiting three days after open cholecystectomy.*

- trauma
- inflammation
  - appendicitis
  - pancreatitis
  - cholecystitis
  - salpingitis

- congestive heart failure
- pneumonia
- renal colic
- renal failure
- leaking abdominal aortic aneurysm
- low serum potassium
- drugs, e.g. morphine
- spinal lesions
- infection
- vascular occlusion
- long-standing intestinal obstruction.

The degree of distension of bowel may vary considerably from a short length of dilated small bowel to distension of the entire intestinal tract. When there is distension of both small and large bowel the appearances cannot usually be distinguished on plain radiographs from low large bowel obstruction. When there is local inflammation, such as pancreatitis, cholecystitis or appendicitis, the ileus may affect only one or two adjacent loops of small bowel – **sentinal loops** – but the appearances are non-specific and in some cases may have features indistinguishable from small bowel obstruction.

LARGE BOWEL PSEUDO-OBSTRUCTION

Pseudo-obstruction is a condition that clinically and radiologically mimics true intestinal obstruction. It is more commonly seen in elderly patients. It may be acute and self-limiting, for example when associated with pneumonia or myocardial infarction, or may be chronic in patients with myxoedema or abnormalities of the musculature of the bowel. Plain radiographic appearances can be dramatic showing very dilated colon and sometimes distended small bowel as well (Fig. 2.28). A contrast enema is usually required to exclude mechanical obstruction so preventing an unnecessary laparotomy. Sometimes, however, the caecum may exceed the critical diameter of 10 cm when perforation is imminent, and a caecostomy or right-sided colostomy may be required to prevent perforation.

PNEUMOPERITONEUM

The presence of free intra-abdominal gas almost always indicates that perforation of a viscus has occurred (Fig. 2.29). The commonest cause is the **perforation of a peptic ulcer**. Other less common causes are perforation of a diverticulum and malignant tumour (Fig. 2.30). Around 70–80 per cent of perforated ulcers will demonstrate free intra-abdominal gas but free gas is almost never seen in perforated appendicitis. By experimenting on himself, Rosco Miller demonstrated that as little as

Figure 2.28 *Pseudo-obstruction seen on supine abdomen. This 58-year-old patient developed abdominal distension and obstructive bowel sounds seven days after a pin and plate operation for a fracture through the femoral neck. The distension settled following the insertion of a rectal tube and conservative treatment.*

Figure 2.29 *Pneumoperitoneum seen on erect chest. A small amount of free intra-abdominal gas is clearly visible under the right hemidiaphragm.*

1 ml of free gas can be detected on an erect chest or left lateral decubitus abdominal film. Studies on patients with free intra-abdominal gas following surgery have demonstrated that a patient should remain in position

Figure 2.30 *Large pneumoperitoneum seen on erect chest. On the right side the raised hemidiaphragm with free gas beneath it simulates a thickened lesser fissure. A large pneumoperitoneum can sometimes be more difficult to diagnose than a small one.*

Figure 2.31 *Pneumoperitoneum and Chilaiditi's syndrome. A small triangle of gas (arrow) can be identified beneath the right hemidiaphragm adjacent to the hepatic flexure of the colon.*

for 5–10 minutes prior to the horizontal ray radiograph being taken, to ensure that any free gas present has time to rise and accumulate in the highest point (Fig. 2.31).

If a perforated viscus is suspected, then a horizontal ray radiograph – either an erect chest or left lateral decubitus abdomen – is mandatory. On the erect chest radiograph, gas is relatively easy to detect under the right hemidiaphragm, but, on the left side, free gas can be difficult to differentiate from stomach and colonic gas. In the left lateral decubitus position, free gas is readily demonstrated lying between the liver and the lateral abdominal wall (Fig. 2.32).

Horizontal ray radiographs may be difficult to obtain in some patients, particularly those who are unconscious, who have suffered trauma or are critically ill. It

(a)

(b)

Figure 2.32 *Pneumoperitoneum seen on (a) erect chest and (b) left lateral decubitus abdomen. A small amount of gas (difficult to ascertain whether it is intraluminal or free) lies beneath the right hemidiaphragm on the erect chest radiograph (arrow). The left lateral decubitus radiograph taken after the patient had been lying on their left side for 10 minutes clearly demonstrates the pneumoperitoneum. (Source: S. Field, in D.J. Nolan (ed.),* A radiological atlas of gastrointestinal disease; *published by John Wiley, Chichester, 1983.)*

Figure 2.33 *Pneumoperitoneum seen on supine abdomen. Streaks and bands of linear gas can be identified in the right subhepatic region (arrows) in this patient with perforated duodenal ulcer. (Source: S. Field in D.J. Nolan (ed.), A radiological atlas of gastrointestinal disease; published by John Wiley, Chichester, 1983.)*

is, therefore, important to be able to recognize the signs of a pneumoperitoneum on supine radiographs, particularly as perforation of a viscus may be clinically silent and be overshadowed by other serious medical or surgical conditions. A supine abdominal film, often taken using portable equipment, may be the only radiograph that can be obtained in these situations.

In nearly 60 per cent of patients with a pneumoperitoneum, gas may be detectable on the supine radiograph as:

- right upper quadrant gas
  - perihepatic
  - subhepatic
  - Morrison's pouch
  - visible fissure for the ligamentum teres
- Rigler's (double wall) sign
- ligament visualization
  - falciform (ligamentum teres)
  - umbilical (inverted 'V' sign)
- triangular air sign

Figure 2.34 *Pneumoperitoneum ('Rigler's sign') seen on supine abdomen. Both sides of the bowel wall can clearly be identified in the distended small bowel loops. There is also free gas in the right upper quadrant. (Source: S. Field in Patrick C. Freeney and Giles W. Stevenson (eds),* Margulis and Burhenne's alimentary tract radiology; *published by Mosby, St Louis, 1994.)*

- cupola sign
- football or air-dome sign
- scrotal air (in children).

Almost half the patient with free gas will have an oval or linear collection of gas visible in the right upper quadrant adjacent to the liver lying mainly in the subhepatic space and hepatorenal fossa (**Morrison's pouch**) (Fig. 2.33). The liver shadow appears darker when it is surrounded by free gas. A less common sign of free gas on a supine radiograph is the visualization of the outer wall of a loop of bowel (**Rigler's sign**) (Fig. 2.34). However, this sign may be misleading if several loops of bowel lie close together or if fat lies outside the bowel wall. The visualization of the falciform (Fig. 2.35) or umbilical ligaments may be demonstrated by the free gas lying on each side of these ligaments. Air in the fissure for the ligamentum teres may produce a band of air in the right upper quadrant. Free gas between loops of bowel may take on a triangular configuration and large amounts may accumulate under the diaphragm (**cupola sign**) or anterior abdominal wall simulating an American football.

PNEUMOPERITONEUM WITHOUT PERITONITIS

Rarely patients who present with vague clinical symptoms have unequivocal evidence of a pneumoperitoneum on chest or abdominal radiographs:

Figure 2.35 *Pneumoperitoneum, and falciform ligament seen on supine abdomen. The falciform ligament is clearly identified by the large amount of free gas which lies on either side of it (arrows). Small extra luminal bubbles of gas lie in multiple intraperitoneal abscesses in this case of perforated gastric ulcer.*

- silent perforation of a viscus which has sealed itself in:
  - the elderly
  - patients on steroids
  - unconscious patients
  - patients being ventilated
  - presence of other serious medical conditions
- postoperative
- peritoneal dialysis
- perforated jejunal diverticulosis
- perforated cyst in pneumatosis intestinalis
- tracking down from a pneumomediatinum
- stercoral ulceration
- leakage through a distended stomach (e.g. endoscopy)
- vaginal – tubal entry of air.

However, clinical examination may demonstrate that there is no evidence of peritonitis or indication for immediate surgery. Most of these patients will have perforated a viscus which has released gas and then sealed itself. Other causes of a pneumoperitoneum under these circumstances include pneumatosis intestinalis, recent abdominal surgery and other iatrogenic causes, such as fallopian tube insufflation or peritoneal dialysis. Embolization of an intra-abdominal viscus has also been implicated and some physical activities in women, such as water skiing, are also well documented causes.

PSEUDOPNEUMOPERITONEUM

There are a number of rare but important conditions which on first appearances may look remarkably similar to a pneumoperitoneum and these must be considered in every doubtful case:

- intestine between liver and diaphragm (Chilaiditi's syndrome)
- subphrenic abscess
- curvilinear supradiaphragmatic pulmonary collapse
- subdiaphragmatic fat
- diaphragmatic irregularity
- cysts in pneumatosis intestinalis.

An error of interpretation may lead to an unnecessary laparotomy in search of a perforated viscus. The commonest of these is interposition of bowel between the liver and the diaphragm on the right side, **Chilaiditi's syndrome** (Fig. 2.36). Although this occurs in a small number of people with chronic lung disease or with postnecrotic cirrhosis of the liver and ascites, it is most commonly an incidental finding. **Subdiaphragmatic fat** can usually be distinguished from air by the slightly more lateral situation of the curvilinear radiolucent lines. Small amounts of gas giving this appearance are normally found under the highest point of the diaphragm. A thin band of curvilinear **pulmonary**

Figure 2.36 *Pseudopneumoperitoneum (Chilaiditi's syndrome). Gas-filled loops of predominantly large bowel beneath both hemidiaphragms simulate a pneumoperitoneum.*

Figure 2.37 *Pseudopneumoperitoneum and curvilinear pulmonary collapse seen on erect chest. A band of curvilinear pulmonary collapse (arrows), with aerated lung beneath it, exactly simulates a small pneumoperitoneum.*

Figure 2.38 *Pseudopneumoperitoneum and double diaphragmatic hump seen on erect chest. The gastric fundal air shadow seen through an uneven diaphragm simulates a pneumoperitoneum. (Source: S. Field, in Patrick C. Freeney and Giles W. Stevenson (eds),* Margulis and Burhenne's alimentary tract radiology; *published by Mosby, St Louis, 1994.)*

atelectasis, situated just above and parallel to the diaphragm with a band of normally aerated lung between the atelectasis and the diaphragm can simulate a pneumoperitoneum almost exactly (Fig. 2.37). Gas within a **subphrenic abscess** can also simulate a pneumoperitoneum. When the left hemidiaphragm is slightly irregular, the stomach fundal gas shadow may be seen between two humps, and the crescent of gas thus formed simulate a pneumoperitoneum (Fig. 2.38). Gas cysts in pneumatosis intestinalis lying between the diaphragm shadow and the intestinal wall may also form a trap for the unwary.

THE POSTOPERATIVE ABDOMEN

The same general principles for diagnosis apply for the postoperative as to the preoperative abdominal radiograph. However, because of recent surgical intervention, the radiological signs may be modified and more difficult to interpret. **Postoperative paralytic ileus** is common and may simulate and coexist with obstruction. Sometimes obstruction from adhesions may occur within a few days of a laparotomy.

Around 60 per cent of all postlaparotomy patients will have evidence of a **pneumoperitoneum** and this will take 1–24 days to be reabsorbed. However, normally, postoperative gas is absorbed within three days. The patient's body habitus is the most important factor influencing the occurrence and duration of postoperative pneumoperitoneum. Gas is absorbed more rapidly in obese patients who normally have no

residual gas after the fourth postoperative day. Providing an identical radiographic technique is used and adequate time is spent in the position for the horizontal ray radiograph (usually 10 minutes), any increase in the amount of gas occurring postoperatively indicates either an anastomotic leak or the perforation of a viscus. Very rarely, gas may track into the peritoneal cavity along an abdominal drain.

RETROPERITONEAL PERFORATION

Retroperitoneal perforation of a viscus occurs most commonly secondary to duodenal ulceration or diverticular disease. In the latter condition gas may track down into the leg.

INTRAPERITONEAL FLUID

Usually fluid within the peritoneal cavity collects in the most dependent part, namely the pelvis. As more fluid

Figure 2.39 *Ascites seen on supine abdomen. Fluid density within the pelvis obliterates the fat line of the superior part of the bladder. Fluid within the flanks displaces the ascending and descending colon medially. The diagnosis was spontaneous intraperitoneal haemorrhage after childbirth. (Source: S. Field in Patrick C. Freeney and Giles W. Stevenson (eds),* Margulis and Burhenne's alimentary tract radiology; *published by Mosby, St Louis, 1994.)*

accumulates it passes up the paracolic gutter on each side and on the right reaches the subhepatic and subphrenic spaces.

The first radiological sign of fluid is a soft-tissue density lying within the pelvis or 'dog ears' – soft-tissue masses visualized lateral to the rectal gas shadow. More fluid causes the ascending and descending colon to be displaced medially and separate from the flank fat stripe (Fig. 2.39). As fluid enters the subhepatic space it causes loss of visualization of the hepatic angle and, finally, when large amounts of fluid are present, separation of small bowel loops, which move centrally, and thinning of the flank stripes may occur. Large amounts of intra-abdominal fluid causes a generalized haze over the abdomen resulting in poor visualization of normal structures such as the psoas and renal outlines.

INFLAMMATORY CONDITIONS

ACUTE APPENDICITIS

Acute appendicitis is the commonest acute surgical condition in the developed world and has an overall mortality of around 1 per cent. When the clinical history and findings are typical, abdominal radiographs are not indicated. However, in a number of patients, particularly the young and old, clinical features may be obscure and the diagnosis difficult or sometimes impossible without further investigations, including a laparotomy. In complicated appendicitis, radiographs may play a significant role in suggesting the diagnosis.

There are no specific plain radiographic signs of acute appendicitis but features which frequently may be found include:

- appendix calculus 5–60 mm (appendolith);
- sentinel loop (dilated atonic ileum containing fluid level);
- widening of properitoneal fat line;

Figure 2.40 *Acute appendicitis seen on supine abdomen. An appendix calculus can be identified in the right side of the pelvis overlying the caecum (arrow). There is also small bowel distension.*

Figure 2.41 *Acute cholecystitis seen on supine abdomen. The gallbladder is full of faceted calcified stones. In addition, several calculi to the right of L2 lie within the common bile duct (arrow).*

Figure 2.42 *Empyema of the gallbladder seen on supine abdomen. Several calcified gallstones can be identified, some containing gas ('Mercedes' sign). One calculus lies over the neck of the right 12th rib and lies in Hartmann's pouch. Two others lie some distance away in the fundus of the gallbladder. An estimate of the gallbladder size can be made from the separation of the gallstones.*

- blurring of properitoneal fat line;
- right lower quadrant haze owing to fluid and oedema;
- scoliosis concave to the right;
- mass indenting the caecum.

Unfortunately many of these features are relatively non-specific. The radiographic signs result from localized inflammatory change leading to an associated paralytic ileus. The signs may change if the appendicitis leads to perforation and abscess formation. The abscess may result in the indentation of the caecum on its medial border and, when the inflammation permeates into the adjacent fat, may lead to loss of the lower part of the properitoneal fat line and the right psoas muscle shadow. Small bowel obstruction may occur as several loops of bowel become matted together or stuck to the inflamed appendix. An appendix calculus, which can often be identified as an oval calcific ring shadow often with multiple rings, is associated with appendicitis, particularly in children (Fig. 2.40). Although air may be seen within the appendix in acute appendicitis, this may also be seen in normal subjects, large bowel obstruction and paralytic ileus, particularly when the appendix is high and retrocaecal in position.

The use of other imaging techniques for the diagnosis of appendicitis is discussed on pages 103–4.

ACUTE CHOLECYSTITIS

Plain radiographic signs of acute cholecystitis include:

- gallstones, visualized in only 20 per cent;
- right hypochondrial mass owing to enlarged gallbladder;
- duodenal ileus;
- ileus of hepatic flexure of colon;
- gas within the biliary system.

About 90 per cent of cases of acute cholecystitis are associated with gallstones (Fig. 2.41). Acute cholecystitis is usually caused by a stone obstructing the cystic duct (Fig. 2.42). However, only around 20 per cent of gallstones contain sufficient calcium to be visible on plain radiographs, and only rarely does the wall of the

Figure 2.43 *Empyema of the gallbladder seen on supine abdomen. The greater omentum containing large amounts of fat was found to surround the inflamed gallbladder. This has rendered the distended gallbladder visible on the plain film (arrows).*

gallbladder itself calcify. Occasionally stones have gas within them forming a star-shaped pattern giving rise to an appearance known as the 'Mercedes' sign. The majority of patients with gallstones, however, never develop acute cholecystitis. It is uncommon to identify a normal sized gallbladder on plain films because it is not surrounded by fat and has the same radiographic density as the adjacent structures. However, if the gallbladder enlarges owing to obstruction of the cystic duct, it may then be visualized by the displacement of adjacent gas-filled structures (Fig. 2.43). In acute cholecystitis the duodenum and hepatic flexure of the colon may show a localized paralytic ileus secondary to inflammation. However, in most patients with acute cholecystitis the plain films may be completely normal or only demonstrate minimal dilatation of small or large bowel.

Scintigraphy using ⁹⁹ᵐTc-labelled derivatives of iminodiacetic acid (IDA) is a simple and reasonably accurate method of diagnosing acute cholecystitis. However, enthusiasm for the technique is variable and usually ultrasound is performed (see p. 151).

Tenderness of the gallbladder as it lies immediately beneath the ultrasound transducer is also a very reliable sign that the gallbladder is acutely inflamed – the **ultrasound Murphy's sign**.

ACUTE PANCREATITIS

The pathological changes occurring in acute pancreatitis include oedema, haemorrhage, infarction of the pancreas, fat necrosis and sometimes acute suppuration. The inflammatory process may extend into the gastrocolic ligament or the paraduodenal area, or follow the root of the mesentery or extend into the anterior pararenal space. The clinical diagnosis of acute pancreatitis can be difficult and often rests on the exclusion of other conditions such as a perforated peptic ulcer. Pancreatitis is usually confirmed by finding a markedly elevated serum amylase level. However, this test has a number of well recognized limitations as the amylase levels may also be raised in perforated peptic ulcer, acute cholecystitis and intestinal obstruction.

A plain abdominal radiograph is frequently taken in patients suspected of having acute pancreatitis. Although a large number of radiological signs have been described, many of these are of little or no value in the diagnosis of acute pancreatitis.

- **Most common and sometimes useful**
  - gas-filled duodenal cap and loop
  - single dilated small bowel loop (sentinel loop)
  - small bowel ileus
  - dilated colon, particularly transverse and ascending
  - dilated terminal ileum
  - loss of the left psoas outline
- **Rare but diagnostic**
  - gas within the pancreas
  - faint mottling owing to fat necrosis

Gas in the duodenum is best demonstrated in the left lateral decubitus position. A dilated transverse colon and isolated dilated loops of proximal small bowel

Figure 2.44 *Acute pancreatitis and pancreatic calcification.*

(sentinel loops) are frequent findings but they are non-specific. A gasless abdomen may be caused by persistent vomiting. Occasionally pancreatic calcification is identified in those patients who also have chronic pancreatitis (Fig. 2.44).

Demonstration of gas within the pancreas, usually seen as multiple small bubbles giving a mottled appearance, is diagnostic of a pancreatic abscess heralding a grave prognosis. In acute pancreatitis ultrasound may demonstrate an oedematous pancreas but gas-filled loops of small bowel resulting from the paralytic ileus may make ultrasound difficult or impossible. In these circumstances CT may demonstrate the pancreas but both CT and ultrasound may be normal in the early stages of acute pancreatitis. Complications of acute pancreatitis such as a pancreatic abscess or pancreatic pseudocyst may produce plain film findings such as a soft-tissue mass but such complications are usually diagnosed by ultrasound or CT scanning (see p. 165).

Pleural effusions, mainly left-sided, may occur in acute pancreatitis. The presence of a left-sided effusion in a patient with proven acute pancreatitis indicates a more severe disease process with a worse prognosis.

INTRA-ABDOMINAL ABSCESSES

Abscesses act as mass lesions displacing adjacent structures, for example elevation of a hemidiaphragm by a subphrenic abscess or displacement of the colon by a paracolic abscess. Abscesses are of soft-tissue density but frequently they contain gas. This gas may form single or multiple small bubble-like radiolucencies, produce radiolucent bands following fascial planes or outline an anatomical space. Sometimes there is a single or loculated large gas/fluid collection in the abscess giving an air–fluid level on an erect film. The inflammatory process and oedema usually cause ill-defined tissue margins and loss of fat lines outlining the adjacent anatomical structures. Plain film diagnosis of abscesses depends on a number of factors but a detailed knowledge is essential of the peritoneal reflections and spaces together with the normal anatomical landmarks. Meticulous attention to detail in viewing the radiograph is also needed as recognition of small bubbles of gas outside the bowel lumen, often unchanged in position on sequential films, strongly suggests an abscess. Although a high proportion of abscesses, particularly if large, may be identified on plain films, ultrasound, CT or radionuclide scanning with labelled leucocytes are more sensitive techniques (see p. 116).

SUBPHRENIC ABSCESS

A subphrenic abscess is nearly always a consequence of surgery (Fig. 2.45). Subphrenic abscesses can be

Figure 2.45 *Subphrenic abscess seen on erect chest. The left hemidiaphragm is raised and there is a left-sided pleural effusion associated with some collapse and consolidation in the left lower lobe. The gas-filled abscess is clearly visible beneath the left hemidiaphragm. The radiograph was taken 10 days following a Hartmann's procedure for diverticular disease.*

expected to show a raised hemidiaphragm on the affected side in 80 per cent of cases; about 70 per cent will show evidence of basal pulmonary consolidation or collapse and 60 per cent will have an associated pleural effusion. In postlaparotomy patients, a subphrenic abscess is the commonest cause of unilateral pleural effusion. Abscesses may be identified as a soft-tissue mass, which may contain irregular pockets of gas and a gas–fluid level on the erect film.

PARACOLIC ABSCESS

Usually a paracolic abscess lies close to the causative lesion. Right paracolic and left paracolic abscesses most commonly follow appendicitis and diverticulitis (Figs 2.46, 2.47). Sometimes, however, infection may spread away from its origin and produce an abscess elsewhere either within the pelvis or in the subphrenic space. Soft-tissue masses, often containing bubbles of gas and causing colonic displacement, are the most common plain film findings.

(a)

(b)

Figure 2.46 *Left paracolic abscess secondary to perforated diverticular disease seen on (a) supine abdomen and (b) contrast enema. Multiple small gas bubbles can be identified in the abscess on the plain film (arrow). The contrast enema clearly demonstrates leak outside the bowel lumen.*

PELVIC ABSCESS

The pelvis is the most dependent part of the abdomen and is the commonest site of abscesses in postlaparotomy patients. A pelvic abscess may occur following localized pelvic inflammatory disease or following appendicitis or diverticulitis. A soft-tissue mass sometimes containing gas may be identified superior to the bladder outline, and the fat interface between the mass and the bladder is usually absent.

GAS WITHIN THE BOWEL WALL

CYSTIC PNEUMATOSIS (PNEUMATOSIS INTESTINALIS)

In this uncommon condition cyst-like collections of gas are seen both subserosally and submucosally in the intestine, with the colon being most commonly affected (**pneumatosis coli**) (Fig. 2.48). Pneumatosis intestinalis is a relatively benign condition usually occurring in the middle-aged and elderly and associated most commonly with chronic obstructive airways disease. The gas-filled cysts in the bowel vary in size from 1 cm to 3 cm, and symptoms include vague abdominal pain, diarrhoea, constipation and mucus discharge. The plain film findings are characteristic: the gas-containing cysts give rise to an appearance quite different from normal gas shadows. Occasionally these cysts rupture producing a chronic pneumoperitoneum without evidence of peritonitis.

INTERSTITIAL EMPHYSEMA

In this rare condition linear bubbles of gas can be identified in the bowel wall and there is often associated oedema of the bowel. It occurs in ischaemia, severe infections or inflammatory bowel disease and in these situations it is associated with bowel necrosis and perforation.

Neonates, especially if premature, can develop severe inflammation of the gut – **necrotizing enterocolitis**. The diagnosis is based on clinical and radiological signs. The infants typically develop abdominal distension, vomiting and bloody diarrhoea. Generalized bowel dilatation, wall thickening and bowel loop separation

(a)

(b)

Figure 2.47 *Left paracolic abscess following perforated diverticular disease seen on (a) abdomen and (b) CT scan. On the plain film the abscess is identified as a large gas-filled viscus overlying the left iliac bone. On the CT scan its close association with the sigmoid colon is demonstrated. In addition the muscles of the abdominal wall have become involved and are being destroyed by the infective process.*

Figure 2.48 *Pneumatosis coli seen on supine abdomen. Numerous ring shadows of varying size can be identified arising from most of the large bowel in this patient aged 87 with abdominal pain and diarrhoea.*

INFECTIONS WITH GAS-FORMING ORGANISMS

Many bacteria are capable of producing gas but those most commonly responsible in humans are *Escherichia coli*, *Clostridium welchii* and *Klebsiella aerogenes*. Such infections usually give rise to severe constitutional disturbance and toxaemia with a high mortality rate; they produce a localized abnormal collection of gas in the abdomen or pelvis. However, over half of all gas-forming infections occur in diabetics when the infecting organism is usually *E. coli*; in this group the constitutional disturbance is usually less than in non-diabetics.

EMPHYSEMATOUS GASTRITIS

Emphysematous gastritis is a severe infection resulting in a contracted stomach with frothy or mottled radiolucencies visible within the stomach wall in the left upper abdomen.

EMPHYSEMATOUS CHOLECYSTITIS

Emphysematous cholecystitis is caused by a gas-forming infection of the gallbladder which results in gas in the

are early plain film findings. Later a foamy gas pattern and a linear or crescentic appearance caused by gas may be seen in the bowel wall when mucosal necrosis and autolysis have developed.

Figure 2.49 *Emphysematous cholecystitis seen on prone abdomen following oral cholecystographic contrast media. Linear gas shadows can be identified within the wall of the gallbladder (arrows) in this diabetic patient aged 62. (Source: S. Field in R.G. Grainger and D.J. Allison (eds),* Diagnostic radiology; *published by Churchill Livingstone, Edinburgh, 1991.)*

Figure 2.50 *Emphysematous cystitis seen on supine abdomen in a 78-year-old diabetic with* E. coli *urinary tract infection. The bladder is distended and linear streaks of gas can be clearly identified within its wall. (Courtesy of Dr A.R. Carter.)*

lumen and/or wall of the gallbladder (Fig. 2.49). It tends to occur in older patients, half of whom are diabetic, and with clinical findings suggestive of acute cholecystitis. It occurs with equal frequency in males and females and, unlike ordinary cholecystitis, gallstones may be absent.

EMPHYSEMATOUS CYSTITIS

Emphysematous cystitis causes gas cysts and linear gas streaks within the wall of the urinary bladder and is sometimes associated with gas within the lumen of the bladder (Fig. 2.50). The condition is most common in diabetics. Emphysematous cystitis must be distinguished from gas confined to the lumen of the bladder caused by a **vesicocolic fistula** which is not associated with gas within the wall of the bladder.

EMPHYSEMATOUS PYELONEPHRITIS

Emphysematous pyelonephritis is recognized by the demonstration of bubbles of gas within the kidney or linear streaks of gas beneath the renal capsule. The condition occurs in uncontrolled diabetics or in patients with obstructive uropathy.

RENAL COLIC

A proportion of patients admitted with acute abdominal pain have acute ureteric obstruction. Although the calculus may be situated in any part of the ureter it is frequently found at its lower end. Although nearly 90 per cent of all ureteric calculi causing obstruction are radiopaque, they are often extremely small and difficult to identify on plain radiographs alone or, if identified, impossible to establish as being located within the ureter. **Phleboliths** within the pelvis are a source of potential confusion but their radiolucent centre and smooth spherical outline help to distinguish them from ureteric stones which are frequently oval, slightly irregular in outline and without a radiolucent centre. The pain of renal colic often leads to air swallowing and an associated paralytic ileus which results in dramatic gas-filled loops of small and large bowel that may also contain fluid levels.

An emergency intravenous urogram is usually required to make a diagnosis and identify the point of obstruction; in many centres this is performed as an emergency soon after hospital admission. Occasionally ureteric colic is complicated by the spontaneous rupture of the renal pelvis, leading to a retroperitoneal accumulation of urine known as a **urinoma**. This can be identified on plain radiographs as a soft-tissue mass with loss of the renal and psoas outline and is often associated with marked paralytic ileus. Diagnosis is usually only confirmed following emergency urography or CT.

LEAKING ABDOMINAL AORTIC ANEURYSM

Signs include:

- soft-tissue retroperitoneal mass;
- curvilinear calcification in the wall;
- loss of psoas outline;
- loss of renal outline;
- displacement of kidney.

A leaking abdominal aortic aneurysm usually presents as an acute abdomen and may sometimes simulate renal colic. The clinical diagnosis may be obvious and, if the patient is in a state of shock, resuscitation followed by urgent surgery is indicated; further investigations are not usually required. If confirmation of a leaking aneurysm is required then ultrasound or CT (*see* pp. 124, 659) will establish the diagnosis of an aneurysm and may demonstrate a retroperitoneal haematoma. However, sometimes a leaking aneurysm is not suspected clinically and chest and abdominal radiographs taken to investigate the pain may show an aneurysm as a central soft-tissue mass obscuring the psoas or renal shadows, particularly on the left side. Curvilinear calcification is a useful observation as it will indicate the size of the aorta and the presence of an aneurysm. Aortic calcification may be seen on an AP radiograph but is best detected on a lateral view. A soft-tissue mass identified outside the calcified aneurysm indicates haematoma caused by the leaking aneurysm. Loss of psoas or renal outlines or displacement of a kidney are strong presumptive evidence of a leak from the aneurysm (Fig. 2.51). An aneurysm is sometimes detected following emergency urography for suspected ureteric colic. The enlarging aneurysm causes displacement and compression of the ureter with resulting back pressure changes in the kidney. There is often an associated secondary paralytic ileus associated with the

Figure 2.51 *Leaking aortic aneurysm seen on supine abdomen. The calcified wall of the aneurysm can be identified on the right (arrows) but the psoas margin can be seen. There is a soft-tissue mass on the left with obliteration of renal and psoas outlines and bulging in the flank. There was a left-sided leak with 5 litres of blood in the left retroperitoneal region.*

leaking aneurysm and the dilated bowel may completely obscure the aneurysm itself.

FURTHER READING

Baker, S.R. and Cho, K.C. 1999: *The abdominal plain film with correlative imaging* (2nd edition). Stanford: Appleton and Lange.

Myers, M.A. 1998: *Dynamic radiology of the abdomen. Normal and pathologic anatomy* (4th edition). New York, NY: Springer-Verlag.

3

Gastrointestinal tract

RICHARD FARROW, GILES W. STEVENSON

INTRODUCTION: TECHNIQUES AVAILABLE

PLAIN RADIOGRAPHS

Plain abdominal radiographs retain an important role in the evaluation of suspected obstruction, perforation, infection, inflammatory bowel disease and calcifications, but often the information available from the radiograph is not specific enough to permit a full diagnosis. A wide array of techniques is available either to supplement the plain film, or in many cases to serve as the initial imaging study. One of the challenges facing radiologists is to identify those patients in whom newer techniques should replace plain abdominal radiographs as the initial imaging examination.

CONTRAST FLUOROSCOPY

The first contrast examination of the upper gastrointestinal (GI) tract using metallic salts introduced into the stomach of guinea-pigs was published in 1896, only months after the initial description of the X-ray by Roentgen. Initially clinical studies of the upper and lower GI tract used a single contrast technique with dense heavy metal salts. Attempts to obtain a more detailed mucosal view by means of a double contrast technique date back to 1906 when a combination of bismuth and effervescent agents was used to visualize the stomach. Publications from Sweden and Japan led to the gradual acceptance of the double contrast

technique in most departments around the world for both upper and lower GI studies. Initially air was used as the negative contrast agent for the colon, but more recently CO_2 has been used in an attempt to reduce postprocedural pain. For double contrast studies the ideal barium is non-flocculating, non-toxic, cheap, has a high radiographic density, gives good mucosal coating and is palatable and easy to administer. For single contrast the radiographic density must be much lower and a premium is placed on non-sedimentation of the barium suspension, which is achieved by the use of more uniform and smaller barium particles.

Barium is an excellent contrast agent for the GI tract provided that is where it stays. Barium aspirated into the lungs is usually harmless and can be expectorated either spontaneously or with help from a physiotherapist. If there is a suspicion that the contrast will not remain within the lumen of the GI tract, because of the presence of a fistula, sinus, perforation or anastomotic leak, a water-soluble contrast agent should be used, since intraperitoneal barium can cause a peritoneal reaction and adhesions, even if sterile. The peritoneal reaction is largely due to the silica content of the barium preparation, which was high in the past but is low in modern barium preparations. The first water-soluble contrast agents were both ionic and of high osmolality, but more recently low osmolar ionic and non-ionic agents have become available. The high osmolar agents retain a place where leaks are suspected but there is no risk of aspiration into the lungs. These high osmolality agents are pneumotoxic, and, in situations where aspiration is a possibility, a low osmolar agent should be used.

In infants the low osmolar agents should be used in all situations to reduce fluid shifts from the intravascular to extravascular spaces that occur owing to the osmotic effect of the high osmolar agents. The exception to this rule is when contrast is being introduced as a therapeutic measure in cases of neonatal meconium ileus. In this situation, the fluid shift caused by the high osmolality of the contrast agent within the bowel is an asset. The shift of fluid into the bowel lumen helps to soften the meconium and makes it easier to pass, but scrupulous attention to fluid balance is then required.

IMAGING EQUIPMENT

There have been many changes in equipment since the early days of GI radiology when the available X-ray tubes produced only a low and inconsistent output. Today high definition digital techniques are used that allow the fluoroscopic image to be stored and printed, with good spatial resolution, without the need for the additional radiation required for a conventional radiographic exposure (Fig. 3.1). When high detail resolution is required, a radiographic exposure can be made in the usual way (Fig. 3.2), and this image can then be further manipulated digitally. Most paediatric and interventional work can be done with the stored fluoroscopic images, with reductions in radiation dose

Figure 3.2 *Normal upper GI study demonstrating normal areae gastricae. Areae gastricae are not always visible on a barium study. Areae over 4 mm in size are statistically associated with duodenal ulcer disease and probably with* Helicobacter pylori *infection.*

Figure 3.1 *Fluoro-record image (to minimize patient radiation dose) from a water-soluble enema study demonstrating a microcolon (small black arrow) and caecum (white arrow), and an abrupt termination to the ileum (long black arrow) owing to ileal atresia.*

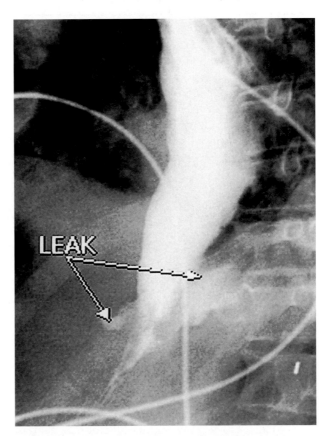

Figure 3.3 *Postoperative anastomotic leak demonstrated using non-ionic contrast swallow. Image annotation at the digital work station has been used to indicate the abnormality.*

of up to one half. The future will see a revolution in digital imaging as TV monitors become more common in hospitals and outside clinics. Original images and images annotated by the radiologist (Fig. 3.3) will become available in operating theatres, outpatient clinics and on the wards. The images can also be combined into a electronic teaching archive or incorporated into Web-based tutorials.

COMPUTED TOMOGRAPHY

By 1975 whole body CT scanners capable of abdominal scanning were available. Further advances reduced scan times, enabling a single CT axial image to be acquired during the space of one breath-hold. More recently spiral scanners have become available which have produced a dramatic reduction in scan times, such that the whole of the abdomen can now be imaged in one breath-hold. This allows a detailed assessment of hollow abdominal organs, in particular the colon. If a full cleansing bowel preparation is given, the colon can be distended with gas, and mucosal disease detected (Fig. 3.4). This technique of CT colography or CT pneumocolon has the potential to replace barium enema studies and diagnostic colonoscopy in many situations and may have a role in colon cancer screening programmes. Currently this technique is being largely used as a problem-solving tool in patients with equivocal results from barium studies or following incomplete colonoscopy. CT pneumocolon can be very useful if

there is a distal colonic carcinoma that is causing marked luminal narrowing preventing adequate barium studies and endoscopy. The CT is used to assess the more proximal colon for synchronous disease and also allows visualization of the liver for metastases.

When the alimentary tract is assessed with CT, the bowel must be distended and opacified, usually with dilute water-soluble contrast or 1 per cent barium, given in divided doses. The first dose is designed to opacify the large and lower small bowel, and a second dose of contrast is given just before the scan to opacify the stomach and upper small bowel. If this oral contrast is not given, loops of bowel may be misdiagnosed as abscess, lymphadenopathy or tumour. Regular barium is not used to opacify the bowel as the high density causes image artefact and degradation of the image. Barium remaining within the bowel from a previous contrast study causes similar problems. CT is useful in the diagnosis and staging of alimentary tract tumours, and in the assessment of inflammatory bowel disease and complications of GI disease or surgery, such as fluid collections and abscesses. In general, CT is at its best in patients with sufficient body fat to delineate all the abdominal organs, both solid and hollow (Fig. 3.5), in contradistinction to ultrasound where excess fat may make examination difficult.

Figure 3.5 *CT scan of the caecum. The caecum has been distended with air, in order to evaluate the ileocaecal valve. Barium enema (after a failed colonoscopy) had shown a large valve with a differential diagnosis of cancer or fatty infiltration. The CT scan shows a prominent valve due to fatty infiltration (arrow) and no evidence of tumour.*

Figure 3.4 *CT pneumocolon showing a pedunculated polyp. The colon is distended with carbon dioxide. There is no faecal residue following the thorough bowel preparation.*

ULTRASOUND

The Japanese, in 1949, were the first to report a medical use for ultrasound, describing falx localization to detect shift of intracranial midline structures. General

Figure 3.6 *Bowel wall thickening. The thickened wall of the transverse colon is demonstrated on ultrasound (the bowel wall thickness is measured with the calipers). This thickening was due to extensive pseudomembranous colitis, but thickening can also be seen with Crohn's disease, ulcerative colitis, ischaemia,* Campylobacter *infection and diverticulitis.*

acceptance of ultrasound awaited the introduction of high-resolution, hand-held, grey-scale scanners which provide a real-time image of the structure under evaluation. Ultrasound is readily available with machines that are both relatively inexpensive and mobile, and uses no ionizing radiation. These advantages mean that ultrasound should generally be considered the initial cross-sectional examination in most patients with suspected abdominal pathology. The use of graded compression with real-time scanning allows evaluation of both bowel wall movement and wall thickness (Fig. 3.6). This, combined with the sensitivity of ultrasound to assess fluid collections and free fluid within the abdomen, has led to its use in a wide range of diseases affecting the bowel and mesentery. Endoscopic ultrasound now provides accurate tumour staging in the upper GI tract and can also be used to guide transoesophageal fine needle aspiration biopsy of mediastinal nodes. Intraoperative probes are becoming available for both open and laparoscopic surgery, and therapeutic focused ultrasound for tumour ablation is moving from the laboratory to the operating theatre, and will in due course move to the radiology department's interventional suite.

RADIONUCLIDE IMAGING

Radionuclide imaging provides images which are of lower spatial resolution than those provided by other imaging techniques but does provide information on

function, which may be impossible to achieve by other means. Most studies are now performed using technetium-99m as the radionuclide; ^{99m}Tc is incorporated into a variety of compounds to provide information on motility and the presence or extent of disease. The labelling of tumour-specific antigens is still being developed but raises the possibility of diagnostic scans for a specific primary tumour and also for assessment of involved but normal-size lymph nodes.

MAGNETIC RESONANCE IMAGING

MRI has traditionally had a very limited place in the assessment of the GI tract. This is largely due to the long scan times required and the intrinsic motility of the bowel, which leads to poor resolution. In addition there is little difference in signal between the bowel wall and bowel contents on scans taken without contrast. Both of these difficulties are being resolved and spectacular images of the small bowel can now be produced. MRI is of proven value in pelvic inflammatory disease and the relationship of fistulae to the sphincter complex (Fig. 3.7).

Figure 3.7 *Perianal abscess. This abscess is seen as an area of high signal (curved arrow) in this pelvic MR scan which uses a fat suppression sequence. Connecting with this abscess is a fistula, seen as a high signal track (straight arrow) which communicates with the skin by the ischiorectal fossa. (Courtesy of S. Somers.)*

ENDOSCOPY

Endoscopy provides an alternative technique to contrast studies in the assessment of the GI tract. It provides indirect but highly detailed visual assessment of intestinal mucosa and also permits therapeutic interventional procedures and biopsies. Both endoscopy and barium studies can detect lesions missed by the other technique. Sensitivity for detecting tumours, polyps and ulcers is operator-dependent for both methods but is generally slightly better for endoscopy. Endoscopy does allow a better assessment of erythematous and angiodysplastic lesions. However, endoscopy has a higher morbidity and mortality than the corresponding barium study, and the need for sedation and postprocedural care are further relative disadvantages. There is less patient movement required for endoscopy and this can be an important consideration in patients with reduced mobility from whatever cause; older patients, for example, tend to prefer endoscopy. Selection between endoscopy or a barium study will thus depend on mobility of the patient, the local availability and quality of the two procedures and on the exact question that needs to be answered in any particular patient.

UPPER GI TRACT (OESOPHAGUS, STOMACH AND DUODENUM)

EXAMINATIONS AVAILABLE

Three different fluoroscopic examinations may be performed to evaluate the upper GI tract, each with some variations depending on the nature of the clinical problem. This section is organized to illustrate the role of each of the examinations: the swallowing assessment, the barium swallow and the barium meal.

SWALLOWING ASSESSMENT

This study is used to assess patients who have difficulty with swallowing, and those who choke on or aspirate food.

The normal process of swallowing is complex and incorporates oral, pharyngeal and oesophageal phases, which link together in a coordinated fashion to propel the food bolus from the mouth to the stomach. This process requires the coordination of many muscles, six cranial nerves (V, VII, IX, X, XI, XII) and the first, second and third cervical nerves. Afferent information is processed within the medulla, with the motor response coordinated through the motor ganglia of the appropriate cranial nerves. Thus neuronal or muscular dysfunction at many levels can result in eating difficulties.

Pharyngeal dysfunction may present with drooling, choking, a nasal voice, cough, recurrent chest infections and hoarseness as well as dysphagia, and it may be difficult to decide the most appropriate specialty for patient management. This has led to the introduction of a multidisciplinary team approach in the evaluation and treatment of these patients, with input from various specialties including speech therapy, radiology, gastroenterology, thoracic surgery and ENT. The presence of a speech therapist during the radiological assessment provides vital information on the exact clinical problems

so that the examination can be tailored to answer the relevant questions. The radiologist and speech therapist should work as a team, issuing a joint report on the findings and the therapeutic implications. The speech therapist can get immediate feedback on the success of any therapeutic manoeuvres instigated. Video (which has largely replaced cine-radiology) is an important component of pharyngeal fluoroscopy and allows the image to be frozen for more detailed assessment, as well as slow-motion viewing. Pharyngeal rings and webs may only be visible for a few frames on a long study and can be missed without slow-motion review. The swallowing assessment is performed mainly in the lateral and AP projections. Barium sulphate is the usual contrast agent and is made up to a variety of viscosities to simulate different foodstuffs. In addition barium can be incorporated into, for example, biscuit and pasta to allow a full assessment of swallowing of both liquids and solids.

Swallowing can be divided into five separate but interconnecting stages. The first is oral control of the bolus and control at the junction of mouth and pharynx, followed in sequence by closure of the palatopharyngeal isthmus, compression of the bolus by the tongue base and the constrictor muscles, closure of the larynx and finally opening of the pharyngo-oesophageal segment. Deficiency at any of these sites initially leads to compensation either by a modification of the type of food eaten or by changes in body habitus (head flexion to compensate for failure of pharyngo-oesophageal opening) or by changes in the action of the involved muscles (tongue and larynx displaced posteriorly to compensate for failure of the constrictor muscles to compress the bolus). Decompensation occurs when compensatory mechanisms no longer suffice. At this point there may be retention of the bolus. The bolus may be retained in the valleculae or piriform sinuses owing to a suboptimal tongue push, weakness of the stripping wave or a relative obstruction such as a pharyngeal web or prominent cricopharyngeus. Alternatively, instead of retention, leakage may occur in one or more of the following ways:

- Weakness, atrophy or resection of the tongue, paralysis of the soft palate or missing teeth can lead to leakage of food from the mouth.
- Nasal regurgitation can occur due to weakness of the soft palate or superior constrictor.
- Penetration, which is the presence of contrast in the laryngeal vestibule or ventricle, or aspiration, defined as contrast in the trachea, may both occur from poor epiglottic tilt, poor elevation of the larynx or poor laryngeal closure.

In infants with suspected pharyngeal dysfunction, tracheo-oesophageal fistula without atresia (the H-type fistula) must be considered and investigated first with low osmolar contrast agents (Fig. 3.8). A nasogastric

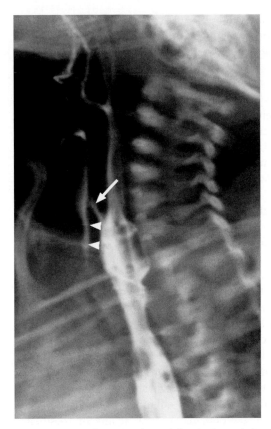

Figure 3.8 *Tracheo-oesophageal fistula (arrow) demonstrated with a low osmolar contrast swallow in a 2-week-old girl who had symptoms of pulmonary aspiration following repair of an oesophageal atresia. A little contrast is seen in the trachea (arrow heads). (Courtesy of Dr K.E. Halliday.)*

feeding tube is positioned in the distal oesophagus and the infant placed prone. Non-ionic contrast is injected as the tube is withdrawn and lateral fluoroscopy will show any tracheo-oesophageal fistula that is present. With this technique, any contrast seen in the bronchial tree must be due to an 'H' fistula, as pharyngeal aspiration has been excluded.

BARIUM SWALLOW

When a barium swallow is requested the radiologist will usually perform a barium meal since diseases in stomach and duodenum may cause or exacerbate oesophageal symptoms. The exception is where the examination is being tailored to a specific question such as the presence or not of an oesophageal perforation. Both barium swallow and endoscopy may be falsely negative in patients with dysphagia. Barium swallow is the best initial examination as it is a very safe procedure and allows detailed assessment of the pharynx as well as the oesophagus. The double contrast study should aim to achieve an oesophagus that is well distended throughout its length and will detect oesophageal webs, which are often missed at endoscopy, and will diagnose the presence of pharyngeal pouches, which may increase the risk of endoscopic

perforation. If no abnormality is seen on the standard views the patient should be asked to swallow a food bolus; barium tablets are available for this purpose but a small marshmallow is probably more convenient. This food bolus can demonstrate subtle strictures not seen on the initial study. Typically the food bolus sticks at the level of the stricture supporting a column of contrast above it and reproduces the patient's symptoms.

Oesophageal symptoms include heartburn, globus, dysphagia, odynophagia and chest pain. It is important that the radiologist be aware of these symptoms so that appropriate modifications in technique can be made.

The routine study includes images of the whole length of the oesophagus in single contrast, in mucosal relief (barium-coated but collapsed and empty) and in double contrast. It is important to achieve good oesophageal distension when barium studies are made, as webs, rings and strictures may otherwise be missed. Conversely the length of strictures may be overestimated, if the distal normal oesophageal segment is not adequately distended. In addition the oesophagus should routinely be assessed in the prone or supine position, which can give valuable information on oesophageal motility.

In the presence of globus, films and video of the pharynx in the AP and lateral projections may reveal webs and epiglottic abnormalities. In dysphagia, if the routine films are normal, fluoroscopy while the patient swallows a 15 mm marshmallow, acting as a solid food bolus, followed by liquid barium, can highlight the site of stricture. In odynophagia (pain on swallowing), additional double contrast views are taken to detect oesophagitis. With heartburn, a more detailed assessment of motility and reflux is carried out. With chest pain, a detailed assessment of motility and reflux is made, and a provocative drug, such as edrophonium chloride, may be used for diffuse spasm or nutcracker oesophagus.

If there is a concern about perforation, owing either to trauma or secondary to endoscopy or surgery, a water-soluble contrast should be used initially followed by barium. This subject is discussed further in the section on postsurgical complications (p. 104).

There are five types of contractile activity that can be observed in the oesophagus, two are peristaltic and three non-peristaltic.

- **Primary peristalsis** starts with a swallow and travels smoothly down the oesophagus taking about 7 s, stripping all the contents into the stomach. Normal individuals may have a very small amount of contrast left behind around the level of the aortic arch on two or three out of five swallows (a phenomenon called **proximal escape**).
- **Secondary peristalsis** is the same type of contraction, but is initiated in mid oesophagus by distension.
- **Tertiary contractions** are of low amplitude manometrically, and radiologically are non-lumen-

obliterating and non-peristaltic contractions, most commonly seen in reflux disease.

- **Lumen-obliterating, non-peristaltic contractions** (higher amplitude) also occur in reflux disease, especially in old age, and are also seen in diffuse spasm, nutcracker oesophagus and in vigorous achalasia.
- **Transient transverse ripples** in the oesophagus are called the feline oesophagus, because the oesophagus in the cat constantly has such striations. These are seen mainly in people with reflux disease, moments after an episode of reflux, but may also occur in normal people.

BARIUM MEAL

With a double-contrast or multiphasic examination of the stomach, CO_2-forming granules are given as well as high-density barium and the patient is rolled to achieve good coating of the gastric mucosa by the barium. With the stomach distended with gas, supine, oblique and lateral views are taken to show all parts of the stomach in both barium-filled and double contrast modes. The radiologist also compresses the accessible parts of stomach and duodenum, as this is a sensitive way of detecting small polypoid and marginated lesions. Once views of the stomach have been obtained, sufficient barium to coat the duodenum is run through the pyloric canal. A smooth muscle relaxant, such as 20 mg of hyoscine-N-butyl bromide (Buscopan) or 0.1 mg of glucagon, may be given by intravenous injection, which has the effect of causing duodenal hypotonicity, relieving any spasm and allowing better distension. Magnified spot views of the duodenal cap are then obtained in various degrees of obliquity. At least one film is taken showing the whole of the duodenal loop and proximal jejunum to detect the occasional distal abnormality, such as unexpected coeliac disease or giardiasis. An adequate examination should include not less than four views of the stomach, two of the duodenal bulb and the whole of the duodenal loop.

OESOPHAGEAL DISORDERS

Gastro-oesophageal reflux

This is the most common motility disorder involving the oesophagus and can cause all of the symptoms described above. Endoscopy is the best method to assess mild oesophagitis, but barium studies provide a broader view of the disease, associated motility disturbances and complications. Either investigation is adequate but endoscopy will overlook the pharyngeal changes associated with globus symptoms, minor strictures and Schatzki rings, and does not provide such a good view of the motility dysfunction, though this is seldom important in deciding treatment.

When acid is instilled into the normal oesophagus, the resting tone of the cricopharyngeus rises. Patients with reflux disease show a variety of abnormalities of the cricopharyngeus, such as incomplete relaxation, delayed relaxation, premature contraction after a bolus passes, and transient mini-Zenker's diverticula. The relation of these changes to globus symptoms is not yet clear, but they often coexist. The primary oesophageal peristaltic wave often becomes inefficient in reflux disease resulting in major proximal escape, and both tertiary contractions and lumen-obliterating non-peristaltic activity can be seen. In old age the latter is sometimes so marked as to cause a corkscrew appearance and may be called presbyoesophagus. This is probably one of the manifestations of reflux disease.

While most patients with severe gastro-oesophageal reflux do have a coexisting hiatus hernia, many patients are seen with hiatus hernia but no reflux, and many with reflux but no hiatus hernia. The primary abnormality in gastro-oesophageal reflux is in the lower oesophageal sphincter which exhibits inappropriately frequent and prolonged transient relaxations, and in severe disease reduced resting tone. The para-oesophageal variety of hiatus hernia makes up only 1 per cent of the hernias seen and is not associated with reflux. Radiologically, the presence of a sliding hiatus hernia is assessed by observing the position of the diaphragmatic hiatus, which can be seen to compress the intrahiatal structures if the patient gives a sniff. This is compared to the position of the gastro-oesophageal junction.

Gastro-oesophageal reflux itself is also assessed with barium studies but the presence of reflux does not correlate well with the presence of reflux oesophagitis. Only 40 per cent of patients with endoscopic evidence of oesophagitis have reflux demonstrated on barium studies. To check for reflux the patient is given barium to drink and the lower oesophagus is visualized with the patient lying supine. If no reflux is seen in this position, the patient is rolled slightly on to the right side to bring the pool of barium in direct contact with the gastro-oesophageal junction, and the patient given sips of water (the water siphon test). This test can demonstrate slight reflux even in normal patients but, if marked reflux is seen, the test is positive. The test also permits the assessment of clearance of refluxed liquid.

In patients with reflux oesophagitis, 50 per cent have abnormal oesophageal motor function resulting in delayed clearing of the barium within the oesophagus and an increase in non-peristaltic contractions seen on the supine swallowing assessment. The best way to assess reflux in difficult cases, or for research purposes, is 24-hour monitoring with a pH probe in the lower oesophagus. Reflux may also be assessed dynamically with a food bolus labelled with a radiopharmaceutical, usually technetium. This can provide semi-quantitative data on reflux as well as oesophageal motility and gastric emptying. With the use of labelled solid and liquid boluses, data on differential handling of these can be obtained.

When gastro-oesophageal reflux is complicated by moderate to severe reflux oesophagitis, morphological changes can be seen on the barium study in 80–90 per cent of patients. Changes are usually not seen in patients with mild superficial oesophagitis. The changes of oesophagitis seen on barium swallow are those of irregularity in the outline of the oesophagus, thickened longitudinal folds with linear ulceration, transverse oesophageal folds, strictures and inflammatory polyps at the top of gastric rugal folds (Fig. 3.9). The inflammatory **gastro-oesophageal polyps** are an indication of chronic reflux disease and appear as a continuation of a single prominent mucosal fold that originates in the gastric fundus and extends into the distal oesophagus. These **folds** are inflammatory and have no malignant potential, but cannot be distinguished radiologically from neoplasm, and therefore have to be biopsied.

Strictures are seen as a complication in 10–20 per cent of patients with reflux oesophagitis, and may be

(a)

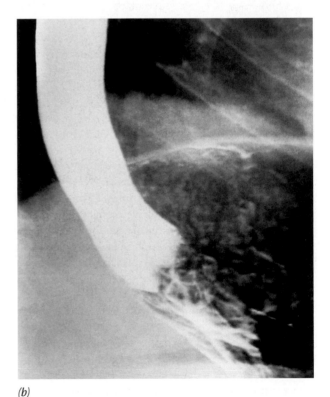

(b)

Figure 3.9 *Gastro-oesophageal reflux. Double contrast barium swallow showing a stricture and oesophagitis. Note the linear folds and scarring. This appearance can occasionally be caused by carcinoma. Endoscopic biopsy should be postponed until the oesophagitis has healed to facilitate endoscopic and histological interpretation.*

Figure 3.10 *Peptic stricture (a). Double contrast upper GI study in a patient with dysphagia shows a possible narrowing in the distal oesophagus (b). A marshmallow swallowed with a mouthful of barium lodges at the site of the stricture. The stricture supports a column of barium and reproduces the patient's symptoms, confirming the stricture which was shown to be a peptic stricture as a cause of the patient's dysphagia.*

(a)

(b)

Figure 3.11 *Peptic stricture (a) in a patient with dysphagia (b). A small (7 mm) marshmallow was used to size the stricture. The marshmallow stuck at the stricture, which supports a column of barium and reproduced the patient's symptoms.*

circumferential and symmetrical (Fig. 3.10) or asymmetrical with sacculation and irregular borders (Fig. 3.11). When seen just above a hiatus hernia, a smoothly tapering stricture is virtually pathognomonic of a benign reflux-associated stricture. However, when all of these features are not present, endoscopic biopsy is advisable to rule out a malignant lesion. Chronic reflux may lead to a change in the distal oesophageal mucosa, from the usual squamous type to a columnar type known as **Barrett's oesophagus**. The columnar epithelium may be of the gastric type, or be specialized columnar or a junctional type: all three types can coexist at the same level. The presence of Barrett's oesophagus predisposes to the development of dysplasia and this can progress to frank adenocarcinoma (Fig. 3.12). The risk of malignant transformation in a Barrett's oesophagus is 1 per 300 patient years. The presence of Barrett's oesophagus should be suspected when there is oesophagitis, an oesophageal stricture or a punched-out ulcer at a distance from the gastro-oesophageal junction, especially if this is seen in the presence of a hiatus hernia and reflux. A distinctive reticular pattern is described on double contrast barium examination, but is not always seen. If a Barrett's oesophagus is suspected, endoscopy with brushings and biopsies of the oesophagus should be performed, both to establish the diagnosis and to allow an assessment of dysplasia.

Figure 3.12 *Adenocarcinoma. Double contrast barium swallow showing narrowing and mucosal irregularity in the lower oesophagus some distance from the gastro-oesophageal junction in a patient with Barrett's oesophagus. The area of narrowing and mucosal abnormality (arrow) is due to adenocarcinoma.*

Oesophageal motility disorders

These may be of striated muscle or smooth muscle. Striated muscle is only present above the aortic arch where myasthenia and Eaton–Lambert syndrome are the main considerations, though these conditions are very rare.

There is a zone of transition where both types of muscle are present, and in the lower two thirds of the oesophagus, there is only smooth muscle. There may be too much motility as in **diffuse spasm** and **nutcracker oesophagus** in which chest pain and dysphagia coexist. Nutcracker oesophagus is hard to diagnose radiologically being characterized by fluoroscopically normal peristalsis with very high amplitude contractions (up to 1200 mmHg) with delayed relaxation, and sometimes with associated non-peristaltic activity, which can be seen spontaneously or provoked with edrophonium chloride. Diffuse spasm characteristically exhibits severe lumen-obliterating non-peristaltic activity, but it may be episodic and therefore overlooked. Manometry is a better way to diagnose these two disorders.

Diminished peristalsis may be seen in **achalasia**. In the early phase, vigorous achalasia may be seen. This condition is halfway between diffuse spasm and achalasia, and shows vigorous lumen-obliterating contractions as well as a poorly or non-relaxing lower oesophageal sphincter. The characteristic finding in established achalasia is marked reduction or absence of the primary peristaltic wave from the aortic arch downwards, and failure of relaxation in the lower oesophageal sphincter. This soon leads to dilatation of the oesophagus above the lower oesophageal sphincter, and the oesophagus may contain a considerable volume of food residue leading to a risk of aspiration and chronic recurrent chest infections. On barium studies there is slow emptying of the barium from the oesophagus into the stomach with the tight lower oesophageal sphincter producing a bird's beak appearance to the lower oesophagus (Fig. 3.13). Administration of gas granules will usually force open the sphincter and allow rapid emptying of the oesophagus in patients with primary achalasia. While these features are diagnostic of achalasia, they do not distinguish between

(a)

(b)

Figure 3.13 Achalasia. (a) Proximal dilatation of the oesophagus with tortuosity and narrowing of the distal oesophagus in this patient with dysphagia. The distal oesophagus is tapered and there is hold-up of barium. (b) When gas granules are given, the distal oesophagus opens and allows the barium to pass into the stomach. There is no primary oesophageal peristalsis. A careful examination of the fundus is important to exclude secondary achalasia due to tumour.

primary and secondary achalasia. **Secondary achalasia** is caused by gastric adenocarcinoma, or metastatic tumour, such as from breast carcinoma, infiltrating the submucosal oesophageal neural plexus and producing nonrelaxation of the sphincter and diminished peristalsis. This may be suspected radiologically by the demonstration of a mass in the fundus, by the failure of the lower oesophageal sphincter to open with a gas-granule bolus by mouth, or by failure of the lower oesophageal sphincter to relax when the patient sniffs amyl nitrite. Endoscopy and biopsy are required to exclude or document such a secondary achalasia. Achalasia itself predisposes the oesophagus to malignant transformation with the risk of oesophageal squamous carcinoma being approximately 10 times greater than in a control population. The appearances of secondary achalasia may also be due to scleroderma, which causes oesophageal dilatation and reduced peristalsis. The gastro-oesophageal junction is patulous and this predisposes to reflux oesophagitis that may lead to a smooth distal oesophageal peptic stricture. **Chagas' disease** can also give appearances on barium studies indistinguishable from achalasia. This disease is largely confined to South America and is caused by the protozoan *Trypanosoma cruzi*. In this disease the organism responsible was isolated and classified before the disease itself was recognized.

Oesophageal dysmotility may also occur in **scleroderma**, which involves the oesophagus in approximately 80 per cent of cases. The smooth muscle of the oesophagus is replaced by collagen, which results in reduced or absent lower oesophageal peristalsis and a low resting lower oesophageal sphincter tone. These abnormalities lead to marked gastro-oesophageal reflux, reflux oesophagitis and stricture formation. These radiological findings, in combination with the reduced primary peristalsis seen on fluoroscopy, suggest the diagnosis of scleroderma. Radiologists should ask about Raynaud's phenomenon in any patient with severely reduced primary peristalsis. It is important to differentiate between scleroderma and idiopathic reflux disease: patients with scleroderma respond badly to fundoplication because the feeble peristalsis cannot push food through the wrap.

The dermatological skin conditions of **epidermolysis bullosa dystrophica** and **pemphigoid** can also affect the oesophagus. Oesophageal involvement with epidermolysis bullosa dystrophica is a disease of childhood that should be investigated with double contrast barium studies because endoscopy carries an unacceptable risk of perforation. The study may show bullae involving the oesophageal mucosa, which appear as discrete filling defects within the oesophagus. These may be extensive and produce areas of ulceration in the mucosa when they burst. Disordered motility also occurs and, in severe cases, strictures develop (Fig. 3.14). Pemphigoid is a disease affecting older patients in whom bullae may also rarely be observed but the more usual finding is

Figure 3.14 *Tight smooth oesophageal stricture secondary to epidermolysis bullosa dystrophica. (Courtesy of Dr W.H. Smith.)*

superficial ulceration. At a later stage strictures develop in the upper oesophagus.

Oesophageal webs and rings

Webs and rings may be found as incidental findings but may also produce dysphagia. The most common abnormal oesophageal ring in the lower oesophagus is at the gastro-oesophageal junction, and was described by Richard Schatzki (Fig. 3.15). The symptomatic **Schatzki ring** is associated with a hiatus hernia and responds well to balloon dilatation. The characteristic history is of intermittent dysphagia for meat in a patient with mild to moderate reflux symptoms. Luminal narrowing to below 12 mm causes dysphagia in almost all cases, while narrowing above 20 mm rarely causes symptoms. The rings are only visible on maximal distension, which is why the mild ones are readily overlooked at endoscopy and on barium studies unless a marshmallow bolus is used. It is unknown why some patients with reflux disease develop extensive oesophagitis with stricture but no ring, and others develop a Schatzki ring with little or no oesophagitis.

Oesophageal webs may be idiopathic, or part of the **Paterson–Kelly–Plummer–Vinson syndrome**. Webs are 1–2 mm thick structures, usually occurring in the cervical oesophagus in older patients. The idiopathic

Figure 3.15 *Schatzki ring causing dysphagia, demonstrated on the single contrast phase of a barium swallow.*

variety is very common, being seen in up to 8 per cent of patients referred for barium examination of the oesophagus. In some patients the webs contain heterotopic gastric mucosa leading to the possibility of peptic ulcer disease. Isolated patches of gastric mucosa are often observed in the cervical oesophagus endoscopically but their significance is unknown. Other webs are seen in the lower oesophagus associated with gastro-oesophageal reflux. The association of cervical oesophageal webs, iron-deficiency anaemia and pharyngeal or oesophageal carcinoma in the Paterson–Kelly–Plummer–Vinson syndrome remains controversial.

Non-reflux oesophagitis

Oesophagitis is most frequently due to gastro-oesophageal reflux, but there are many other causes.

Infectious oesophagitis usually presents with odynophagia in contrast to the heartburn or dysphagia of reflux disease. Infectious oesophagitis may be caused by a wide range of pathogens, the most common being candida, herpes simplex and cytomegalovirus (CMV) but tuberculosis, diphtheria, cryptococcus and other organisms are occasionally responsible. Cases of infectious oesophagitis are most often seen in patients with reduced immunocompetence owing to diabetes mellitus, chemotherapy, radiotherapy and treatment with steroids or antibiotics. Increasingly, infectious oesophagitis is encountered in patients immunosuppressed following transplantation or with depressed T-cell function due to HIV infection.

By far the most common cause for infectious oesophagitis is candidal infection, usually from *Candida albicans*, but surprisingly only 50 per cent of affected patients have oral lesions. At endoscopy, adherent white plaques are seen on a background of erythematous, friable mucosa. Double-contrast barium studies have a sensitivity of 90 per cent in the diagnosis of candidal oesophagitis. The appearance of multiple well-defined slightly raised nodules that run in a longitudinal fashion, interspersed between normal-looking mucosa, is a highly suggestive pattern. Other patterns include a cobblestone appearance due to coalescing plaques, and prominence of the longitudinal oesophageal folds or granular pattern due to oedema. In more severe cases pseudomembrane formation and deeper ulceration lead to a shaggy appearance of the oesophagus or even a double-barrelled oesophagus owing to undermining of the mucosa (Fig. 3.16). Areas of narrowing are usually

Figure 3.16 *Candida oesophagitis. Patient with lymphoma undergoing chemotherapy showing shaggy appearance of the oesophagus from ulceration. (Courtesy of S.S. Amar.)*

due to oedema, but true strictures can occur and tend to be long and smoothly tapering.

Herpes oesophagitis causes small vesicles, which later burst leaving a shallow ulcer. In a more advanced state, pseudomembrane formation occurs giving a similar appearance to that seen with candida. In 50 per cent of patients with endoscopic herpes oesophagitis, double contrast barium studies show discrete ulcers, usually in the mid oesophagus. These ulcers are often surrounded by a ring of surrounding oedema giving a halo appearance on the barium study.

CMV oesophagitis appears endoscopically as discrete ulceration with normal surrounding mucosa. On double contrast barium studies CMV may appear as large superficial ulcers measuring a few centimetres in diameter, a finding rarely seen with the other forms of infectious oesophagitis. Less common are superficial ulcers similar to those seen with herpes. Granular mucosa and thickened longitudinal folds from CMV infection occasionally mimic reflux oesophagitis.

Oesophagitis leading to stricture formation may also be caused by **ingestion of drugs** particularly doxycycline, tetracycline, potassium chloride and quinidine, especially when tablets remain in the oesophagus for longer than usual. This prolonged transit may be due either to reduced motility or because tablets are taken in the supine position or without a water chaser. The oesophagitis is usually mid-oesophageal as this is where tablets tend to stick because of the slight narrowing caused by external compression from the aorta and left main bronchus, and also because this is the site of least effective peristalsis, the point where striated and smooth muscle merge and where the manometric pressure during peristalsis is lowest. A large left atrium can cause a further area of oesophageal compression and predispose to tablet hold-up and subsequent oesophagitis. On double contrast barium studies there are ulcers usually in the mid oesophagus. The ulcers are often shallow and may be single or multiple.

Radiotherapy to the thorax used in the treatment of malignancy affecting the lung, mediastinum or thoracic spine can also lead to oesophagitis. The oesophagitis presents with substernal burning pain, dysphagia or odynophagia, 2–3 weeks after the radiotherapy. The symptoms may last several weeks or subside over a 48-hour period. Most patients are treated empirically but if double contrast barium studies are performed in the acute phase they will demonstrate superficial ulceration in the segment corresponding to the radiation field. With higher radiation doses the appearance may be more striking, with large ulcers and areas of mucosal sloughing and the possible development of fistula formation. The fistulae are usually to the left main bronchus and are caused by radiation necrosis owing to end arteritis obliterans. Disordered motility can occur 1–2 months after the completion of therapy. Stricture formation within the irradiated segment may occur

Figure 3.17 *Long oesophageal stricture with some linear ulceration corresponding to the previous radiotherapy field.*

later, usually 4–8 months after the radiotherapy (Fig. 3.17).

Sclerotherapy is another cause of oesophageal injury, occasionally leading to an incompetent lower oesophageal sphincter, reflux, severe ulceration and stricture.

Corrosive chemicals, such as acids, alkalis and phenols, when ingested, can cause injury to the oesophagus. The damage caused by alkalis tends to be more severe than that seen with acids. The oesophagitis progresses through an acute necrotic stage followed by ulceration and sloughing of necrotic mucosa, which then heals with granulation tissue. Later there is fibrosis with resultant strictures, which are smoothly tapering and occur in the region of the carina, although the whole oesophagus may be involved. Steroids, antibiotics and prophylactic dilatation are used, but despite these measures up to 40 per cent of patients proceed to stricture formation. In the patients who do proceed to stricture there is an increased risk of oesophageal carcinoma.

Nasogastric (NG) tube placement of between 3 and 15 days can also cause oesophagitis and subsequent stricture usually after a delay of 1–4 months. The NG tube may cause damage from gastro-oesophageal reflux owing to the effects of the tube being placed across the gastro-oesophageal junction, direct trauma or an irritant effect by the tube. Patients typically present with heartburn or odynophagia secondary to oesophagitis before it progresses over several weeks to dysphagia as

Figure 3.18 *Long irregular oesophageal stricture secondary to nasogastric tube placement. Dysphagia developed in this patient 3 months after a hospital admission.*

Figure 3.19 *Irregular oesophageal stricture with marked nodularity and shouldered margins from a squamous cell carcinoma.*

the stricture develops. On double contrast barium studies the initial oesophagitis typically appears as a long segment with marked ulceration. The oesophageal stricture develops over a short period of time and tends to involve a long segment of distal oesophagus (Fig. 3.18). Treatment is problematic but relief of dysphagia can be obtained by serial dilatations.

Neoplasms

Dysphagia with or without weight loss may be the presenting symptom of oesophageal malignancy, which is squamous cell carcinoma in 90 per cent of cases. Adenocarcinoma accounts for about 10 per cent, particularly in the presence of Barrett's oesophagus, and carcinosarcoma about 1 per cent. Oesophageal carcinomas occur in the distal oesophagus in 40 per cent, in the mid oesophagus in 40 per cent and in the proximal oesophagus in 20 per cent. Tumours can be detected on the mucosal relief phase of a barium study but the best method is with double contrast. On barium studies early oesophageal carcinomas may appear as an area of mucosal irregularity, a sessile polyp or a zone in the oesophagus which does not distend as well as the rest. Barium swallow is not a reliable method to detect early and asymptomatic carcinoma. Cytology appears to be the most sensitive technique for early lesions. Barium swallow, properly performed, remains a sensitive investigation for those carcinomas that are causing dysphagia. Large tumours may give the appearance of irregular

sessile polyps often with ulceration, or as an apple-core stricture. Advanced tumours may appear as smoothly tapering strictures, irregular strictures (Fig. 3.19) or as coarse nodular lesions. A varicoid variety resembling oesophageal varices may also be seen.

Once the diagnosis is established, a CT scan provides information with regard to staging (Fig. 3.20), but CT is not completely reliable for the detection of aortic invasion or for local lymph node involvement. Endoscopic ultrasound is an alternative test, which in good hands provides accurate local staging information. Prognosis is good for patients with early stage disease, but such patients are very rare. By the time dysphagia is present there is little hope of cure, with 5-year survival figures remaining stubbornly below the 5 per cent level.

The oesophagus can be involved by **secondary malignant disease** either by direct invasion, invasion from adjacent lymph nodes or by blood-borne metastases. Bronchogenic carcinoma is the most common primary to affect the oesophagus. With direct invasion the appearances are similar to those seen in primary malignant disease. Nodal involvement causes focal narrowing usually of the anterior oesophageal wall in the mid oesophagus.

Benign tumours of the oesophagus can cause dysphagia, although most are detected as incidental findings on barium studies performed for other indications. The most common benign tumour is the **leiomyoma** accounting for about 50 per cent of benign

(a)   *(b)*

Figure 3.20 *Carcinoma of the oesophagus. (a) The tumour is causing marked thickening of the wall of the oesophagus (arrows). (b) A more cranial section shows tumour (arrows) extending alongside the trachea (T) and dilated oesophagus (O).*

tumours. Leiomyomas predominantly occur in middle-aged men and histologically they resemble uterine fibroids in appearance. Leiomyomas develop in the smooth muscle of the muscularis externa usually in the distal two thirds of the oesophagus. Leiomyomas in the oesophagus are usually between 1 and 6 cm in size, although they can grow very large and weigh up to 5 kg. Despite this, they rarely ulcerate and so are seldom a cause of blood loss. The leiomyoma may be seen as a soft-tissue density mass projecting from the wall of the oesophagus and, with double contrast barium studies, these submucosal lesions appear as a filling defect.

Foreign bodies

Dysphagia, odynophagia or chest pain may be caused by intraluminal obstruction secondary to a swallowed foreign body. This is most often seen in infants, children or patients with psychiatric problems. Smooth foreign bodies such as coins, buttons and batteries may pass freely into the stomach but if they do lodge in the oesophagus they tend to do so in areas of normal narrowing, at the thoracic inlet, the aortic arch and the diaphragmatic hiatus. These swallowed foreign bodies may stick elsewhere in the oesophagus, particularly if there is an underlying and perhaps subclinical stricture. Sharp foreign bodies do not lodge in such a predictable fashion and may snag at any level. The most common swallowed foreign body causing dysphagia is a partially chewed **meat bolus**. **Metallic foreign bodies** are easily seen on a plain film (Fig. 3.21), but for other objects contrast studies may be needed. Again the use of a marshmallow swallow can be very useful for showing small, otherwise hard-to-demonstrate foreign bodies. If there is any chance of a perforation caused by the swallowed foreign body water-soluble contrast should be

Figure 3.21 *Metallic foreign body in the oesophagus. The patient had swallowed a razor blade.*

used initially. Water-soluble contrast has been recommended if the patient is having an endoscopy on the same day, as barium tends to clog the suction and biopsy channels of an endoscope. If barium has been used, preliminary work suggests that a combination of metoclopramide and effervescent agents after completion of the barium study can allow endoscopy to be performed safely. The use of atropine to relax the oesophageal musculature or of glucagon to relax the lower oesophageal sphincter may help to encourage the passage of a lodged foreign body, as will swallowed gas granules in selected patients.

Trauma

The oesophagus may be perforated spontaneously by vomiting, iatrogenically during endoscopy, and sometimes by closed or penetrating trauma. Vomiting causes gastric fundal mucosa to intussuscept into the lower oesophagus, which may cause a tear in the mucosa of either the oesophagus or the stomach. This is the **Mallory–Weiss tear**, which presents with haematemesis. These longitudinal tears are almost impossible to see on barium swallow and are best diagnosed by endoscopy. Vomiting against a closed throat or with a full stomach may cause a tear in the oesophagus that is full thickness (**Boerhaave's syndrome**). Typically this tear occurs in the left posterior wall of the lower 5 cm of the oesophagus, and leads to a leak that goes directly between the leaves of the inferior pulmonary ligament, where it may be contained for a while, appearing on the plain film as a triangular-shaped air collection behind the heart. Once the ligament gives way, gastric contents escape into the left pleural cavity as well as up into the mediastinum. Plain films may be sufficient for diagnosis but, if there is doubt, a water-soluble contrast swallow will reveal the leak.

GASTRIC AND DUODENAL DISEASE

Barium meal, endoscopy, ultrasound and CT can be used to examine the stomach and duodenum. Both barium and endoscopy miss about 5 per cent of lesions over 1 cm in diameter, but endoscopy is far more accurate for small lesions. Erosive gastritis can be detected readily on good barium meals, and severe gastritis and duodenitis can also be diagnosed with some reliability. Endoscopy also has the advantage of permitting biopsies but has a higher associated morbidity and mortality. The inability to visualize oesophageal motility limits the endoscopic assessment of reflux disease by comparison with a barium study. Thus young mobile adults will have most serious pathology adequately demonstrated on a good barium meal, and barium study provides the best overall initial assessment of gastro-oesophageal reflux disease. On the other hand, patients with GI bleeding, or previous gastric surgery as well as those who are elderly or immobile are best assessed for gastroduodenal disease with endoscopy. Overall, endoscopy is more sensitive than barium for gastric and duodenal pathology; and is easier to perform

well in the old and immobile, so that it is the initial examination of choice for suspected gastric and duodenal disease.

Disease of the stomach and duodenum may present with dyspepsia, abdominal pain, weight loss, anorexia, vomiting or symptoms of acute or chronic blood loss.

Dyspepsia which affects up to 40 per cent of the population, may be defined as pain or discomfort in the upper abdomen or chest, which is relieved or exacerbated by eating. Many would insist that it should be present for not less than 3 weeks before any investigation is performed. Dyspepsia has numerous causes including gastro-oesophageal reflux disease, oesophageal and gastric motility disorders, peptic ulcers, gastric carcinoma, pancreatitis and biliary pathology. Patients with these symptoms are often investigated with barium studies or endoscopy of the upper GI tract together with abdominal ultrasound. Performing all of these investigations on the 40 per cent of the population with symptoms would be a huge financial drain and also result in a large number of deaths on the basis of current postendoscopy mortality data (1 death in 10 000 procedures). The main concern with not investigating these patients is that a gastric carcinoma will be missed, but a carcinoma is rare in patients under the age of 50 years and in those without weight loss or anaemia. A rational approach is to treat with a trial of H_2-receptor or proton pump blockers those patients suffering dyspepsia for 3 weeks in whom the suspicion of gastric carcinoma is low, i.e. those without weight or blood loss. Further investigation may be confined to patients with little or no response after 10 days and those whose symptoms have improved but not resolved at 10 weeks.

The discovery of the key role of *Helicobacter pylori* as the cause of peptic ulcer disease and as a Class 1 carcinogen for gastric cancer has modified this approach. The British Society of Gastroenterology has issued guidelines on the investigation of patients with dyspepsia, which broadly follow those outlined but incorporate a serological test for *H. pylori* for patients under the age of 45 years. If this test is positive, the patient should be investigated even in the absence of worrying symptoms such as weight loss. The serological test for *H. pylori* is less accurate in older patients and these patients also have a higher risk of gastric carcinoma, so the guidelines suggest investigating all patients with dyspepsia over the age of 45 years.

Gastritis and duodenitis

Inflammation of the stomach and duodenum has numerous causes, but a major discovery of the 1980s was that the organism, *H. pylori* infects the stomach of perhaps 40 per cent of the population in developed countries and 85 per cent of the population in less developed countries. Children living in poor or

Figure 3.22 *Large areae gastricae. Enlarged areae gastricae in the antrum are associated with duodenal ulcer disease and this is now known to arise on the basis of* H. pylori *infection and increased gastrin production.*

Figure 3.23 *Heterotopic gastric mucosa in the base of the duodenal cap seen as small polygonal filling defects (arrow). Originally described radiologically as a normal variant, they are now readily visible endoscopically. Such heterotopia is often associated with* H. pylori *infection, but the strength of this association is unknown.*

overcrowded conditions acquire the infection during the first few years of life. *H. pylori* is a gram negative, spiral bacillus isolated from biopsy of the upper GI tract at endoscopy in up to 95 per cent of patients with chronic antral gastritis. *H. pylori* is also found in 80 per cent of patients with gastric ulcers and in virtually all patients with duodenal ulcers. *H. pylori* causes an acute antral superficial gastritis, increased gastrin output, hyperchlorhydria, and duodenal or gastric ulceration. It sometimes causes a hypertrophic gastritis, progressing to Ménétrier's disease; it may also cause a lymphoid response in antral mucosa progressing to lymphoid hyperplasia and mucosa-associated lymphoid tissue (MALT) lymphoma. In some patients the gastritis progresses to atrophy and intestinal metaplasia. The organism count then declines as it cannot live on intestinal cells, but the metaplasia may progress on to dysplasia and carcinoma. There is therefore considerable interest in treatment aimed at eradication of *H. pylori*. However, eradication is not entirely without risk, and there have been deaths from pseudomembranous colitis in patients on drug therapy. The treatment is expensive and often with minor side effects but the cost of eradication is substantially less than that of repeated treatment for recurrent duodenal ulceration. Radiologically, *H. pylori* infection may be suspected when antral gastritis is diagnosed on the basis of thickened folds and/or erosions in the antrum in the absence of non-steroidal anti-inflammatory drugs (NSAIDs) or aspirin (Fig. 3.22). Findings of duodenitis, such as thickened folds, poor coating and erosions in the absence of Crohn's disease and coeliac disease, are also suggestive of *H. pylori* infection, as is the recognition of heterotopic gastric mucosa in the duodenal bulb (Fig. 3.23).

There are other important causes of gastritis. Erosive gastritis and duodenitis occur in over 20 per cent of patients with Crohn's disease, but disease in these sites is rarely the cause of initial presentation. Sarcoidosis and certain infectious agents, in particular tuberculosis and syphilis, cause gastritis. Eosinophilic gastritis, usually in the antrum, is associated with a blood eosinophilia, but is seldom an isolated lesion, and is usually seen in association with ulceration or strictures in the small bowel. Ulcerations and erosive gastritis may be idiopathic or due to a direct toxic action on the stomach by corrosives, certain medications and following radiotherapy.

Ménétrier's disease presents clinically with epigastric pain, weight loss and peripheral oedema secondary to protein loss from the stomach. On barium studies it is characterized by marked thickening of the gastric folds (Fig. 3.24) but involvement of the antrum does not preclude the diagnosis. The mucosal detail is often poor because of the copious amounts of mucus seen in this condition. It is associated with low or absent acid production in 75 per cent of patients and represents a late stage of *H. pylori* infection.

Pyloric stenosis classically presents with projectile non-bilious vomiting in a 2–8-week-old, usually male, infant. Although examination by an experienced clinician can make the diagnosis in the majority of patients, based on a combination of history and the clinical

Figure 3.24 *Ménétrier's disease. Double contrast seen on barium meal as thick rugal folds. Thick folds may also be seen in Crohn's disease, lymphoma and Zollinger–Ellison syndrome. Patients with thick folds should have an upper GI endoscopy with biopsy to obtain the definitive diagnosis and to test for* H. pylori.

finding of an epigastric smooth mass, there is increasing use of radiology in diagnosis. Single contrast barium studies have been the traditional way to image this condition. This shows gastric outlet obstruction and either a single or double strand of barium within a narrowed elongated pyloris. Ultrasound is being increasingly used for diagnosis (Fig. 3.25). The stomach is often fluid filled but, if not, fluid should be given to the patient to distend the stomach. The pyloric canal is thickened and elongated with a muscle thickness more than 4 mm and a length greater than 15 mm.

Peptic ulcer disease

Duodenal ulcers are almost always benign but both benign and malignant gastric epithelium may ulcerate.

Both gastric and duodenal ulcers are typically seen as round collections of barium usually less than 1 cm in diameter, and mucosal folds radiating outward indicate some degree of chronicity. During healing, ulcers sometimes become serpiginous or linear. In the past **gastric ulcers** were often larger on initial presentation but now with earlier treatment large ulcers are rare in countries where there is ready access to medical care. When giant gastric ulcers, defined as larger than 3 cm, are seen, they are associated with a higher complication

(a)

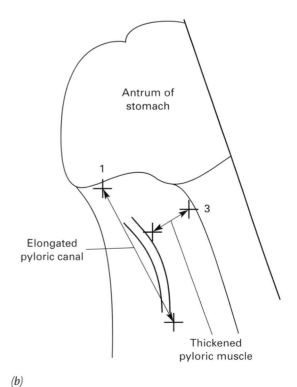

(b)

Figure 3.25 *Ultrasound scan showing an elongated and thickened pyloric canal in a neonate with pyloric stenosis.*

rate from perforation and bleeding but not with a higher malignancy rate. Most gastric ulcers occur on the lesser curve or the posterior wall of the antrum or body and the distribution tends to be more distal in young patients, since gastric ulcers occur in transitional epithelium. The level of the junctional epithelium migrates up the stomach with increasing age, so that the elderly often have their gastric ulcers high on the lesser curve near the cardia. Benign ulcers in the fundus or in the proximal part of the greater curve are very rare, and any ulcer in this position should be biopsied in case of malignancy. Most ulcers are single but multiple ulcers are seen in 20 per cent of cases and each of the ulcers must be assessed individually to determine the aetiology, as benign and malignant ulcers can coexist.

Duodenal ulcers are seen in the cap in 95 per cent of cases and most postbulbar ulcers are seen proximal to the ampulla of Vater (Fig. 3.26). The anterior wall of the duodenal bulb is the site of 50 per cent of duodenal ulcers and is the area most difficult to examine radiologically. Duodenal ulcers distal to the papilla are infrequently seen and suggest the diagnosis of Zollinger–Ellison syndrome. Multiple ulcers are also suggestive of the Zollinger–Ellison syndrome but are seen in up to 15 per cent of patients with peptic ulcer disease. Duodenal ulcers heal quickly with appropriate treatment but may lead to bulbar deformity or an ulcer scar with radiating folds originating at the site of the original ulcer crater. The ulcer scar may have a small central depression, which, when seen with surrounding radiating folds, can be mistaken for an active ulcer. When bulbar deformity is produced through scarring, the unaffected parts of the duodenal cap balloon outward as pseudodiverticula. When these pseudodiverticula are multiple, the classic 'cloverleaf' appearance of the duodenal cap is produced. Scarring from ulcers in the pyloric canal, distal antrum and postbulbar region can lead to outflow obstruction. Endoscopy is the preferred examination in dyspeptic patients with previous duodenal ulcer disease.

When gastric ulcers are being assessed as benign or malignant, it is important to obtain images of the ulcer in profile and *en face*. The profile views are often improved by imaging the patient erect and the *en face* views by the use of compression. Benign ulcers penetrate through the gastric mucosa and cause more extensive destruction in the submucosa leading to an undermining of the overlying mucosa. In malignant ulceration, the ulcer occurs within an area of malignant epithelium. Ulcers which penetrate beyond the wall of the stomach are likely to be benign but this can be seen with early gastric carcinoma. The radiating folds with benign ulceration tend to be regular and are seen up to the edge of the ulcer crater, while in malignant disease the radiating folds end before reaching the ulcers and are irregular or amputated in appearance. Two careful studies have shown that a gastric ulcer which has the characteristic radiological features of a benign ulcer is

Figure 3.26 *Duodenal ulcer with narrowing of the pylorus shown on water-soluble contrast study to rule out perforation. Endoscopy is not required for ulcers that are clearly in the duodenal cap (bulb), but is prudent for pyloric channel ulcers, which may represent ulceration in a distal gastric carcinoma.*

histologically benign. Ulcers of indeterminate status on radiological criteria (about 25 per cent of which prove to be malignant) and ulcers that are clearly radiologically malignant (about 95 per cent confirmed as malignant) should be biopsied without delay. Since gastric ulcers should be followed to complete healing in order to reduce the likelihood of relapse, it makes sense to make endoscopy the follow-up procedure to assess for healing, and to biopsy for dysplasia and *H. pylori*. An ulcer that fails to heal on treatment must be biopsied.

Peptic ulcers can also lead to **perforation**, which may be free or confined. Free perforation occurs when an ulcer erodes into the peritoneal cavity, which typically occurs with ulcers on the anterior wall of the stomach or duodenum. Anterior gastric wall ulcers are rare and most free perforations are caused by duodenal ulcers. If there is free peritoneal air on plain films, then no further imaging is usually required, but when there is a suspicion of perforation but no free air, water-soluble contrast studies or CT may be indicated. When there has been a perforation but there is no free air, the perforation is not shown on a contrast examination in 50 per cent of cases because of spontaneous sealing. Of those in whom perforation is shown, 50 per cent show a free leak into the peritoneal cavity and the other 50 per cent a contained leak within a walled-off cavity. Posterior wall ulcers occasionally perforate through to the lesser sac or into the anterior pararenal space. Water-soluble contrast studies can show these leaks, but the extent of any abscess formation is better assessed by abdominal CT or ultrasound examination. Confined perforation of posterior wall ulcers involves the pancreas in up to 75 per cent of cases but may also penetrate surrounding organs to produce an abscess in the liver, spleen or transverse mesocolon. These confined leaks show as abnormal gas collections on plain films or cavities on water-soluble contrast examination in 50 per cent of cases. CT can demonstrate the presence of the abscess cavity even after the leak has sealed off and should be considered whenever there is a deep posterior wall ulcer. Fistulae may develop secondary to peptic ulcer disease and include gastroduodenal (seen as a double-channel pyloric canal on barium studies), gastrocolic, gastroperi-cardial, duodenocolic, choledochoduodenal and duodeno-renal fistulae. Barium studies can usually determine the site, size and communication of the fistulous track.

Zollinger–Ellison syndrome should be suspected when postbulbar ulcers and ulcers in the fourth part of the duodenumn or jejunum are demonstrated either on barium meal or endoscopy, especially if accompanied by large quantities of resting fluid in the stomach and duodenum. The syndrome is caused by hypersecretion of gastrin either from an autonomous tumour or, rarely, from primary G-cell hyperplasia which results in the production of large quantities of gastric acid. The tumour is usually malignant and is situated in the pancreas in 75 per cent of cases, in the duodenum in 15 per cent and in other sites in 10 per cent. Some 25 per cent of gastrin-omas are associated with multiple endocrine neoplasia (MEN type 1) and are seen in combination with tumours of the parathyroids, pituitary and adrenal. The large quantities of gastric acid leads to peptic ulcers in 90 per cent of patients and the volume of gastric secretions produces diarrhoea in 50 per cent. The ulcers are often multiple and resistant to treatment with H_2-receptor blockers although proton pump inhibitors can lead to healing. When the Zollinger–Ellison syndrome is strongly suspected on biochemical and clinical grounds, the patient should be assessed for metastatic disease using ultrasound, CT or MRI. When there is no widespread metastatic disease and surgical cure is being considered, radiology may help with tumour localization. In addition to the cross-sectional imaging, additional information may be obtained preoperatively by endoscopic ultra-sound and selective angiography. This may be supple-mented by arterial stimulation with secretin and venous sampling for gastrin. During surgery intraoperative ultra-sound is an excellent localization technique and should increasingly be used in these complex cases.

Benign tumours

Gastric polyps are hyperplastic in 75–90 per cent of cases. **Hyperplastic polyps** have no malignant potential and if positively identified require no further follow-up. They appear radiologically as smooth sessile lesions, usually measuring less than 1 cm in size, and occur mainly in the gastric fundus or body. When in the dependent part of the barium pool, they appear as

Figure 3.27 *Pedunculated polyp arising close to the pyloric canal (arrows). On this image the polyp is lying within the antrum, but on other images it was seen to prolapse into the duodenal cap. Histology confirmed an adenomatous polyp.*

filling defects but, when seen on the non-dependent surface, they are outlined by a ring or crescent of barium at the junction between the polyp and the normal mucosa. Hyperplastic polyps can grow larger, and then may be pedunculated or lobulated, in which case the diagnosis of a hyperplastic polyp cannot be made with certainty and endoscopic excision biopsy is required. There is evidence in some cases that hyper-plastic polyps regress following eradication of *H. pylori*.

Adenomatous polyps do have malignant potential, with carcinomatous foci being found in 50 per cent of those greater than 2 cm in size. They occur most commonly in the antrum appearing as filling defects in the dependent barium pool and may be sessile or pedunculated (Fig. 3.27). Adenomatous polyps tend to be more lobulated than hyperplastic polyps and are usually larger measuring over 1 cm. In view of the malignant potential adenomatous polyps should undergo endoscopic excision biopsy. Adenomatous polyps are also found in the stomach and duodenum in both familial polyposis coli and Gardner's syndrome, but most gastric polyps in these conditions are hyper-plastic and occur in the gastric fundus (Fig. 3.28).

In Peutz–Jeghers' syndrome, the gastric polyps are **hamartomas** with almost no malignant potential and appear as sessile or pedunculated polyps measuring up to 3 cm in size. Hamartomatous polyps are also seen in juvenile polyposis. Cronkhite–Canada and Cowden's syndrome also have gastric hamartomatous polyps and these have a small malignant potential. Cronkhite–Canada syndrome in contrast to the others is character-ized by a carpet of small, subcentimetre, gastric polyps.

Leiomyomas account for about 40 per cent of benign gastric tumours and may cause problems owing to

Figure 3.28 *Hyperplastic gastric polyps in a patient with familial polyposis coli. The polyps spare the antrum and are benign.*

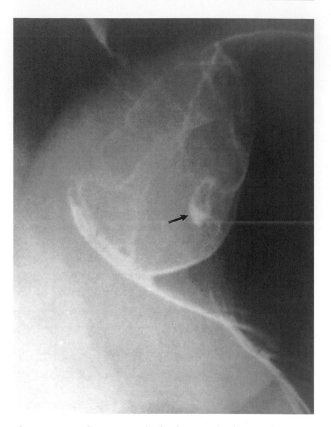

Figure 3.29 *Leiomyoma. The barium study shows a large smooth mass at the cardia with a central depression containing a pool of barium (arrow). The patient presented with a haematemesis because of bleeding from the ulcer.*

haemorrhage, a palpable mass, nausea or, in the case of pedunculated tumours, gastric outflow obstruction from prolapse into the antrum or duodenum. Leiomyomas may rarely be recognized on plain films as a soft-tissue mass but are more commonly picked up on barium studies of the stomach or by endoscopy. Small leiomyomas are covered with normal gastric mucosa, indent the normal gastric outline and have well-defined margins when seen *en face*. With larger tumours there is often ulceration, seen radiographically as a barium-filled crater on the surface of the tumour mound (Fig. 3.29).

Ectopic pancreatic rests can mimic leiomyomas. They are usually single, measure up to 3 cm in size and are located on the greater curve of the gastric antrum or between the duodenal cap and the ampulla of Vater (Fig. 3.30). Like leiomyomas, they may have a central puddle of barium. This is due to a rudimentary ductal system producing a dimple on the surface of the rest. If the duct system is more advanced it may appear as multiple small pouches filled with barium and this appearance is pathognomonic of ectopic pancreatic rests.

MALIGNANT TUMOURS

Gastric carcinoma has been in decline over the last fifty years but in those who have the disease the outlook remains poor with a 20 per cent 5-year survival rate. Gastric carcinoma is predominantly a disease of middle-to-old age but the proportion of young patients affected is increasing. The fundus, body and antrum are affected

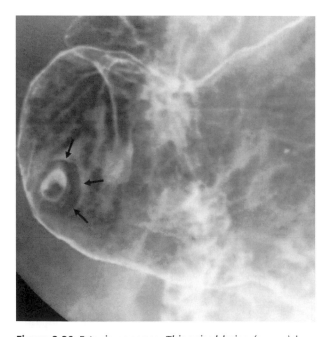

Figure 3.30 *Ectopic pancreas. This raised lesion (arrows) in the antrum with central depression could be an ulcer, an ulcerated carcinoma or, most likely at this site, ectopic pancreas, which was the final diagnosis. Endoscopy is required to confirm the diagnosis.*

equally with about 10 per cent of tumours being diffusely infiltrating. Over 90 per cent of cases are due to adeno-carcinoma and most are detected in an advanced stage, i.e. they have invaded the muscularis propria. There are two types of the disease: a diffuse (signet cell) type which affects younger people and has an incidence that has not changed over the years, and an intestinal type that is associated with intestinal metaplasia and is due largely to *H. pylori* infection and its sequelae. Pernicious anaemia and the associated autoimmune gastritis is also associated with gastric carcinoma but *H. pylori* is no more common in these patients than in the general population. Gastric carcinoma remains common in several countries and the precise role of genetic and environmental factors, including *H. pylori*, remains unclear, although the World Health Organisation has now accepted *H. pylori* as a primary carcinogen for gastric cancer. Partial gastrectomy, particularly the Bilroth II variety, is associated with later development of gastric carcinoma in the gastric remnant.

The Japanese Endoscopy Society has classified early gastric carcinoma (Table 3.1). Type I lesions are seen on barium studies as polypoid masses projecting into the lumen of the stomach. These may be of considerable size and still be early carcinoma histologically, because many of these lesions represent malignant change in an adenomatous polyp. Type II lesions may appear as areas of mucosal irregularity, nodularity or loss of the normal mucosal pattern, and may be slightly elevated or depressed. Type III lesions are areas of ulceration with barium pooling, but, in contrast to the features seen with benign ulcers, the Type III early gastric cancers tend to have shallow ulcers with radiating folds which stop abruptly at some distance from the ulcer. The radiating folds may be fused or clubbed.

Early lesions, particularly in the region of the cardia, are not easily demonstrated and subtle changes in the gastric fold pattern should be sought. Lesions under 1 cm are usually missed, and even 1–2 cm Type II lesions are very hard to detect unless ulcerated.

Table 3.1 *Early gastric cancer (Japanese Classification)*

Type	Description	Appearance
I	Polypoid (> 0.5 cm in height)	
IIa	Superficial, elevated (< 0.5 cm in height)	
IIb	Superficial, flat or minimal elevation	
IIc	Superficial, depressed	
III	Excavated	

Endoscopy is a little more sensitive than barium for detection of small early gastric carcinomas, but the flat non-ulcerated lesions are still very easily overlooked.

Advanced carcinomas are more obvious on double-contrast studies, and Borrmann has described four types:

Type 1: A non-ulcerating polypoid mass which projects into the lumen of the stomach. These lesions may become very large (Fig. 3.31) but are usually well-differentiated (Fig. 3.32). When the mass lies in the barium pool in the dependent portion of the stomach, it appears as an irregularly polypoid, nodular filling defect and, when on the non-dependent surface, it is outlined by a ring of barium.

Type 2: A fungating tumour that is closely related to a Type 3 lesion.

Type 3: An ulcerating gastric carcinoma that may show tumour nodules in the surrounding mucosa. The folds radiating out from the ulcer are fused, clubbed and amputated, stopping at a distance from the actual ulcer crater.

Type 4: A scirrhous carcinoma that infiltrates the stomach producing a shrunken or non-distensible stomach known as linitis plastica or water-bottle stomach. There is often antral sparing with the tumour seen as an area of non-distensibility in the body and/or fundus (Fig. 3.33). Adequate gaseous distension is needed if this is to be recognized. Scirrhous tumours may also produce slight mucosal irregularity or nodularity.

Figure 3.31 *Carcinoma of the cardia (arrows) invading the oesophagus. The prevalence of carcinoma at this site is increasing, possibly owing to short segment Barrett's disease.*

Figure 3.32 *Malignant gastric polyp shown on CT examination in an elderly patient with anaemia as a filling defect in the contrast-filled stomach (arrow). (Courtesy of E. Jurriaans.)*

Figure 3.34 *Normal variants are common and can be confusing. This 'polyp' (arrow) at the apex of the duodenal bulb is normal and is produced by bulking of mucosa at the acute angle between the distended first and second parts of the duodenum.*

Figure 3.33 *Advanced gastric carcinoma. Lack of local distensibility draws attention to a tumour of the greater curve of the stomach. There is also compression of the lesser curve. CT scan showed that this was due to simple liver cysts and not to metastases.*

CT and endoscopic ultrasound are used to stage gastric carcinomas, with assessment of direct and lymphatic spread. CT findings of enlarged local nodes or local invasion are unreliable and do not necessarily indicate advanced disease. CT is more accurate at showing distant metastatic disease, but minor findings should not be accepted without biopsy confirmation. With these provisos, CT scanning might be useful in surgical planning for these patients, especially in directing the approach to a palliative rather than curative resection.

Figure 3.35 *Adenomatous polyp in the third part of the duodenum (arrows). Barium study performed with Buscopan as hypotonic agent.*

(a)

(b)

Figure 3.36 *Chronic pancreatitis. (a) Barium meal and (b) CT scan in 49-year-old patient with vomiting and elevation of serum alkaline phosphatase. The compression of the duodenum could be due to pancratitis or carcinoma. CT scan was chosen to confirm the pancreatic origin of the mass (black arrow), and to guide percutaneous biopsy. Note the anterior abdominal wall skin markers as an aid to biopsy (white arrow). Biopsy was negative for cancer and the clinical course remained consistent with chronic pancreatitis.*

OTHER DUODENAL LESIONS

The duodenum may be affected by disease of neighbouring organs, such as the pancreas, and there are also uncommon duodenal primary tumours, such as leiomyoma, leiomyosarcoma, neurofibroma and carcinoma. These neoplasms may present with bleeding or obstruction and are readily shown on barium studies, but they must be distinguished from pseudopolyps, which are due to redundant mucosa when there is acute angulation of the intestine, most commonly at the junction of the first and second parts of the duodenum (Fig. 3.34). Lesions that appear primarily duodenal require endoscopy and biopsy (Fig. 3.35) while extrinsic compression or invasion is best assessed by CT examination (Fig. 3.36).

An unusual cause of vomiting occurs in **obstruction of the third part of the duodenum** by the root of the superior mesenteric artery. This occurs in patients who have lost a great deal of weight, and once it has developed, the obstruction leads to further weight loss. Enteral or parenteral nutrition and regaining weight will cure the condition in those who do not have a serious underlying disease. Barium study shows a dilated second and third part of duodenum with vigorous peristalsis and sudden cut-off in front of the aorta (Fig. 3.37). Turning the patient prone results in flow of barium past the obstruction, indicating that it is not a stricture.

Figure 3.37 *Superior mesenteric artery syndrome. Abrupt termination to the barium column in the third part of the duodenum is seen in a patient with marked weight loss secondary to an eating disorder. There was active peristalsis in the more proximal duodenum. Following the passing of a jejunal tube for feeding and weight gain, the obstruction in the third part of the duodenum resolved.*

Figure 3.38 *Normal small bowel meal. (a) Digital image of the whole abdomen with the patient prone. Spot views of the terminal ileum are obtained in single (b) and double contrast (c). The mucosa in the terminal ileum is shown in exquisite detail.*

(a)

(b)

LOWER GI TRACT

SMALL BOWEL

Examination

Only the first and last 15 cm of the small bowel are within reach of the endoscopist. Investigation relies heavily on barium-based studies either single or double contrast, though ultrasound and CT are proving to have an increasingly valuable role. Examination of the stomach and duodenum requires a relatively small volume of high-density barium and the injection of an agent to reduce motility (such as Buscopan), while investigation of the small bowel requires a large volume of low-density barium and often the oral administration of metoclopramide to shorten transit time. The examination of the stomach and duodenum therefore has requirements that are in direct contrast to those needed for adequate examination of the small bowel.

Clinical findings should be used to decide whether to request a barium meal or a small bowel study. Examination of the small bowel may be by means of a small bowel meal or by a small bowel enema, otherwise known as **enteroclysis**. Both examinations have strengths and weaknesses. The small bowel meal is

(c)

quicker, easier to perform, is less uncomfortable for the patient and has minimal complications. Enteroclysis allows better evaluation of the exact site of pathology and gives more bowel distension, facilitating assessment of adhesions.

For a **small bowel meal** the patient drinks a mixture of low-density barium and metoclopramide syrup, and plain films of the abdomen are obtained at intervals until the barium has reached the colon. Once contrast has reached the colon, spot views of the terminal ileum are taken. The rest of the small bowel is also carefully examined fluoroscopically with compression applied to separate loops of bowel and to assess for tethering. Following this an attempt may be made to view the distal ileum in double contrast by inserting a small tube into the rectum and insufflating carbon dioxide until it refluxes around the colon into the ileum (Fig. 3.38).

Optimal distension of the small bowel requires a high barium flow rate which can be achieved by **enteroclysis**. Rapid delivery of fluid to the stomach or duodenum increases the risk of gastro-oesophageal reflux and pulmonary aspiration. These risks are minimized by infusing barium directly into the jejunum. The patient's nose and throat are anaesthetized and intravenous sedation (e.g. midazolam) may also be administered. The tube is placed into the patient's nostril and advanced into the jejunum, with the help of a stiffening wire and changes in patient position. Once in the jejunum a balloon at the end of the catheter may be inflated to further reduce reflux. Enteroclysis can be performed as a single contrast study using dilute barium (Fig. 3.39) or as a double contrast study using higher density barium and a methylcellulose chaser. The column of barium is visualized using fluoroscopy as it advances through the small bowel and images are recorded for later study. The procedure is unpleasant for the patient but serious complications such as perforation are extremely rare.

The small bowel can be imaged with **transabdominal ultrasound**. The bowel can be assessed for peristalsis and wall thickening, which is greatly helped by the use of a graded compression technique. Focal or generalized bowel wall thickening may be detected particularly if the appropriate clinical history and physical signs are given to guide the conduct of the examination.

CT examination is used in the assessment of the small and large bowel. A double dose of oral contrast is needed to opacify both distal and proximal intestine in order to distinguish intestinal loops from pathology. The first dose is given approximately 60 minutes before the CT examination and the second dose 10 minutes before. Rectal and vaginal contrast is sometimes useful if the large bowel, or particularly the pelvis, is being examined. Intravenous contrast is important if an abscess is suspected or if demonstration of mesenteric vessels is required to distinguish them from lymph nodes or metastases.

Figure 3.39 *Normal small bowel enema (enteroclysis) demonstrating normal valvulae conniventes and good distension of the small bowel. The use of a low-density barium and a high kilovoltage ensures that overlapping loops of bowel are not obscured.*

One of the most common indications for investigation of the small bowel is the diagnosis or follow up of inflammatory bowel disease, in particular Crohn's disease (*see* p. 87).

DISEASES OF THE SMALL BOWEL

Malabsorption

When **malabsorption** is suspected or demonstrated on clinical grounds, endoscopically directed biopsy of the second or third part of the duodenum is extremely useful for obtaining a diagnosis, particularly of coeliac disease. Endoscopic biopsies have now largely replaced the peroral biopsy technique under fluoroscopic guidance, such as the Crosby capsule. Malabsorption may be due to a primary disorder of the bowel such as coeliac disease or may be secondary to infection or altered immunity. Barium studies remain helpful in equivocal cases to assess the extent of disease and to investigate for complications of the underlying disease. Tropical sprue shows similar appearances on barium studies to those seen with coeliac disease although the aetiology is very different.

Coeliac disease is particularly prevalent in northern Europe and is due to a sensitivity to alphagliadin. The complications of malabsorption include osteomalacia and there may be radiological evidence of this on the abdominal radiograph. The barium study is abnormal in 90 per cent of patients and shows dilatation of the

Figure 3.40 *Coeliac disease. Small bowel meal in a patient with anaemia. There is small bowel dilatation and ileojejunal fold reversal. The left upper quadrant loops have fewer valvulae (like ileum), while those in the right lower quadrant have closely packed valvulae (like jejunum). Dilatation is the most common finding and often the only abnormality, but fold reversal is not uncommon and is diagnostic.*

jejunum, especially the more distal part. The valvulae conniventes are most often normal but, owing to the dilatation of the bowel, the margins may lose their rounded appearance and appear rather square (Fig. 3.40). Rarely, in advanced coeliac disease the valvulae may be completely absent. This is known as the 'moulage sign'. More commonly the number of valvulae increases in the ileum and decreases in the jejunum to the extent that there is a reversal of the normal pattern of distribution. The hypersecretion of fluid seen in coeliac disease may give the barium a rather granular appearance but the classic radiological sign of flocculation is rarely seen with the new barium preparations. Complications of coeliac disease may also be shown, including enteroenteric intussusception, lymphoma and carcinoma, which may affect the small bowel or the oesophagus.

Intestinal infections such as **giardiasis** can also cause malabsorption. Giardiasis is usually an acute illness but may become chronic with inflammation of the proximal small bowel. If it is suspected, diagnosis is by endoscopy and jejunal fluid aspiration. On barium studies there is thickening of the valvulae conniventes, spasm of the bowel and oversecretion of fluid, giving the barium a rather granular appearance. This abnormal appearance is confined to the jejunum and definitive diagnosis may be obtained from stool culture or distal duodenal/jejunal biopsies obtained at endoscopy.

Whipple's disease is a rare disease with a wide range of presenting complaints. The patient may present with gastrointestinal symptoms of malabsorption with steatorrhoea or non-gastrointestinal tract symptoms of arthralgia and fever. The disease is mostly seen in northern Europe and the USA in male patients. Endoscopy with duodenal biopsies will establish the diagnosis showing the lamina propria filled with periodic acid-Schiff positive macrophages and bacilli. The bacilli, *Tropheryma whippelii*, are also seen in the extracellular spaces and are the cause of the disease. Symptoms respond well to antibiotics, which need to be continued for several months, and follow-up biopsies show clearance of the *Tropheryma whippelii*. Small bowel barium studies show nodules predominantly in the jejunum measuring 1–2 mm in size. In uncomplicated Whipple's disease the folds are of normal thickness but the malabsorption can lead to hypoalbumenaemia causing a diffuse and smooth thickening of the folds. On CT there may be nodal disease in the peritoneum and retroperitoneum; characteristically these have a high fat content and appear as low attenuation masses (Fig. 3.41).

Figure 3.41 *Whipple's disease. CT scan showing multiple low attenuation masses in the peritoneum and retroperitoneum owing to fatty infiltration of enlarged nodes.*

In **eosinophilic gastroenteritis**, there is a mucosal infiltration of eosinophils which can be idiopathic or related to a food allergy. As the stomach is almost always involved the diagnosis is confirmed by gastric biopsy. If there is predominantly mucosa involvement, patients present with diarrhoea, vomiting and sometimes malabsorption. The barium studies show fold thickening in the stomach and small bowel (Fig. 3.42), and there may be nodularity also. The disease is patchy and there is usually intervening normal bowel between the involved segments. The disease may predominantly involve the muscularis which leads to a

Figure 3.43 *Primary intestinal lymphangiectasia showing diffuse small bowel fold thickening in a 3-year-old patient who presented with severe protein-losing enteropathy.*

Figure 3.42 *Eosinophilic gastroenteritis showing fold thickening in the proximal jejunum with gastric and jejunal involvement. Gastric biopsy showed marked mucosal infiltration with eosinophils.*

different clinical picture of obstruction owing to muscle thickening and luminal narrowing. This typically occurs in the gastric antrum but it can affect the small bowel. Barium studies show the area of focal narrowing and proximal bowel dilatation secondary to the obstruction; the bowel is otherwise normal.

Intestinal lymphangiectasia may be primary and due to a congenital abnormality of the lymphatics draining the bowel or secondary to lymphatic obstruction most often from abdominal carcinoma or lymphoma. The lymphatic obstruction leads to malabsorption of fat and to an increased protein loss from the bowel. On barium studies multiple small nodules are seen together with fold thickening (Fig. 3.43). In secondary lymphangiectasia the underlying cause of the lymphatic obstruction is superimposed on these findings, and the extent of the abdominal disease can be assessed by CT.

Systemic mastocytosis is the systemic extension of urticaria pigmentosa and involves an increase in mastocytes in the affected organs. Patients may have symptoms of peptic ulcer disease and diarrhoea with malabsorption, owing to histamine release from the mast cells stimulating increased acid production. Small bowel involvement can produce nodules or target lesions on barium studies.

Jejunal diverticulosis can cause malabsorption secondary to bacterial overgrowth. The increased number of bacteria make use of vitamin B12, reducing its availability for distal absorption. The bacteria also increase the deconjugation of bile salts leading to reduced micelle formation and fat absorption. The deconjugated bile salts also act as direct intestinal

irritants leading to watery diarrhoea. The jejunal diverticula protrude from the site of entry of the vasa recta and bulge between the leaves of the mesentery. The malabsorption can usually be controlled by intermittent courses of antibiotics, but surgery may be required if this fails to control symptoms or if there are other complications such as bleeding. On small bowel barium studies the diverticula are usually easily seen as smooth walled outpouchings (Fig. 3.44). CT has little to add unless there is a suspicion of perforation and abscess formation.

Figure 3.44 *Jejunal diverticulosis with multiple narrow necked jejunal diverticula on the mesenteric border. Some of the diverticula are arrowed.*

Scleroderma can involve the small bowel and present with malabsorption owing to stasis and bacterial overgrowth. Plain films show distended proximal bowel loops, which can be misinterpreted as small bowel obstruction. Barium studies mirror these changes but may demonstrate this luminal dilatation in combination with crowding of the valvulae conniventes owing to muscle loss and replacement by collagen; this gives the 'hidebound' appearance characteristic of scleroderma. Barium studies may also show sacculation of the small bowel; this can be differentiated from jejunal diverticulosis by the broad mouths of the sacculations and the fact that they arise from the antimesenteric border.

Amyloidosis can affect the gastrointestinal tract and give symptoms of malabsorption or obstructive symptoms. The amyloid protein can be deposited in any of the layers of the bowel leading to ischaemia, muscle loss and subsequent dysmotility and malabsorption from mucosal involvement. On barium studies there may be surface nodularity with multiple nodules measuring 3–4 mm in size, fold thickening, luminal narrowing and bowel wall thickening.

Tumours

These are much less common than those of the large bowel and are of different cell types.

Intestinal lymphoma constitutes about one third of all small bowel malignant tumours and is most commonly of the non-Hodgkin variety. Lymphoma is also seen with an increased frequency in patients with AIDS and possibly in patients with Crohn's disease. Small bowel lymphoma has a variety of appearances on barium studies:

- Thickening of the bowel wall is the most common appearance from lymphomatous infiltration. When this is diffuse, the abnormal bowel merges into normal bowel with no clear margin of transition. In the abnormal segment the mucosal folds may be absent or thickened. Bowel wall involvement and extramural disease are recognized by the separation of adjacent bowel loops, as only the lumen is filled with barium. Often there are slight strictures within the involved segment of bowel. Alternatively the involvement can be more localized and circumferential with well-defined margins.
- Mucosal abnormalities are produced by lymphomatous infiltration of the bowel and appear as loss of the valvulae and nodularity. The involved segment may be of normal diameter, narrowed or dilated. A lymphomatous mass may ulcerate, the ulceration appearing on barium study as a pool of contrast. The ulceration may be so extensive as to leave only a thin rim of viable lymphomatous cells at the base of the ulcer and in this case the barium study often shows

Figure 3.45 *Lymphoma showing bowel wall thickening. On this CT scan there is marked bowel wall thickening (arrow) in one of the ileal loops with contrast confined to the lumen. The stomach and a few other bowel loops also showed wall thickening from lymphomatous involvement.*

a focally dilated segment of bowel. If the lymphoma is predominantly intraluminal it appears as a polypoid filling defect and can lead to obstruction. Less commonly, lymphoma causes multiple nodules that may carpet the bowel. These nodules may ulcerate and show a central depression filled with barium.

- Extramural spread may lead to fistulous connections between the affected bowel and adjacent normal loops of bowel. If the lymphoma is predominantly extramural and affecting the mesenteric nodes, the bowel outlined by barium may have a scalloped margin from the external indentation. Although barium studies, particularly enteroclysis, show small bowel lymphoma to good effect, the extent of the disease, bowel wall thickening and involvement of regional lymph nodes are best seen with abdominal CT (Fig. 3.45). These advantages make CT an excellent technique for following the progress of the disease and its response to treatment. Follow-up scans should be performed to a set protocol so that direct comparisons can be made with previous studies.

Adenocarcinoma may arise in the small bowel, the frequency decreasing with distance from the ligament of Treitz, with most tumours seen in the duodenum and jejunum. As in the colon, small bowel adenocarcinomas arise from malignant transformation within an adenoma. In families with Lynch II hereditary non-polyposis colon cancer the incidence of small bowel adenocarcinoma is 50 times greater than in the general population. On barium studies an adenocarcinoma commonly appears as a well-defined region of luminal narrowing with loss of the normal mucosal pattern and overhanging edges. The narrowing causes progressive obstruction with dilatation of the bowel proximal to the

Figure 3.46 *Carcinoid. CT scan in a patient with diarrhoea showing a soft-tissue mass and multiple radiating soft-tissue strands (arrows) extending into the mesentery. This spoke wheel pattern indicates a desmoplastic reaction and is most commonly seen in carcinoid.*

Figure 3.47 *Metastatic disease throughout the peritoneal cavity causing diffuse small bowel fold thickening and nodularity seen throughout the small bowel.*

carcinoma. The bowel wall thickening and involvement of regional lymph nodes may be seen to good effect with abdominal CT. Histological diagnosis is often postponed until surgery but can be obtained by biopsy via an enteroscope or, rarely, by radiologically guided percutaneous core or fine needle aspiration biopsy.

Carcinoid tumour most often originates in the bowel with 40 per cent occurring in the appendix and about 30 per cent in the small bowel. The histology of these tumours does not correlate well with the behaviour of the tumour. Tumours less than 1 cm in diameter are unlikely to have distant metastases. On barium studies the tumours are often small and appear as nodules often in the distal ileum. The tumour can induce a fibrotic reaction in the adjacent mesentery resulting in kinking or acute angulation of bowel loops with straight segments of intervening bowel similar to that seen with postoperative adhesions. The bowel lumen may be narrowed either as a result of the desmoplastic reaction or from compression by a mesenteric tumour mass. CT is proving useful in the assessment of carcinoid tumours, and the liver can also be imaged for the presence of metastases (Fig. 3.46).

Metastases can spread from distant tumours to involve the small bowel via the blood, through the peritoneal cavity, by direct invasion from adjacent tumours or via lymphatics (Fig. 3.47). Although malignant melanoma is a rare tumour it frequently spreads to involve the bowel. The metastases appear as multiple polypoid luminal filling defects, but there is often a sizeable extraluminal component as well. In the stomach and duodenum these intraluminal polyps show central depressions which fill with a pool of barium but this feature is rarely seen in the jejunum and ileum. These polypoid masses can act as a lead point for an intussusception (Fig. 3.48). Tumour nodules can also occur in the mesentery which cause external compression on the bowel. Metastatic melanoma can also appear as a large mass, in which ulceration can occupy almost the entire volume of the tumour resulting in a dilated segment of bowel which is prone to haemorrhage.

Figure 3.48 *Melanoma. The patient was known to have a melanoma and presented with an acute abdomen. The CT scan shows a large filling defect (long arrow) in the contrast-filled bowel from an intussusception that contains oral contrast in its centre (small arrow). At surgery the patient had a melanoma metastasis as the lead point of the intussusception. (Courtesy E. Jurriaans.)*

Benign tumours of the small bowel are often asymptomatic but may cause bleeding or act as a lead point for an intussusception.

Leiomyomas arising in the submucosa appear on barium studies as smooth filling defects with stretched but otherwise normal mucosal covering. If they arise in the subserosa then there may be no intraluminal component but adjacent loops of bowel will be displaced. On CT the leiomyoma is seen as a mass in which there may be central necrosis.

Adenomas account for about 25 per cent of benign tumours and can arise throughout the small bowel but are most often seen in the duodenum and proximal jejunum.

Lipomas constitute the only other common small bowel benign tumour and they usually arise in the ileum. Lipomas appear as rounded filling defects on barium studies and it may be possible to change their shape by manual compression on the abdomen. The appearance on CT is a mass related to the small bowel, which has the attenuation value of fat.

LARGE BOWEL

Examination

Detailed imaging of the large bowel is by means of colonoscopy, contrast enema, CT, ultrasound and MRI. **Endoscopy** allows biopsy material to be obtained but is a more lengthy procedure with an associated higher morbidity and mortality. For routine colonoscopy and barium enema the patient must have bowel preparation so that the colonic mucosa can be well visualized. The bowel preparation is achieved by means of oral laxatives taken the day before the procedure. The routine radiographic study is the double contrast barium enema using high density barium. An anti-spasmodic agent such as Buscopan may be used if there is colonic spasm. Carbon dioxide or air is insufflated through the rectal tube once enough barium has been introduced and the patient is turned repeatedly to achieve double contrast views of the entire colon. Traditionally air has been used as the negative contrast agent but there may be considerable postprocedural pain which is largely abolished by the use of carbon dioxide. The double contrast barium enema examination provides excellent mucosal detail of the colonic mucosa but does require considerable agility on the part of the patient. Simplified techniques have been described to facilitate double contrast examinations in frail patients but alternative techniques, particularly abdominal CT (Fig. 3.49), can often provide the necessary information with less patient discomfort.

The strengths of endoscopy and the double contrast barium enema can be combined by a biphasic examination using flexible sigmoidoscopy and a modified double contrast barium enema. Flexible sigmoidoscopy

(a)

(b)

Figure 3.49 *Carcinoma of the colon. (a) CT scan shows an area of thickened bowel wall (arrows) in the ascending colon with marked narrowing of the lumen. (b) CT scan on the same patient shows low attenuation lesions in the liver representing metastases from the colonic primary. Thus, with a single examination, the patient's primary tumour and the metastases were diagnosed.*

can image the sigmoid and descending colon, sometimes to the splenic flexure. This is less painful for the patient than formal colonoscopy and can be performed without the need for intravenous analgesia and sedation. It also permits mucosal biopsy and the detection of subtle vascular changes associated with colitis in the distal colon. Immediately following the flexible sigmoidoscopy, a modified double contrast barium enema is performed. This allows assessment of the colon not visualized by endoscopy, around to the caecum. As the sigmoid has already been visualized, this area can be omitted from the barium study and the radiologist can concentrate on the remainder of the colon.

Patients with perianal disease, particularly Crohn's, may have exquisite local tenderness, such that barium enema, colonoscopy or even simple digital rectal examination may be impossible because of pain. A caudal block administered by an anaesthetist takes only five minutes to perform and will provide at least half an hour of complete perianal anaesthesia, allowing comfortable radiological and endoscopic examinations that would otherwise require a general anaesthetic.

Faeces, air bubbles, mucus or foreign bodies can cause confusing filling defects on double contrast barium enema which may resemble a polyp. These can generally be moved along the bowel by flowing barium or gas over them and can thus be differentiated from a true polyp. Diverticula can also have appearances similar to a polyp but can usually be filled with barium or be seen on an oblique view projecting outside the bowel rather than into the lumen.

The advent of spiral scanning allows **CT assessment** of colonic mucosal disease. This requires the patient to have a full cleansing bowel preparation as for a barium enema or colonoscopy, and the whole abdomen is then scanned in a single breath-hold after the colon has been distended with gas via a rectal catheter. Most investigators perform this study with the patient in the prone position and intravenous contrast enhancement can be helpful. The acquired images can then be viewed as axial cuts to detect polyps, carcinomas, metastases or other pathology (Fig. 3.50). The images can also be manipulated on a workstation to produce a 3D dataset, and this can be viewed as a virtual colonoscopic image. The manipulation of the data to produce this colonoscopic image is time-consuming and so an alternative strategy is to assess the axial images and limit 3D reconstruction to areas of concern or uncertainty.

In a case of suspected large bowel obstruction the diagnosis can be confirmed using a single contrast technique that requires no bowel preparation and much less patient movement than the double contrast technique. Dilute barium is run in until it reaches the obstruction or is seen refluxing into the terminal ileum. If a perforation is suspected, water-soluble contrast should be substituted for the barium. If pseudo-obstruction (**Ogilvie's syndrome**) is suspected, the diagnosis is best made using a water-soluble single contrast enema. Pseudo-obstruction can be treated by decompression which can be either colonoscopic or fluoroscopic using specially designed coaxial catheters.

DISEASES OF THE LARGE BOWEL

Adenoma and adenocarcinoma

Most adenocarcinomas arise in pre-existing adenomas. The presence of a familial polyposis syndrome greatly increases the risk that one of the polyps present will

Figure 3.51 *Adenoma. Three adenomas in the right colon of a 48-year-old man, who also had a 5 mm rectosigmoid polyp. When a colonic adenoma is discovered there is a 34–53 per cent chance of further adenomas being present. Thus the finding of one polyp should stimulate the search for more.*

Figure 3.50 *CT pneumocolon showing both a pedunculated polyp (P) and annular colonic carcinoma (C). The left iliac aneurysm (A) was an incidental finding. (Courtesy of Dr G.F. Maskell.)*

progress to an adenocarcinoma but these cases account for only 1 per cent of all colonic carcinomas. Hereditary non-polyposis colon cancer is responsible for about 5 per cent of colorectal cancer, and hereditary factors play a part in a further 15 per cent of cases with family clusters of colonic adenocarcinoma. A further risk factor is total ulcerative colitis. After the first 10 years of colitis, the risk increases with about 10 per cent of patients developing carcinoma in 25 years.

Both adenomas and carcinomas are most commonly found in the rectosigmoid area, although with increasing age there is a shift of this distribution, with more lesions being seen in the ascending colon. Adenomatous polyps are often multiple and, if one is found, there is an approximately 50 per cent chance that a further synchronous polyp will be present (Fig. 3.51). If more than a dozen polyps are found, it is likely that the patient has a polyposis syndrome. Carcinomatous foci may be present in adenomatous polyps that are macroscopically indistinguishable from benign adenomas. The size of the lesion is the single most important predictor of malignancy. Carcinoma is virtually unknown in polyps smaller than 5 mm, is present in 1 per cent of polyps measuring between 5 and 10 mm and in 50 per cent of those larger than 2 cm. Polyps larger than 5 mm seen on barium studies should be removed, especially if the polyp is lobulated or has an irregular outline. Patients with adenomas less than 5 mm in diameter are statistically at no increased risk for later development of carcinoma. Detection of lesions of this size is therefore not of clinical importance. Only about 40 per cent of these small polyps are detected on double contrast barium enema examinations while colonoscopy detects about 60 per cent. Polyps larger than 1 cm have a 90 per cent detection rate by colonoscopy and 75–85 per cent rate by double contrast barium enema.

Cancer detection rates can be as high as 98 per cent by both techniques, but this is rarely achieved in practice. Most cancers missed on double contrast barium enema are visible on the films. Double reading of films provides the best chance of avoiding diagnostic error.

Polyps appear on double contrast barium studies as sessile plaques, sessile hemispheres, pedunculated spheres or as carpet lesions (Fig. 3.52). Carpet lesions, which are often tubulovillous adenomas, are flat, may be quite large and produce a change in the normal mucosal pattern of the bowel. The plaque-like lesions appear as slight elevations of the bowel wall when seen tangentially. The sessile hemispheres are seen as larger protrusions into the bowel lumen. This can be confused with a diverticulum although the diverticulum points away from the bowel lumen, whereas the polyp points into the bowel lumen. Seen *en face* the sessile hemispheric polyp appears as a ring of barium (Fig. 3.53). Pedunculated polyps when seen in profile appear as a polypoid mass attached to a stalk of variable length. When seen *en face*

Figure 3.52 *Adenoma. Subtle flat adenoma in the transverse colon (arrow). When this quality of display can be provided, barium enema will miss fewer lesions than colonoscopy in the right colon, but endoscopy has better sensitivity in the sigmoid colon. (Courtesy A. O'Donovan.)*

the appearance of a pedunculated polyp with a short stalk is that of a 'Mexican hat' or 'target'.

Some **adenocarcinomas** have a large intraluminal component while others infiltrate deeply with a smaller intraluminal mass. In both cases narrowing occurs and there is replacement of normal colonic mucosa by tumour, which often ulcerates. As the tumour advances around the circumference of the bowel, it resembles a saddle but, with further growth, the advancing edges meet, causing a circumferential stricture of the classic applecore type (Fig. 3.54). Polypoidal tumours can be very difficult to recognize if they are oblique to the X-ray beam, i.e. neither seen *en face* nor in profile. In this situation the only clue to their presence may be a fine line of barium paralleling the bowel wall. The appearance in patients with ulcerative colitis is often atypical, with carcinomas appearing as smooth, apparently benign-looking strictures. These strictures should be biopsied in all cases.

	En face	Profile
Sessile	◯	⌒
Pedunculated	○	⌇

Figure 3.53 *The appearances of polyps.*

Figure 3.54 *Carcinoma showing an applecore stricture at the hepatic flexure.*

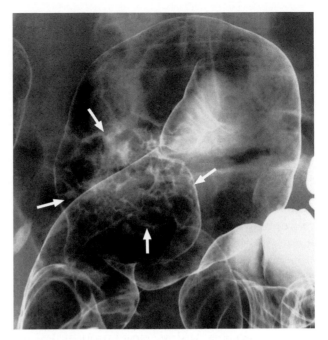

Figure 3.55 *Villous adenoma. Double contrast barium enema showing an area of diffuse mucosal abnormality with rather irregular barium coating (arrows). The individual fronds of the tumour are coated with barium.*

Staging of colorectal cancer requires the determination of the depth of invasion of the tumour, presence of lymph node metastases and the presence of other remote metastases, particularly to the liver. With rectal cancer, local invasion is best assessed by endorectal ultrasound; with more proximal tumours, assessment is best by CT. However, the sensitivity of CT is only 50–60 per cent for local extension. For distant spread, either CT or MRI can be used, but immunoscintigraphy is more sensitive than either of these for nodal and peritoneal metastases. When metastatic liver disease is assessed, ultrasound is often used as an initial investigation, but CT and MRI are more sensitive. Intraoperative ultrasound may show lesions that have been overlooked by the preoperative evaluation.

Villous adenomas appear as areas of mucosal irregularity or a frond-like mass, with the individual fronds of the tumour covered in barium (Fig. 3.55). True villous lesions tend to occur in the rectum and caecum and can cause diarrhoea with electrolyte loss owing to the large surface area of these tumours. Villous adenomas often secrete mucus, which may be inadequately cleared by bowel preparation. The mucus coats poorly with barium and these tumours may, therefore, easily be overlooked, if the possible significance of an area of poor coating and mucus is not recognized at fluoroscopy. A villous adenoma is 10 times more likely to harbour carcinoma than is a tubular adenoma.

There are a number of hereditary and non-hereditary polyposis syndromes. The best known is **adenomatous polyposis coli** in which there is hereditary transmission, multiple polyps and the development of colonic carcinoma in untreated individuals. The mode of transmission is autosomal dominant with high penetration but about one third of cases occur as a result of new mutations. The polyps vary in size from under 1 mm to 1 cm or more, and are more numerous in the descending colon and rectosigmoid than in the more proximal colon. The whole colon can be affected such that no normal mucosa can be identified and the bowel is carpeted by multiple polyps. The colonic polyps develop before the age of 20 in most patients, but polyps can appear for the first time in older individuals. The polyps develop into colonic carcinomas after about 15 years. Double contrast barium studies are useful for diagnosis, to assess the extent of the disease and the presence of carcinoma. As all of these patients eventually develop colonic carcinoma, a prophylactic colectomy should be performed, which can usually be deferred without penalty until the patient has reached the late teens. Patients with adenomatous polyposis coli may also develop hyperplastic and adenomatous polyps in the stomach, duodenum and small bowel. These patients have a higher incidence of duodenal carcinoma than non-polyposis-affected individuals. If adenomatous polyposis coli is associated with certain extracolonic manifestations, such as soft tissue tumours, skeletal osteomas and retroperitoneal fibrosis, the condition is given the eponym of **Gardner's syndrome**.

Other non-adenomatous polyposis syndromes include **Peutz–Jeghers syndrome**, which is an autosomal dominant disease with cutaneous pigmentation and hamartomatous GI polyps. The cutaneous pigmentation usually consists of small brown macules around the lips and occasionally on the palms of the hands or soles of the feet. The GI presentation is often obstruction secondary to intussusception with one of the hamartomatous polyps as a lead point. Polyps are seen in the small bowel in a majority of patients and also seen in the colon and stomach in about 30 per cent of patients. Although the small bowel polyps do cause intussusception and obstruction which may require surgery, they are not premalignant. The colonic polyps may be adenomatous rather than hamartomatous and are thus prone to undergo malignant transformation. Peutz–Jeghers syndrome is also associated with an increased risk of other malignancies, including pancreas, uterine and breast carcinomas. Radiologically polyps appear as small well-defined filling defects in the stomach and colon, but the whole of the small bowel can be carpeted in tiny 1–2 mm polyps.

A further hamartomatous condition is **Hamartoma syndrome**, otherwise known as **Cowden's disease**. This is a rare autosomal dominant condition. The major features are mucocutaneous lesions, abnormalities of thyroid, gland, breast carcinoma and multiple hamartomatous polyps of the GI tract. The GI lesions have little or no malignant potential. They are most often seen in the rectosigmoid as small sessile lesions and are best imaged with a high quality double contrast study. Less commonly lesions are seen in the oesophagus and stomach, but endoscopy may be required to show these small lesions.

Cronkhite–Canada syndrome is a rare non-familial polyposis syndrome. Patients usually present with abdominal pain, weight loss and diarrhoea, and later develop abnormalities outside the GI tract, including alopecia, skin hyperpigmentation and dystrophic changes in the nails. The GI polyps are found in the stomach, small bowel and colon. The polyps are small to moderate size sessile lesions. In all sites they are multiple, but the stomach is the site where there is most often complete carpeting of the mucosa by these lesions. In the stomach there may be associated rugal hypertrophy.

Juvenile polyposis can take one of several forms. An isolated juvenile polyp is the most common colonic tumour in childhood and usually presents with rectal bleeding. Polyps number between one and five and can be distributed anywhere in the rectum or colon. They vary from a few millimetres to several centimetres in size and can be sessile or pedunculated. There is usually no family history. Most of these polyps are hamartomatous, but there is a chance that any individual polyp could be adenomatous and thus have malignant potential. If there are multiple polyps these should be removed, but a single polyp is probably best followed for a year or so as many spontaneously resolve. If there are six or more juvenile polyps in the colon, the condition is termed 'juvenile polyposis'. This is much less common than isolated juvenile polyps. The majority of cases are non-familial but some do show autosomal dominant transmission. Juvenile polyposis is a precancerous condition and there is also an increased risk of malignancies in the stomach, duodenum and pancreas.

Metastatic disease

This can involve the large bowel either by direct extension, peritoneal implantation or the haematogenous route. **Direct invasion** from contiguous tumours occurs most frequently from an ovarian primary in females and from a prostatic carcinoma in males. In females a primary tumour of the left ovary can extend to involve the inferior margin of the sigmoid colon. On barium examination this appears as sharp angulation of the sigmoid loops with spiculation and tethering of the mucosa. With involvement from a prostatic primary, the rectum is the involved segment of bowel. Initially a prostatic primary will extend superiorly to involve the seminal vesicles, and at this point may appear as an extrinsic mass indenting the outline of the rectosigmoid but causing no mucosal derangement. With further posterior extension, the anterior rectal mucosa is involved and will appear on barium studies as spiculation and tethering of the mucosal folds. With more advanced disease the tumour can completely encircle the rectum, mimicking both the symptoms and the radiological appearance of a primary rectal carcinoma. On barium examination this is seen as a circumferential rectal narrowing with enlargement of the presacral space but there is, in addition, spiculation of the mucosa, which differentiates the condition from a primary rectal tumour. CT and MR scans of the pelvis can be very helpful to differentiate between primary bowel tumours and secondary involvement. Tumours can also involve the bowel via **extension** along a peritoneal fold. In this way pancreatic carcinoma can spread to the inferior surface of the transverse colon along the transverse mesocolon, whereas gastric carcinoma spreads along the gastrocolic ligament to involve the superior surface of the transverse colon. In both cases the affected border of the transverse colon shows evidence of fixation, irregularity and spiculation while the uninvolved border may appear sacculated.

Blood-borne metastases may also involve the bowel. Secondaries from a breast primary are the most common but are usually small and asymptomatic, appearing on barium studies as an area of nodularity. Less often breast secondaries cause strictures of the bowel with irregular mucosa on barium examination. **Melanoma** can also involve the large bowel and usually appears as a mass protruding into the bowel lumen covered with normal colonic mucosa that is frequently

Figure 3.56 *Serosal metastases causing narrowing of the sigmoid colon from invasion by drop metastases from the stomach. The serrated edges are characteristic. The appearances should not be mistaken for diverticulitis. Note the absence of diverticula.*

ulcerated. A similar appearance can, however, be seen with **lymphoma**, **Kaposi's sarcoma** and **carcinoid tumour**. Intraperitoneal seedlings, most commonly from ovarian carcinoma, may also be detected on double contrast barium studies (Fig. 3.56). They may appear as an external mass on the large bowel but with more extensive disease there is angulation of bowel loops, tethering and spiculation of the mucosa and scalloping of ileal loops. CT is useful in confirming omental involvement and may also demonstrate the primary tumour and the extent of other secondary disease.

Endometriosis

A change in bowel habit, a reduction in stool calibre and abdominal pain may also be the presenting symptoms in endometriosis. This is a disorder affecting women between the ages of 20 and 45 years who most frequently present with dyspareunia, dysmenorrhoea and infertility. It is due to heterotopic endometrium in extrauterine locations. This endometrium remains under hormonal control and secretes and proliferates with the menstrual cycle, producing cysts filled with new and old blood, so-called 'chocolate cysts'. Involvement of the bowel affects the rectosigmoid in 95 per cent of cases but may be seen in any part of the large or small bowel or even rarely the stomach. On double contrast barium enema examination, the endometrial implants appear as submucosal or serosal deposits with intact overlying mucosa. It is often difficult to distinguish confidently between endometriosis and metastatic disease to the bowel, but sometimes MRI can help in this respect. Metastatic disease is generally low signal on T1 sequences and high signal on T2 sequences. Endometriomas are often multilocular containing both

solid and cystic areas. The signal on MRI varies characteristically depending on the age of the blood.

Diverticular disease

This is the most common disease affecting the colon in the western world, primarily as a result of the low fibre content of diets in these countries. It affects about 5 per cent of the population under the age of 40, but this figure has increased to over 50 per cent by the age of 80. The sigmoid colon is mainly affected with the curious exception of Japan where the right colon is affected more frequently than the left. Complications occur in approximately 5 per cent of all patients with diverticula and require surgical or radiological intervention in 0.5 per cent. The out-pouchings from the bowel contain mucosa and submucosa and occur at the site where the nutrient arteries pass through the submucosa. On double contrast barium studies viewed in profile, the diverticula appear as protrusions from the bowel filled with a variable amount of barium. *En face* they appear as a ring shadow or as a hat, the dome of which points away from the bowel lumen. Diverticula may be mistaken for polyps especially if they invert into the bowel lumen. Changes in the calibre of the bowel are often seen in the presence of diverticular disease and may appear before true diverticula develop. Calibre changes are usually due to thickening of the circular muscle layer with shortening of the taenia. On barium enema radiographs, deep haustral clefts are seen arising from both sides of the bowel which interdigitate with each other to produce a concertina appearance to the bowel.

Diverticulitis occurs in 20 per cent of patients with diagnosed diverticular disease (Fig. 3.57). Inflammation

Figure 3.57 *Barium enema shows narrowing of the sigmoid, compression of the adjacent diverticula (arrow) and an absence of mucosal destruction. These features are suggestive of acute diverticulitis. CT scan provides a much better overall picture of the colon and adjacent organs in the assessment of acute diverticulitis.*

and mucosal erosion at the apex of a diverticulum may progress to erosion of the muscle wall of the diverticulum causing perforation and abscess formation either in the wall of the bowel or more commonly in the pericolic fat. This can subsequently lead to frank perforation, haemorrhage, fistula formation or a pericolic abscess. The radiological signs of diverticulitis depend on the demonstration of deformed diverticular sacs, extravasation of contrast or of the presence of an abscess, and CT is the examination of choice in a sick patient with diverticulitis. Deformity of the sac is an early sign of diverticulitis but may also be due to the presence of previous disease causing fibrosis around the sac, so that although sometimes useful it is by no means a specific sign. The demonstration of extravasation of contrast material is a more useful sign and easier to recognize. The leak of contrast may be into an abscess cavity or may connect with another pelvic organ such as the bladder. The contrast may also appear as a track running parallel to the long axis of the colon. In this situation the contrast is situated in a subserosal abscess and often connects up with several diverticular sacs, giving a double lumen appearance to the bowel. The diagnosis of a pericolic abscess is often difficult with barium investigation, although the abscess may sometimes be identified as an indentation in the outline of the colon. These abscesses are more reliably demonstrated using CT, which may also show thickening of the bowel wall or small fluid collections in the paracolic spaces. Ultrasound is less useful for full assessment of acute complicated diverticulitis, as pathological details are frequently obscured by gas. CT and ultrasound can also be used to guide interventional procedures. Diverticulitis also causes strictures and obstruction. These strictures may resemble a carcinoma radiologically but the margin between narrowed and normal calibre bowel is more tapering in nature than that seen with malignant strictures. Also with a diverticular stricture the mucosa is intact and the diameter of the narrowed lumen is more variable. A diverticular sac in the middle of a narrowed segment is strong evidence against a carcinoma as the cause of the narrowing. Carcinomatous strictures tend to be less than 7 cm long. In the final analysis double contrast barium enema is not a reliable method to exclude carcinoma in the presence of suspected acute diverticulitis and any suspicious stricture should be biopsied for histological confirmation. Diverticulitis and cancer can coexist.

A further complication of diverticulitis is bleeding, which can be very brisk. Angiography has shown that in many cases the actual source of the bleeding is an angiomatous malformation rather than the diverticulitis itself. Angiography allows the site of the bleeding to be identified, permitting either embolization of the bleeding source or a localized surgical resection. A giant sigmoid diverticulum, which is in fact a large cyst, can also arise as a complication of diverticulitis, and clinically these present with abdominal pain and a mass. On plain films a pelvic mass is seen which may have an air–fluid level. On barium studies contrast enters the cyst in almost 70 per cent of cases and the cysts are associated with radiologically demonstrable diverticula in 80 per cent of patients.

RECTUM

Examination

The rectum may be affected by the same inflammatory, infective and malignant processes as the rest of the large bowel and the appearance of these disorders is covered elsewhere. However, the presence of the anal sphincters makes the demonstration of bowel fistulae particularly important in this area. Fistulae can be investigated by injecting water-soluble contrast into the sinus tract or into the rectum. Often a more detailed assessment of a fistula, including the relationship to the internal and external sphincters, is required, but this is difficult to provide with traditional contrast studies, as the position of the sphincters is not visualized. Anorectal ultrasound can be very useful for demonstrating fistulous tracts and their relationship to the bowel wall and the surrounding sphincters. MRI is also useful, particularly as most of these patients have a very tender perineum and the introduction of an anorectal ultrasound probe can cause considerable discomfort. The fistulous tract has a high signal on T2-weighted and fat-suppression scans, and the entry points on to the two epithelial-lined surfaces may be clearly demonstrated. MRI can provide images in any plane which is a great advantage over CT.

Rectal disorders

Constipation and incontinence
Constipation is a term that may be used loosely by patients to refer to symptoms that may result from either delayed transit or difficulty with evacuation. Tumours and metabolic disorders should be considered, but the majority of patients have transit disorders or pelvic floor dysfunction. Most patients respond to simple management. For those who do not respond, it is useful to assess colonic transit in order to detect major transit problems. Patients who are shown to have major transit delay may not need detailed assessment of pelvic floor function. A convenient transit study is a shape study in which the patient swallows each day for 5 days a capsule containing 24 radiopaque rings. A single abdominal radiograph on day 6 allows determination of bowel transit time (Fig. 3.58). With the patient on a usual diet, a transit time of up to three days is acceptable, corresponding to 72 shapes on the radiograph.

Pelvic floor dysfunction leading to problems with defecation is predominantly seen in female patients who

Figure 3.58 *Colon transit study in 27-year-old woman with 'constipation'. The finding on day 6, that 91 of 120 shapes remain within the patient, indicates a transit time of almost 4 days. Moreover, as the majority of the shapes are in the right colon there is probably segmental dysmotility.*

comprise about 80 per cent of the referred population. Patients may present with incontinence, which can take the form of a constant leak of faeces or an ability to hold only a small volume of stool before defecation occurs with little or no warning. Alternatively patients can present with constipation which can take the form of excessive straining to initiate or complete defecation, difficulty in starting defecation or inability to completely empty the rectum. Imaging evaluation of these patients depends largely on defecating proctography but this is complemented by endorectal ultrasound and MRI, which provide exquisite anatomical detail of the sphincter musculature.

To perform **defecating proctography** the small bowel should first be opacified with oral water-soluble contrast. Thick barium paste is instilled into the rectum and, in female patients, the vagina is also opacified using a contrast–gel mixture. Fluoroscopic imaging is carried out with the patient sitting on a radiolucent commode. The patient is asked to contract the pelvic floor musculature, which decreases the anorectal angle and increases the anal canal length. When the patient strains (without defecating), the anorecal angle increases, the anal canal lengthens and the anorectal junction descends. Measurements of anorectal angle

and pelvic floor excursion have not been found to be associated consistently with any disease entities in recent reports. Imaging is performed during defecation. Patients who need to adopt various positional changes or use digital techniques to defecate are filmed while performing these procedures.

Rectocoeles are relatively common in the normal population, but are large in some patients with weakened pelvic floors and then are often associated with other abnormalities. They usually appear on defecating proctography as anterior outpouchings of the rectal mucosa. These may be associated with rectal intussusception which usually starts 5–10 cm above the anal canal. The intussusception is usually anterior and can descend to obstruct the anal canal causing symptoms of obstruction or of the solitary rectal ulcer syndrome.

Patients may also show evidence of an **enterocoele**, which appears as a separation between the vagina and the anterior wall of the rectum during straining and defecation. This gap might fill with opacified loops of small bowel descending into the pouch of Douglas (Fig. 3.59).

Figure 3.59 *Enterocoele. Defecogram in a patient with constipation demonstrates a large enterocoele (E) with contrast-filled loops of small bowel separating the vagina (small arrow) from the rectum. There is also a rectal intussusception with a linear filling defect (long arrow) in the column of rectal contrast caused by the intussuscepting rectal wall.*

In patients with constipation but with normal colonic transit, abnormalities of the puborectalis muscle are not uncommon. On straining and defecation there may be either no change or a decrease in the anorectal angle instead of the normal increase. Alternatively, the puborectalis muscle may relax normally but there is no relaxation of the external anal sphincters. This is often associated with painful anal conditions such as anal fissure or painful haemorrhoids, but can also be secondary to central neuronal abnormalities often caused by compressive lesions within the spinal canal or demyelination.

Defecating proctography may also be useful in patients with **incontinence** from rectal prolapse; the incontinence in this condition may be partly due to dilatation of the external sphincter by the prolapsing mucosa. When this is present on the barium study the patient may benefit from rectopexy or posterior anal repair. When the incontinence is due to sphincter trauma, the defecating proctogram is less useful as it merely documents a lax and leaking anal canal without indicating the cause. In such patients anorectal ultrasound is the examination of choice, as it can demonstrate the location of the damage and thus determine whether the sphincters are completely disrupted or whether there is focal damage that is more likely to be amenable to surgical repair.

HIRSCHSPRUNG'S DISEASE

Hirschsprung's disease usually presents in the neonatal period with abdominal distension, vomiting and delayed passage of meconium. The symptoms are due to colonic obstruction secondary to an aganglionic colon segment in which there is an absence of ganglia in Auerbach's and Meissner's plexus. The disease always affects the distal bowel and can extend in continuity for a variable distance proximally, rarely affecting the whole colon. Hirschsprung's disease is associated with an increased incidence of malrotation which predisposes to volvulus and ischaemia with subsequent intestinal atresia. Hirschsprung's disease is usually seen as an isolated finding, although there may be other neural crest abnormalities and the disease occurs with a higher incidence in patients with Down's syndrome.

The diagnosis can usually be made if an adequate history and clinical examination are obtained. A history of abnormal stool passage dates from birth and the rectum is empty on clinical examination. Despite this the diagnosis is occasionally delayed until later life when patients present with constipation and proximal colonic dilatation.

If the diagnosis remains in doubt, despite a thorough history and examination, rectal manometry showing failure of reflex relaxation of the internal anal sphincter can be useful. Rectal biopsy remains the gold standard for the diagnosis of Hirschsprung's disease, demonstrating the absence of ganglia.

Radiological findings are those of colonic obstruction on the plain abdominal film, and contrast studies are performed to exclude other causes of distal obstruction, such as meconium impaction or an atretic segment. The barium study is performed using a small lumen catheter

Figure 3.60 *Short segment Hirschsprung's disease showing colonic dilatation (c) above the affected narrowed segment in the rectum between the arrows. (Courtesy of Dr S.V. Thorogood.)*

with the patient in the left lateral position. The typical appearance is of dilated colon above the affected segment and a smooth tapered narrowing down to the diseased segment (Fig. 3.60). As little barium as possible should be used in an attempt to reduce the chance of barium impaction. A lateral film after the enema catheter has been removed shows the most distal segment to best effect. Patients with total colonic involvement demonstrate slightly different radiology with the plain film suggesting distal ileal or caecal obstruction, and the barium study demonstrating rapid filling of a non-dilated colon with reflux into the terminal ileum. The colonic appearances can be modified by the coexistence of colitis, which is a not uncommon complication of Hirschsprung's disease. In these patients the colon has a spiculated appearance above the narrowed segment.

Initial treatment is to decompress the bowel, which is usually by means of a defunctioning colostomy. Definitive surgery to remove or bypass the aganglionic segment is usually delayed until the colon has decompressed and the patient is older, usually at about one year.

HERNIA

Hernias rarely need radiological investigation but occasionally patients present with symptoms suggestive of an inguinal hernia but in whom no hernial sac can be felt clinically. **Herniograms** in these patients can detect small symptomatic hernias or prevent unnecessary exploratory surgery when no evidence of a hernia is shown. Herniography may also be helpful in the assessment of recurrent hernias following surgical repair. The examination is contraindicated when an incarcerated hernia is suspected, because the examination will fail to show a hernial sac.

To perform herniography, the peritoneal cavity is opacified with water-soluble contrast. Five folds can be identified, the median umbilical fold, two medial umbilical folds and two lateral umbilical folds. These divide the inguinal area into six fossae, three on each side of the midline comprising a supravesical fossa, and a medial and lateral inguinal fossa. Direct inguinal hernias originate from the supravesical fossa or from the medial inguinal fossa, while indirect inguinal hernias are seen as outpouchings from the lateral inguinal fossa. Femoral hernias have narrower necks than inguinal hernias and appear as pear-shaped protrusions. Generalized weakness of the groin can also be identified at herniography, and is a condition that affects young athletes as well as older men. Rare hernias may require tailored examinations (Fig. 3.61).

INFLAMMATORY BOWEL DISEASE

CROHN'S DISEASE

Crohn's disease was originally known as terminal ileitis, but it is now recognized that any part of the bowel from the mouth to the anus can be involved, and there may be widespread manifestations in non-intestinal body systems. The disease is uncommon on a worldwide basis with a prevalence of between 10 to 70 per 100 000, but the incidence has been increasing by up to 400 per cent in the last 40 years. The highest incidence is in Western Europe, the United States and Israel and it is very rare in Africa. The sex distribution is equal but Crohn's disease is more common in Caucasians and Jews. Patients typically present between the ages of 15 to 25 years or between 50 to 80 years. Crohn's disease can present with a variety of symptoms, the most common of which are abdominal pain, bleeding and diarrhoea. Abdominal pain is a symptom in 75 per cent of patients on initial presentation. This can be a lower abdominal colicky pain or a more severe pain in the right iliac fossa, mimicking appendicitis. Rectal bleeding is seen in about 50 per cent of patients when the disease is active, but profuse bleeding or blood mixed with mucus is more suggestive of ulcerative colitis. Physical examination may reveal an abdominal mass and/or tenderness, and sigmoidoscopy often shows areas of inflammatory change interspersed with normal mucosa. As well as involvement of the bowel there are many extraintestinal diseases associated with Crohn's disease, some of which can precede the bowel-related symptoms, such as low back pain from an associated sacroiliitis. Skin complaints such as pyoderma gangrenosum, erythema nodosum, dermatitis herpetiformis or vitiligo are also seen. The cardiovascular system can also be affected with thrombophlebitis or cardiac failure resulting from myocarditis or a cardiomyopathy. Finger clubbing

(a)

(b)

(c)

Figure 3.61 *Spigelian hernia. (a) The hernia is seen as a focal outpouching in the sigmoid colon. (b) The hernia was reducible with digital pressure by the patient's thumb (arrow). (c) The hernia was identified at surgery and repaired. (Courtesy Dr J. Gately.)*

Figure 3.62 *^{99m}Tc-leucocyte scan in a patient with known Crohn's disease showing uptake in the terminal ileum (arrow) and caecum, indicating recurrence of disease.*

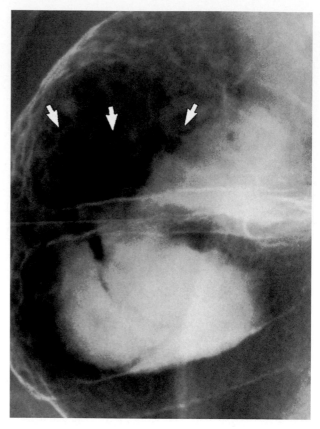

Figure 3.63 *Aphthous ulceration. Double contrast barium examination of the rectum in a patient with Crohn's disease, showing ring and dot lesions; the dots (arrows) represent tiny ulcers.*

occurs in up to 40 per cent of patients particularly with proximal small bowel involvement, and can be associated with hypertrophic osteopathy with periosteal reaction seen on plain radiographs of the wrist.

Crohn's disease can affect the whole of the GI tract. Small bowel involvement, in particular the terminal ileum, is the commonest site of involvement but pure colonic involvement is also seen. Disease of both colon and terminal ileum is common but the stomach, duodenum and oesophagus can also be affected. Involvement of the bowel is characteristically patchy in nature with segments of normal bowel being interspersed between diseased segments ('skip lesions'). Even in areas of disease, bowel involvement is usually asymmetrical with disease on the mesenteric border predominating, leaving the antimesenteric border relatively spared. As the small bowel is the commonest involved site, small bowel investigations are frequently requested. These can visualize the small bowel in single contrast and the terminal ileum in double contrast by means of a pneumocolon technique. Active disease can be assessed by a nuclear medicine-labelled white cell scan when regions of bowel with active inflammation show increased activity (Fig. 3.62).

Radiological changes of Crohn's disease

Mucosal granularity and enlargement of the lymphoid follicles

These are early changes which appear as nodular sessile protrusions into the bowel lumen. Lymphoid follicles

are, however, seen as a normal finding in young patients, and in this population great care must be taken to avoid overdiagnosing disease.

Ulceration

Larger lymphoid nodules may develop mucosal ulceration producing aphthoid ulcers. These appear as small barium-filled craters measuring 1–2 mm in diameter surrounded by a lucent halo produced by the lymphoid nodule. The appearance is that of ring and dot lesions, where the ring represents a meniscus of barium around a follicle and the dot represents the ulcer crater (Fig. 3.63). These lesions are known as **aphthous ulcers** and are difficult to see on single contrast views of the small bowel even with a meticulous compression technique. They may be more clearly seen when a pneumocolon technique demonstrates the terminal ileum in double contrast. Aphthous ulcers may also be seen in the colon on double contrast barium enemas, and in the stomach or duodenum on barium meal examination. These aphthous ulcers may occur singularly or in groups, and tend to occur at the edge of more severe established disease. The surrounding mucosa in the colon is usually normal in contrast to ulcerative colitis.

The ulcers may remain unchanged for long periods but can also be seen to enlarge or to regress completely. Alternatively the ulcers may coalesce to give a wide area of lattice-type ulceration, in which the ulcers are surrounded by inflamed oedematous bowel. It is the combination of the ulceration and the raised surrounding mucosa that gives a cobblestone appearance to the bowel. The areas surrounding the ulcers appear as raised irregular areas and, as the ulceration extends, the islands of inflamed but non-ulcerated mucosa give a false appearance of polyps. The inflammation in Crohn's disease spreads to involve the full thickness of the bowel wall, although this is usually asymmetrical and can affect only part of the circumference of the bowel. When the active episode of Crohn's disease remits, the ulcerated mucosa begins to heal and inflamed hyperplastic mucosa may remain as post-inflammatory pseudopolyps. These may be small and round or oval in shape but long filiform polyps may also occur. Fronds of proliferating mucosa can be seen which may be mistaken for a villous adenoma.

Bowel wall thickening

During an acute flare-up of the disease, the oedema and inflammation leads to bowel wall thickening which, on barium studies, is seen as separation of adjacent loops of bowel (Fig. 3.64). The barium-filled lumen of normal loops of bowel are closely applied or can be made to approximate with abdominal compression, whereas the barium in an inflamed section of diseased bowel may be separated from adjacent loops by a distance of several centimetres.

These areas of bowel wall thickening are more directly shown by CT (Fig. 3.65) or by ultrasound; the latter shows a target lesion when the bowel is imaged in transverse plane. Separation of bowel loops can also be due to fibrofatty infiltration into the mesentery, which becomes thickened from oedema and fibrous tissue; it is seen on CT as streaky high attenuation areas in the normally low attenuation mesentery. CT with oral contrast is an excellent initial radiological examination in a patient with an acute flare-up of Crohn's disease showing the mucosal thickening as well as abscess formation.

Strictures

Strictures are seen in approximately 20 per cent of cases of Crohn's disease owing to oedema and inflammatory tissue or to fibrosis. The narrowing can be very marked and result in the 'string sign', the narrowed segment containing only a string-like thread of barium. A stricture can be associated with a fistula, which tends to originate at the proximal end of the narrowed segment. Fibrotic strictures can be very tight and are irreversible and often require surgical resection. These strictures can be long or short and there are frequently segments of normal-calibre bowel interspersed between the stric-

Figure 3.64 Crohn's disease. Small bowel meal in a patient with jejunal Crohn's disease, demonstrating some thickened valvulae conniventes (long arrow) and patchy wall thickening (small arrow). The distal bowel appears normal.

Figure 3.65 Crohn's disease showing thickened bowel wall in loops of distal ileum (arrow). This patient has active disease but there is no dilatation of the proximal bowel loops to suggest obstruction.

tures (Fig. 3.66). The ends of these strictures can be very abrupt and can mimic malignant strictures in the colon. In these cases biopsy is usually required for diagnosis.

Figure 3.66 *Crohn's disease. Small bowel meal showing multiple strictures of varying lengths in the small bowel.*

Abscess

The detection of an abscess is very important as clinical diagnosis is often difficult, especially as many of these patients are on steroids. On CT with intravenous contrast enhancement abscesses characteristically show a non-enhancing centre composed of necrotic tissue with an enhancing wall, while phlegmonous masses enhance more uniformly. While abscesses can occur spontaneously they are often related to surgery and occur in about 20 per cent of Crohn's disease patients at some point. They can occur in the abdominal wall, between loops of bowel or in the retroperitoneum. CT is also helpful in planning the most appropriate skin access site for percutaneous drainage.

Fistula

A wide range of imaging tests may be required to assess the full extent of fistulae depending on their site. For **ileo-ileal fistula**, small bowel barium investigation often shows the site and course, but detailed compression views of suspicious areas may be needed. **Ileocolic fistulae** can be shown in an antegrade fashion using a small bowel barium technique, or retrogradely by means of a barium enema. **Enterocutaneous fistulae** can be demonstrated by a sinogram. It is important to take the time to manoeuvre the sinogram catheter as deeply as possible into the sinus tract in order to demonstrate a fistula and to show all significant connections. **Vaginal fistulae** may be demonstrated by barium enema techniques but occasionally require a vaginogram.

Perianal and **perineal fistulae** are difficult to demonstrate using conventional contrast studies. CT is a very useful technique to investigate this area and can demonstrate about 90 per cent of lesions. CT provides information not only on the site of fistulous tracks but also on the presence of any associated abscesses.

Endorectal ultrasound can be useful in identifying the presence of a perianal track and its relationship to the sphincters. An alternative examination is MRI which can show the fistulous track as a high signal on the T2-weighted and fat-suppression sequences and can sometimes provide additional information in the region of the ischiorectal fossa.

Remote complications of Crohn's disease

A non-erosive **arthropathy** can occur in peripheral joints as part of the extraintestinal manifestations of Crohn's disease. About one fifth of patients are affected at some time and this type of arthritis usually occurs at or soon after the onset of intestinal symptoms. Patients can also develop a symmetrical bilateral sacroiliitis similar to that seen in ankylosing spondylitis and 75 per cent of patients are HLA B27 positive. Radiographically the sacroiliac joint space appears irregular with erosions particularly affecting the iliac side of the joint; sclerosis is also seen at the joint margins. With time there may be complete fusion of the joint. Late changes are easily seen on a plain radiograph of the pelvis and can usually be seen on an abdominal film taken because of bowel symptoms. Early changes are harder to visualize but a limited number of narrow section CT scans through the sacroiliac joints can detect these subtle changes (Fig. 3.67). The radiation dose from a conventional three-view radiographic examination of the sacroiliac joints is approximately three times that of the thin-section CT mini-series.

Extraintestinal manifestations of Crohn's disease may be secondary to **malabsorption** caused by the diseased bowel and include weight loss, anaemia of chronic disease and a fatty liver appearing hyperechoic on ultrasound and with a low attenuation on CT.

Figure 3.67 *Sacroiliitis showing erosions (arrow) and sclerosis on this CT scan of a patient with inflammatory bowel disease. A sacroiliitis CT protocol provides excellent definition of the sacroiliac joints at a lower radiation dose than from a conventional sacroiliitis plain film series. (Courtesy L. Friedman.)*

Gallstones occur in up to 50 per cent of patients especially following terminal ileal resection and are best imaged with upper abdominal ultrasound. **Pericholangitis** is also seen but usually follows a benign course. **Sclerosing cholangitis** is uncommon. **Amyloidosis** affecting the liver and kidneys is also seen resulting in enlargement of these organs.

Urinary calculi occur in 5–10 per cent of patients. These are most often urate stones because of fluid loss, particularly in patients with an ileostomy that may lead to an increased risk of dehydration and acidosis. **Oxalate stones** also occur; oxalate is usually bound to calcium in the small bowel. In malabsorption fatty acids bind the calcium and soluble sodium oxalate enters the colon where it is passively absorbed.

Patients with Crohn's disease have an increased incidence of small and large bowel **carcinoma**, though less than that of chronic total ulcerative colitis. The tumours frequently develop in surgically bypassed loops of large or small bowel and tend to occur at an earlier age than carcinomas which are not Crohn's related. The carcinomas are usually of colloid or mucinous type. There are problems with the diagnosis of carcinoma in Crohn's disease, as strictures are in most cases the result of the Crohn's disease rather than a complicating tumour. The incidence of **lymphoma** and **leukaemia** in patients with Crohn's disease is also increased.

ULCERATIVE COLITIS

Ulcerative colitis is most common in westernized countries where there is an incidence of 1 in 1000. Presentation below the age of 5 years or above the age of 75 is rare and most cases present between the ages of 15 and 25 years. Up to 25 per cent of patients have a close relative who is also affected by the disease. Patients typically present with bloody diarrhoea with or without mucus, and may also complain of weight loss, abdominal pain and extraintestinal problems with joint pain, skin and eye complaints.

An assessment of the extent of the disease is important in regard to complications but it is known that double contrast barium enema underestimates the extent of disease compared to both colonoscopy and histology. Barium enema examination is unable to detect the loss of vessel pattern that is the earliest endoscopic pattern of ulcerative colitis. Colonoscopy also underestimates the extent of disease compared with histology. In the 1960s Goligher showed that disease extending to the hepatic flexure on barium studies should be assumed to be an extensive colitis causing histological change throughout the colon.

It is important to distinguish between Crohn's disease and ulcerative colitis and this distinction may be made in most cases by a careful consideration of all of the clinical, radiological and histological data, but approximately 10 per cent of cases show intermediate features preventing a clear separation. In acute disease the macroscopic pathological features as displayed in radiographs may be more helpful in differentiation than the histology, which can be difficult to analyse in the face of an acute colitis, the histology becoming more reliable in the quiescent phase. The bowel in ulcerative colitis is affected in a uniform fashion both circumferentially and continuously, in contrast to the discontinuous disease involvement characteristic of Crohn's colitis. The diseased segment in ulcerative colitis usually extends from the rectum proximally but, in patients on treatment, the rectum may be normal endoscopically and radiologically in the presence of active proximal disease. The distribution and extent of active disease can be assessed with a labelled leucocyte scan. A small group of patients appear to progress over the space of a few years from classic ulcerative colitis to classic Crohn's disease, both radiologically and histologically.

Radiological changes in ulcerative colitis

Granularity and ulceration

On double contrast barium enema the early changes of ulcerative colitis are those of mucosal granularity (Fig. 3.68). The normal smooth pencil-thin line of barium

Figure 3.68 *Ulcerative colitis showing a granular mucosa in the transverse and descending colon.*

coating is replaced with multiple rings of barium, representing focal mucosal elevation, and dots of barium from superficial ulceration. This combination of small rings and dots gives the appearance of mucosal granularity when seen *en face* and of a slightly fuzzy appearance to the barium coating when seen tangentially. In the majority of patients the colon is the only part of the bowel to be affected, with disease extending proximally for a variable distance from the rectum.

During a more severe acute attack of ulcerative colitis, extensive superficial ulcerations occur with more marked focal oedema giving a stippled and nodular appearance to the mucosa on barium studies; linear ulcers may also be seen. In contrast to Crohn's disease these changes are circumferential and affect the bowel in continuity without skip lesions. The ulcers tend to be shallower than those seen with Crohn's disease.

Terminal ileal changes

In total ulcerative colitis the terminal ileum may show abnormalities in up to 40 per cent. These include a granular mucosa, giving a diagnosis of backwash ileitis (Fig. 3.69), but the most common change is of a patent

Figure 3.69 *Ulcerative colitis. Double contrast barium enema showing typical granular mucosal change and narrowing in the colon. There is also a patulous ileocaecal valve and granular terminal ileum owing to backwash ileitis.*

ileocaecal valve and a dilated terminal ileum. The more proximal small bowel is not affected. Ulceration does not, however, occur in the terminal ileum in ulcerative colitis, and ulceration extending into the small bowel therefore prompts the search for an alternative diagnosis, such as Crohn's disease, or a secondary diagnosis of superadded infection, such as tuberculosis, yersinia or campylobacter.

Polyps

Various types of polyps are seen in ulcerative colitis. **Inflammatory polyps** and pseudopolyps occur during an acute attack of ulcerative colitis, and postinflammatory polyps in the quiescent phase. Inflammatory polyps appear as filling defects on a granular mucosa and are typically multiple. **Pseudopolyps** are seen during severe acute attacks of ulcerative colitis. The polyps are in fact islands of oedematous mucosa surrounded by areas in which the colon has been denuded of mucosa by extensive confluent ulceration. Once an acute severe attack has subsided, postinflammatory polyps can develop and are seen in approximately 10 per cent of patients with ulcerative colitis. These **postinflammatory polyps** may be sessile or may project into the bowel lumen as finger-like processes known as filiform polyps. Clues to the postinflammatory nature of these polyps are usually provided by other changes in the mucosa but occasionally these polyps are seen on a background of normal mucosa.

Shortening and narrowing of the colon with loss of haustra

This develops in total chronic ulcerative colitis, an appearance sometimes called the 'lead pipe' colon.

Presacral thickening

This occurs when there is an increase in the gap between the anterior margin of the sacrum and the posterior wall of the rectum on lateral radiographs of the pelvis. This gap is known as the **presacral space** and in normal patients is usually less than 1 cm in size.

Strictures

Strictures are common in chronic ulcerative colitis, usually benign in aetiology and may be reversible or permanent. Reversible strictures are due to muscle hypertrophy but appear similar to permanent strictures on barium studies with smoothly tapering ends and smooth mucosa. Differential diagnosis should be made between benign and malignant strictures and, particularly when multiple strictures are present, from cathartic colon.

Megacolon

Ulcerative colitis is an important but not the sole cause of toxic megacolon which can also be seen in Crohn's disease, ischaemic colitis, Behçet's disease and infective causes including amoebiasis and pseudomembranous colitis. Toxic megacolon is an important condition to recognize because of the high associated mortality. The diagnosis rests on a combination of clinical and radiological findings. Clinically the patient presents with abdominal pain, fever, raised white cell count and acute phase proteins. On plain abdominal films the striking abnormality is colonic dilatation beyond the 6 cm upper limit of normal. It is important to perform a

(a)

(b)

(c)

Figure 3.70 *Double contrast barium enema in a patient with a past history of ulcerative colitis showing (a) multiple filiform polyps (long black arrow), (b) a dysplasia-associated lesion (open arrow) and (c) a carcinoma (small black arrow). The presence of a dysplasia-associated lesion means that there is a strong likelihood of a co-existing carcinoma.*

plain film before embarking on barium studies as barium enema can precipitate colonic perforation. The dilatation of the colon is secondary to transmural inflammation with neuromuscular degeneration. Perforation, which usually occurs in the sigmoid colon, is not uncommon in toxic megacolon and is associated with a very high mortality.

Colonic tumours

These can complicate ulcerative colitis and, as in Crohn's disease, tend to be of the colloid or mucinous type. The risk of tumour development increases with an early onset of disease and can be recognized in patients with extensive or pancolitis who have had ulcerative colitis for 10 years. On double contrast barium studies dysplastic changes appear as irregularity and nodularity of the mucosa and nodular filling defects (Fig. 3.70). Dysplastic areas may herald and/or progress to carcinoma. These dysplastic changes are, however, difficult to demonstrate unless the bowel preparation is optimal, and may be difficult to differentiate from active disease. It is not possible to exclude a carcinoma in a stricture which appears radiologically benign. For several years routine colonoscopic surveillance of patients with ulcerative colitis at high risk for colon cancer has been recommended, but the usefulness of this has recently been questioned, and there is still no clear evidence that surveillance improves survival. However, colonoscopic biopsy of suspicious lesions seen on barium studies is very useful, particularly for those patients with radiologically visible areas of dysplasia.

Remote manifestations of ulcerative colitis

Ulcerative colitis is also associated with extraintestinal disease:

- anaemia, common from blood loss, malnutrition and the effects of drug therapy;
- deep venous thrombosis or pulmonary emboli;
- iritis and uveitis, often in combination with skin and joint symptoms;
- pyoderma gangrenosum or erythema nodosum, often coinciding with an acute attack of colonic disease;
- symmetrical sacroiliitis and spinal changes identical to ankylosing spondylitis, sometimes antedating the onset of colonic symptoms;
- arthritis, occurring with a peripheral joint involvement, which typically migrates from one joint to another;
- liver abnormalities, occurring in about 5 per cent of patients with ulcerative colitis and including fatty change secondary to malnutrition. Pericholangitis, sclerosing cholangitis and cholangiocarcinoma also occur, sclerosing cholangitis predisposing to cholangiocarcinoma.

ISCHAEMIC BOWEL DISEASE

Ischaemia of the bowel may be due to arterial or venous causes and can be generalized or localized to a short segment of bowel.

ACUTE OCCLUSIVE ISCHAEMIA

This is usually caused by embolic occlusion in the territory of the superior mesenteric artery and is particularly common in the elderly population. The extent of the ischaemia may include the whole of the small bowel as well as the right side of the colon. Patients usually present with ill-defined abdominal pain. Rectal bleeding, acidosis, pyrexia and a raised white cell count may also occur, but are similarly non-specific. The high mortality of up to 90 per cent from this type of ischaemia is largely due to the frequent delay in diagnosis. Plain-film findings in acute mesenteric ischaemia tend to occur late. They include a generalized ileus and bowel wall thickening. More specific signs such as air in the wall of the bowel and air in the portal vein are only seen in later stages when there is bowel necrosis. Air in the portal vein visible on plain film carries a very poor prognosis.

CT scanning is diagnostic in about a third of cases and can demonstrate relatively early on the non-specific signs of dilated bowel loops, thickened bowel wall and ascites. When a loop of affected bowel is imaged in cross-section, a double halo appearance can be seen due to low-attenuation bowel content and wall oedema separated by a ring of hyperaemic enhancing bowel wall. Intramural gas and portal vein gas can also be identified at an earlier stage than is possible with plain films. Air may be seen in the mesenteric vessels and is a highly specific sign of acute mesenteric ischaemia.

Ultrasound can also provide clues to the diagnosis by demonstrating thickened bowel wall and ascites. Barium examinations have little place when acute ischaemia is suspected because the findings are non-specific and more importantly residual barium within the bowel lumen interferes with the other imaging modalities.

CT is often useful as a screening procedure in a patient with an acute abdomen in whom bowel ischaemia is just one of several possibilities. However, the sensitivity of CT and ultrasound is low and, when the clinical likelihood of acute intestinal ischaemia is high, angiography should be performed urgently. Angiographic assessment includes aortography and selective superior mesenteric arterial injection. At angiography the occlusion may be complete or partial. When complete the vessel is seen to come to an abrupt end (Fig. 3.71) and, when partial, an intraluminal filling defect is seen. Emboli tend to lodge distal to the first three centimetres of the superior mesenteric artery, whereas thrombi tend to occur within the first two centimetres of the origin of the superior mesenteric artery. The occlusion from both emboli and thrombi

leads to a reflex vasoconstriction of the distal mesenteric vessels, which can mimic non-occlusive mesenteric ischaemia. This distal vasoconstriction is probably responsible for the progression of bowel ischaemia and bowel infarction that may develop, despite a technically successful surgical embolectomy. Therefore, surgery should be supplemented with transcatheter papaverine infusion to treat the mesenteric vasoconstriction. The papaverine infusion should start at the time of the angiography and continue during and after surgery.

ACUTE NON-OCCLUSIVE MESENTERIC ISCHAEMIA

This is the most common type of mesenteric ischaemia and carries a high morbidity particularly if diagnosis is delayed. In this condition there is no evidence of vessel occlusion but ischaemia occurs owing to marked mesenteric vasoconstriction. The differentiation of occlusive from non-occlusive mesenteric ischaemia is important as surgical treatment is usually required for the former but not for the latter, unless bowel infarction has occurred. Non-occlusive mesenteric ischaemia is usually secondary to a low cardiac output from a variety of causes. The reduced cardiac output leads to a reflex vasoconstriction of the mesenteric vessels causing bowel hypoxia. As this progresses, further bowel necrosis may occur leading to septicaemia and a further reduction in cardiac output. This condition can also develop in patients on vasopressive drugs owing to the vasoconstriction they cause.

Patients in whom non-occlusive mesenteric ischaemia is the likely diagnosis should have an initial chest and abdominal plain film to exclude other pathology, followed by early angiographic assessment consisting of an aortogram, followed by selective superior mesenteric arterial injection. These images should be carefully studied to exclude a proximal obstructing thrombus or embolus, as distal vasoconstriction is commonly seen secondary to occlusive mesenteric ischaemia.

The angiographic diagnosis of non-occlusive mesenteric ischaemia is made when there is diffuse mesenteric vasoconstriction in the absence of proximal occlusive disease. Systemic hypotension or vasopressive agents will also cause this appearance and therefore correction of hypotension is vital before the angiogram is performed. The diagnosis should also be made with much caution if the patient is on vasopressive medication. The vasoconstriction in non-occlusive mesenteric ischaemia appears as vessel narrowing. Once the diagnosis has been established, treatment is by transcatheter infusion of a vasodilator and correction of the underlying abnormality leading to the low-flow state. Papaverine is the most commonly used vasodilator and is infused directly into the superior mesenteric

Figure 3.71 *Superior mesenteric artery embolism secondary to atrial fibrillation. The selective mesenteric arteriogram shows an abrupt cut-off (arrow) to the contrast a few centimetres from the origin of the vessel. (Courtesy of J. Mernagh.)*

artery. The infusion can be continued for up to 5 days, but 24 hours is usually enough to reverse the vasoconstriction provided that supportive measures are implemented to correct the underlying abnormality. Digoxin and vasopressive agents should be avoided if at all possible in these patients. Despite optimal treatment some patients do progress to bowel necrosis and urgent surgery will be required.

CHRONIC MESENTERIC ISCHAEMIA

This is due to arterial narrowing and is also hard to diagnose; however, the urgency of diagnosis is not so great. The typical presenting complaint is upper abdominal pain starting approximately 15 minutes following food and lasting for about 2 hours. Weight loss is a frequent consequence as patients reduce the frequency of food intake. The cause of the ischaemia is usually atherosclerotic stenosis of the mesenteric vessels causing ischaemia at times of maximal flow following meals. The rich collateral blood supply to the bowel and the slow progressive nature of the vessel narrowing usually protects against ischaemia until at least two of the mesenteric vessels are affected by at least a two thirds reduction in blood flow. Unfortunately many asymptomatic patients both young and old have flow reductions on ultrasound, which limits the usefulness of this technique as a screening tool. Angiography is usually required when the diagnosis is suspected clinically in order to demonstrate the exact extent of the flow reduction. Traditionally treatment has been surgical, but it carries a significant morbidity and mortality and angioplasty is increasingly being used. Usually only one vessel needs to be dilated to produce a clinical improvement.

MESENTERIC VEIN ISCHAEMIA

This is a rare cause of mesenteric ischaemia and was probably confused with non-occlusive mesenteric ischaemia in the past. Patients present with gradually increasing abdominal pain, which may be associated with other pathology, such as trauma, portal hypertension or hypercoagulable states. Selective superior mesenteric arterial injection may show a diffuse vasoconstriction with marked opacification of the small intramural vessels. Non-visualization of the venous phase of the study is also suggestive of the diagnosis, but intravenous filling defects are more specific (Fig. 3.72).

ISCHAEMIC COLITIS

This is an important cause of colitis in the elderly population. The cause is unclear in most cases but is

Figure 3.72 *Superior mesenteric vein thrombosis demonstrated during an i.v. contrast-enhanced CT. The thrombus is seen as a filling defect (arrow) in the superior mesenteric vein. (Courtesy G. Gill.)*

thought to be due to a combination of a low-flow state and small vessel disease. Most patients are over the age of 60 and present with abdominal pain or rectal bleeding. The region of the splenic flexure is most commonly involved as it is a watershed zone between the superior mesenteric artery and inferior mesenteric artery territories. The left colon and sigmoid are not uncommonly involved and no part of the colon is immune.

Ischaemic colitis mostly affects the mucosa but can be transmural increasing the risk of gangrene and perforation. The ischaemic episode may be self-limiting resulting in complete healing which occurs in about a third of cases. An intermediate group of patients develop strictures or chronic colitis. Plain films may show no abnormalities or a non-specific ileus. More specific signs, such as submucosal haemorrhage and oedema, visible as thumbprinting, are sometimes seen (Fig. 3.73). The diagnosis can be established in most cases with a double contrast barium enema. If there is a clinical suspicion of perforation or gangrenous bowel, barium is contraindicated. When barium enema is performed early in the course of the disease, the most common finding is thumbprinting, seen as smooth polypoid filling defects which protrude into the bowel lumen. Another sign is thickened parallel folds running in a transverse fashion in the affected segment owing to oedema and accentuated by the spasm which frequently coexists. At a later stage there may be sloughing of the necrotic mucosa and a barium examination at this stage will show evidence of ulceration. The ulcers tend to run in a longitudinal fashion and can mimic the ulcers of inflammatory bowel disease, but ischaemic ulcers change over a few weeks as the disease progresses. These ulcers may heal completely or persist as chronic ulcerative ischaemic colitis with persistent symptoms. Alter-

Figure 3.73 *Thumbprinting at the splenic flexure. Single contrast barium examination in a patient with rectal bleeding. The appearance may be due to haemorrhage or oedema secondary to ischaemic colitis, intramucosal haemorrhage (as in Henoch–Schönlein syndrome) and less likely pseudomembranous colitis, ulcerative colitis, Crohn's disease and amoebic colitis.*

natively the ulceration can heal leaving a stricture. Strictures can be seen as early as 3 weeks after the acute ischaemic episode; they are usually smooth in outline on barium studies with tapering ends but there may be associated lobulated out-pouchings. The strictures may be seen without a clear history of precipitating ischaemia but rarely give rise to obstructive symptoms.

INFECTIVE BOWEL DISEASE

Tuberculosis

Tuberculous infection of the GI tract is a rare occurrence in western countries, but may be expected to rise with the increase in tuberculous disease at other sites which is now being reported, especially in the USA. Pulmonary disease accompanies GI involvement in about 20 per cent of cases and the terminal ileum remains the area most commonly affected. At all sites tuberculosis is often accompanied by weight loss, loss of appetite and malaise. Malignant

disease is usually the initial clinical diagnosis.

Oesophageal disease tends to affect the upper third and results in shallow ulcers and mucosal thickening causing disruption of the normal primary and secondary peristaltic waves. In the stomach the antrum is most frequently involved and ulceration and fibrosis predominate. In both oesophagus and stomach, fibrosis and luminal narrowing occur and may mimic carcinoma. Occasionally a large mass, a **tuberculoma**, appears as a filling defect on barium studies. Caseating lymph nodes around the stomach can be identified on both CT and ultrasound and may help in the diagnosis. In the duodenum and small bowel ulceration, wall thickening and fistulae can develop, but a common final stage is fibrosis with narrowing. These features are best demonstrated with enteroclysis but even then are hard to separate from the findings in Crohn's disease.

The terminal ileum and caecum are by far the most common sites for intestinal tuberculous disease and require examination with both double contrast barium enema and small bowel meal with pneumocolon technique for complete evaluation. In the early stages the terminal ileum may show spasm but, later, deep ulcers, which are partially or completely circumferential, develop, as well as fibrosis leading to a narrowed ulcerated terminal ileum with a widely patent, gaping ileocaecal valve. The combination of strictures in the caecum and terminal ileum can lead to partial or complete obstruction with dilatation of the proximal loops of bowel, usually in association with caecal distortion and shortening of the right side of the colon. Enteroliths may develop proximal to these strictures and are seen on plain films of the abdomen as small or lamellated areas of calcification within the bowel.

Peritonitis can also develop, which is initially associated with ascites (Fig. 3.74) with bowel wall and mesenteric thickening, best shown on ultrasound or CT. Later there is lymphadenopathy particularly in the right iliac fossa. The nodes tend to mat together and central

Figure 3.74 *Tuberculous peritonitis. Ultrasound of the abdomen showing multiple fibrous peritoneal strands giving a lattice-like appearance. (Courtesy V. Patel.)*

caseation develops, which causes adhesions and often a degree of bowel obstruction.

AIDS

Clinical acquired immunodeficiency syndrome (AIDS) is diagnosed when a patient with human immunodeficiency virus (HIV) develops an opportunistic infection or tumour. These infections or tumours often present as GI tract disease and GI tract pathology is common in patients who have developed AIDS.

A 'flu-like illness can signal HIV seroconversion and can present with nausea and diarrhoea or, less commonly, with odynophagia or dysphagia related to oesophageal ulceration. Diarrhoea is not uncommon in patients with HIV infection and should trigger a thorough search for opportunistic infection. When no evidence of an opportunistic infection is found in these patients, a diagnosis of HIV enteropathy can be made.

Candida

Infection with candida usually presents with sore throat or odynophagia. The typical white plaques can be seen within the oral cavity and brushings can be taken. Oesophageal candidal infection is best diagnosed by endoscopy with brushings but the barium findings are often characteristic and can spare the patient with odynophagia an endoscopic examination. Early disease appears as diffuse oesophageal irregularity on barium studies sometimes with fold thickening. With more advanced disease the irregularity becomes more pronounced and a cobblestone-type appearance is seen, with barium filling the irregular spaces between the candidal plaques. Ulceration can be seen with severe disease but this is rarely seen in isolation. Any ulceration that is present is superimposed on the background changes of candidal plaques.

Cytomegalovirus

Cytomegalovirus (CMV) infection is common in patients with AIDS. It can affect most parts of the GI tract from the oesophagus to the colon. The radiological appearance of oesophageal CMV on barium studies is different from that seen with candidal infection. With CMV infection there are usually large oesophageal ulcers often greater than 2 cm in size with normal mucosa seen between the ulcerated areas.

In the stomach CMV can cause gastritis with aphthoid ulcers appearing as ring and dot lesions on double contrast barium studies. This is a non-specific appearance and endoscopy with biopsy allows microscopy to assess for viral inclusion bodies.

The small bowel is rarely affected but occasionally isolated ulceration or terminal ileitis is present. In patients with terminal ileitis the disease is usually an extension of infection in the caecum and right colon. Early colonic and terminal ileal disease is seen as lymphoid nodular hyperplasia with discrete, well defined, small elevations in the mucosa. As the disease advances, multiple small ulcers are seen. As in the oesophagus, the ulceration occurs on a background of normal mucosa. In severe disease the ulceration is deeper and this is associated with thickening of the bowel wall. This thickening can be seen on barium studies, CT or ultrasound. There may be haemorrhage into the bowel wall in the late stages when the disease is associated with a high mortality.

Herpes

Herpetic infection is largely confined to the mouth, oesophagus and anorectal areas, but only in the oesophagus do barium studies have a significant place in diagnosis and assessment of disease progression. Like CMV, herpetic oesophagitis has an appearance that is distinct from that seen with candidal oesophagitis. On double contrast barium studies herpetic oesophagitis appears as multiple, scattered, discrete, small ulcers on a background of normal oesophageal mucosa. Herpetic oesophagitis can be suggested as the diagnosis by these appearances, but this should be confirmed by endoscopy with biopsy of the affected region.

Cryptosporidium

Cryptosporidium infection usually presents with diarrhoea, which can be very severe. The infection affects the small bowel and on barium studies the folds may be normal, and the only finding is dilution of the barium owing to the marked intestinal secretion. However, fold thickening may be seen and tends to affect the proximal small bowel and duodenum, although with severe disease the whole of the small bowel can be affected. Endoscopic biopsy of the affected bowel shows partial villous atrophy with marked inflammatory changes.

Mycobacterium tuberculosis

TB is an uncommon cause of GI tract infection in AIDS patients but does cause oesophagitis and colitis. In the oesophagus infection is due to spread from adjacent infected mediastinal lymph nodes causing the oesophageal wall thickening best shown by CT. Fistulous tracts can also occur between the oesophagus and the mediastinum or bronchi, and, if this is suspected clinically, a swallow should be performed with a low osmolar, non-ionic contrast agent.

As in patients without AIDS, TB colitis preferentially affects the ileocaecal region with wall thickening and luminal narrowing. The colitis can spread distally to affect much of the right colon and is usually associated with right iliac fossa lymphadenopathy. These lymph nodes may have central necrosis and appear as a low attenuation mass at CT and show central hypoechogenicity at ultrasound.

Mycobacterium avium-intracellulare (MAI)

Patients with MAI infection usually present with diarrhoea and weight loss from small bowel involvement. The bowel wall is infiltrated with macrophages with results similar to that seen in Whipple's disease. As with Whipple's disease, there is irregularity and thickening of the small bowel folds on small bowel studies, which usually affects most of the small bowel. MAI infection can be associated with local lymphadenopathy which can have central necrosis.

Kaposi's sarcoma

Kaposi's sarcoma (KS) can affect any part of the GI tract but skin involvement usually antedates any GI tract symptoms. Early lesions are best seen at endoscopy as violacious macules but biopsy of these lesions is often not rewarding because of the submucosal location of disease. As the disease advances, the macules grow to become raised papular lesions, which are then visible on high-quality double contrast barium studies. These papules are smooth and well defined but the characteristic central umbilication is frequently not present. Disease advancement is characterized by growth in size and number of the lesions, which can cause intussusception or gastric outlet obstruction. These complications together with assessment of tumour bulk can be well shown by CT. On CT the nodular thickening can be seen, provided that adequate bowel contrast is given, and these areas show marked enhancement with intravenous contrast. This nodular thickening can usually be distinguished from infective causes, because of its focal distribution, and from lymphoma, because of the paucity of associated lymphadenopathy. Bleeding from these vascular lesions can occur with advanced disease.

Lymphoma

Abdominal lymphoma is not uncommon in patients with AIDS. It is usually associated with lymphadenopathy, which is usually bulky. Isolated GI tract lymphoma can present with intussusception, perforation or acute appendicitis owing to obstruction of the appendiceal lumen by tumour.

POSTRADIOTHERAPY CHANGES

Radiotherapy can be complicated by both acute and chronic injury to any part of the GI tract. Complications are more likely with higher doses covering large areas at short intervals. Previous surgery increases the chance of complications as the bowel is less mobile, because of adhesions resulting in the same part of the bowel being exposed to each radiation fraction. Chemotherapy also increases the chance of injury, as do conditions which compromise the blood supply to the bowel, such as diabetes or cardiac failure.

The acute radiation changes are rarely investigated radiologically and resolve by 6 weeks. Chronic damage can occur due to small vessel injury and patients may present months to years later. Acute damage to the **oesophagus** usually presents with odynophagia, although it is rarely investigated. Barium studies show mucosal fold thickening and abnormal motility. Chronic radiation damage to the oesophagus can present with dysphagia owing to stricture, which must be differentiated from tumour recurrence. Radiotherapy strictures are smooth in appearance on double contrast barium studies with gently tapering margins, while tumour recurrence is typically irregular in outline. Endoscopy and multiple biopsies are often needed to make the distinction. Ulceration may occur in the oesophageal wall and these ulcers can progress to fistula formation. Fistulae most often communicate with the bronchus but can also involve other mediastinal structures.

Radiation damage to the **stomach** leads to a higher incidence of peptic ulcer disease. Narrowing and fibrosis of the antrum can lead to outflow obstruction, and endoscopy and biopsy are usually necessary to differentiate the effects of radiation from tumour, lymphoma, tuberculosis and Crohn's disease.

Acute radiation damage to the **small bowel** usually leads to malabsorption and diarrhoea. In the long term, patients can present with abdominal pain, diarrhoea,

Figure 3.75 *Radiotherapy changes. A small bowel enema shows dilated proximal small bowel loops and narrowed loops in the pelvis, which are fixed and show fold thickening. The appearances are secondary to previous pelvic radiotherapy for ovarian disease.*

which is often bloody, and obstruction. The terminal ileum and pelvic loops are most frequently involved and on small bowel meal examination or enteroclysis the loops of bowel are relatively fixed with sharp angulation instead of the usual smooth turns (Fig. 3.75). Smooth tapering strictures can also be seen with dilatation of loops of proximal bowel. Fistulae can develop either between adjacent loops of bowel or to the skin or pelvic organs, and abscesses are not uncommon. Thickened bowel wall, fistulous tracks and abscesses can be demonstrated on CT.

Acute **colonic involvement** is common and presents with diarrhoea. Chronic involvement can also present with diarrhoea and abdominal pain. A double contrast barium study may show narrowing with smoothly tapering margins (Fig. 3.76). The underlying mucosa may be normal or show thick folds and thumbprinting secondary to oedema and haemorrhage from ischaemia. Fistulae can develop either to the skin, the bladder or the vagina.

Rectal perforation from a balloon enema tip is more likely in a patient with fragile narrowed bowel secondary to radiotherapy. It is therefore very important that the clinician inform the radiologist about previous radiotherapy if a patient is referred for barium enema, so that an appropriate enema catheter can be selected. The same considerations make endoscopy hazardous.

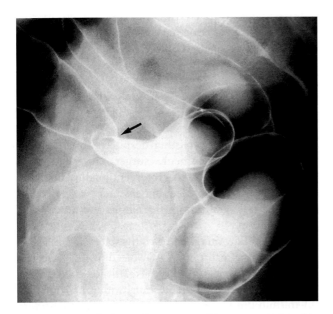

Figure 3.76 *Radiation stricture. Smoothly narrowed sigmoid loop (arrow) without shouldering or evidence of mucosal disease. This is characteristic of chronic radiation ischaemia: in this case it is associated with treatment for carcinoma of the cervix. The small bowel is often also involved and the ischaemia may cause ulceration and long-standing minor blood loss.*

CATHARTIC COLON

In patients with chronic laxative abuse a cathartic colon can develop which, in its later stages, mimics the features seen in ulcerative colitis. The first changes in laxative abuse are colonic dilatation and lengthening, but, after many years, haustra are lost and the colon shortens and narrows. The colon shows shallow ulcers seen as small pools of contrast on barium studies. In contrast to ulcerative colitis the caecum and right side of the colon are predominantly affected with cathartic colon. Multiple narrowed segments are seen in motility dysfunction, but they are permanent with cathartic colon. Multiple narrowed fibrotic strictures may also be present. The differentiation from ulcerative colitis can usually be made on barium studies combined with appropriate clinical information, and may be supported by melanosis seen on endoscopy.

GI BLEEDING

Acute gastrointestinal bleeding may require immediate resuscitative measures before any diagnostic tests can be brought to bear. Bleeding, however, may be chronic, necessitating infrequent but repeated blood transfusion and/or oral iron. Chronic blood loss is often more difficult to diagnose owing to the slow nature of the haemorrhage. The investigative strategy is usually similar in both cases, and begins with endoscopy but, when this is not diagnostic, close liaison with the radiology department is essential in order to optimize the sequence of investigations needed. Acute GI bleeding carries a mortality rate of 8–10 per cent. This figure has changed little over the past fifty years despite the advances in diagnostic and therapeutic techniques, partly because many people with GI bleeding have severe associated medical conditions, and perhaps also because of the increasing age of the population.

ACUTE

Acute upper GI bleeding

The type and severity of the bleed dictate the choice and timing of the first investigation. If there is haematemesis of either bright blood or 'coffee grounds' and/or melaena, it is likely that the bleeding source is from the upper GI tract, proximal to the jejunum. Conversely, if there is rectal bleeding, which is not black and tarry (melaena), then the bleeding is likely to be coming from the lower GI tract or from a huge upper GI bleed when associated haematemesis may be expected, but is not always present. GI bleeds that appear to be small should

Figure 3.79 *Meckel's diverticulum (arrow) found on peroral pneumocolon at the end of a small bowel meal examination. These small sacs are seldom obvious on routine films.*

Figure 3.80 *Meckel's diverticulum. ^{99m}Tc-pertechnetate scan showing an isolated area of uptake in ectopic gastric mucosa in a Meckel's diverticulum in the right iliac fossa (arrow) occurring at the same time as normal uptake of radionuclide in the stomach.*

ing enteroclysis for those patients with a negative small bowel meal. Some authorities recommend omitting the small bowel meal and proceeding directly to enteroclysis, claiming this is more sensitive for the detection of small tumours, but this approach does subject all such patients to the more invasive procedure.

Nuclear medicine studies can also be used at this stage, using either a red cell-labelled scan to detect the site of intermittent blood loss or a pertechnetate scan to look for ectopic gastric mucosa within a Meckel's diverticulum (Fig. 3.80). Ectopic gastric mucosa can lead to peptic ulceration and blood loss particularly in younger patients. If the site of haemorrhage still remains obscure a contrast enhanced abdominal CT scan should be performed to look for bowel-related masses and involvement of the mesentery. Finally angiography may be performed. The inferior mesenteric artery should be examined first before the bladder fills with contrast, followed by the superior mesenteric and coeliac arteries. Superselective catheterization may be required to show a small lesion. If angiography also fails to show a bleeding site, consideration should be given to provocative testing, which needs careful discussion with all involved parties (surgeon, patient and radiologist) as it is not without risk, but it can provide the answer when all else has failed. Provocative testing involves pretreating the patient with heparin and then performing the angiogram. Enteroscopy is a relatively new and very invasive procedure in which a narrow non-steerable endoscope is passed through the nose and manoeuvred into the small bowel. In one study enteroscopy revealed the source of bleeding in one third of patients in whom

all other tests had been negative. Its place in clinical practice is not yet clear and probably awaits further technical improvements.

THE ACUTE ABDOMEN

Patients presenting with an 'acute abdomen' present a formidable diagnostic challenge. A detailed history and examination, combined with blood tests and plain radiographs of the chest and abdomen may lead to a specific diagnosis. More often a list of possible diagnoses is formulated. Often the most pressing decision is whether the patient needs immediate operation based on the patient's condition and the likely diagnosis. Additional imaging can help to narrow the differential diagnosis and aid in this decision process in a select group of patients. While conventional contrast studies still have a place, the most useful additional investigations in these patients are abdominal and pelvic ultrasound and CT. Disease affecting any of the abdominal systems may cause or contribute to an acute abdomen, and these include pancreatic, renal, gynaecological, hepatic, splenic and alimentary tract disease. Non-abdominal causes also need to be considered, in particular cardiac and pulmonary disease, and specifically lower lobe infection. Diseases causing a generalized disturbance, such as the vasculitides, can affect multiple end organs and present with an acute abdomen; more obscure pathology such as familial Mediterranean fever can also present in this way.

PERFORATION

Patients with a suspected perforation, which is not confirmed on plain radiographs, may benefit from water-soluble contrast studies which can show a small free leak or the cavity of a contained perforation. CT scanning is also useful to confirm small amounts of extraluminal gas, particularly in the retroperitoneum where the ability to show the location of this gas can help in determining the site of the perforation. The perforation is likely to be from the sigmoid, if free gas is seen low in the abdomen and from the duodenum if seen only in the upper abdomen.

TRAUMA

CT with intravenous contrast enhancement is particularly useful in patients with solid organ trauma but can also be helpful in the identification of bowel trauma. Bowel trauma produces focal bowel wall thickening or soft-tissue density collections around the site of traumatized bowel due to local haematoma. Air in the peritoneal cavity or in the retroperitoneum is detected with a greater sensitivity than on plain radiographs. Air is, however, not always seen in the presence of a small perforation and oral water-soluble contrast is, therefore, advisable. This may confirm a leak by appearing in an extraluminal location and can also localize the site of the perforation. A haemoperitoneum appears as high attenuation fluid collection with the peritoneum, which differentiates it from serous fluid, which has a low attenuation. Haemoperitoneum is usually the result of solid organ damage but can also be seen with damage to the hollow viscera.

OBSTRUCTION

In cases of obstruction the clinical findings and plain films usually provide the diagnosis but CT can sometimes be useful by showing a transition zone between proximal dilated loops of bowel and collapsed bowel distally. Thus the site of the obstruction is usually demonstrated, and the cause for the obstruction may often be shown by the demonstration of a bowel-related mass or a more specific finding such as intussusception.

If findings suggest a distal colonic obstruction, an enema should be performed to differentiate mechanical obstruction from pseudo-obstruction (**Ogilvie's syndrome**). A single contrast enema suffices and in pseudo-obstruction barium flows freely past the site of apparent obstruction. With a colonic obstruction a single contrast study is usually quite adequate to detect an obstructing lesion. In the middle-to-old-age adult population obstruction is usually due to diverticular disease and/or carcinoma, but the differentiation

Figure 3.81 *Abscess as a complication of diverticular disease. The abscess is seen as a low attenuation mass lesion (arrow) on this pelvic CT scan. Air within sigmoid diverticula is also seen. The abscess was drained percutaneously under CT guidance. (Courtesy A. O'Donovan.)*

between them is not always possible on the barium study.

DIVERTICULAR DISEASE

Diverticular disease can present in a variety of ways, including an acute abdomen. A barium enema examination will confirm the presence of diverticular disease and, in patients without clinical evidence of complications, may be all that is required. Barium studies are not very accurate in the evaluation of collections around the colon and, in patients in whom an abscess is suspected on clinical findings, a CT scan is the preferred examination (Fig. 3.81); this will confirm the presence of colonic diverticula but will also demonstrate the size, shape and position of any pericolonic collection. Patients with single or few distinct abscess collections may benefit from initial percutaneous abscess drainage under ultrasound or CT control.

APPENDICITIS

Imaging may also help in the diagnosis and treatment of appendicitis and suspected appendicitis. Traditionally it has been prudent to operate to remove an appendix suspected of being the cause of an acute abdomen. There is, however, often uncertainty about the cause of right lower quadrant pain especially in young female patients in whom a gynaecological origin for the pain must also be considered. Transabdominal or transvaginal ultrasound is the preferred examination when the

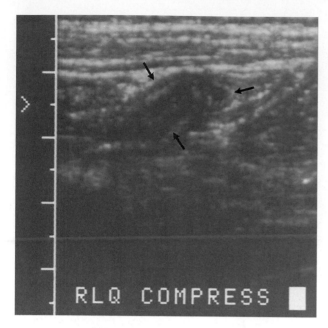

Figure 3.82 *Appendicitis. Ultrasound carried out on a child with abdominal pain reveals a blind-ending oedematous loop of bowel (arrows), almost a centimetre in diameter, that was not compressible – the diagnostic ultrasound features of appendicitis.*

differential includes a gynaecological cause for the pain, as the visualization of the uterus, ovaries and adnexae is superior to that from CT. The appendix itself is examined using the technique of graded ultrasound compression. Bowel loops in the right lower quadrant are imaged and compressed using the ultrasound transducer as a pressure device. Normal bowel will compress but an inflamed appendix will show minimal compression and be greater than 7 mm in diameter while being compressed (Fig. 3.82). The wall will be hypoechoic and the lumen hyperechoic, so giving a target appearance on transverse section; when seen in longitudinal section, the thickened bowel appears as a tube-like structure of varying length.

An **appendicolith** may also be seen as a highly reflecting focus within the appendix, which casts an acoustic band seen as a dark shadow lying behind the bright appendicolith reflection.

If no abnormality is detected in the right iliac fossa the rest of the abdomen should be examined for other causes of abdominal pain. This includes the pelvis, the upper abdomen and an assessment of free fluid. Ultrasound is about 90 per cent accurate in the diagnosis of acute appendicitis, but problems arise with retrocaecal appendix and in patients with large amounts of subcutaneous fat, which causes considerable image degradation. In these cases and when there is a clinical suspicion of an appendix abscess, a CT scan is the preferred examination.

INTUSSUSCEPTION

Intussusception usually presents in babies between the ages of 3 months and 2 years with abdominal pain, vomiting, and blood and mucus in the stools. The commonest type of intussusception is the ileocolic when small bowel invaginates into the colon. The diagnosis may be made on plain films. Ultrasound shows a mass with a hyperechoic centre surrounded by concentric hyper- and hypoechoic rings. The radiologically guided intussusception reduction should only be attempted if the clinical history is short and there are no signs of peritonitis. An attempt can be made with a longer clinical history if the symptoms are intermittent. A surgeon should be involved at an early stage, as the attempt at intussusception reduction can be complicated by perforation. The patient should be rehydrated and stabilized prior to the attempted reduction, which can be performed using barium, water or air, but carbon dioxide reduction is the technique of choice. A small catheter is placed in the rectum and the patient placed prone or supine, carbon dioxide is insufflated with the pressure maintained at between 80 and 120 mmHg. Pressures below 80 mmHg are unlikely to reduce the intussusception, while pressures over 120 mmHg increase the risk of perforation. The carbon dioxide must be given through the correct apparatus to ensure that the pressure can be controlled, and this equipment should include a pressure-release device, which prevents the development of pressures over 120 mmHg (Fig. 3.83).

THE POSTSURGICAL PATIENT

Patients are often referred for radiological assessment of the GI tract following surgery, either as a precautionary measure or to determine the cause of a postoperative complication. The radiological technique employed will depend on the type of surgery performed and the question to be addressed. It is extremely helpful if the surgeon provides the radiologist with a detailed diagram of the surgery undertaken so that the postsurgical anatomy is known. If the radiologist has this knowledge the examination can be devoted to answering the clinical question rather than working out the anatomy. The contrast agents used in the immediate postoperative period are generally water-soluble. Patients in whom perforation has not been shown on water-soluble contrast studies may then require a barium study to provide better anatomical detail.

THE OESOPHAGUS

Tumour surgery

Various palliative surgical procedures are employed for oesophageal carcinoma all of which may require

(a)

(b)

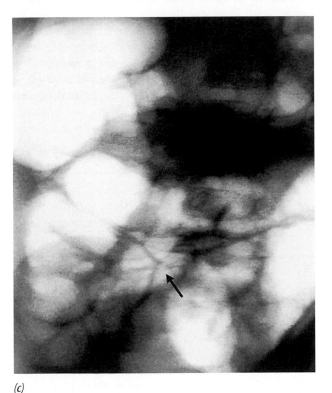

(c)

Figure 3.83 *Intussusception. (a) Ultrasound showing concentric hyperechoic and hypoechoic rings in an infant with abdominal pain. A diagnosis of intussusception was made and a carbon dioxide enema (b) shows the colon filled with gas, with a large filling defect (arrows) in the ascending colon representing the partially reduced intussusception. (c) Keeping the pressure of CO_2 between 80 and 120 mmHg, the intussusception was completely reduced and gas was seen to enter the small bowel (arrow). The two fluoroscopy images were obtained using a fluororecord technique keeping radiation dose to the absolute minimum. The images were manipulated so that gas appears white.*

postoperative imaging. One week after oesophagogastrectomy a routine non-ionic contrast study is usually performed. The oesophagogastrectomy may be combined with an antireflux procedure and complications from both parts of the operation may therefore be present simultaneously. Ideally the patient drinks the contrast in various positions, as an **anastomotic leak** may only be demonstrated when the site of the leak is on the dependent part of the oesophagus, although such an examination is not always possible owing to patient discomfort or immobility. As well as contrast leaks, aspiration into the trachea may be demonstrated. There may also be **obstruction**, either at the anastomosis from oedema or haemorrhage, or at the distal part of the intrathoracic stomach. Such distal obstructions may be due to oedema, around the site of the antireflux procedure, or gastric volvulus. Many of these patients present with dysphagia after an interval, and this may be due to tumour recurrence or a benign stricture, either at the anastomosis or in the low neo-oesophagus secondary to reflux oesophagitis. While most of these patients will require endoscopy to provide a histological diagnosis, a preliminary barium study will identify the site of the problem, and lead to a safer and more focused endoscopic examination.

Colonic interposition may also be used as an alternative to oesophagogastrectomy. Complications from colonic interposition are higher than with oesophagogastrectomy, with anastomotic leaks occurring in up to 40 per cent of patients. Mediastinal complications such as haematoma or abscess are also seen and best imaged by CT scans. At a later stage a stricture may develop, particularly at the proximal anastomosis, leading to delay in emptying and dilatation of the interposed colon.

Gastro-oesophageal reflux

The oesophagus may also be operated on in an attempt to reduce gastro-oesophageal reflux. In the postoperative period, dysphagia may occur owing to oedema or haemorrhage at the gastro-oesophageal junction, which appears on contrast studies as a fundal mass with a tapering lower oesophagus supporting a column of contrast. These appearances usually resolve as the oedema subsides over a few weeks, but a persistent narrowing may be demonstrated owing to an overtight fundal wrap.

Achalasia

Patients with achalasia who have had a cardiomyotomy or pneumatic dilatation also require postoperative assessment. Following a cardiomyotomy, perforation is the most frequent immediate postoperative complication. In about 50 per cent of cases the oesophagus is seen to have an eccentric outpouching at the site of the myotomy and it is important that this is not mistaken for a leak. Delayed complications are those of gastro-oesophageal reflux and complications related to reflux.

Patients who have had pneumatic balloon dilatation have a perforation risk of up to 4 per cent. A limited water-soluble contrast swallow and a chest X-ray are usually performed, as some of these perforations can be clinically silent. If no leak is seen on this initial study, a barium contrast study should be performed to assess the anatomy of the area more thoroughly and to detect subtle leaks. There is considerable oedema immediately following balloon dilatation and small leaks can therefore be missed. A contrast study should be repeated if the patient's condition deteriorates in the postoperative period. If a contrast swallow is negative in a patient in whom there is a high index of suspicion of an oesophageal leak, an urgent CT should be organized.

THE STOMACH AND DUODENUM

Common to almost all surgery to the stomach and duodenum is the risk of postoperative **perforation** which varies depending on the particular type of surgery performed. The radiological investigation depends on the presentation. When a leak is suspected a single contrast water-soluble study is helpful, with careful attention being taken to ensure that the patient is examined in several positions.

Fever, leucocytosis and/or pain occurring a few days following surgery suggest an **abscess**. Ultrasound is an excellent tool to investigate this potential complication although the presence of a postoperative ileus may result in too much bowel gas for proper evaluation. In this setting a CT scan of the upper abdomen is indicated with intravenous contrast to determine the size and site of the collection (Fig. 3.84). Most abscesses are suitable

(a)

(b)

Figure 3.84 *Postoperative abscess. (a) An abdominal film 5 days after laparoscopic fundoplication shows a gas collection in the mediastinum (arrow). (b) CT scan revealed that the abscess (arrow) involved the upper abdomen, and further cuts showed that it extended into the mediastinum. The abscess was drained percutaneously with an approach through the left lobe of the liver and the catheter tip was later manoeuvred up into the mediastinum.*

for percutaneous drainage and again ultrasound or CT may be used to guide the drainage procedure. In patients with an abscess after surgery a contrast study is also indicated to detect a continuing leak.

In patients who have had operations for peptic ulceration, recurrent **ulcers** can occur. These are best investigated by endoscopy, as is local recurrence in patients who have had surgery for carcinoma. Due to the distorted anatomy, adequate endoscopic evaluation is not always possible and in this situation a barium study may provide valuable information. Double contrast barium examination of the postoperative stomach is more difficult than in a native stomach due to problems of flooding of the distal bowel. Postoperative problems are similar for patients who have had surgery for peptic ulcer disease or gastric carcinoma, and the complications also overlap; the following discussion therefore applies to both groups.

Barium studies are useful to assess anastomotic strictures which can lead to outlet obstruction. Gastric emptying can be quantified using a radiolabelled solid and/or liquid feed by recording the gastric activity over time. The radionuclide study is usually reserved for patients who have symptoms of **gastric outflow obstruction**, but no structural abnormality on barium studies or at endoscopy. Gastric stasis is not uncommon after gastric surgery and may lead to problems with bloating, vomiting and weight loss, in a similar fashion to that seen with mechanical obstruction. Gastric outlet obstruction can also occur due to intussusception of gastric remnant mucosa, or the entire gastric wall thickness may prolapse through the anastomosis. Outflow obstruction in the immediate postoperative period may be due to stomal oedema which may persist for two to three weeks. At endoscopy the stoma appears oedematous and closed, but once the endoscope has been passed through it, gastric drainage often improves. Pancreatitis is another cause of postoperative outflow obstruction, and clinical features guide the diagnosis.

Patients can also develop **retrograde intussusception** of the small bowel into the gastric remnant, which typically involves the efferent loop. This can be seen in the immediate postoperative period but tends to occur as a delayed complication after many years. If seen in the immediate postoperative period the presentation is usually dramatic with upper abdominal pain, an upper quadrant mass, vomiting and haematemesis. Plain radiographs are often unrewarding but barium studies show a mass lesion within the gastric remnant consisting of jejunal loops which have oedematous compressed folds giving a coiled spring appearance. In the delayed form symptoms are less severe, the intussusception is often intermittent and barium studies give the greatest yield if performed during an acute attack.

Gastric surgery may also be complicated by the **dumping syndrome** but this is generally a clinical diagnosis and imaging has little to offer. Radionuclide studies however can quantify the speed of gastric emptying.

Malabsorption can also occur as a postoperative complication in patients who have had gastric surgery. Malabsorption can occur because of bacterial overgrowth secondary to stasis in an afferent loop, which can be diagnosed by carbon-14 breath tests. Alternatively the malabsorption can be due to coeliac disease, which can be precipitated by gastric surgery. The diagnosis of malabsorption may be made by the appearance of the small bowel loops during barium studies, but the diagnosis is confirmed with endoscopic biopsy of the distal duodenum or jejunum. Malabsorption may also occur from an inadvertent gastroileal anastomosis at surgery when a gastrojejunal anastomosis was intended. This is uncommon and tends to occur when the surgery has been particularly difficult.

Patients may also develop **obstruction of the afferent loop** leading to vague pains relieved by vomiting. This is difficult to investigate with routine barium studies because in 20 per cent of normal postoperative patients the afferent loop is not opacified. Ultrasound can be useful in demonstrating a dilated loop of bowel in the upper abdomen. A CT scan with oral contrast is an alternative technique demonstrating a U-shaped dilated loop of bowel containing no contrast; this may be associated with dilated bile ducts.

Gastric surgery is also performed as a weight control procedure in patients with morbid obesity, using either a stapling procedure to reduce the volume of the stomach or a bypass operation. **Gastritis** or **ulceration** at the suture or staple line may occur. The gastritis and proximal ulceration is best assessed endoscopically but ulceration within the narrowed gastric channel may be difficult to evaluate and, in this situation, double contrast barium techniques might show the ulcer crater. Outlet obstruction is not a rare complication in the immediate postoperative period from oedema, and generally settles without investigation or specific treatment. In the immediate postoperative period the anastomosis may leak causing an abscess.

In the later postoperative period following any gastric surgery, **small bowel adhesions** can cause obstruction. There is a paucity of good data on the merits of CT, small bowel meal and enteroclysis in these patients but practice is moving toward CT in the acute situation (Fig. 3.85) and enteroclysis in chronic recurrent obstruction (Fig. 3.86). Enteroclysis may not be possible with some types of gastric surgery because of difficulty in cannulating the jejunum. CT with oral water-soluble contrast demonstrates a transition zone between dilated proximal and normal distal bowel, with acute angulation of bowel loops at the site of the adhesion. Barium meal examination or enteroclysis can show a sharp angulation of bowel loops, and often reproduces the patient's symptoms when a large volume of barium reaches the diseased segment.

Figure 3.85 *Small bowel obstruction due to adhesions. The CT scan shows multiple loops of dilated small bowel but a collapsed terminal ileum (arrow) and caecum. No bowel-related masses were seen at the transition point.*

Figure 3.86 *Adhesions. Spot film from a small bowel enema in a patient with repeated adhesions with postprandial pain and distension. The kink (arrow) in the distal ileum was constant and due to an adhesion. Surgical lysis of this adhesion stopped the attacks.*

THE SMALL BOWEL

Surgery on the small bowel can be complicated by **postoperative leak** which should be investigated by water-soluble contrast delivered as close to the leak as possible. The initial administration of contrast should be through a nasogastric, nasojejunal tube or by

ileostomy, depending on whether the leak is thought clinically to be from proximal or distal small bowel. When clinical suspicion persists after a negative or suboptimal fluoroscopic examination, abdominal CT following oral water-soluble contrast will often show both the leak and any associated abscess.

In patients with **enterocutaneous fistula**, a sinogram can be performed using a small-bore feeding tube passed from the skin opening deeply into the track with water-soluble contrast to demonstrate any connection with the bowel.

Feeding jejunostomy tubes can be placed for long- or short-term feeding. The position of the feeding tube can be checked before starting feeding by injecting water-soluble contrast to confirm that the tube is within the bowel lumen and that the contrast flows freely into distal loops. If there is tube displacement, either initially or due to later tube migration, the contrast will be seen to enter a cavity or outline a track. The tip of the tube may be seen to lie outside of the bowel loops. If the tube has migrated it is often possible to reposition it using catheters and guide-wires under radiological control and thus avoid a repeat operation. Small bowel obstruction distal to the feeding tube can also be investigated by injecting barium down the tube.

Ileostomies may not function well in the immediate postoperative period or develop problems later. Most abnormalities occur close to the ostomy and include adhesions or stenosis causing obstruction. Herniation around the stoma can also occur, as can disease recurrence in the remaining small bowel. These problems are best investigated by retrograde barium studies. Ileal stenosis close to the ostomy site can cause obstruction and appear as a narrowed segment of bowel with proximal dilatation. This can occur very close to the ostomy site so it is important not to pass catheters too far into the bowel or these lesions will be missed. Recurrent disease usually gives similar findings to those seen with the primary disease. Insufflation of CO_2 or air to obtain a double contrast study of the distal bowel can be very helpful in recurrent mucosal disease, especially with Crohn's disease. Alternatively an endoscope can be passed retrogradely through the ostomy, which has the advantage of allowing biopsies of suspicious areas. Adhesions can also cause obstruction and may appear as sharply angulated loops of bowel associated with dilatation proximal to the adhesion. If para-ileostomy herniation is suspected, CT is probably the best imaging modality, and only limited thin sections are required through the site of the ostomy. Para-ileostomy herniation is seen as a loop of bowel lying beside the stoma and protruding out of the abdominal cavity into the subcutaneous tissues.

Patients with small bowel surgery may also develop a **blind loop** or **pouch syndrome** and present with malabsorption, diarrhoea and abdominal pain. The malabsorption, which is due to bacterial overgrowth in the blind loop or pouch, can be investigated by carbon-14 breath tests. The anatomy of these loops can be demonstrated with a barium meal, although enteroclysis often provides more detailed information.

Patients with a small bowel **bypass operation** frequently develop complications, which are difficult to investigate because of non-opacification of the bypassed loop. Conventional antegrade barium studies can show abnormalities such as stricture and adhesions and thus help in the distinction between structural abnormalities and bypass enteritis. Abnormalities in the diseased segment, such as intussusception, are best evaluated by ultrasound or CT.

Patients may also develop small bowel problems following the formation of a **ileo-anal pouch**. The pouch is initially protected with a proximal ileostomy and, before this is reversed, the pouch is usually checked using water-soluble contrast for anastomotic leaks. These pouchograms are performed with soft catheters and can demonstrate leaks, displacement of the bowel by a collection and abnormal gas collections within an abscess. An abscess can be further studied with contrast-enhanced CT scan. At a later date patients can develop **pouchitis** with diarrhoea and pain. Pouchitis appears on barium studies as mucosal fold thickening within the pouch, associated with spasm. The inflammation in the pouch can also be detected by endoscopy with biopsy or most easily with a technetium-labelled leucocyte scan. The clinical symptoms, however, are sufficiently clear that in many cases antibiotic treatment will be given on clinical diagnosis and no imaging is needed.

THE LARGE BOWEL

Following colorectal surgery, postoperative leaks and fistulae are investigated in similar ways to those used for the small bowel. Recurrent disease and postoperative strictures may be evaluated by double contrast barium studies or endoscopy. Complete obstruction is best studied with a low density single contrast technique as patients are often sick and this technique requires little patient movement. Studies through colostomies are performed in much the same way as for ileostomies. If the defunctioning limb of the colostomy is cannulated and contrast injected, the colon typically appears to have a small lumen and may show features of diversion colitis with nodular mucosa giving the appearance of focal nodular hyperplasia. These patients are generally asymptomatic and the findings are of no clinical significance.

FURTHER READING

British Society of Gastroenterology 1996: *Guidelines in gastroenterology*. London: BSG.

Freeny, P.C., Stevenson, P.C. 1994: *Margulis & Burhenne's alimentary tract radiology*, 5th edn. St Louis, MO: Mosby.

Gore, R.M., Levine, M.S., Laufer, I. 1994: *Text book of gastrointestinal radiology*. Philadelphia, PA: W.B. Saunders.

Laufer, I., Levine, M.S., Rubesin, S.E. 1999: *Double contrast gastrointestinal radiology*. Philadelphia, PA: W.B. Saunders.

Lee, J.K.T., Sagel, S.S., Stanley, R.J., Heikan, D.P. 1998: *Computed body tomography with MRI correlation*, 3rd edition. Philadelphia, PA: Lippincott–Raven.

Rumack, C.M., Charboneau, M.D., Wilson S.R. 1997: *Diagnostic ultrasound*. St Louis, MO: Mosby.

Taveras, J.M., Furrucci, J.T. *et al.* 1998: *Radiology*, Vol. 4. Philadelphia, PA: Williams & Wilkins.

Yamada, T., Alpers, D.H., Laine, L., Owyang, C., Powell, D.W. 1999: *Textbook of gastroenterology*, 3rd edition. Philadelphia, PA: Williams & Wilkins.

4

Peritoneum, mesentery and retroperitoneum

JEREMIAH C. HEALY, RODNEY H. REZNEK

Before the introduction of cross-sectional imaging, the peritoneum, mesentery and retroperitoneal structures could only be imaged with difficulty, often requiring invasive techniques. Ultrasound, and more particularly computed tomography (CT) and magnetic resonance imaging (MRI), have allowed the accurate demonstration of the anatomy of these regions and detailed detection of pathology; even minor changes can be reliably shown.

PERITONEUM

NORMAL ANATOMY

The peritoneum is the largest and most complex serous membrane in the body. In the male it forms a closed sac, whereas in the female it is penetrated by the lateral ends of the fallopian tubes. The peritoneal cavity is the potential space between the visceral and parietal layers of peritoneum, consisting of a main region (termed the greater sac) and a diverticulum (the omental bursa or lesser sac), situated behind the stomach.

The radiological anatomy of the peritoneum is illustrated using axial CT with the peritoneal space demonstrated using positive contrast medium (Fig. 4.1).

PERITONEAL SPACES

The peritoneal cavity is divided into two main compartments by the transverse colon and its mesentery, which connects the colon to the posterior abdominal wall (Fig. 4.2); the

- **supramesocolic compartment**
- **inframesocolic compartment**.

Supramesocolic compartment

The supramesocolic compartment can be divided into right and left peritoneal spaces, which in turn are arbitrarily divided into a number of subspaces; these are normally in communication, but often become separated by adhesions:

The right supramesocolic space has three subspaces:

- The **right subphrenic space** extends over the diaphragmatic surface of the right lobe of the liver to the right coronary ligament postero-inferiorly and the falciform ligament (Fig. 4.1a) medially, which separates it from the left subphrenic space.
- The **right subhepatic space** (Fig. 4.1b) can be further divided into anterior and posterior compartments. The anterior subhepatic space (Fig. 4.1b) is limited

(a)

(b)

(c)

(d)

(e)

Figure 4.1 *Normal anatomy shown on CT after intraperitoneal injection of contrast medium. (a) CT with intraperitoneal contrast, at the level of the porta hepatis, demonstrating the right subphrenic space (small black arrows), the left anterior subphrenic space (white arrow), the left posterior subphrenic space (open white arrow) and the falciform ligament (curved black arrow). (b) CT with intraperitoneal contrast, at the level of the renal hilum, demonstrating the lesser sac (curved black arrow), anterior right subhepatic space (small black arrow), Morrison's pouch (large black arrow) and the left posterior subphrenic space (white arrow). Fat lies within the greater omentum (open white arrows). (c) CT with intraperitoneal contrast, just above the aortic bifurcation, demonstrating the right paracolic gutter (curved white arrow), left paracolic gutter (curved black arrow) and right infracolic space (small black arrows). (d) CT with intraperitoneal contrast, at the level of the iliac crests, demonstrating the left infracolic space (small black arrows). (e) CT with intraperitoneal contrast, at the level of the uterus (u) and bladder (b), demonstrating the paravesical (small black arrows), uterovesical (white arrow) and rectovesical (large black arrow) spaces.*

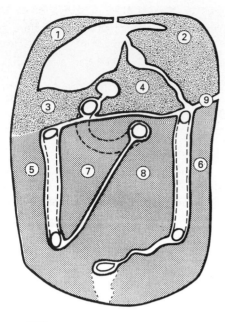

☐ Supramesocolic compartment
☐ Inframesocolic compartment

Figure 4.2 *Diagram to show the posterior peritoneal spaces and the peritoneal attachments to the posterior abdominal wall. (1) Right subphrenic space; (2) left subphrenic space; (3) right subhepatic space; (4) lesser sac; (5) right paracolic gutter; (6) left paracolic gutter; (7) right infracolic space; (8) left infracolic space; (9) the phrenicocolic ligament.*

inferiorly by the transverse colon and its mesentery. The posterior subhepatic space (Fig. 4.1b), also known as the **hepatorenal fossa** or **Morrison's pouch**, extends posteriorly to the parietal peritoneum overlying the right kidney. Superiorly the subhepatic space is bounded by the inferior surface of the right lobe of the liver. The right subphrenic space and right subhepatic space communicate freely with the right paracolic gutter (Fig. 4.2).

- The **lesser sac** extends behind the stomach, anterior to the pancreas, communicating with the rest of the peritoneal cavity through a narrow inlet, the **epiploic foramen** (foramen of Winslow). A prominent oblique fold of peritoneum is raised on the posterior wall of the lesser sac by the left gastric artery, dividing it into two major recesses. The smaller superior recess completely encloses the caudate lobe of the liver. It extends superiorly deep into the fissure for the ligamentum venosum and lies adjacent to the right diaphragmatic crus. The larger inferior recess (Fig. 4.1b) lies between the stomach and the visceral surface of the spleen. It is bounded inferiorly by the transverse colon and its mesentery, but can extend for a variable distance between the leaves of the greater omentum.

The left supramesocolic space has four arbitrary communicating subspaces:

- The **left anterior perihepatic space** (Fig. 4.1b) is bounded medially by the falciform ligament, posteriorly by the liver surface, and anteriorly by the diaphragm.
- The **left posterior perihepatic space**, also called the gastrohepatic recess, follows the inferior surface of the lateral segment of the left hepatic lobe.
- The **left anterior subphrenic space** (Fig. 4.1a) lies between the anterior wall of the stomach and the left hemidiaphragm, communicating inferiorly with the left anterior perihepatic space.
- The **posterior subphrenic (perisplenic) space** (Fig. 4.1a) covers the superior and inferolateral surfaces of the spleen.

The **phrenicocolic ligament** (Fig. 4.2), extending from the splenic flexure of the colon to the diaphragm, partially separates the perisplenic space from the rest of the peritoneal cavity. It forms a partial barrier to the spread of fluid from the left paracolic gutter into the left subphrenic space, explaining why left subphrenic collections are less common than right-sided collections.

Inframesocolic compartment

The inframesocolic compartment (Fig. 4.2) is divided into two unequal spaces by the root of the small bowel mesentery, as it runs from the duodenojejunal flexure in the left upper quadrant to the ileocaecal valve in the right lower quadrant:

- The smaller **right infracolic space** (Fig. 4.1c) is bounded inferiorly by the small bowel mesentery, extending from the duodenojejunal flexure to the ileocaecal valve.
- The larger **left infracolic space** (Fig. 4.1d) is in free communication with the pelvis except where it is bounded by the sigmoid mesocolon.

The **paracolic gutters** are the peritoneal recesses on the posterior abdominal wall lateral to the ascending and descending colon. The right paracolic gutter (Fig. 4.1c) is larger than its counterpart on the left (Fig. 4.1c) and is continuous superiorly with the right subhepatic and subphrenic spaces. Both paracolic gutters are in continuity with the pelvic peritoneal space.

Inferiorly the peritoneum is reflected over the fundus of the bladder, the anterior and posterior surface of the uterus in females, and on to the superior part of the rectum. The urinary bladder subdivides the pelvis into right and left **paravesical spaces** (Fig. 4.1e). In men there is only one potential space for fluid collection posterior to the bladder, the **rectovesical pouch**. In women there are two potential spaces posterior to the bladder, the **uterovesical pouch** (Fig. 4.1e), and posterior to the uterus, the **rectouterine pouch** (pouch of Douglas) (Fig. 4.1e).

PERITONEAL REFLECTIONS

In early fetal life as the abdominal cavity divides into the retroperitoneum and peritoneum, the parietal peritoneum is reflected over the peritoneal organs to form a series of supporting ligaments, mesenteries and omenta. Consequently a natural connecting pathway for the extension of intra-abdominal disease is formed between the retroperitoneum and structures enveloped by peritoneum, which has been termed the **subperitoneal space**.

The small bowel mesentery, sigmoid mesocolon, and greater omentum are frequently involved in disease processes, and can sometimes be identified in normal anatomy.

- The **small bowel mesentery** (Fig. 4.3) is a broad fan-shaped fold of peritoneum connecting the loops of jejunum and ileum to the posterior abdominal wall, extending obliquely from the duodenojejunal flexure to the ileocaecal valve.
- The **sigmoid mesocolon** is a fold of peritoneum that attaches the sigmoid colon to the posterior pelvic wall.
- The **greater omentum** (Fig. 4.1b) is the largest peritoneal fold in the abdomen. It descends from the

Figure 4.3 *T1-weighted coronal MRI demonstrating the liver (L), the normal small bowel mesentery (small black arrows), the right iliac crest (IC) and the superior mesenteric artery to the small bowel (curved black arrow).*

stomach and proximal duodenum, passing inferiorly, anterior to the small bowel, before turning superiorly again to insert into the anterosuperior aspect of the transverse colon.

PERITONEAL FLUID

Fluid collections are by far the commonest imaging finding in pathological processes affecting the peritoneum. Free fluid, or ascites, within the abdomen may result from a variety of underlying conditions.

ASCITES

Ascites results from increased fluid production in, or reduced fluid removal from, the peritoneal cavity. The fluid may be a transudate, for example, secondary to hypoproteinaemia, congestive heart failure and cirrhosis. Alternatively it may be an exudate, for example, secondary to carcinomatosis, peritonitis and pancreatitis. The fluid may also be haemorrhagic or chylous in nature. Peritoneal fluid collects initially within the pelvis. As more fluid collects, flow occurs in a cephalad direction in either paracolic gutter to reach the subphrenic and subhepatic spaces. Ascites is more common in the right subphrenic and subhepatic spaces as flow to the left subphrenic space from the left paracolic gutter is impeded by the phrenicocolic ligament.

Plain film radiography is an insensitive technique for the detection of ascites. The topic is discussed on p. 39.

Ultrasound is an extremely sensitive technique for detecting free fluid in the peritoneal cavity, detecting as little as 10 ml of free fluid in the pouch of Douglas. Uncomplicated ascites is typically echo-free and mobile within the peritoneal cavity. The gas-containing bowel loops float anteriorly within this fluid, which consequently may obscure the para-aortic and retroperitoneal structures. If the ascites is due to infection or malignant neoplasm, the fluid may become loculated by adhesions from bowel and peritoneal ligaments tethered to the abdominal wall. The mesentery may be thickened and bowel peristalsis may be diminished or abolished. Infective or malignant ascites may contain echoes owing to pus, other cellular material or septa.

CT can also demonstrate very small amounts of ascites and allows visualization of fluid within the leaves of the mesentery and lesser sac, a relatively blind spot for ultrasound. The distribution of ascites varies according to aetiology: transudate ascites usually has a smaller lesser than greater sac component; carcinomatosis has similar sized collections in both sacs, and pancreatitis gives large lesser sac collections, which may extend into the greater omentum or even into the mediastinum.

(a)   (b)

Figure 4.4 *Perirenal urinoma. (a) Axial CT showing a markedly dilated right renal pelvis prior to excretion of contrast (small arrow). Fluid has accumulated in the perirenal space medially and laterally as a large right-sided perirenal urinoma (curved arrows). (b) More superior axial CT scans following intravenous contrast show contrast in the upper pole collecting system (small arrow), and in the perirenal urinoma posteriorly (large arrow).*

On MRI, most fluid has a low signal on T1-weighted images and a very high signal on T2-weighted images. Infective and malignant fluid often has a higher protein content than transudate ascites, and therefore may have recognizably higher signal on T1-weighted images. However, the MRI appearances are not specific, and needle aspiration, which can be guided by ultrasound, is needed to confirm the nature of the ascites.

INTRAPERITONEAL HAEMORRHAGE

Haemorrhage secondary to anticoagulation, a bleeding diathesis or visceral trauma can be specifically identified on CT owing to the high attenuation value of fresh blood. Within several days, however, clot lysis occurs and the attenuation of the haemorrhage decreases, approaching the density of water by 2–4 weeks.

The haemorrhagic fluid may appear inhomogeneously dense on CT due to irregular clot formation and resorption, or because of intermittent bleeding. In the case of haemoperitoneum due to trauma, contrast-enhanced CT helps to identify the injured viscera.

PERIRENAL URINOMAS

These usually occur in the retroperitoneum, but can occur intra-abdominally if the tissue planes are disrupted by trauma or surgery (Fig. 4.4). Delayed contrast-enhanced CT may show filling of the urinoma with iodinated contrast (Fig. 4.4b).

CHYLOUS ASCITES

This can occur as a consequence of disruption to the lymphatic vessels by tumour or surgery. Occasionally on CT the Hounsfield numbers of chylous ascites may be negative owing to its high fat content, thus allowing a specific diagnosis to be suggested by imaging.

INTRAPERITONEAL BILOMAS

These occur following trauma, surgery and spontaneous rupture of the biliary tree. Bile elicits a low-grade inflammatory reaction that walls off the collection within the mesentery and omentum. On CT most bilomas have low attenuation except when complicated by infection or haemorrhage. They are usually located in the right upper quadrant, but can be found in the left upper quadrant in 30 per cent of cases.

INFECTION

Peritoneal cavity infection may be generalized (**peritonitis**) or localized (**peritoneal abscess formation**). The response of the peritoneum to infection is consistent, producing oedema and inflammation, followed by a fibroblastic exudate forming adhesions between peritoneal surfaces in an attempt to contain the infection.

(a)

(b)

Figure 4.5 *Intra-abdominal tuberculosis. (a) CT with intravenous contrast showing ring enhancing low density lymph nodes at the porta hepatis (straight arrows). Note also focal abnormalities in the spleen (curved arrows). (b) CT showing nodular soft-tissue thickening in the greater omentum (arrowed).*

PERITONITIS

Peritoneal inflammation may be secondary to bacterial or granulomatous infection, or to a variety of chemical substances, as in biliary peritonitis.

In the presence of peritonitis ultrasound may identify free fluid in the peritoneal cavity and the mesenteric fat may appear very echogenic but visualization may be obscured by free gas and distended loops of bowel.

On CT there may be thickening of the mesentery, increased density in the mesenteric fat, and ascites.

Tuberculous peritonitis is rarely encountered in the developed world, but there is an increased incidence in patients with AIDS and in immigrant populations. On CT, the following signs are highly suggestive of tuberculous peritonitis:

- enlarged lymph nodes with central low density due to caseous necrosis (Fig. 4.5a), seen in up to 40 per cent of patients in the mesenteric and peripancreatic areas;
- nodular thickening of the peritoneal surfaces (Fig. 4.5b);
- associated ascites, which is characteristically of relatively high density owing to its high protein content (Fig. 4.6).

Classically three forms of TB peritonitis are described, although there is frequently overlap in the appearances:

- 'wet' type, with free or loculated ascites which is seen most frequently in 90 per cent of cases. The attenu-

ation value of the ascites may be high (25–45 HU), reflecting the high protein and cellular content of the fluid;
- 'fibrotic-fixed' type, with mass formation in the omentum and matting together of bowel loops seen in 60 per cent of cases;
- 'dry/plastic' type, which presents with small bowel obstruction from fibrous adhesions and is seen in 10 per cent of cases.

Associated features of intra-abdominal tuberculosis may also be present, such as thickening of the bowel

Figure 4.6 *CT showing high density ascites (black arrows) and soft-tissue thickening in the mesenteric fat (white arrows) in this patient with tuberculosis. Also notice the inflammatory thickening of the perirenal fascia bilaterally (open white arrows).*

wall, particularly the terminal ileum, focal abnormalities in the liver or spleen due to granulomata (Fig. 4.5a), and occasionally adrenal pathology. The chest radiograph is abnormal in only 50 per cent of patients with tuberculous peritonitis.

Meconium peritonitis is a sterile chemical peritonitis occurring *in utero* following perforation of the bowel as a consequence of small or large bowel obstruction. The perforation seals *in utero* owing to the resultant inflammatory response. Obstetric ultrasound may show polyhydramnios, fetal ascites or dilated bowel. The plain film on delivery shows marked intraabdominal calcifications scattered throughout the peritoneal cavity with distended bowel indicating obstruction. If the obstruction involves the lower small bowel, a barium enema examination may reveal a microcolon as the colon is underused.

Figure 4.7 *Longitudinal ultrasound in the right upper quadrant, showing the liver (L), the kidney (K) and the diaphragm (D). There is a hypoechoic right subphrenic collection (arrowed) above the liver and right kidney, consistent with an abscess.*

INTRAPERITONEAL ABSCESS

Intraperitoneal abscess remains a major cause of morbidity and mortality following surgery, despite modern surgical techniques and antimicrobial therapy. The symptoms and signs are usually non-specific and thus early diagnosis and effective management are essential.

Prompt diagnosis depends on understanding the dynamic anatomy of the peritoneal spaces and the peritoneal reflections (pp. 110–113). The most common sites for abscess formation include the pelvis, the right subphrenic and the right subhepatic spaces.

Plain film diagnosis is discussed on page 43. If a fistula or sinus has formed to the skin surface, opacification with an iodinated contrast agent will visualize the abscess cavity.

The accuracy of ultrasound for the detection of intraperitoneal abscess is not as high as CT, since successful ultrasound examination depends on the patient's body habitus and abscesses are often obscured or confused with bowel loops. However, ultrasound is a rapid, inexpensive and readily available first-line technique. It is best suited for diagnosing abscesses in the right and left upper quadrants, especially subphrenic collections (Fig. 4.7), because the ability to image in the longitudinal plane allows easy distinction between fluid above and below the diaphragm. It is also very good for detecting pelvic collections using the distended bladder as an acoustic window. The ability to perform portable ultrasound examinations on the ward or on ITU in critically ill patients is a major benefit.

On ultrasound the abscess cavity may appear echofree, mimicking a cyst, or it may contain low level echoes or solid elements. The margin of the collection is usually thick and irregular depending on its age. As ultrasound is completely reflected at soft tissue-air interfaces, the abscess may be obscured if it contains bubbles of gas. Similarly, abscess collections within the mesentery are poorly visualized as they are obscured by the surrounding loops of bowel containing gas.

CT, which is much less operator-dependent than ultrasound, is the most sensitive technique for the detection of intraperitoneal abscess. The entire abdomen and pelvis can be surveyed. The CT appearances depend to some extent on the age of the abscess. In the earliest stages the abscess may appear as a mass, representing the swollen tissues or viscera colonized by neutrophils and bacteria. As the process advances, its centre undergoes liquefactive necrosis, producing a region of fluid attenuation, the margin of which enhances following intravenous contrast enhancement. About 30 per cent of abscesses contain air, which appears as dark bubbles on CT or produces an air–fluid level. Displacement of adjacent structures and thickening or obliteration of adjacent fat planes accompanies abscess formation. Most abscesses are round or oval in shape on CT, but those adjacent to solid organs may be lenticular or crescenteric in configuration. The CT appearances may suggest the cause of the abscess; for example, a right lower quadrant mass containing a calcific density is likely to represent an appendix abscess with an associated appendicolith.

The accuracy of CT for detecting abscesses in the subphrenic spaces and pelvis is similar to ultrasound. Subphrenic abscesses have the same features on CT as abscesses elsewhere. However, it can occasionally be extremely difficult to determine whether fluid lies above or below the diaphragm. Spiral CT, which allows longitudinal reconstruction, allows this distinction to be made with greater ease (Figs 4.8a,b). CT is much better than ultrasound for detecting collections centrally within the abdomen and those closely related to bowel. Additionally, unlike ultrasound, CT is not dependent on body habitus and the position of drains and dressings. In addition the CT appearances may suggest the cause of the abscess.

- **Acute appendicitis** can be diagnosed on unenhanced CT by identification of the appendix, periappendiceal inflammation, and an appendix abscess with an associated appendicolith.

(a)

(a)

Figure 4.8 *Subphrenic abscess on spiral CT. (a) Axial CT showing the liver (L) and a large encapsulated fluid collection containing a pocket of air, consistent with a right subphrenic abscess (A). The abscess contains a drain (arrowed). (b) Sagittal reformation from axial spiral CT showing the liver (L) and a right subphrenic abscess (A).*

- **Acute diverticulitis** is identified on CT by ill-defined inflammation in the pericolic fat and sigmoid mesocolon, in association with colonic diverticula and thickening of the colonic wall.
- CT also demonstrates marked bowel wall thickening with mural stratification and often a target or double halo sign in **Crohn's disease** (Fig. 4.16, p. 121).

Both ultrasound and CT have significant roles to play in needle aspiration and percutaneous drainage of abscesses, thus reducing the morbidity of reoperation. Radionuclide imaging using gallium-67 or leucocytes labelled with indium-111 is quite sensitive for detecting intraperitoneal abscess formation; however, the specificity of this technique is much poorer than CT or ultrasound. Even when radionuclide imaging is positive, ultrasound or CT is required to localize collections anatomically.

MRI does not offer any benefit over ultrasound and CT for the diagnosis of intraperitoneal abscess. At present, MRI of the abdomen is degraded by respiratory and peristaltic bowel movement and fluid in the bowel can be difficult to differentiate from extraluminal collections. Also MRI contrast opacification of the bowel is not as effective as in CT.

TRAUMA

CT is essential in the diagnosis and management planning of abdominal trauma, which has significantly reduced the number of negative exploratory laparotomies. Peritoneal fluid seen on CT after trauma may represent blood, urine or bowel contents.

Haemoperitoneum is seen in approximately two thirds of all intraperitoneal solid-organ (hepatic or splenic) injuries but it is not seen if the injury does not extend to the organ surface, or if there is no capsular disruption. A haemoperitoneum is also seen in vascular injuries, especially of the pelvic vessels, in association with skeletal fractures. Following trauma the only sign of active haemorrhage on enhanced CT is focal or diffuse high attenuation areas (> 90 HU), representing extravasated intravascular contrast mixed with blood.

Intraperitoneal bladder rupture is usually associated with high attenuation fluid collections as a consequence of excreted intravenous contrast material. This extravasation is best detected on delayed images.

In the absence of visceral or bony injury, large amounts of free intraperitoneal fluid, free intraperitoneal air and intense bowel wall enhancement suggests bowel rupture. However, this is relatively rare, occurring in about 5 per cent of patients who have laparotomy for blunt abdominal trauma. Bowel injury is almost always associated with a large mesenteric haematoma.

Abdominal CT provides global evaluation of the abdomen and retroperitoneum and organ specific information. However, it is a relatively expensive test and it requires transfer to the scanning suite. Diagnostic peritoneal lavage (DPL) is fast, comparatively inexpensive and may be as sensitive as CT in screening for serious intraperitoneal injury. Sonography is also a fast, accessible method for detecting haemoperitoneum, but it suffers from being both operator- and patient-dependent, resulting in a poorer sensitivity than CT or peritoneal lavage for detecting serious peritoneal trauma.

NEOPLASMS

METASTASES

The most common malignant process involving the peritoneum is metastatic disease. Peritoneal metastases usually originate from intra-abdominal primary neoplasms, including the stomach, colon, ovary and pancreas. Prior to the advent of CT, peritoneal metastases were not radiographically detectable until late in the disease, when they displaced adjacent organs, caused intestinal obstruction, or produced radiological signs from massive ascites on plain films. Conventional barium studies only provide indirect signs of peritoneal and mesenteric disease owing to displacement of bowel, mucosal tethering, or invasion into the bowel itself. Abnormal findings on CT often eliminate the need for a barium study, or at least suggest the region to examine in detail.

In patients with large amounts of ascites, ultrasound is capable of demonstrating superficial peritoneal and omental tumour nodules as small as 2–3 cm, but ultrasound will not detect small peritoneal deposits if there is only minimal ascites. Also ultrasound will not identify centrally located tumour deposits as these are obscured by bowel gas and by the increased acoustic impedance of mesenteric fat.

Although MRI may offer superior soft-tissue contrast to CT, the spatial resolution of the technique, at present, is diminished by movement artefact caused by bowel peristalsis and respiration. Therefore CT is the imaging procedure of choice for evaluating patients known to have, or suspected of having peritoneal or mesenteric neoplasms.

Metastatic neoplasms disseminate throughout the peritoneum in four ways:

- direct spread along the peritoneal ligaments, mesenteries and omenta;
- intraperitoneal seeding through the ascitic fluid;
- lymphatic extension;
- embolic haematogenous spread.

However, it must be stressed that none of these appearances is specific for the malignancies mentioned and can be mimicked by other metastatic tumours, primary peritoneal tumours such as mesothelioma, and inflammatory conditions, such as pancreatitis and tuberculous peritonitis. Also many of the distinct patterns of metastatic disease described often coexist.

Peritoneal spread of neoplasms

Intraperitoneal seeding of neoplasms depends on the normal flow of fluid within the peritoneal cavity. This flow is facilitated by gravity, and in the upper abdomen by changes in intra-abdominal pressure caused by respiration. The pouch of Douglas, the lower small bowel mesentery near the ileocaecal junction, and the right paracolic gutter are the most common sites for pooling of ascites, and subsequent fixation and growth of peritoneal metastases.

On barium examination, peritoneal metastases may produce angulation and kinking of bowel loops and spiculation and tethering of their mucosal folds.

On CT early peritoneal involvement produces increased density within the fat adjacent to the primary neoplasm. Subsequently, a mass contiguous with the primary neoplasm may be seen extending along the expected course of the peritoneal reflection. As these peritoneal reflections are in continuity with the posterior abdominal wall, spread may also occur to the retroperitoneum. Neoplastic infiltration of the greater omentum can produce soft-tissue nodular thickening within the omental fat (Fig. 4.9). Early in the disease, this will appear as an ill-defined loss of the normal clarity of the fat. With more advanced disease, a large mass may separate the colon from the anterior abdominal wall in a phenomenon known as 'omental caking' (Fig. 4.10). Widespread peritoneal metastases and omental caking, which occasionally calcify, are most frequently associated with metastatic ovarian cancer.

Specific neoplasms often spread by anatomically predictable routes and give characteristic CT appearances:

- Malignant neoplasms of the stomach, colon, pancreas and ovary can spread directly along the visceral peritoneal reflections to affect other peritoneal structures.
- Neoplasms of the colon, stomach and pancreas use the transverse mesocolon and greater omentum as conduits for spread.
- Gastric malignancies can spread to the spleen via the gastrosplenic ligament.
- Neoplasms of the pancreatic tail spread via the phrenicocolic ligament to the splenic flexure of the colon.
- Biliary and hepatic malignancies usually spread via the lesser omentum and hepatoduodenal ligaments.
- Ovarian cancer spreads along all of its adjacent mesothelial surfaces to produce marked peritoneal thickening, nodularity and rounded masses (Fig. 4.11). It also frequently produces cake-like masses and cystic mesenteric masses.

Figure 4.9 *CT showing ascites (open arrows) lateral to the liver (L) and soft-tissue stranding in the omental fat (solid arrows) in this patient with disseminated ovarian cancer.*

Figure 4.11 *CT showing diffuse peritoneal deposits (white arrows) and ascites (black arrows) from ovarian cancer. The irregular liver surface is also due to peritoneal disease (curved white arrow).*

Figure 4.10 *CT showing diffuse soft-tissue nodules in the mesentery (black arrows) and omental caking (white arrows) in this patient with peritoneal metastases from colonic cancer.*

- Carcinoid and lymphoma produce marked soft-tissue thickening in the small bowel mesentery, with shortening of the mesentery, perivascular soft-tissue encasement and tethering of the bowel.
- Pancreatic, breast and colonic metastases commonly produce stellate masses, with radiating mesenteric extensions along the vessels.

Lymphatic dissemination

Lymphatic spread is the primary route of metastasis for lymphoma. Approximately 50 per cent of patients with non-Hodgkin's lymphoma have enlarged mesenteric lymph nodes at presentation. These nodes may be confluent producing large mass lesions in the mesentery. Characteristically, these nodal masses surround and encase vessels, particularly the superior mesenteric vessels. It is important to note, however, that enlargement of mesenteric lymph nodes can be due to inflammatory causes such as Crohn's disease, Whipple's disease and tuberculosis. In these conditions individual lymph nodes generally remain more discrete and rarely become a conglomerate mass.

Embolic metastases

Metastases may spread via the mesenteric arteries to the antimesenteric border of the bowel, where malignant cells can implant and subsequently grow into submucosal nodules. On barium studies these deposits appear as 'bull's eye' or 'target' lesions with central ulceration as the deposit outgrows its blood supply. This type of deposit is characteristic of malignant melanoma metastases. Embolic metastasis to the stomach may produce a 'linitis plastica' appearance on barium meal examination, with marked narrowing of the lumen and scirrhous thickening of the bowel wall. This type of appearance is seen particularly with embolic breast metastases. On CT these metastases produce thickening of the adjacent mesenteric leaves or focal bowel wall thickening with associated ulceration.

Pseudomyxoma peritonei

In pseudomyxoma peritonei the peritoneal surfaces become diffusely involved with large amounts of mucinous material as a consequence of rupture of a mucinous cystadenocarcinoma or cystadenoma, usually of the ovary or appendix. It occurs more frequently in females than in males. On CT there may be low attenuation masses surrounded by discrete walls, which may contain calcification. The low attenuation masses may contain septa and often fill the peritoneal spaces, causing scalloping of the liver margins (Fig. 4.12). The inability of the bowel to float anteriorly in this gelatinous material, along with the other CT features, are characteristic of the condition.

PRIMARY NEOPLASMS

Primary neoplasms of the peritoneum are rare and are usually of mesenchymal origin.

Mesothelioma

Mesothelioma (Fig. 4.13) arises in the serosal lining of the pleura, peritoneum and pericardium associated with asbestos exposure. Peritoneal involvement may occur alone or in combination with pleural involvement. On CT there is marked thickening of the peritoneum, mesentery and omentum, which may show an irregular or nodular appearance. Peritoneal calcification (which may be seen on plain films) and associated ascites are seen on CT. The amount of ascites may be disproportionately small in relation to the peritoneal disease when compared to other peritoneal neoplasms. The mesenteric involvement may produce a stellate appearance caused by thickening of perivascular bundles. These appearances, however, are not specific for mesothelioma and may be indistinguishable from metastases, lymphoma or tuberculous peritonitis. The diagnosis is strongly suggested if there is concomitant thickening

and calcification of the pleura in a patient with a history of asbestos exposure (Fig. 4.13).

Lipomatous tumours

These occasionally involve the peritoneal cavity and have typical CT and MRI appearances. Benign lipomas are well-defined and composed entirely of fat except for very thin septa. Liposarcomas (Figs 4.14, 4.15) are distinguished from lipomas by the presence of soft-tissue elements within the fatty material and their locally invasive nature.

MESENTERY

CT, with appropriate bowel contrast opacification, is the best modality for identification of mesenteric abnormalities because of the presence of a relatively large amount of fat in the normal mesentery. Pathological conditions infiltrating the mesentery increase the attenuation of the fat, obscure the mesenteric vessels and distort the associated bowel loops.

Currently MRI is less valuable for detecting and characterizing mesenteric pathology because respiratory and peristaltic bowel movements degrade the images.

OEDEMA

Mesenteric oedema may be a consequence of many pathologies, including hypoalbuminaemia, cirrhosis,

Figure 4.12 *Contrast-enhanced CT showing low density masses (arrowed) causing characteristic scalloping of the liver (L) margin in this patient with pseudomyxoma peritonei.*

Figure 4.13 *CT through the lung bases (L) and upper abdomen, showing peritoneal deposits (white arrows) and ascites (black arrows) in this patient with peritoneal mesothelioma; note also the bilateral pleural plaques (curved white arrows).*

Figure 4.14 *Liposarcoma. CT showing a well-defined retroperitoneal liposarcoma (arrowed) intimately related to the right perirenal space, containing soft-tissue stranding.*

Figure 4.15 *Liposarcoma. CT showing a massive mesenteric liposarcoma; note that some parts have the attenuation of normal fat (curved white arrows), but other regions have soft-tissue density and fluid density (straight arrows).*

nephrosis, heart failure, tricuspid disease, constrictive pericarditis, portal hypertension, portal vein thrombosis, mesenteric artery and vein thrombosis, vasculitis, Budd–Chiari syndrome, inferior vena cava obstruction and trauma. Some of these conditions, such as heart failure and portal hypertension are frequently encountered clinically, and can sometimes present difficulty in differential diagnosis with other frequent conditions, such as peritoneal carcinomatosis.

On CT, mesenteric oedema increases the density of the mesenteric fat, which has a normal range of −100 to −160 HU, and has similar density to subcutaneous fat to values of −40 to −60 HU. In addition, the mesenteric arteries and veins are not clearly visualized as they course to the bowel wall, and there may also be associated ascites.

If the mesenteric oedema is secondary to a systemic disease, such as heart failure, it is accompanied by a

generalized increased density in the retroperitoneal and subcutaneous fat secondary to generalized oedema. In cirrhosis, where mesenteric oedema is secondary to portal hypertension, CT may also demonstrate serpiginous varices in the retroperitoneum, greater and lesser omentum, and mesentery.

Mesenteric oedema secondary to arterial or venous thrombosis tends to be more focal in nature but can sometimes be diffuse. Superior mesenteric vein thrombosis is an important cause of intestinal ischaemia. The typical appearance of chronic superior mesenteric vein thrombosis is enlargement of the vein, with a central low density surrounded by a higher density wall. The thrombus may be of high attenuation in the acute state. If bowel infarction is present, CT will show intramural bowel gas and gas within the portal and mesenteric veins. CT is also of great value in establishing an underlying local cause of venous thrombosis, such as pancreatic cancer, pancreatitis or Crohn's disease.

CROHN'S DISEASE

Crohn's disease is identified on CT as bowel wall thickening of 1–2 cm. CT also identifies extramural abnormalities in the mesentery, including abscess formation, phlegmon, fibrofatty proliferation and enlarged mesenteric lymph nodes. Fibrofatty proliferation, also known as creeping fat of the mesentery, is the most common cause of separation of bowel loops. On CT, the sharp interface between bowel and mesentery is lost and the attenuation is increased owing to the influx of inflammatory cells and fluid. The mesentery is often hypervascular, with vascular dilatation, and wide spacing of

Figure 4.16 *Crohn's disease. Post-contrast CT showing prominence of the vasa recta on the mesenteric border (black arrows) known as the 'comb' sign. Note also the 'target' sign of acute Crohn's disease (white arrow) with intense enhancement of the ileal mucosa and muscularis propria-serosa.*

the vasa recta, which is known as the 'comb sign'. The bowel wall may be thickened, and marked enhancement of the mucosa and the bowel wall may occur, giving rise to an appearance known as the 'target' sign (Fig. 4.16).

A phlegmon is an ill-defined inflammatory mass in the mesentery or omentum which may resolve completely or progress to an abscess. On CT, a phlegmon produces a loss of definition of surrounding organs and a smudgy or streaky appearance of the adjacent fat. CT, with adequate bowel contrast, can also demonstrate the course of fistulae and sinus tracts. Demonstrating these changes in the mesentery on CT may help to distinguish between causes of inflammatory bowel disease, as mesenteric complications do not occur in ulcerative colitis.

TUMOURS AND CYSTS

DESMOID TUMOUR

Mesenteric desmoid tumours (aggressive fibromatosis) are infiltrating fibroblastic proliferations, which do not show the features of an inflammatory response or neoplasia. They occur in 9–18 per cent of patients with familial adenomatous polyposis. In this condition, desmoid tumours arise either in musculoskeletal sites or in the mesentery. Unlike muscular desmoids which seldom cause symptoms, mesenteric desmoids are potentially life-threatening. On CT, the earliest changes are an ill-defined loss of clarity of the normal mesenteric fat, which with time acquires a 'whorled' appear-

ance, as linear soft tissue is interleaved with fat. This retractile mesenteritis results in tethering, angulation and then encasement of bowel. Finally, this desmoplastic response results in an irregular mass-like lesion often encasing loops of bowel (Fig. 4.17a), which is also well-demonstrated on barium follow through examination. Depending on the stage of development, these masses vary in size between 2 and 20 cm. Up to 50 per cent of the masses will be 10 cm or larger at the time of presentation. The infiltrative nature of desmoids commonly results in obstruction of, or damage to, local bowel loops and vascular structures, as well as the urinary tract. On MRI, desmoid tumours generally have low signal on T1- and T2-weighted scans (Fig. 4.17b) due to their large fibrous component.

MESENTERIC/OMENTAL CYSTS

Mesenteric and omental cysts can be lymphatic hamartomas, lined by mesothelial cells with serous or chylous fluid within them, or enterogenous cysts, derived from a sequestered intestinal diverticulum. The radiological appearance is the same irrespective of the aetiology. They appear as centrally placed soft-tissue masses displacing adjacent bowel around them on the plain abdominal film. On ultrasound they are well-defined, echo-free fluid collections in the central abdomen. On CT they are well-defined, single (occasionally multiple) fluid-filled structures found most commonly in the small bowel mesentery. Occasionally, if there is a significant amount of chylous fluid present, there may be a fat–water fluid level within them. On MRI mesenteric cysts show the typical signal characteristics of fluid,

(a)

(b)

Figure 4.17 *Mesenteric desmoid tumours. (a) CT showing an ill-defined mesenteric desmoid tumour (white arrows) encasing a loop of small bowel centrally (curved black arrow). (b) Axial T1-weighted MRI, at the same level of the CT scan, showing an ill-defined mesenteric desmoid of low-signal intensity (arrowed).*

namely low signal intensity on T1-weighted images and very high signal intensity on T2-weighted images.

LYMPHADENOPATHY

Lymphatic dissemination plays a minor role in the dissemination of intraperitoneal metastatic carcinoma, but is the primary mode of spread of lymphoma to mesenteric nodes. Approximately 50 per cent of patients with non-Hodgkin's lymphoma have mesenteric node involvement at presentation, as opposed to 5 per cent with Hodgkin's disease. On CT these nodes range from small discrete nodules in the mesenteric fat to large confluent masses surrounding the superior mesenteric vessels. Non-neoplastic causes of mesenteric lymphadenopathy include Crohn's disease, sarcoidosis, Whipple's disease, tuberculous peritonitis, giardiasis and AIDS.

RETROPERITONEUM

NORMAL ANATOMY

The retroperitoneal space is bounded anteriorly by the parietal peritoneum, posteriorly by the transversalis fascia and laterally by the lateral conal fascia. It is largest posteriorly but continues anteriorly as the properitoneal fat compartment. It extends from the diaphragm to the pelvic brim. The retroperitoneum contains the true retroperitoneal organs (the adrenal glands, kidneys, ureters and pancreas), and those structures that are closely applied to the posterior abdominal wall and only covered in part by parietal peritoneum (the aorta, the inferior vena cava, portions of the duodenum and colon, lymph nodes and nerves).

The retroperitoneal space can be divided into five separate components:

- a poorly defined space surrounding the aorta, inferior vena cava, their branches and tributaries;
- the psoas spaces;
- the kidneys and perirenal spaces;
- the posterior pararenal spaces;
- the complex anterior pararenal space produced by fusion of the dorsal mesenteries of the stomach, duodenum, and colon with the posterior body wall.

Plain radiography only identifies advanced pathology in the retroperitoneal space indirectly by its effect on adjacent structures, e.g. loss of the psoas shadows, erosion of the adjacent lumbar vertebrae and deviation of the calcified wall of the aorta.

Cross-sectional imaging, in the form of ultrasound, CT and MRI, allows exquisite, non-invasive imaging of the normal and pathological retroperitoneal anatomy.

THE GREAT VESSELS

The aorta, inferior vena cava, their branches and their tributaries course within a loosely defined space just anterior to the vertebral bodies. This space is in continuity with the posterior mediastinum and thus pathological processes can spread between these regions. The **abdominal aorta** begins at the hiatus of the diaphragm and extends inferiorly to its bifurcation into the common iliac arteries at the fourth lumbar vertebra. The calibre of the aorta decreases as it progresses caudally to its bifurcation. At the level of the diaphragmatic crura, the aorta measures up to 2.5 cm in diameter on imaging, tapering to 1 cm at the bifurcation. Ultrasound demonstrates the aorta well in thin patients, but bowel gas may obscure some portions especially in the lower abdomen. The major branches including the coeliac trunk, the superior mesenteric, the renal, and the very proximal inferior mesenteric arteries can sometimes be identified on ultrasound, but are more consistently demonstrated on contrast-enhanced CT.

The **inferior vena cava** (IVC) is formed by the two common iliac veins at the level of the fifth vertebral body. It ascends to the right of the aorta to the level of the diaphragm, initially adjacent to the lumbar vertebrae but, as it moves in a cephalad direction, it becomes more ventral in position. Its calibre varies greatly depending on the phase of respiration. The IVC is well seen on both ultrasound and CT. Ultrasound is particularly well-suited to demonstrating the intrahepatic portion of the IVC but the infrahepatic portion of the IVC is obscured by bowel gas in as many as 30 per cent of cases. However, the accuracy of ultrasound exceeds that of CT in demonstrating the intrahepatic and supradiaphragmatic portions of the IVC. Demonstrating patency of the IVC on CT requires intravenous contrast medium. MRI identifies the aorta and IVC as flow voids on spin-echo techniques (Fig. 4.18), whereas with other motion-sensitive sequences these vessels can be shown as high signal structures.

Variants of IVC anatomy are relatively common, because of its complex embryological development from several primitive segments. Awareness of these variations is important to avoid misdiagnosing pathology in the retroperitoneum. A left-sided IVC occurs in 0.2 per cent of the general population and may be confused with lymph node enlargement. The usual form consists of a left cava draining into a large left renal vein that crosses in front of the aorta to a normal caval segment above the renal vein.

Para-aortic and paracaval lymphatics and lymph nodes accompany these vessels in their entire course. In

Figure 4.18 *Coronal T1-weighted MRI scan showing a signal void of flowing blood in a patent aorta (curved black arrow) and IVC (straight black arrow). Note the large right-sided renal tumour (curved white arrow).*

Figure 4.19 *Coronal T1-weighted MRI scan showing the upper parts of normal psoas muscles (arrowed).*

normal patients these nodes are usually less than 1 cm in short axis dimension on CT; however in the retro-crural location 6 mm is taken to be the upper limit for normal nodes.

THE PSOAS MAJOR AND MINOR MUSCLES

The relationship of these muscles to nerves, lumbar arteries and the sympathetic trunks, are best demonstrated on CT and MRI (Fig. 4.19) rather than on ultrasound.

RETROPERITONEAL SPACES

On CT and MRI, the normal retroperitoneal spaces are well demonstrated. The posterior renal fascia is seen in continuity with the lateral conal fascia, which extends anteriorly just lateral to the ascending or descending colon. The thinner less well-defined anterior renal fascia intersects with the posterior renal fascia at an acute angle. Lateral to the lateral conal fascia, posterior to the renal fascia, but within the transversalis fascia, lies the **posterior pararenal space**, continuous with the pro-peritoneal fat stripe. It contains no organs but is closely related to the posterior surfaces of the ascending and descending colon. Consequently inflammatory conditions from the large bowel can extend into this area.

The dorsal mesenteries of the stomach (pancreatic tail and splenorenal ligament), duodenum (mesoduo-denum and head of the pancreas), and ascending and descending colon fuse to form the **anterior pararenal space**. This space contains duodenum, ascending colon, descending colon and pancreas. CT and MRI can elegantly demonstrate pathologic processes affecting any of these organs and the retroperitoneal space.

AORTIC ATHEROSCLEROSIS, ANEURYSM RUPTURE AND DISSECTION

ATHEROSCLEROSIS AND AORTIC ANEURYSMS

These can be detected on plain radiographs in a large number of cases by identifying mural calcification. Ultrasound is the diagnostic procedure of choice in confirming the diagnosis of a clinically suspected aortic aneurysm, as it is relatively inexpensive and readily available. It allows differentiation of aneurysmal dilatation from a tortuous atheromatous aorta of normal diameter, a hyperdynamic aorta in a thin patient, and transmitted pulsation from a para-aortic mass. Unlike angiography, which measures the lumen of flowing blood only, ultrasound demonstrates both the size of the lumen and any associated thrombus. An aneurysm with a true diameter ≥ 5 cm has an increased risk of rupture. Progressive enlargement of an aneurysm, which is easily followed on ultrasound, at a rate less than 1 cm per annum is often regarded as an indication for surgery.

(a)

(b)

Figure 4.20 *Aortic aneurysm on spiral CT. (a) Contrast-enhanced CT showing a large aortic aneurysm (white arrows) with calcification in its wall (arrowhead) and intraluminal thrombus (black arrows). Incidental note is also made of bilateral simple renal cysts (curved white arrows). (b) 3D CT reformation of the aortic aneurysm in the same patient (white arrows), arising below the superior mesenteric artery (black arrow).*

Ultrasound sometimes allows visualization of the renal arteries, which is important because their relationship to the aneurysm affects the surgical treatment and the associated morbidity and mortality. The exact extent of an aortic aneurysm and its relation to any branches, however is most accurately demonstrated using dynamic contrast-enhanced spiral CT (Figs 4.20a,b).

ACUTE RUPTURE

Acute rupture of the aorta is a surgical emergency with a high mortality, and imaging studies are not usually appropriate as they serve only to delay surgery. Imaging is useful in subacute or chronic rupture. On ultrasound a pulsating haematoma or a periaortic collection extending into the flanks may be seen.

AORTIC DISSECTION

This gives a characteristic ultrasound appearance with a 'flapping' inner wall representing the intimal flap. However, CT is a more accurate technique as it is less operator-dependent than ultrasound and surveys the entire abdominal aorta, an important factor in the evaluation of aortic rupture or dissection. The accuracy of CT for detecting both abdominal aortic dissection and extension of thoracic dissection into the abdominal aorta is high, comparable to aortography. Initial non-contrast CT scans may help to detect medial displacement of intimal calcification, but the definitive CT finding of aortic dissection is a contrast-filled double channel with an intervening intimal flap. If one channel is completely thrombosed, differentiating a dissection from a fusiform aneurysm with adherent clot may be

difficult. Associated findings in dissection are intraluminal thrombosis, dilatation of the aorta with compression of the true lumen, irregular contour of the contrast-filled part of the aorta, and differential flow to the kidneys. CT, preferably with a spiral scanning technique and dynamic contrast enhancement, can demonstrate false aneurysms, retroperitoneal haematomas and even contrast leaking from a rupture. Ultrasound and CT can also effectively evaluate the postoperative complications of aortic grafts, which include occlusion, infection, false aneurysm formation, haemorrhage and aorto-enteric fistula. Infection is particularly well evaluated on CT as pockets of air can be identified in the aortic lumen (Fig. 4.21).

Figure 4.21 *CT showing an infected aortic graft, with bubbles of air in the anterior wall and in the posterior thrombus (black arrows). Note the periaortic ill-defined soft tissue consistent with inflammation (white arrows).*

MRI is rapidly becoming an accurate investigation for examining abdominal aortic disease. It is at least as accurate as CT and aortography for the diagnosis of aortic dissection. Furthermore the diagnosis can be made reliably without the use of iodinated contrast material, an important advantage for a patient who risks complications from iodinated contrast injection. However, MRI generally remains a less clinically useful investigation than ultrasound or CT because it is still relatively expensive and time-consuming, and there are also considerable difficulties in monitoring critically ill patients.

INFERIOR VENA CAVA THROMBOSIS

Tumoral and non-tumoral thrombosis of the IVC can be identified using ultrasound from the level of the renal veins to the right atrium. Below this level the IVC is usually obscured by bowel gas. On ultrasound, thrombosis within the IVC is highly reflective and the IVC is distended. Fresh thrombus, however, may have lower echogenicity. Doppler ultrasound allows characterization of flow or lack of flow within the IVC. It also aids the identification of recanalization following anticoagulant treatment.

Contrast-enhanced CT demonstrates the entire abdominal IVC and its tributaries. On CT a fresh thrombus distends the IVC and has a density similar to circulating blood; an older thrombus is of lower density. When the occlusion is complete, the involved segment does not enhance on postcontrast images. Ultrasound is more accurate than CT in defining the superior limit of the intracaval thrombus. The IVC is invaded in approximately 10 per cent of patients with renal cancer and the superior extent of tumour thrombus must be determined since it influences the surgical approach. The distinction between tumour thrombus and bland non-tumour thrombus is seldom possible. CT and ultrasound are both relatively inaccurate for predicting invasion of the wall of the IVC by tumoral thrombus.

Venous thrombosis produces intraluminal signal on spin-echo MRI sequences with focal dilatation of the IVC similar to the findings on CT and ultrasound. MRI is as accurate as CT in displaying normal flow and thrombus within the IVC. Its major advantage is that it does not need intravenous contrast enhancement. It can therefore be used in patients with contraindications to iodinated contrast agent administration, or when CT and ultrasound are equivocal. CT, MRI and Doppler ultrasound can also be used to document the patency of portocaval or mesocaval shunts.

LYMPHADENOPATHY

CT is the most widely used method of detecting retroperitoneal lymph node pathology and is the

Figure 4.22 *Contrast-enhanced CT showing enlarged retroperitoneal lymph nodes (arrowed) in this patient with non-Hodgkin's lymphoma.*

standard method for staging disease in patients with **lymphoma** and **testicular tumours**. In these diseases CT demonstrates all the enlarged nodes and also demonstrates any extranodal pathology. For tumours such as renal cell, cervical and prostatic carcinoma, CT can rapidly evaluate the primary site, any lymph node metastases and the liver in one examination. It is, therefore, the first choice investigation for oncologic staging and for follow-up after treatment or surgery.

As with ultrasound and MRI, CT relies on an increase in size to diagnose nodal pathology. Retroperitoneal nodes are considered enlarged on CT if they measure over 10 mm in their shortest axis. In the retrocrural area, nodal enlargement is diagnosed when the shortest axis is over 6 mm (Fig. 4.22). On CT, malignant nodal enlargement may follow one of the following patterns: discrete lymph node enlargement, conglomerate lymph node enlargement or large masses in which separate nodes are no longer visible. Massive enlargement of the retroaortic or retrocaval nodes may cause anterior displacement of the aorta and vena cava.

The accuracy of CT for detecting intra-abdominal and pelvic lymphadenopathy in malignant disease is reported to be as high as 90 per cent. Difficulty in interpretation can result from non-opacified bowel or vessels, which can be resolved with meticulous attention to bowel opacification and vascular enhancement. False-positive results largely relate to lymph-node enlargement from other causes, for example infection. False-negative results occur when infiltrated lymph nodes are not enlarged. CT is extremely useful in following response of nodal disease to treatment and in diagnosing remission, especially in lymphoma. However, patients with massive lymphadenopathy at presentation may not revert completely to normal, as bulky fibrosis may persist within the successfully treated lymph nodes following

Figure 4.23 *Coronal T1-weighted MRI showing a large nodal metastasis to the left psoas (arrowed) from ovarian cancer.*

Figure 4.24 *Transverse abdominal ultrasound scan showing enlarged hypoechoic retroperitoneal lymph nodes in this patient with metastatic carcinoid (arrowed). These lie to the right of the aorta (A) and anterior to the vertebral body (V). Nodes are also seen lying posterior to the left lobe of the liver (L).*

chemotherapy and radiotherapy, particularly in Hodgkin's disease and testicular tumours. Biopsy of such masses can be achieved using CT guidance.

On **MRI**, abnormal nodes are diagnosed on the basis of size rather than by any alteration in signal intensity. They are best seen on T1-weighted sequences as their signal intensity is usually higher than that in muscle but lower than in fat (Fig. 4.23). On T2-weighted sequences nodes may be difficult to distinguish from surrounding fat, which can be of similar signal intensity. Generally, abnormal nodes show homogeneous signal intensity but they may appear inhomogeneous when calcified or necrotic.

MRI is as accurate as CT for evaluating the retroperitoneum for lymphadenopathy, but at present is not as good a survey technique for the rest of the abdomen. The images may be degraded by movement artefacts from respiration or peristalsis, and inadequate bowel opacification may cause confusion in separating bowel from lymph node masses. Also poorer spatial resolution may compromise visualization of minimally enlarged lymph nodes. Similarly, a cluster of normal-sized nodes that are readily defined by CT as discrete normal structures may be misdiagnosed as a solitary enlarged node on MRI. MRI thus offers no substantial benefit over CT for routine staging and follow-up. However, MRI is a useful problem-solving technique in certain situations. It can, for example, distinguish vascular structures as flow voids without the use of iodinated contrast agents, and thus may help to separate nodes from vessels in difficult areas, such as the internal iliac nodal area. Surgical clips do not degrade MRI images to the same extent as they degrade CT images, and thus MRI may be useful in follow-up after surgery.

On **ultrasound**, enlarged nodes typically show uniformly low echogenicity, sometimes appearing almost echo-free (Fig. 4.24). Ultrasound can detect abnormal nodes as small as 1.5 cm and can be used to direct needle biopsy. However, with the inability to

Figure 4.25 *Delayed lymphangiogram film showing normal opacified nodes on the right of the spine (closed arrows). On the left the nodes are abnormal as they are enlarged and show multiple filling defects (open arrows).*

penetrate bowel gas, which may obscure the retroperitoneum in about a third of cases, ultrasound is not a useful survey technique.

Gallium scintigraphy has proved disappointing for identifying abdominal malignant lymph nodes, with a true positive rate of only 48 per cent.

Bipedal **lymphangiography** was previously used universally to investigate possible lymph-node abnormalities (Fig. 4.25). The procedure is often time-consuming, sometimes difficult to perform, and uncomfortable for the patient. It does not demonstrate all nodal groups, and lymph nodes totally replaced by disease may not be opacified. However, bipedal lymphangiography is of some value in the investigation of patients whose cross-sectional imaging is equivocal, as lymphangiography can detect abnormality in normal-sized nodes that would otherwise be overlooked.

Figure 4.27 *Axial T1-weighted MRI following contrast enhancement showing a left-sided malignant fibrohistiocytoma (arrowed) occupying the left psoas and erector spinae muscles, invading the spinal canal and displacing the left kidney (K) laterally.*

TUMOURS

Approximately 80 per cent of retroperitoneal tumours are malignant. In adults, most are mesenchymal in origin, the commonest being **liposarcoma, leiomyosarcoma** (Fig. 4.26) and **malignant fibrohistiocytoma** (Fig. 4.27). They tend to be quite large at presentation, only producing symptoms when they compress adjacent structures. Plain films will identify these neoplasms at an advanced stage by detecting erosion of lumbar vertebrae or displacement of the renal shadows and psoas outlines. Diagnosis is readily achieved on CT even when these tumours are quite small.

CT illustrates the extent and effect on adjacent structures and may suggest the histological diagnosis. Retroperitoneal lipomas appear as sharply marginated,

homogeneous masses with a CT attenuation value equivalent to normal fat. The other tumours are predominantly of soft tissue density though they may show calcification. Liposarcomas may, however, have areas of low attenuation consistent with normal fat, especially when well-differentiated (Fig. 4.17a). Leiomyosarcomas often have areas of necrosis and cystic degeneration which appear as areas of fluid density on CT. Other retroperitoneal neoplasms include neurogenic tumours such as neurofibromas (Fig. 4.28), extra-adrenal phaeochromocytomas and paragangliomas. Neurogenic tumours sometimes extend through a

Figure 4.26 *Contrast-enhanced CT showing a retroperitoneal leiomyosarcoma arising from the IVC (arrowed). Incidental note is made of a scarred atrophic right kidney (K).*

Figure 4.28 *Axial CT showing a low-density left retroperitoneal neurofibroma at the left L2 exit foramen (arrowed).*

widened neural foramen into the extradural space, where they can produce nerve root or cord compression.

In children the commonest retroperitoneal tumours are rhabodmyosarcomas, neuroblastoma and teratomas. On CT most of these tumours show soft-tissue density; neuroblastomas classically also have diffuse stippled calcification within their substance. Teratomas may have areas of fatty density and calcifications within them. MRI in general offers little additional information but can be useful in selected cases. For example, it can diagnose lipomas and liposarcomas on the basis of their signal characteristics, as fatty tumours have very high signal on T1-weighted images. MRI may be more useful than CT in differentiating neoplastic tissue from normal psoas muscle; this can help to exclude psoas invasion. The psoas muscle is well demonstrated on MRI and has a lower signal intensity than retroperitoneal tumours on T2-weighted images. MRI may also be of value in identifying extension of retroperitoneal tumours into the spinal canal (Fig. 4.27), as the intrathecal space, spinal cord, and nerve roots are exquisitely demonstrated on MRI.

UNDESCENDED TESTES

The testes originate as paired retroperitoneal structures, arising from the gonadal ridge on the medial aspect of the mesonephros and descend into the scrotum during the eighth month of gestation. Normal testicular descent may be arrested at any point along a path extending from the renal hilum to the scrotum.

About 80 per cent of maldescended testes are found distal to the inguinal ring and thus can be palpated. However, 20 per cent are not palpable either because of congenital absence, as happens in 4 per cent, or because they are located within the abdominal cavity.

The undescended testis is 12–40 times more likely to harbour foci of malignancy than a normal testis, therefore finding a testis within the abdominal cavity is important. Several series show that both CT and MRI are sensitive techniques for preoperative localization in non-palpable undescended testes. The accuracy of both techniques is greater for the identification of low-lying than it is for high intra-abdominal testes. Accurate localization requires careful attention to pelvic anatomy, as the undescended testis is typically smaller and more elliptical than the normally descended testis and is most frequently identified near the inguinal ring adjacent to the iliac vessels. On CT, atrophic and dysplastic testes appear as small foci of soft tissue similar in density to the adjacent abdominal wall musculature. MRI provides distinct advantages over CT in detection due to its multiplanar imaging capabilities. Undescended tests are usually of high signal on T2-weighted images, but may be of low signal if atrophic.

FLUID COLLECTIONS

RETROPERITONEAL ABSCESSES

The common sites for retroperitoneal abscesses are the psoas muscle and perirenal spaces. Many retroperitoneal abscesses are due to direct extension of infection from contiguous structures, such as the spine, kidney, bowel and pancreas. Most are due to pyogenic bacterial pathogens, but occasionally they can be tuberculous in nature (Fig. 4.29).

CT best demonstrates the extent of the abscess and any associated abnormalities in contiguous structures. On CT the psoas muscle is enlarged, usually having lower density centrally, representing the abscess. Visualization of the abscess is made more conspicuous by intravenous contrast enhancement, which enhances the rim of the abscess (Fig. 4.29). Gas bubbles may be seen within the abscess if it is caused by a gas-forming organism or if it communicates with the bowel.

Figure 4.29 *Tuberculous abscess. Contrast-enhanced CT showing a rim-enhancing tuberculous abscess occupying the right psoas muscle (arrowed).*

Ultrasound can demonstrate psoas abscesses in the upper retroperitoneal space as echo-free areas within the psoas muscle surrounded by an irregular thick wall. However, if gas is present, the abscess may be obscured as ultrasound is completely reflected at soft-tissue–gas interfaces.

MRI shows psoas abscesses to have a very high signal on T2-weighted images but, in general, does not offer any substantial advantage over CT or ultrasound for detection or management. However, MRI may demonstrate spinal pathology more elegantly, using sagittal and coronal scanning planes.

(a)

(b)

Figure 4.30 *Retroperitoneal fibrosis. (a) Axial contrast-enhanced CT showing the aorta (black arrow) surrounded by periaortic retroperitoneal fibrosis (white arrows). (b) Axial T1-weighted MRI showing a signal void in the aorta (arrowhead), and low-signal periaortic retroperitoneal fibrosis (straight arrows). There is dilatation of the left renal pelvis (curved arrow).*

RETROPERITONEAL HAEMORRHAGE

Retroperitoneal haemorrhage is usually due to anticoagulant therapy, trauma or bleeding from an aortic aneurysm or retroperitoneal tumour. Spontaneous psoas haemorrhage may also occur in patients with a bleeding diathesis such as haemophilia. CT is the most accurate, non-invasive technique for detecting retroperitoneal haemorrhage. The exact location depends on the cause of the haemorrhage, for example a haematoma from a leaking aneurysm will surround the aorta before extending into the adjacent retroperitoneum. The attenuation value depends on the age of haemorrhage. **Acute haematomas** show higher attenuation than circulating blood, because clot formation and retraction causes a greater concentration of haemoglobin. A **chronic haematoma**, which may have associated calcification, appears as a low density mass as clot lysis takes place. The appearance of a subacute or chronic haematoma can thus be confused with a retroperitoneal tumour, abscess, lymphocoele or cyst.

Ultrasound shows acute haematomas as echo-free fluid collections. Chronic haematomas may appear as complex multiseptate structures or even solid masses. The appearance of haemorrhage on MRI is complex and depends on the field strength of the magnet and the age of the haemorrhage. It may have a characteristic appearance on MRI, but occasionally bleeding into a tumour or abscess may be indistinguishable from a simple bleed.

RETROPERITONEAL CYSTS

Retroperitoneal cysts are rare and include lymphatic cysts, inclusion cysts, embryonic gastrointestinal cysts and genitourinary tract remnants. Their imaging features are similar, namely a well-defined, thin-walled, fluid-filled mass.

FIBROSIS

Retroperitoneal fibrosis is characterized by fibrous tissue proliferation along the posterior aspect of the retroperitoneal cavity, generally confined to the central and paravertebral regions. The tissue is sharply delineated and tends to envelop rather than displace adjacent structures, such as the ureters and blood vessels. The histological features range from an active inflammatory process to a more acellular, hyalinized reaction. Most cases are idiopathic but retroperitoneal fibrosis can be secondary to certain drugs (such as methysergide), primary and secondary tumours, aneurysms and aneurysm surgery.

On **intravenous urography** there is medial deviation and obstruction of the ureters, typically at about L4/5 bilaterally.

On **ultrasound** an ill-defined echo-poor mass of fibrous tissue can sometimes be identified together with any associated hydronephrosis.

CT, however, offers the best delineation of the process, demonstrating a periaortic soft-tissue mass of similar attenuation to muscle (Fig. 4.30a), which may show enhancement following intravenous contrast. Retroperitoneal fibrosis tends to encase the aorta anteriorly and laterally, distinguishing it from retroperitoneal malignancy, which may occur behind the aorta displacing it anteriorly. Retroperitoneal fibrosis most commonly encases the infrarenal aorta and common iliac arteries and is often predominantly left-sided. Hydronephrosis is well demonstrated on CT when the ureters are obstructed. Insidious disease progression is the general rule. Shrinkage of retroperitoneal fibrosis in response to treatment with steroids is sometimes demonstrated using CT; however residual periaortic tissue is common following treatment and CT has no value in determining disease activity in such circumstances. It may not always be possible to distinguish retroperitoneal fibrosis from other retroperitoneal masses and CT can be used to guide percutaneous biopsy, which should be generous in size to differentiate from malignancy.

MRI is as accurate as CT in demonstrating retroperitoneal fibrosis. The soft tissue is of low signal intensity on both T1- (Fig. 4.30b) and T2-weighted imaging. As with ultrasound and CT, hydronephrosis is readily demonstrated.

FURTHER READING

Bennett, H.F., Balfe, D.M. 1995: MR imaging of the peritoneum and abdominal wall. *Radiology Clinics of North America* **3**(1), 99–120.

Birnbaum, B.A., Balthazae, E.J. 1994: CT of appendicitis and diverticulitis. *Radiology Clinics of North America* **32**(5), 885–98.

Brooks, A.P., Reznek, R.H., Nugent, K., Farmer, K.C.R.,

Thompson, J.P.S., Phillips, R.K.S. 1994: CT appearances of desmoid tumours in familial adenomatous polyposis: further observations. *Clinical Radiology* **49**, 601–7.

Enkelgen, J.D., Ros, P.R. 1997: Retroperitoneal MR imaging. *Magnetic Resonance Imaging Clinics of North America* **5**(1), 165–78.

Gore, R.M., Balthazar, E.J., Ghahremani, G.G., Miller, F.H. 1996: CT features of ulcerative colitis and Crohn's disease. *American Journal of Roentgenology* **167**, 3–15.

Guest, P.J., Reznek, R.H., Selleslag, D., Geraghty, R., Slevin, M. 1992: Peritoneal mesothelioma: the role of computed tomography in diagnosis and follow-up. *Clinical Radiology* **45**(2), 79–84.

Healy, J.C., Reznek, R.H. 1998: The peritoneum, mesenteries and omenta: normal anatomy and pathological processes. *European Radiology* **8**, 886–900.

Lee, J.K., Hiken, J.N., Semelka, R.C. 1998: Retroperitoneum. In Lee, J.K., Sagel, S.S., Stanley, R.J., Heiken, J.P. (eds). *Computed body tomography with MRI correlation* Philadelphia, New York: Lippincott-Raven, 1023–85.

Meyers, M.A. 1994: Intraperitoneal spread of infections. In Meyers, M.A. (ed.), *Dynamic radiology of the abdomen: normal and pathologic anatomy* (4th edition). New York: Springer-Verlag, 55–113.

Meyers, M.A., McGuire, P.V. 1995: Spiral CT demonstration of hypervascularity in Crohn's disease: 'vascular jejunization of the ileum' or 'comb sign'. *Abdominal Imaging* **20**, 327–32.

Mindelzun, R.E., Brooke Jeffrey, R., Lane, M.J., Silverman, P.M. 1996: The misty mesentery on CT: differential diagnosis. *American Journal of Roentgenology* **167**, 61–5.

Raptopoulos, V. 1994: Abdominal trauma: emphasis on computed tomography. *Radiology Clinics of North America* **32**(5): 969–87.

Rubin, G.D., Silverman, S.G. 1995: Helical (spiral) CT of the retroperitoneum. *Radiology Clinics of North America* **33**(5), 903–32.

Sivit, C. 1996: CT scan of mesentery-omentum peritoneum. *Radiology Clinics of North America* **34**(4), 863–84.

(a)   (b)

(c)   (d)

Figure 5.1 *Normal liver anatomy on CT. (a) Scan through the superior aspect of the liver showing middle (curved arrow), left (arrowhead) and right (arrow) hepatic veins. (b) Scan through the level of the portal vein (P) showing the left portal (arrow) and right portal (curved arrow) veins. The inferior aspect of the ligamentum teres (arrowhead) separates the medial and lateral segments of the left lobe. (c) Scan through the caudate lobe of the liver (C) separated from the lateral segment of the left lobe of the liver by the ligamentum venosum (arrow). (d) Scan through the gallbladder fossa (curved arrow). A line joining the inferior vena cava (I) divides the liver into right and left lobes at this level. The ligamentum teres (arrow) divides the left lobe into medial and lateral segments at this level.*

Readily visible landmarks for all segments are not visualized on every section. However, when the scan is taken as a composite, highly accurate segmental landmarks can be established.

DIFFUSE HEPATOCELLULAR DISEASE

CIRRHOSIS AND FATTY CHANGE

Ultrasonography

Because of the opposing effects of fatty change and fibrosis, the liver is either enlarged or of normal size in the early stages of cirrhosis. A small, shrunken liver is seen only in advanced stages. Criteria for the sonographic diagnosis of cirrhosis include increased parenchymal echogenicity, decreased beam penetration through the liver and poor depiction of intrahepatic portal vein walls. Similar findings are encountered with fatty change and therefore, in the early stages, fatty change cannot be distinguished from cirrhosis. In more advanced cirrhosis, the left lobe is relatively preserved or enlarged, the caudate lobe hypertrophied, and both are relatively large compared to the right lobe. Advanced cirrhosis results in contour indentations, nodularity and occasionally regenerating nodules, usually 0.5–1.5 cm in diameter, which are isoechoic with the parenchyma.

Figure 5.2 *Severe fatty change in a liver of normal size shown on CT. The presence of a marked amount of fat has lowered the density of the liver to such an extent that the blood vessels appear of higher density than the liver parenchyma (arrows).*

Computed tomography

Fatty liver is the most common CT feature in early cirrhosis and results in lowering of the CT density of the liver parenchyma, usually to below 40 Hounsfield units (HU) (Fig. 5.2). Hepatomegaly is frequent but the liver contour is normal. In advanced cirrhosis, an overall decrease in liver volume is accompanied by atrophy of the right lobe and medial segment of the left lobe, and hypertrophy of the caudate lobe and lateral segment of the left lobe (Fig. 5.3). Caudate lobe enlarge-

Figure 5.3 *Cirrhosis with portal hypertension shown on CT after intravenous injection of contrast medium. There is atrophy of the right lobe and medial segment of the left lobe with hypertrophy of the caudate and lateral segment of the left lobe. The liver surface is irregular and there is a small amount of ascites. Large collateral vessels are seen in the region of the splenic hilum, around the gastro-oesophageal junction and along the lesser curve of the stomach (arrows).*

ment is present early in cirrhosis and roughly parallels the degree of cirrhosis thereafter. Regenerating nodules cause nodularity of the liver contour (Fig. 5.4). Non-uniform attenuation, often striking, can result from chronic fatty infiltration or fibrosis.

(a)

(b)

Figure 5.4 *Cirrhosis of the liver. (a) Scan without intravenous contrast medium showing a small shrunken liver containing multiple small nodules. A large amount of ascites (A) is seen. (b) Scan taken after intravenous injection of contrast medium, showing irregularity of the liver contour and inhomogeneous attenuation due to multiple regenerating nodules. A collateral vessel due to portal hypertension is seen anteriorly (arrow).*

Magnetic resonance imaging

Common findings in MRI, as with other cross-sectional imaging modalities, include contour nodularity, relative right lobe atrophy and hypertrophy of the left and caudate lobes. Vascular distortion is better demonstrated on MRI than ultrasound or CT. Available data on the signal characteristics are conflicting, and clear-cut, clinically useful, diffuse alterations in signal intensity induced by cirrhosis have yet to be elucidated.

PORTAL HYPERTENSION

In most cases, portal hypertension is secondary to liver disease, and imaging of the liver is helpful in providing confirmatory evidence of diffuse pathology. Where the cause of portal hypertension is uncertain, imaging of the portal venous anatomy is crucial.

Portal or splenic vein enlargement, or both, is easily detected on CT or ultrasound. Portosystemic collaterals are often readily seen as tortuous, tubular or round masses of soft tissue attenuation on unenhanced scans; scans after injection of a bolus of contrast medium may be necessary to confirm their vascular nature (Fig. 5.3). **Oesophageal varices** can be suggested on CT by a thickened oesophageal wall with a lobulated outer contour and a scalloped lumen with intraluminal protrusions that exhibit marked contrast enhancement.

Assessment of portal vein size and patency can also be made sonographically. A portal vein exceeding 16 mm in diameter on deep inspiration in the supine position has been shown to be diagnostic of portal hypertension in a high percentage of cases. Lack of the normal distension of the portal, splenic or superior mesenteric veins on deep inspiration, and loss of the normal respiratory fluctuation in the Doppler signal are other signs indicating portal hypertension. Indirect signs such as splenomegaly, the opening of collaterals and ascites are also reliably demonstrated by ultrasound.

Portal or splenic vein thrombosis is seen on contrast-enhanced CT scans as a lucent blood clot surrounded by an enhanced vessel wall together with inhomogeneous enhancement of the periportal parenchyma (Fig. 5.5). When the vein is occluded and enlarged, it is likely that tumour thrombus is present – hepatocellular carcinoma, cholangiocarcinoma, pancreatic carcinoma and gastric carcinoma are the likely causes. Numerous **collateral veins** by-passing the occluded portal vein are recognized on CT by the appearance of serpentine, opacified collaterals in the hepatoduodenal ligament.

In most cases, ultrasound can demonstrate portal vein thrombosis in the main portal vein or its larger branches as echogenic material within the vascular lumen. In older thrombus, when the obstruction is complete, and the lumen entirely filled with echogenic material, it may be difficult to identify the vein at all.

Conventional spin-echo MRI is comparable to CT and arterial portography for demonstrating the presence or absence of portosystemic collaterals and portal vein thrombus. MR angiography can also provide images of the thrombosed portal vein. The exact signal characteristics of the thrombus will vary with age, pulse sequence and field strength.

Direct preoperative demonstration of the portal venous anatomy is now best achieved by **arterial portography** which has replaced the traditional technique of splenoportography as it is safer and gives additional information about the vascular tree. Selective catheterization of the splenic, hepatic and superior mesenteric arteries gives a full demonstration of the arterial supply to the liver as well as showing the portal venous anatomy. The position and patency of the mesenteric, splenic and portal veins, IVC and renal veins can be assessed in order to help decide which form of shunt to use.

BUDD–CHIARI SYNDROME

Ultrasound, CT and MRI will almost invariably show ascites, hepatomegaly and mild splenomegaly in Budd–Chiari syndrome. Caudate hypertrophy with right lobe atrophy and left lobe hypertrophy is common. Thrombus within the hepatic veins in the acute phase, or non-visualization in the chronic phase, can be detected on ultrasound (with or without Doppler), CT or MRI, as can intrahepatic and extrahepatic venous collaterals. In chronic cases of Budd–Chiari syndrome, the typical CT pattern is inhomogeneous enhancement due to a mixture of normal or hypertrophied hepatic parenchyma with regions of liver atrophy (Fig. 5.6).

Hepatic scintigraphy may demonstrate a characteristic pattern in Budd–Chiari syndrome: a central region of normal activity (appearing 'hot') in the caudate lobe, the rest of the liver showing greatly diminished activity. This characteristic pattern is seen only when the veins draining the caudate lobe (which enter separately into the vena cava) are spared.

FOCAL LIVER DISEASE

METASTATIC NEOPLASMS

Signs and symptoms of metastases occur in only 50 per cent of patients with hepatic metastases. Biochemical hepatic function tests can be misleading: they may be normal in 25–50 per cent of cases with metastases and

Figure 5.5 *CT and ultrasound in portal vein thrombosis. (a) CT scan taken after intravenous injection of contrast medium showing a filling defect within the portal vein (arrow). (b) A scan at a level superior to (a) shows extension of the filling defect into the left portal vein (arrows) which is also expanded. (c) CT scan at a level superior to (b) showing a defect in the enhancement of the parenchyma in the left lobe (arrows) due to the presence of thrombus. (d) Longitudinal ultrasound scan in the same patient showing numerous echoes within the portal vein (arrows) consistent with thrombus. The normal common duct is seen lying anterior to the portal vein in this projection (open arrows). (e) Transverse ultrasound scan showing thrombus within the left portal vein (arrows). A patent vein is shown in the right lobe of the liver, free from any internal echoes (open arrow).*

(a)

(b)

Figure 5.6 *Budd–Chiari syndrome on CT. (a) CT scan after intravenous contrast medium showing inhomogeneous enhancement of the liver parenchyma with focal areas of increased and decreased enhancement. Thrombosis can be seen within the inferior vena cava (arrows). (b) Scan taken slightly superior to (a) showing relative sparing of the left lobe and extension of the thrombus superiorly. The hepatic veins are not opacified.*

elevated in numerous benign abnormalities. Carcinoembryonic antigen measurements and visual inspection of the liver at laparoscopy or surgery are also generally considered insufficiently sensitive or specific for detecting metastases.

Radionuclide liver/spleen scanning has significant false-negative and false-positive rates ranging from 15 to 25 per cent. Lesions less than 2 cm are rarely detected and central lesions greater than 2 cm can be missed frequently. Although tomography has brought about improvement, ultrasound, CT and MRI predominate in the evaluation for metastatic disease in most institutions.

Ultrasound

High-resolution, real-time ultrasound is a highly sensitive and specific modality for detecting small liver metastases. Drawbacks remain, such as the unfavourable body habitus of some patients and the poor visibility of small lesions near the dome of the liver and the liver surface. Also, the segmental anatomy is more readily appreciated on CT or MRI for liver resection evaluation.

Metastases can be hyperechoic, hypoechoic or isoechoic compared to the surrounding parenchyma. A thin hypoechoic rim may be seen (the 'halo' sign) (Fig. 5.7). Multiple, large, poorly demarcated hyperechoic masses are usually metastases from colorectal carcinoma.

The development of high frequency transducers has led to the use of ultrasound for intraoperative use. Intraoperative sonography, performed immediately before metastectomy, has been shown to yield additional information compared with preoperative CT and ultrasound.

Computed tomography

CT is the preferred single imaging technique for screening the abdomen for metastatic disease. Incremental bolus dynamic CT (rapid liver scanning after intra-

Figure 5.7 *Multiple liver metastases shown on a longitudinal ultrasound scan. Multiple hyperechoic lesions are seen in a patient with colonic carcinoma. A typical lucent 'halo' is seen around most of the lesions (open arrows).*

(a)   (b)

Figure 5.8 *Liver deposits best demonstrated on CT after intravenous injection of contrast medium. (a) A CT scan through the liver without contrast medium showing no obvious focal abnormality. (b) After intravenous injection of contrast medium, a scan at the same level as (a) shows two small focal abnormalities enhancing to a lesser extent than the adjacent normal liver parenchyma (arrows).*

venous injection of a bolus of contrast medium) is a very accurate means of detecting focal liver masses over 1 cm in size but its sensitivity for lesions less than 1 cm is only about 50%.

Most hepatic metastases are hypovascular and therefore hypodense on contrast-enhanced scans (Fig. 5.8). Calcification can occur within liver deposits, particularly in patients with colon carcinoma (Fig. 5.9). Computed tomographic hepatic arteriography and CT arterial portography maximize differential contrast enhancement between liver parenchyma and metastases and thus improve the detection of liver metastases by as much as 50 per cent when compared with routine contrast-enhanced CT. These are, however, invasive procedures requiring catheter placement in the hepatic, superior mesenteric or splenic artery, and are only justified in evaluating patients being considered for major hepatic surgery.

Magnetic resonance imaging

MRI is having an increasing impact on the evaluation of the liver in both the screening and staging of malignant disease, and may eventually become the definitive method for the evaluation of hepatic metastases. Comparisons of MRI with both ultrasound and CT are sparse but it is difficult to distinguish statistically significant differences between the accuracies of CT and MRI. Most metastases, being hypovascular, exhibit a low-to-intermediate signal intensity on T1-weighted images and an increased signal on T2-weighted images. The use of MRI liver contrast agents, including those targeted specifically at the reticuloendothelial system or taken up by hepatocytes, is likely to increase the sensitivity of MRI in detecting focal liver pathology.

Figure 5.9 *A CT scan without intravenous injection of contrast medium showing the typical appearance of calcification within a focal liver deposit (arrow) in a patient with colonic carcinoma.*

Arteriography

Since the introduction of ultrasound and CT, arteriography of the liver has a very limited role in diagnosis. However, therapeutic manoeuvres can be conducted through a catheter placed percutaneously in the hepatic artery. This method has been effectively used, for example, in metastatic carcinoid tumours.

Figure 5.10 *CT scan showing a unifocal hepatocellular carcinoma (arrows) in a patient with cirrhosis. The tumour can be seen to enhance inhomogeneously after intravenous injection of contrast medium and to contain abnormal vessels (arrowheads).*

Figure 5.11 *CT scan after intravenous injection of contrast medium showing a multifocal hepatocellular carcinoma. The liver lesions are seen to enhance to a lesser extent than the adjacent normal liver parenchyma. There is also tumour extension into the inferior vena cava (arrow).*

PRIMARY LIVER TUMOUR (HEPATOCELLULAR CARCINOMA)

Plain films may show generalized hepatomegaly or a localized bulge in the contour of the diaphragm. Calcification may be seen on the plain film but is very unusual in untreated hepatocellular carcinoma.

The appearance of hepatocellular carcinoma on ultrasound, CT and MRI is variable but can be divided into three major categories that correlate well with pathological data. The most common appearances are discrete lesions (solitary or multiple), diffuse parenchymal infiltration and a combination of the discrete and diffuse hepatic patterns.

Ultrasound

On ultrasound, discrete lesions are usually hypoechoic, only occasionally isoechoic, and detected by a thin, hypoechoic halo. The diffuse pattern results in disorganization of the normal echo pattern with multiple areas of increased and decreased echogenicity without distinct masses. Unfortunately, these ultrasound patterns can also be seen with other entities such as metastases, fatty liver, cirrhosis or lymphoma, making guided biopsy necessary for definitive diagnosis. Ultrasound demonstration of venous involvement favours hepatocellular carcinoma over metastases, as it has a propensity to invade the portal and hepatic veins. Such features, including ascites and splenomegaly, are well demonstrated on ultrasound.

Computed tomography

On CT, discrete solitary or multiple lesions are seen as well-defined low-density areas of decreased attenuation, usually 20–30 HU lower than adjacent normal liver (Fig. 5.10). Foci of calcification may be seen within the tumour. Most primary liver tumours enhance after intravenous injection of contrast medium owing to their hypervascularity, but they still show a lower CT number than the normal enhanced liver parenchyma (Fig. 5.11). As with ultrasound, the solitary or multiple discrete pattern of hepatocellular carcinoma cannot be distinguished from metastases. Diffuse parenchymal infiltration results in irregular, poorly defined areas of decreased density within the liver. After intravenous injection of contrast medium, they enhance inhomogeneously and to a lesser extent than the surrounding normal parenchyma (Fig. 5.12).

The sensitivity of ultrasound and CT for detecting hepatocellular carcinoma is similar and both exceed 80 per cent. CT is, however, useful for early detection of extrahepatic metastases, most commonly to the lung. Metastases to the adrenal glands, peritoneal cavity, lymph nodes and skeleton are also readily detected by CT. Thus, when hepatocellular carcinoma is being staged, it is important to use the two techniques in conjunction. CT surpasses ultrasound in showing the distribution of the tumour within the liver as well as extrahepatic spread, while ultrasound is superior in the evaluation of the portal and hepatic veins.

Magnetic resonance imaging

The MRI appearance depends on the type of disease (solitary, multiple or diffuse), degree of fibrosis, the

Figure 5.12 *Diffuse parenchymal infiltration owing to a hepatocellular carcinoma, shown as an irregular 'geographical' area of abnormal enhancement after intravenous injection of contrast medium (arrows).*

Figure 5.13 *Transverse ultrasound scan through the posterior segment of the right lobe of the liver showing a well-defined area of uniformly increased echogenicity (arrows).*

possibility of necrosis or haemorrhage and the sequences used. Typically, lesions are of decreased signal intensity on T1-weighted images and moderately increased on T2-weighted images. Data are not yet available on the accuracy of MRI for the detection or staging of hepatocellular carcinoma.

HAEMANGIOMAS

Haemangiomas are found in up to 3 per cent of patients undergoing routine CT scanning of the liver and can often be confused with other focal liver pathology. The majority are small, **capillary lesions** and are seen on ultrasound as clearly defined, highly reflective lesions close to the periphery of the liver (Fig. 5.13). **Cavernous haemangiomas** are less common and have a varied appearance, being hyper- or hypoechoic. Duplex or colour Doppler sonography has not contributed significantly to establishing the diagnosis. Most haemangiomas do not change substantially over time, although a few may become less echogenic. In about 55 per cent of cases, haemangiomas will display specific morphological findings on CT allowing a diagnosis to be made with close to 90 per cent probability, namely lowdensity compared to normal liver on the precontrast scan, peripheral contrast enhancement on the immediate postcontrast phase and progressive 'fill-in' on delayed scans up to 30 minutes following intravenous administration of contrast medium, until the haemangioma becomes the same density as the adjacent normal parenchyma (Fig. 5.14). This pattern can, however, also be seen in 5 per cent of metastases and, if the patient is known to have a primary malignancy, follow-up is usually advised.

Scintigraphy with ^{99m}Tc-sulphur colloid depicts haemangiomas as non-specific focal regions of decreased activity. Technetium-99m-labelled red blood cell scanning is very specific. Typically, dynamic scanning seconds after injection of a bolus of labelled red blood cells shows hypoperfusion with gradually increasing activity owing to red blood cell accumulation on serial delayed imaging, which peaks within 30 to 50 minutes after injection. This pattern of radioactivity is considered diagnostic of haemangioma.

MRI has also been used in diagnosing haemangiomas. The characteristic appearance is a sharply defined homogeneous hyperintense mass on T2-weighted images and a hypointense appearance on T1-weighting. Unfortunately, there is overlap of the signal characteristics with other conditions, notably necrotic tumours and hypervascular metastases. Gadolinium-enhanced MRI produces a pattern of enhancement similar to that seen with contrast-enhanced CT.

Thus, when typical imaging features are present in a patient with normal liver function tests and no known primary malignancy, the diagnosis of haemangioma is statistically very likely and can be made with a high degree of accuracy. Patients with known primary malignancies are slightly more problematic, especially when the typical CT appearance is not present. If needed, fine-needle aspiration can be performed.

FOCAL NODULAR HYPERPLASIA AND ADENOMAS

Ultrasound, CT and MRI cannot reliably distinguish focal nodular hyperplasia or adenomas from other hepatic masses. The presence of a central fibrous scar, recognized as a central radiolucency on a non-contrast

(a)

(b)

(c)

(d)

Figure 5.14 *Cavernous haemangioma on CT. (a) Precontrast CT scan showing focal area of decreased density in the posterior segment of the right lobe of the liver (arrow). (b) Scan at the same level as (a) taken during intravenous injection of contrast medium showing pools of contrast medium on the periphery of the lesion (arrows). (c) Scan at same level 3 minutes after intravenous injection of contrast medium showing progressive 'filling in' of the lesion with dense contrast medium. (d) CT scan at 30 minutes after intravenous injection of contrast medium showing that the lesion has become the same density as the adjacent liver parenchyma.*

CT scan, an area of increased echogenicity on ultrasound, or a hyperintense area on T1-weighted MR images may strongly suggest the diagnosis of **focal nodular hyperplasia** (Fig. 5.15). However, a similar appearance may be seen in fibrolamellar hepatocellular carcinomas.

The capsule of an **adenoma** may contain an excess of lipid-laden hepatocytes permitting a low-density

Figure 5.15 *Focal nodular hyperplasia. A CT scan without intravenous contrast medium showing a well-defined focal abnormality in the posterior segment of the right lobe. A central stellate radiolucency can be identified (arrowheads) corresponding to a central fibrous scar. Ascites and an irregular liver margin owing to cirrhosis are noted.*

Figure 5.16 *Adenoma of the liver. A large inhomogeneous focal abnormality is seen in the posterior aspect of the right lobe of the liver on an unenhanced CT scan. Areas of high density (arrows) can be seen within it corresponding to a spontaneous bleed within the adenoma.*

peripheral ring to be identified on CT. Areas of increased density on non-contrast scans representing haemorrhage are a common finding on CT in patients whose adenomas have bled (Fig. 5.16).

BENIGN CYSTS

Solitary or multiple congenital liver cysts are a frequent incidental finding. On ultrasound, they appear as rounded, smooth-walled, echo-free areas with distal enhancement owing to the low attenuation of ultra-

sound by the clear fluid within the cyst (Fig. 5.17). The presence of internal echoes should raise the suspicion that the lesion is not a simple cyst. On CT, cysts are seen as sharply defined homogeneous areas, the contents of which have a density nearer to that of water and do not enhance after intravenous injection of contrast medium (Fig. 5.18). The contents of the cyst influences the appearance on MRI, but usually the signal is low on T1-weighted images and high on T2-weighted images. The differential diagnosis of benign congenital cysts includes hydatid disease, abscesses, degenerating tumours and 'cystic' metastases.

Figure 5.17 *Benign liver cyst on ultrasound. A longitudinal ultrasound scan of the liver showing an anechoic lesion (arrows) with a sharp posterior margin and distal enhancement (open arrows).*

Figure 5.18 *Liver cyst on CT. CT scan after intravenous injection of contrast medium showing a well-defined, small, fluid-filled focal lesion that does not enhance (arrow).*

Figure 5.19 *Liver abscess on ultrasound. This longitudinal ultrasound scan shows a large multiseptate fluid collection owing to the presence of a large abscess. The lesion is well-defined from the normal liver parenchyma (arrows).*

Figure 5.20 *Liver abscess on CT. CT scan after intravenous injection of contrast medium showing marked enhancement of the thick-walled liver abscess (arrows). A central non-enhancing area is due to purulent necrosis.*

INFLAMMATORY LESIONS

Abscesses

CT is more sensitive than ultrasound for the detection of abscesses, most of which are solitary and occur in the posterior part of the right lobe of the liver. Their imaging appearance depends on the stage of develop-

ment. At an early stage an abscess appears as a focal area of altered echogenicity on ultrasound, which then liquefies to produce the typical irregular, cavitating lesion (Fig. 5.19). The central portion of such an abscess is purulent material which does not enhance on CT after intravenous injection of a bolus of contrast medium, but the periphery is frequently hypervascular and enhances strongly (Fig. 5.20). About a third of abscesses contain air (Fig. 5.21). In immunocompromised patients, infection with fungi such as *Candida* spp. typically produces multiple small abscesses. On ultrasound these may be seen as multiple minute areas of

(a)

(b)

Figure 5.21 *(a) Multifocal liver abscess on non-contrast CT showing multiple pockets of air (arrows). (b) After contrast medium, an enhancing wall can be demonstrated (arrow).*

(b)

(a)

Figure 5.22 *Candida infection of the liver. (a) Transverse ultrasound scan of the liver showing multiple minute areas of increased echogenicity caused by multiple minute Candida abscesses. (b) Non-contrast CT scan on the same patient as (a) showing multiple focal areas of decreased attenuation corresponding to the Candida abscesses.*

increased echogenicity (Fig. 5.22a) and on CT as areas of decreased density (Fig. 5.22b).

Hydatid disease

Echinococcus granulosus usually presents as a large cystic cavity, most often in the right lobe, whereas *E. alveolaris* frequently resembles an infiltrating tumour. The cysts are readily detected on ultrasound and CT, and in 50 per cent of cases show the pathognomonic appearance of daughter cysts within the larger cyst (Fig. 5.23). Hydatid cysts are often indistinguishable from simple

cysts. Debris within the cyst can be due to dead scolices or to superinfection. Calcification, present in 25 per cent of cases, is most readily seen on CT, but can also be identified on plain radiographs and ultrasound.

HEPATIC TRAUMA

Plain radiographs provide a useful initial assessment of the patient with liver trauma by identifying right-sided rib fractures, local ileus in the right upper quadrant,

(a)

(b)

Figure 5.23 *(a) CT scan after intravenous injection of contrast medium showing a well-defined thick-walled fluid collection (arrows). (b) Obvious serpiginous enhancing strands within the cyst represent collapsed daughter cysts (open arrow). This was due to infection with* Echinococcus granulosus.

(a)

(b)

Figure 5.24 *Hepatic trauma. (a) CT after intravenous contrast medium showing an intrahepatic haematoma of low density, not enhancing with contrast medium (arrows). (b) A scan inferior to (a) showing a large subcapsular haematoma (arrows). Laceration of the margins of the liver can be identified (open arrows). Intraperitoneal blood is seen on both scans.*

elevation of the right hemidiaphragm and perhaps a right pleural effusion. However, trauma to the hepatic parenchyma is best assessed with CT.

Patients who are haemodynamically stable can be assessed by CT, but unstable patients, or those with severe penetrating injuries, may need to go directly to surgery or therapeutic angiography. Hepatic lacerations, intrahepatic and subcapsular haematomas and haemoperitoneum are all well demonstrated on CT (Fig. 5.24). The pelvis is always included because seemingly trivial lacerations with small amounts of blood in the upper abdomen may show surprisingly large amounts of blood in the pelvis.

Hepatic lacerations are the most common hepatic injuries and are seen as linear, round or branching, poorly enhancing regions of low density. Intrahepatic haematomas are usually hypodense relative to the contrast-enhanced parenchyma and may be seen in the absence of true lacerations. Subcapsular haematomas, usually associated with lacerations, are well-circumscribed, lenticular or oval fluid collections of low density that flatten or indent the underlying hepatic parenchyma.

Figure 5.25 *Longitudinal ultrasound scan with the patient in the right anterior oblique position to show the normal common duct (white arrows) lying anterior to the portal vein (P). The right hepatic artery passing between the duct and the portal vein can also be demonstrated (black arrows). The IVC is cut across in an oblique projection.*

BILIARY SYSTEM

IMAGING TECHNIQUES

ULTRASOUND

Ultrasound has revolutionized the approach to biliary tract disease and has replaced routine plain radiogra-

phy, cholecystography and intravenous cholangiography. The gallbladder and biliary tree can be examined without the need for contrast media or ionizing radiation. There are no specific or relative contraindications to ultrasound and it should be the initial imaging approach for any gallbladder or biliary tree problem. Further investigations are largely determined by the ultrasound findings.

Figure 5.26 *Longitudinal ultrasound showing dilatation of the common duct at the level of the porta hepatis (arrows). A normal portal vein is seen posteriorly (p). A mass in the head of the pancreas (M) can be seen narrowing the distal aspect of the dilated duct (open arrows).*

Figure 5.27 *Dilatation of the intrahepatic biliary system demonstrated on a transverse scan through the liver. The dilated ducts (arrows) have a typical branched, stellate appearance and are distinguished from venous structures by their echogenic margins.*

The common bile duct is usually readily identified on ultrasound (Fig. 5.25). The supraduodenal portion within the hepatoduodenal ligament is most frequently seen anterolateral to the portal vein. The retroduodenal portion is less readily seen as it is obscured by gas within the duodenum. The upper limit of normal for the internal diameter of the common bile duct is 5–7 mm. As it is often not possible to identify the insertion of the cystic duct into the common hepatic duct, the common hepatic duct cannot be distinguished reliably from the common bile duct. Hence the term 'common duct' is applied to both structures. The cystic duct itself can be demonstrated sonographically in less than 50 per cent of cases. Dilatation of the intrahepatic and extrahepatic biliary system is reliably detected on ultrasound (Figs 5.26, 5.27). On ultrasound, the gallbladder appears as a sonolucent structure with increased through transmission. The normal thickness of the distended gallbladder wall is 2–3 mm (Fig. 5.28).

Figure 5.28 *Oblique view of the normal gallbladder (GB) on ultrasound lying anterior to the IVC.*

COMPUTED TOMOGRAPHY

CT is used infrequently as the primary approach to a biliary tract problem but is generally reserved for those patients in whom ultrasound proves inconclusive, particularly when bowel gas or obesity has prevented a satisfactory ultrasound examination. Demonstration of the gallbladder is less reliable than with ultrasound, but the lower half of the common bile duct is shown more reliably than with ultrasound. Dilated intrahepatic bile ducts can be detected accurately (Fig. 5.29) and the distinction between medical and surgical causes of jaundice can be made in 90 per cent of cases.

ENDOSCOPIC RETROGRADE CHOLANGIOPANCREATOGRAPHY (ERCP)

ERCP allows direct opacification of the biliary tree and the pancreatic ductal system. The indications include inconclusive ultrasound, for example where ultrasound has failed to reveal the cause of a dilated biliary system, or where ultrasound has shown normal calibre ducts in

(a)

(b)

Figure 5.29 *Choledochal cyst. (a) CT scan after intravenous injection of contrast medium showing marked dilatation of intrahepatic bile ducts. These have the typical low-density, tubular appearance. (b) Scan taken more inferiorly showing the cyst (C) lying along the course of the duct posterior to the normal gallbladder (GB).*

the presence of clinical and biochemical evidence of obstruction. ERCP also plays an important role in the management of choledocholithiasis as, although ultrasound is excellent for demonstrating stones within the gallbladder, it is less accurate for showing bile duct stones. ERCP is also indicated when bile duct stones are shown and sphincterotomy is indicated. Suspected sclerosing cholangitis is a further indication for ERCP. The major contraindication to ERCP is a recent attack of pancreatitis. Complications, notably post-ERCP pancreatitis, occur in 5 per cent of procedures.

MAGNETIC RESONANCE CHOLANGIOPANCREATOGRAPHY (MRCP)

Magnetic resonance cholangiopancreatography uses MRI to visualize fluid in the biliary and pancreatic ducts

(a)

(b)

Figure 5.30 *Magnetic resonance cholangiopancreatography (MRCP). (a) Normal study. A heavily T2-weighted breath-hold study showing the normal intrahepatic and common bile ducts, the pancreatic duct and the fluid-filled duodenum. (b) Choledochal cyst. A saccular dilatation of the common duct at the level of the junction of the left and right hepatic ducts. The normal common duct distal to the cyst is demonstrated. Only a portion of the pancreatic duct joining the common duct is seen on this view.*

as high signal intensity on heavily T2-weighted sequences. Different sequences using both breath-hold and non-breath-hold techniques have been used to obtain MRCP images (Fig. 5.30). The administration of contrast media is not required. The technique is still evolving but at present the spatial resolution seen on ERCP cannot be achieved regularly on MRCP. When compared to ERCP there are limitations. Direct visualization of an abnormal ampulla is not possible, biopsy material cannot be obtained and intervention, such as stent placement, cannot be carried out. MRCP is also less sensitive in identifying choledocholithiasis. Nevertheless, there are certain situations in which MRCP is particularly advantageous. These include patients who are pregnant or who have acute pancreatitis, and for whom an ERCP may be dangerous, and patients with altered gastric anatomy caused by prior surgery. Nevertheless, because contrast agents and sedation are not required, it is free of serious complications and is noninvasive, MRCP is likely to replace diagnostic ERCP as the diagnostic imaging modality of choice for imaging the biliary and pancreatic ducts.

SCINTIGRAPHY

Hepatobiliary scintigraphy involves the use of radiopharmaceuticals, which are excreted into the bile. Technetium-99m-labelled *N*-substituted iminodiacetic acid derivative (IDA) compounds are used, the most frequent being dimethyl IDA (or HIDA). Renal excretion increases with increasing hyperbilirubinaemia making HIDA an unsuitable agent in the presence of jaundice. On a normal scan taken 1 hour after injection, activity will be shown in the liver, major intrahepatic ducts, gallbladder, common bile duct and small intestine. Indications for bile scintigraphy include the diagnosis of acute cholecystitis, the detection of developmental anomalies of the biliary tree, assessing biliary dynamics and showing leaks following biliary duct trauma.

CONGENITAL ABNORMALITIES OF BILIARY TRACT

BILIARY ATRESIA

When investigating a child with biliary atresia, diagnostic imaging is aimed at demonstrating the anatomy and function of the liver and biliary tree, and distinguishing between neonatal hepatitis and biliary atresia. Ultrasonography and scintigraphy are the main imaging modalities. Sonography is used to exclude other causes of obstructive jaundice, e.g. a choledochal cyst; to evaluate the hepatic parenchyma and liver size. Hepatobiliary

scintigraphy with HIDA will differentiate **neonatal hepatitis** from biliary atresia. In biliary atresia, no activity will be seen in the bowel on a HIDA scan. To improve the accuracy of the technique, the baby is pretreated with phenobarbitone for 3 days to increase biliary excretion.

CHOLEDOCHAL CYSTS

A choledochal cyst produces a soft-tissue mass in the right upper quadrant adjacent to the liver with inferior displacement of the duodenal loop and the right kidney. The cyst may be identifiable on plain film but ultrasound is the best imaging modality. Classic findings are a normal size extrahepatic bile duct entering a cystic mass. The cystic mass is usually adjacent to the gallbladder within the porta hepatis or within the pancreatic head. The intrahepatic ducts may be dilated. Biliary sludge or calculi may be detected within the cyst. As there is a greatly increased risk of gallbladder malignancy arising in choledochal cysts in adolescence or childhood, care should always be taken when a choledochal cyst contains debris, because papillary neoplasms are often misinterpreted as debris.

CT is helpful for delineating the size and extent of both intrahepatic and extrahepatic choledochal cysts (Fig. 5.29) and for showing the relationship of the cyst to adjacent intraperitoneal and extraperitoneal structures. MRCP will also provide information on the position of the cyst in the remainder of the biliary tree (Fig. 5.30b).

A **choledochocoele** (Type II choledochal cyst) is a developmental dilatation of the intraduodenal portion of the distal common bile duct. This condition may be suspected first during a barium meal examination, where a negative-filling defect is identified at the ampulla on the medial wall of the duodenum.

Intrahepatic biliary cysts (**Caroli's disease** or Type V choledochal cysts) may be demonstrated on ultrasonography as sonolucent intrahepatic tubular structures converging on the porta hepatis representing the grossly dilated biliary tree. Proving communication between these dilated structures is paramount in distinguishing Caroli's disease from cystic disease of the liver or multiple abscesses. This can best be achieved by ERCP.

GALLSTONES

High resolution, real-time ultrasound has an accuracy of greater than 95 per cent in the detection of gallstones in the gallbladder. The false-negative rate is about 5 per cent and most missed calculi are either smaller than 2 mm or are impacted in the neck of the gallbladder. Problems of

Figure 5.31 *Gallstone. A longitudinal ultrasound scan of the gallbladder containing an echogenic focus (arrows). An absence of echoes (acoustic shadow) is seen distal to the stone.*

Figure 5.32 *Gallbladder sludge. A longitudinal ultrasound seen through the gallbladder showing echogenic material within it, without casting an acoustic shadow.*

interpretation arise at the neck because the valves of Heister characteristically appear strongly echogenic and may mimic gallstones. Ultrasound diagnosis of gallstones depends on several criteria: one or more echogenic foci within the gallbladder lumen; acoustic shadowing arising beyond an echogenic focus; and change in position of this focus with change in the patient's position (Fig. 5.31). With strict application of these criteria, a diagnostic accuracy of 100 per cent can be reached.

The phenomenon of acoustic shadowing is due to a combination of reflection of the incident beam and absorption of sound by the stone, and is independent of calculus composition, shape and surface characteristics. Most stones which do not case acoustic shadows are smaller than 5 mm. Gallbladder 'sludge', which is due to a mixture of calcium bilirubinate and cholesterol, produces homogeneous low or mid-level echoes which form a dependent layer and slowly change position with gravity (Fig. 5.32). Sludge is seen in patients with biliary stasis on an obstructive or non-obstructive basis (such as prolonged fasting, hyperalimentation, haemolysis). However, the presence of sludge can make it difficult to distinguish between sludge and polypoid forms of gallbladder carcinoma. A repeat examination after resumption of eating, after which sludge should disappear, is usually required.

The sensitivity of ultrasound in detecting gallstones within the bile ducts is poor: only some 55–65 per cent of stones will be found. This low rate of detection is partly accounted for by the fact that about one third of patients with duct stones have normal calibre ducts, and

partly because stones are usually impacted in the distal third of the common duct which is often obscured by intestinal gas (Fig. 5.33). If duct stones are thought likely clinically and ultrasound is not confirmatory, then direct cholangiography (Fig. 5.34) is required.

Duct stones are usually easily detected with ERCP or MRCP, which may show the common duct to be dilated or to be of normal calibre. An accepted rule of thumb is that complete obstruction of the common duct shown at ERCP is seldom due to calculi. The only exception is when a calculus becomes impacted at the ampulla. A major advantage of ERCP in the investigation of choledocholithiasis is the potential for

Figure 5.33 *Bile duct calculus. A longitudinal ultrasound scan through the common duct showing an extremely dilated common duct (arrowed) with an echogenic stone (arrowheads) impacted in the distal part of the duct and casting an acoustic shadow.*

Figure 5.34 *A percutaneous transhepatic cholangiogram showing filling defects in the gallbladder and distal common bile duct caused by gallstones (arrows).*

endoscopic sphincterotomy. Most centres quote a success rate of 80 per cent, complication rate of 8 per cent and mortality rate of 1 per cent, the most common complications being perforation, cholangitis, haemorrhage and pancreatitis.

Ultrasound, ERCP, scintigraphy and MRCP all play a role in the investigation of patients with persistent symptoms following cholecystectomy. In the immediate postoperative period, ultrasound or CT can identify haematomata and abscesses in the gallbladder bed, monitor their progression or resolution, and allow drainage under image guidance if necessary. ERCP will allow demonstration of the bile ducts and enable sphincterotomy. Scintigraphy can detect a bile leak and show its extent.

ACUTE CHOLECYSTITIS

ACUTE CALCULOUS CHOLECYSTITIS

Ultrasound and scintigraphy are both useful for 'emergency' diagnosis of acute cholecystitis. Factors

such as the availability of the technique and the cost of the procedure must be taken into account before choosing which test to perform.

High sensitivities, in the range of 85–95 per cent, are reported for both ultrasound and scintigraphy in the diagnosis of acute cholecystitis, but specificities are somewhat lower. The advantages of ultrasonography are speed, more consistent evaluation of adjacent structures, lack of dependence on hepatic excretory function and lower cost. In practice, ultrasound is more frequently requested for confirming a diagnosis of acute cholecystitis.

Ultrasound

The demonstration of gallstones alone is not diagnostic of acute cholecystitis, as gallstones may be present in patients with right upper quadrant pain from other causes. Other criteria must be demonstrated to make the diagnosis, including gallbladder wall thickening, gallbladder wall sonolucency, gallbladder distension and the sonographic Murphy's sign, where maximal tenderness is elicited over the gallbladder on palpation with the ultrasound transducer (Fig. 5.35). With the exception of focal gallbladder tenderness, there are many other causes for these secondary ultrasound signs. For example, gallbladder wall thickening can be seen in chronic cholecystitis, adenomyomatosis, renal failure, portal hypertension, pancreatitis and ascites. Similarly, a lucency within the gallbladder wall has a low positive predictive value for acute cholecystitis, and gallbladder distension can occur in diabetes mellitus, hyperalimentation, narcotic analgesia and other nonobstructive

Figure 5.35 *Acute cholecystitis. Longitudinal ultrasound scan of the gallbladder showing markedly thickened walls (straight arrows), lucency within the thickened gallbladder wall (open arrows) and linear lucency adjacent to the gallbladder wall (curved arrows).*

(a)

(b)

(c)

Figure 5.36 *Acute cholecystitis and perforation of gallbladder. (a) CT scan showing thickening of the gallbladder wall (straight arrow) with a small amount of fluid adjacent to the gallbladder (curved arrow). Bile is also present in the subhepatic space (open arrows) from perforation of the gallbladder. The common duct is dilated. (b) A scan at a level inferior to (a) showing the presence of stones within the gallbladder and common duct (arrows). (c) A scan superior to (a) showing intrahepatic bile duct dilatation and the extent of the bile leak into the subhepatic space.*

causes of diminished gallbladder emptying. Using a combination of findings in an appropriate clinical setting gives a good positive predictive value for sonography. The more findings that are present, the higher the positive predictive value.

Scintigraphy

Cholescintigraphy, using ^{99m}Tc-IDA derivatives, is an accurate and efficacious means of evaluating patients suspected of having acute cholecystitis. When the cystic duct is patent, the gallbladder is visualized by 60 minutes following injection. Normal gallbladder visualization excludes acute cholecystitis with virtual certainty. Over 90 per cent of patients with acute cholecystitis show an absence of gallbladder activity, about 7 per cent show delayed gallbladder visualization and, very occasionally, an obstructive pattern with no activity in the gallbladder, common bile duct or small intestine despite satisfactory liver uptake. False-positive results occur in chronic cholecystitis, acute pancreatitis, alcoholic liver disease and hyperalimentation.

Computed tomography

Although rarely performed with the intention of diagnosing acute cholecystitis, CT is capable of suggesting the diagnosis and occasionally the diagnosis is made with CT when unsuspected clinically (Fig. 5.36). Other than gallstones, the most common CT finding is gallbladder wall thickening, especially when focal or non-uniform. Low-density oedema in the space between the liver substance and the gallbladder is another feature; localized fluid collections adjacent to the gallbladder and in the subhepatic or subphrenic spaces suggest perforation.

Complications of acute cholecystitis

Acute **perforations** are associated with free spill of bile into the peritoneum and associated peritonitis. Subacute perforations are the most common, they tend to wall off and form pericholecystic abscesses. Chronic perforations are associated with fistulous communications with other organs. Ultrasound is best suited to demonstrating the free fluid associated with acute perforations and the irregular fluid collections which are seen in the hepatocholecystic space in subacute perforations.

Empyema of the gallbladder is suggested when findings of acute cholecystitis are accompanied by multiple highly reflective intraluminal echoes on ultrasound without shadowing, layering or gravity dependence. These echoes correspond to purulent exudate and debris within highly viscous bile and are indistinguishable from highly viscous sludge.

Gangrene of the gallbladder can be suggested in the appropriate clinical setting when ultrasound shows extremely shaggy, irregular and asymmetric walls. Intraluminal membranes corresponding to desquamated mucosa are common in gangrenous gallbladders (Fig. 5.37). They are seen as irregular, non-shadowing echoes within the gallbladder lumen, close to and paralleling the wall.

ACUTE ACALCULOUS CHOLECYSTITIS

Sonography alone is often non-specific for diagnosing acalculous cholecystitis but when taken in conjunction with the clinical history, it may be diagnostic. The most suggestive sonographic findings are gallbladder wall thickening less than 4 mm (provided the gallbladder is distended to at least 5 cm in length), intraluminal membranes and pericholecystic fluid in the absence of ascites. Sludge or coarse echoes suggestive of pus within the gallbladder lumen and gallbladder distension (> 8 cm in the long axis of > 5 cm transversely) are abnormal but less specific findings. A normal ultrasound examination of the gallbladder does not exclude acalculous cholecystitis: the sensitivity of ultrasound in acalculous cholecystitis is significantly less than in calculous cholecystitis.

EMPHYSEMATOUS CHOLECYSTITIS

Plain film findings usually become visible only 24–48 hours after the onset of symptoms. Gas may be seen first in the gallbladder wall or lumen (Fig. 5.38). Intramural gas may be seen as a crescentic lucency, a lucent halo or a bubbly necklace around the gallbladder. Ultrasound can also diagnose emphysematous cholecystitis by demonstrating gas in the gallbladder wall or lumen.

Figure 5.38 *Erect plain film showing gas within the gallbladder in a patient with emphysematous cholecystitis. (Courtesy of Dr J.E. Dacie.)*

Figure 5.37 *Gangrene of the gallbladder. Transverse ultrasound scan showing irregular thickening of the gallbladder walls (arrows), which are poorly defined from the adjacent liver parenchyma. Echoes seen within the gallbladder lumen are due to desquamated mucosa.*

Computed tomography in complications of cholecystitis

Although ultrasound is the study of choice, CT can detect complications of acute cholecystitis and is better at diagnosing perforations. This is because CT can depict small pericholecystic gas collections and differentiate them from bowel gas more easily than ultrasound and because CT is better at detecting a gallstone outside the gallbladder.

(a)

(b)

Figure 5.39 *Gallbladder carcinoma. (a) Longitudinal ultrasound scan showing thickening of the gallbladder wall (arrows) containing an inhomogeneous echogenic mass caused by neoplasia. (b) Transverse scan through the central portion of the mass (M) within the gallbladder.*

BILIARY TRACT NEOPLASIA

GALLBLADDER CARCINOMA

Primary carcinoma of the gallbladder is the fifth most common gastrointestinal tract malignancy and represents 1–3 per cent of all malignancies at autopsy. The most common sonographic appearance, seen in 50 per cent of patients, is replacement of the gallbladder by a complex mass (Fig. 5.39). In 20 per cent, there is diffuse or focal irregular thickening of the gallbladder wall. Occasionally, there is an irregular, polypoid mass within the lumen. Ultrasound has a predictive accuracy of about 55–85 per cent in the diagnosis of gallbladder cancer. Many of the false-positive results are due to misinterpretation of inflammatory changes. Ancillary findings are: gallstones within the gallbladder, seen in 50 per cent of cases; biliary duct dilatation owing to invasion of the porta hepatis; liver masses owing to direct extension or metastases; and adenopathy in the peripancreatic region or in the porta hepatis.

Similar features are seen on computed tomography (Fig. 5.40). The most common finding is a mass in the region of the gallbladder fossa that replaces all or most of the gallbladder. Direct extension into the adjacent liver is common. Less common appearances are irregular wall thickening or intraluminal masses. Ancillary findings include gallstones, wall calcification, dilated intra- or extrahepatic bile ducts, hepatic metastases and peripancreatic or para-aortic lymph node enlargement.

Adenocarcinomas account for 85 per cent or more of gallbladder cancers. Other malignancies such as

Figure 5.40 *Gallbladder carcinoma. A CT scan through the gallbladder fossa showing an inhomogeneous mass obliterating most of the gallbladder (arrows). A small remaining portion of the normal gallbladder can be demonstrated (arrowhead).*

spindle cell sarcomas, carcinoids or oat cell carcinomas are radiologically indistinguishable from adenocarcinoma.

MALIGNANCY OF THE BILE DUCTS

Cholangiocarcinoma is an uncommon tumour accounting for only 0.3–0.5 per cent of all malignancies.

Figure 5.42 *Advanced cholangiocarcinoma. CT scan after intravenous injection of contrast medium showing an irregular low-density mass in the region of the head of the pancreas (arrows) from a cholangiocarcinoma. Extension is seen with the gallbladder fossa. There is also enlargement of para-aortic lymph nodes (curved arrows).*

Figure 5.41 *Cholangiocarcinoma. A percutaneous cholangiogram showing an irregular narrowing of the common duct (arrows) with proximal dilatation.*

It originates in the larger bile ducts: about 10 per cent arise in the intrahepatic ducts, 10–26 per cent at the confluence of the hepatic ducts (**Klatskin tumour**), 15–30 per cent in the proximal common duct and 30–36 per cent arise in the distal common duct.

Percutaneous transhepatic cholangiography (Fig. 5.41) and ERCP are the best modalities for depicting bile duct neoplasms. Bile duct carcinoma can be classified cholangiographically as either obstructive, stenotic or protuberant. The obstructive type is the most frequent, occurring in about 70 per cent of cholangiograms and appearing as a U- or V-shaped obstruction with a nipple, rat-tail, smooth or irregular termination. The stenotic type shows a strictured lumen with irregular margins and post-stenotic dilatation (Fig. 5.41). The length of stenosis may be long or short. The polypoid or protuberant type appears as an intraluminal filling defect with irregular margins, attached at one point to the wall.

A specific diagnosis of biliary duct neoplasm can only rarely be made with ultrasound or CT. Ultrasound demonstrates dilatation of the bile ducts proximal to the tumour in the vast majority of cases, but only occasionally can a mass be seen either within or surrounding the duct. The CT manifestations include biliary dilatation, metastatic disease and, least commonly, demonstration of the primary tumour itself. If the tumour is obstructive, the site of the tumour will determine the degree and distribution of bile duct dilatation, and whether the gallbladder is dilated. Local of distant metastatic disease may be seen. Proximal tumours invade the liver or gallbladder, whereas distal tumours may invade the duodenum and pancreas (Fig. 5.42). On both ultrasound and CT, an intrahepatic cholangiocarcinoma is usually indistinguishable from a **primary liver neoplasm**.

While bile duct carcinoma carries a poor prognosis, the outcome is better than for carcinoma of the pancreas. Preoperative imaging studies need to define the anatomical location and extent of the lesion. It may be evident at an early stage that the lesion is unresectable when ultrasound or CT shows extensive local spread, liver or lung metastases. ERCP or percutaneous cholangiography have a major role to play in the preoperative assessment because extension into second order branches of both lobes usually means that the tumour is unresectable.

BENIGN STRICTURES

It must be emphasized that there is great difficulty in radiologically differentiating between benign and malignant strictures of the biliary tree. The commonest causes of benign strictures are chronic pancreatitis and bile duct surgery. Other inflammatory conditions include tuberculosis and stone disease.

If ultrasound or CT indicate that the obstruction is low, then ERCP is the investigation of choice. It usually shows a long smooth stricture of the common bile duct. If it is known from ultrasound that the obstruction is high, then although ERCP may delineate the stricture, percutaneous transhepatic cholangiography should be performed, as such strictures involve first- or second-order branches, and all separately obstructed segments need to be identified.

The secondary effects of long-standing biliary obstruction, such as fibrosis or cirrhosis with portal hypertension and varices, may also be seen on ultrasound or CT.

BILE DUCT INFLAMMATION

PRIMARY SCLEROSING CHOLANGITIS

The hallmark of primary sclerosing cholangitis, a disease of unknown aetiology, is involvement of all or some of the biliary tree by a chronic inflammatory process where any cause of secondary obstruction, such as stones or infection, has been excluded. The disease is associated with a variety of disorders of which ulcerative colitis is the most common, but which includes Crohn's disease, mediastinal and retroperitoneal fibrosis, pancreatitis, orbital pseudotumour and thyroiditis. Currently, the diagnosis is based on imaging findings in the majority of cases. Ultrasound is often normal or inconclusive, although non-specific bile duct wall thickening may be seen. CT may show mild duct dilatation with a distended irregular branching pattern. Characteristically, the ducts do not taper towards the periph-

ery of the liver, as they typically do in other causes of duct obstruction. Direct cholangiography shows irregular, nodular, beaded narrowing of the extra- and intrahepatic biliary systems (Fig. 5.43). ERCP is the preferred approach to visualize the bile ducts as it provides a greater likelihood of success in the absence of intrahepatic duct dilatation. Although the findings are fairly characteristic, a rare multifocal cholangiocarcinoma can give an identical appearance.

AIDS-ASSOCIATED CHOLANGITIS

Because opportunistic organisms such as cryptosporidium, cytomegalovirus and *Candida albicans* may be found in the bile of patients with AIDS, they are implicated in the biliary inflammation seen in some patients suffering from AIDS. Ultrasound often shows severe gallbladder wall thickening in the absence of gallstones and the common bile duct is dilated without any obvious cause (Fig. 5.44). Cholangiography may show findings similar to primary sclerosing cholangitis: intra- and extrahepatic ductal involvement with irregular strictures and mild dilatation. Papillary stenosis is frequently present and is sometimes considered the key feature. The liver may show an increase in periportal echoes.

ACUTE (ASCENDING) CHOLANGITIS

Usually, the role of imaging in acute cholangitis is to define the cause of obstruction and to confirm that no additional findings, such as abscesses, are present. Pus

Figure 5.43 *Sclerosing cholangitis. ERCP showing involvement of the extra- and intrahepatic biliary tree with 'beading' of the common duct and irregular narrowing of ducts.*

Figure 5.44 *Longitudinal ultrasound scan of the gallbladder in a patient suffering from AIDS showing marked thickening of the gallbladder wall (arrows).*

within dilated ducts may be seen at ultrasound as echogenic material or as filling defects on cholangiography.

RECURRENT PYOGENIC CHOLANGITIS (ORIENTAL CHOLANGITIS)

Plain films in recurrent pyogenic cholangitis may show gas in the biliary tree and occasionally may show intrahepatic calcifications, representing biliary stones. Nearly all patients show extrahepatic dilatation on ultrasound and there is often dilatation of the intrahepatic ducts. The detection rate for stones by ultrasound is about 40 per cent. CT readily shows the pattern of duct dilatation, the pneumobilia, stones and concomitant features such as extrahepatic fluid collections, pancreatitis and splenomegaly.

BILIARY PARASITES

In *Ascaris lumbricoides* infestation of the biliary system, intestinal worms are present in 90 per cent of patients. Sonography is reliable for diagnosing the presence of the worm within the lumen of intrahepatic or extrahepatic common duct or gallbladder.

PANCREAS

NORMAL PANCREAS

On **ultrasound**, the normal pancreas displays a homogeneous echogenicity similar to liver in 50 per cent of patients and greater echogenicity than liver in the other half. The pancreas is bounded by the higher echogenicity of the retroperitoneal fat and investing connective tissue (Fig. 5.45). As fat infiltration occurs, the overall echogenicity of the pancreas increases, making identification of the pancreatic boundaries difficult. The major limitation of ultrasound is the inability to image the entire gland in 15–20 per cent of cases.

On **CT**, the normal pancreas has an attenuation that is lower than liver or spleen, and similar to kidney, muscle and blood. It has a relatively homogeneous radiodensity except where it is infiltrated by fat in the obese and the elderly. Its borders are frequently lobulated but may be smooth. Evaluation of the pancreas with CT routinely requires intravenous administration of contrast medium because contrast enhancement improves the rate of tumour detection and demonstrates the relationship of tumour to adjacent vessels. Peak enhancement of the pancreas occurs after about 3 seconds after peak enhancement of the aorta, and thus the best images of the pancreas are

Figure 5.45 *Normal transverse ultrasound scan of the pancreas showing the pancreas lying anterior to the splenic vein (S), the common duct within the head of the pancreas (arrowhead), the uncinate process of the pancreas (arrow), the left lobe of the liver (L), and the falciform ligament (open arrows). Posteriorly lie the aorta (A) and the inferior vena cava (IVC) joined by the left renal vein.*

achieved by rapidly injecting a bolus of 100–150 ml of contrast medium and scanning rapidly either on 'dynamic' or 'spiral' mode. CT has become the leading technique for the evaluation of patients with known or suspected neoplastic and inflammatory disease. The high spatial and contrast resolution of current generation fast scanners permits visualization of pancreatic parenchyma in all patients.

The pancreas is visualized on **MRI** as a medium signal intensity structure surrounded by higher signal intensity fat on T1-weighted images (Fig. 6.1a, p. 177). On fast spin echo T2-weighted images, the pancreas appears hypointense to fat and to the spleen. On fat-suppressed T1-weighted images, the pancreas appears very intense.

Although evaluation of pancreatic size is important for recognizing pancreatic disease, it is difficult to assign precise measurements for normal pancreatic size, which varies with age, patient size, state of respiration, measurement site and measurement technique. Furthermore, various studies differ substantially in their estimates of the upper limit of normal.

The main pancreatic duct appears on **ERCP** as smooth-walled, and tapers gradually from the head to the tail. Intralobular ducts enter at nearly right angles (Fig. 5.46). The normal main pancreatic duct measures up to 4 mm in internal diameter within the head, up to 3 mm within the body and 2 mm in the tail. On CT scans, the greatest normal internal duct diameter is 5 mm in the head and 3 mm in the tail. The main pancreatic duct tends to increase in size with age. The accessory pancreatic duct (of Santorini) drains the

Figure 5.46 *Normal pancreatic duct on ERCP showing filling of intralobular ducts (arrowheads) and the accessory pancreatic duct (arrow).*

upper part of the pancreatic head and penetrates the anteromedial wall of the second part of the duodenum at the junction of its upper and distal thirds. In 10 per cent of individuals, the accessory duct does not communicate with the duct of Wirsung (pancreas divisum).

PANCREATIC NEOPLASMS

PANCREATIC DUCT CELL ADENOCARCINOMA

Duct cell adenocarcinoma accounts for 75–85 per cent of non-endocrine tumours of the pancreas. It is local-ized to the head in 70 per cent of cases, the body in 10 per cent and the tail in 5 per cent. The entire gland is involved in the remaining 15 per cent of cases.

Computed tomography

CT is the single best imaging modality for the detection and staging of pancreatic ductal adenocarcinoma in terms of overall accuracy, reliability and reproducibility. Modern CT scanners show a pancreatic abnormality in close to 99 per cent of patients with cancer. Optimal use of intravenous and oral contrast medium improves evaluation. Thus, if abdominal symptoms are present, a normal CT strongly suggests that these symptoms are not due to duct cell carcinoma.

The most common CT finding is a focal non-calcified mass (Fig. 5.47), although non-focal enlargement has been reported in up to 15 per cent of cases. As in the case of sonography, most duct cell carcinomas are not detected until they are at least 2 cm in size, large enough to alter the size and shape of the gland. Exceptions are small tumours in the head which present with bile or pancreatic duct dilatation (Fig. 5.48). Most tumours will distort the contour of the gland, but some small masses may show more subtle features such as: 'rounding' of the usually wedge-shaped uncinate process (Fig. 5.49); a 'normal'-sized head in an otherwise atrophic gland, and focal loss of the normal 'marbling' of the gland usually seen in the elderly (Fig. 5.48). Almost all carcinomas enhance to a lesser extent than the surrounding pancreatic parenchyma after intravenous injection of a bolus of contrast medium (Fig. 5.50). Occasionally, lucent areas are seen within the mass which may be related to associated pancreatitis rather than to tumour necrosis.

(a)

(b)

Figure 5.47 *Pancreatic carcinoma. (a) Transverse ultrasound scan showing a typical hypoechoic mass in the tail of the pancreas (arrows). The splenic vein is encased by the tumour. (b) CT scan in the same patient after intravenous injection of contrast medium showing a mass of lower density than the normally enhancing pancreas (arrows) encasing the splenic artery.*

(a)

(b)

(c)

Figure 5.48 *(a) CT scan after intravenous injection of contrast medium with a small mass within the head of the pancreas (arrows) showing loss of the normal 'marbled' appearance of the pancreas. (b) Scan through the liver showing intrahepatic bile duct dilatation. (c) ERCP showing the small mass demonstrated in (a) causing a filling defect within the distal pancreatic duct (arrow). A stent has been inserted into the dilated common duct (open arrows).*

Figure 5.49 *Carcinoma of the uncinate process. CT scan after intravenous injection of contrast medium showing a small mass in the uncinate process (arrows). Retroperitoneal lymph node enlargement (curved arrows) and liver secondaries are noted.*

Dilatation of the main pancreatic duct is detected in 50–75 per cent of cases of pancreatic carcinoma (Fig. 5.50). This sign is particularly important in detecting a small duct cell carcinoma of the head of the pancreas or an ampullary carcinoma, because pancreatic duct dilatation may be the only abnormality on CT. Parenchymal atrophy often accompanies duct dilatation.

Carcinoma of the head of the pancreas almost always results in biliary dilatation. Early or incomplete obstruction may be limited to the extrahepatic ducts. The gallbladder is often, but not always, distended, when the level of obstruction is distal to the cystic duct. Typically CT shows a dilated common duct down to the site of the tumour but, unlike benign disease, there is a sudden transition from a dilated duct to no visible duct at all within the tumour.

Ultrasound

In roughly 25 per cent of patients delineation of the pancreas on ultrasound is inadequate, most commonly

(a)

(b)

Figure 5.50 *Small pancreatic carcinoma. (a) Small hypodense lesion is seen in the pancreatic body (arrows) that is not deforming the contour of the pancreas but causing dilatation of the pancreatic duct. (b) oblique view of ERCP corresponding to the CT showing an irregular stricture and duct dilatation proximal to the tumour.*

because of overlying bowel gas. Nevertheless, ultrasound is often the method most frequently used to investigate patients clinically suspected of having pancreatic cancer as it is relatively inexpensive, readily available and can accurately distinguish non-obstructive from obstructive jaundice – the presenting feature in 50 per cent of patients. The fundamental ultrasound finding is focal hypoechoic pancreatic mass (Figs 5.47, 5.51), although pancreatic carcinomas are occasionally isoechoic. Ultrasound may have the advantage of being able to distinguish changes in echogenicity which can make small tumours apparent before they cause a change in contour. A strong clinical probability of pancreatic neoplasm with a normal ultrasound always necessitates further investigation.

ERCP

Given the high accuracy of non-invasive studies, ERCP is used primarily as a technique to further assess patients with ambiguous CT findings or as part of the procedure of stenting. Obstruction of the main pancreatic duct is the most common pancreatographic finding in carcinoma. The obstruction may be difficult to differentiate from that caused by pancreatitis. In carcinoma the ducts distal to the obstruction may show post-stenotic dilatation but are otherwise usually normal, whereas changes consistent with pancreatitis are usually present in obstruction caused by pancreatitis. In carcinoma, the obstruction itself is usually irregular, nodular, rat-tailed or eccentric, and smooth or blunt in pancreatitis. Localized encasement of the main pancreatic duct is the next most common appearance after obstruction (Fig. 5.50). This encasement is generally 1–2 cm in length and is irregular. The distal duct is

Figure 5.51 *Pancreatic carcinoma. Hypoechoic inhomogeneous mass in the body and tail of the pancreas (arrows) resulting in occlusion of the splenic vein (SV). Nodal enlargement is seen to the left of the aorta (A).*

normal, the proximal (upstream) duct is dilated and the transition abrupt. Small side branches near the encasement are frequently compressed by tumour and do not fill. Occasionally a mass lesion can be seen within a dilated pancreatic duct (Fig. 5.48).

STAGING OF PANCREATIC CANCER

The aim of preoperative staging of pancreatic cancer is to identify potentially resectable tumours. Only about 10 per cent of patients have resectable tumours. Conversely,

(a)

(b)

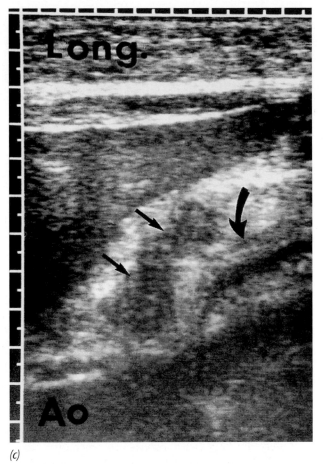

(c)

Figure 5.52 *Encasement of the superior mesenteric artery in pancreatic carcinoma. (a) CT scan after intravenous injection of contrast medium showing low density tumour encasing the superior mesenteric artery (arrows). (b) T1-weighted MRI scan showing the normal signal void encased by tissue of low signal intensity (arrow). (c) Longitudinal ultrasound scan showing encasement of the coeliac (arrows) and superior mesenteric arteries (curved arrow).*

as pancreaticoduodenectomy carries a high morbidity and mortality, imaging is also directed towards identifying those patients in whom the tumour has spread beyond the margins of the gland and is unresectable. The most generally accepted criteria of unresectability are the presence of liver metastases, adenopathy, tumour encasement of the coeliac or superior mesenteric arteries (not splenic artery), and obstruction or invasion of the portal and mesenteric veins.

Computed tomography

CT is the best imaging technique for staging patients with pancreatic cancer. Invasion of major adjacent arteries and veins is a contraindication to surgical resection. Involvement of the coeliac axis and its branches, the superior mesenteric artery or the major veins

(portal, splenic, superior mesenteric) appears as a thickening of the wall of the vessel or as a soft-tissue mantle obscuring the normal sharp interface between the vessel and the renal and the perivascular fat (Fig. 5.52). Veins may be totally obliterated and venous obstruction may be recognized only by collateral vessels. Although the venous changes are generally the result of invasion by a contiguous neoplasm, tumour growth in the perivascular lymphatics is responsible for periarterial 'cuffing'. Because of extrinsic intraparenchymal lymphatic connections, lesions anywhere in the gland can result in perivascular changes in any of the major arteries. As elsewhere in the body, CT can only demonstrate lymph node pathology by showing enlargement, which may be the result either of malignant infiltration or of reactive hyperplasia (Fig. 5.49). Microscopic involvement of nodes without enlargement is fairly common in pancreatic cancer. Invasion of adjacent organs can best be diagnosed on CT when tumour tissue has entered the substance of the affected structure. In the absence of definite evidence of invasion, it may not be possible to decide whether the loss of intervening fat between the tumour and the adjacent organs is the result of invasion or mere contact between the mass and adjacent organs.

The positive predictive value of CT in predicting 'unresectability' of a pancreatic cancer is extremely high at between 90 and 100 per cent; there are very few false-positive predictions of unresectability. The sensitivity of CT in detecting many of the features of unresectability is, however, lower. This is usually due to the failure of CT to detect lymph node metastases, small liver metastases and small peritoneal deposits. There is little difference between CT and angiography in detecting vascular involvement.

Ultrasound

Many of the vascular alterations that occur as a result of pancreatic carcinoma are demonstrable by ultrasonography. Encasement of the coeliac axis or superior mesenteric artery may be seen as thickening of the

periarterial tissues, and venous involvement seen as abrupt change in the calibre of the affected vein (Figs 5.47, 5.52). Duplex Doppler may increase the sensitivity of ultrasound in detecting vascular involvement. Ultrasound is less sensitive than CT in detecting vascular involvement and lymphadenopathy.

Endoscopic ultrasound has proved extremely accurate in detecting local infiltration of the portal vein, adjacent arteries and lymph node infiltration. The technique is, however, limited by not being able to detect liver or peritoneal disease.

Magnetic resonance imaging

The exact role of MRI in staging the local spread of pancreatic cancer has not yet been established. Pancreatic neoplasms, their retroperitoneal spread and venous patency are best evaluated using T1-weighted spin-echo sequences. On heavily T1-weighted images, pancreatic carcinoma typically appears as a mass with low signal intensity. Like CT, MRI is also capable of assessing arterial or venous involvement and lymph node enlargement (Figs 5.52, 5.53).

(a)

(b)

(c)

Figure 5.53 *Pancreatic carcinoma. (a) Low density mass (arrows) on contrast-enhanced CT lying within the head of the pancreas in close proximity to the superior mesenteric vessels. (b) T1-weighted MRI showing the typical appearance of a mass of low signal intensity (arrow). (c) Gradient echo MRI showing the mass encasing the superior mesenteric vessels.*

(a)

(b)

Figure 5.54 *Mucinous (macro) cystadenoma of the pancreas. (a) CT scan showing a typical large cystic mass replacing the body and tail of the pancreas. (b) Transverse ultrasound scan on the same patient showing a large fluid-filled mass. Echogenic septa (arrows) are more readily seen on ultrasound.*

PRIMARY CYSTIC NEOPLASMS OF DUCT CELL ORIGIN

Primary cystic neoplasms of the pancreas, which represent 10–15 per cent of pancreatic cysts in surgical series, are classified as either microcystic adenomas or mucinous cystic neoplasms. These are usually easily distinguished from each other by their imaging characteristics, which correspond to their differing gross morphology.

Microcystic adenoma

The vast majority of these benign tumours occur in females over the age of 60 years. The tumour occupies the head, body or tail of the pancreas, but occasionally occupies the entire gland. Almost all the cysts are less than 2 cm in diameter and the CT appearance is usually a water density mass sometimes containing solid elements. Individual cysts are too small to be identified on CT. Calcification occurs more frequently than in any other pancreatic tumour. The calcification is dystrophic in nature and is seen within a central fibrotic scar that may have a stellate appearance on CT. The tumour does not have a well-developed capsule on CT and is poorly demarcated from the normal gland. Contrast enhancement may be seen, owing to a rich network of capillaries within the tumour. On ultrasound, the most common pattern is a solid-appearing mild to moderately echogenic mass with or without small cystic areas, since almost all the cysts are less than 2 cm in diameter. Bright central echogenic foci with or without shadowing caused by calcification are sometimes visible.

Septations are often better appreciated on sonography than on CT.

Mucinous cystic neoplasms

Like microcystic adenoma, this tumour occurs predominantly in females but, unlike microcystic adenoma, has a malignant potential, developing into a low-grade mucinous adenocarcinoma. On CT, the mass is a well-demarcated, round or oval thick-walled cyst. The mass is generally over 5 cm in diameter (Fig. 5.54) and solid enhancing excrescences can occasionally be seen in the wall, particularly if the tumour is malignant. Dystrophic peripheral calcification is seen in about 15 per cent of cases. The main differential diagnosis is a pancreatic pseudocyst.

ISLET-CELL TUMOURS

The term islet-cell tumour encompasses a range of rare neoplasms of neuroendocrine origin arising in or in close proximity to the pancreas. A small proportion are non-functioning but the majority, approximately 85 per cent, secrete one or more biologically active peptides or amines normally found in the adult pancreas, or other substances not usually present in the pancreas such as gastrin. The role of imaging is to localize these tumours, usually prior to surgery, and to look for evidence of malignancy.

Insulinomas are the most frequent functioning pancreatic tumours accounting for 60 per cent of all islet-cell tumours. They are usually very small: 90 per cent are less than 2 cm, and are located with equal

(b)

(a)

Figure 5.55 *Insulinoma. (a) Transverse ultrasound scan through the pancreas showing small islet-cell tumour (arrow). (b) T1-weighted MRI scan showing typical low signal intensity lesion (arrow) corresponding to the abnormality seen on ultrasound.*

frequency in the head, body and tail of the pancreas; 10 per cent are malignant.

Gastrinomas account for about 20 per cent of all islet-cell tumours, are found in the pancreas and in the proximal duodenal wall, and about 60 per cent are malignant and often multiple. Other functioning islet-cell tumours, such as glucagonomas, VIPomas, somatostatinomas and carcinoid tumours, tend to be several centimetres in diameter at diagnosis and are frequently malignant.

Many imaging modalities are currently available for the investigation of patients with islet-cell tumours, including ultrasound, CT, MRI, arteriography, venous sampling and radionuclide imaging. None has established itself as clearly superior to the others.

Ultrasound is generally the first line of investigation and an islet-cell tumour is usually seen as a well-circumscribed mass of lower echogenicity than the normal pancreas (Fig. 5.55). Tumours as small as 7 mm have been detected. Liver metastases may be seen with malignant tumours and are most often hypoechoic. The sensitivity of transabdominal ultrasound is low, partly due to overlying bowel gas, but also because relatively poor resolution 3.5–5.0 MHz transducers are needed to obtain pictures from a structure positioned deep within the abdomen. **Endoscopic ultrasound** overcomes these problems by allowing the positioning of a high frequency (7.5–10 MHz) transducer in close proximity to the pancreas, obtaining high-resolution images. The early results are extremely encouraging. Intraoperative ultrasound also allows high-resolution examination of the pancreas and can be used as an adjunct to palpation during surgery.

The majority of islet-cell tumours are isodense on non-contrast-enhanced **CT** and cannot therefore be

recognized. On postcontrast CT they are seen as rounded areas that enhance more than the surrounding pancreas (Fig. 5.56). Local nodal and liver deposits may also be seen, usually as enhancing masses. The sensitivity of CT for delineation of these tumours depends on size, but is usually about 65–75 per cent for insulinomas and gastrinomas. Small tumours may also be seen on **MRI**, usually as round, low-signal lesions on T1-weighted images (Fig. 5.55), showing high signal on T2-weighted images.

Arteriography still has a role in localizing islet-cell tumours, particularly when this has not been achieved by less invasive techniques. Selective injections of contrast medium into the coeliac axis and superior mesenteric artery followed by superselective studies of the splenic, dorsal pancreatic, gastroduodenal and pancreaticoduodenal arteries are made. An islet-cell tumour typically appears as a round, well-circumscribed blush in the capillary phase and venous phases. Lesions may be missed on angiography because they are too small or too hypovascular, or because they are obscured by a blush of adjacent bowel or spleen.

Transhepatic portal venous sampling is the most sensitive but most invasive method of localizing functioning tumours, with a significant complication rate of close to 10 per cent. The technique involves transhepatic catheterization of the splenic and portal veins with serial sampling of the splenic, superior mesenteric and portal veins. This technique cannot pinpoint a tumour in the same way as an imaging study but localizes it to a region of the pancreas.

Venous sampling can also be combined with direct stimulation. In this technique, selective arterial catheterization and venous sampling are performed following direct injection of a stimulant such as calcium.

(a)

(b)

Figure 5.56 *Insulinoma. (a) CT scan showing small enhancing lesion (arrowed) owing to insulinoma. (b) Area of increased uptake (arrowed) in octreotide scan from insulinoma corresponding to lesion seen on CT. the normal liver (L), spleen (S) and left kidney (K) are all demonstrated. The patient has a right pelvic kidney.*

A radiolabelled derivative of **octreotide**, ^{111}In-pentatreotide, a synthetic somatostatin analogue, can be used to localize pancreatic endocrine tumours if they express somatostatin receptors (Fig. 5.56).

In practice, in almost all cases, initial imaging is performed with a combination of transabdominal ultrasound and CT or MRI. When these tests are negative or equivocal, arteriography is the next line of investigation. Further investigation depends on local practice and suspected tumour type. Endoscopic ultrasound is rapidly emerging as a technique of high sensitivity. Transhepatic venous sampling and somatostatin receptor imaging have the advantage that they are not dependent on tumour size and are particularly applicable to difficult cases where other imaging modalities are negative.

PANCREATITIS

Pancreatic inflammatory disease can be classified by clinical or pathological criteria into acute or chronic forms. Acute pancreatitis is characterized clinically by the acute onset of abdominal pain and a rise of pancreatic enzymes in the blood. Most patients, although not all, recover without permanent morphological and functional changes in the gland. Chronic pancreatitis is characterized clinically by recurrent or persistent episodes of abdominal pain, usually with evidence of functional pancreatic insufficiency.

ACUTE PANCREATITIS

Imaging has four major roles in patients with acute pancreatitis:
- confirmation of the diagnosis;
- exclusion of other causes of pain where the clinical findings are equivocal;
- assessing the severity of the inflammation;
- the detection of complications.

Imaging

The **plain film** signs associated with acute pancreatitis are discussed on p. 42.

CT is the most sensitive imaging modality for evaluating acute pancreatitis but in very mild cases the pancreas may appear normal. CT is better than ultrasound for detecting the presence of pancreatic necrosis and other complications, and is, therefore, better for predicting the outcome of acute pancreatitis. In most cases the gland is enlarged, the pancreatic contour is irregular and the parenchyma appears inhomogeneous. The peripancreatic fat is usually hazy and shows an increase in density accompanied by fascial thickening (Fig. 5.57). In more severe cases, fluid collections are

Figure 5.57 *Acute phlegmonous pancreatitis. Non-enhanced CT scan in a patient with acute pancreatitis showing swelling of the pancreas and loss of definition of the peripancreatic fat planes. There is extension of the inflammatory process into the left pararenal space (arrows).*

Figure 5.58 *Acute pancreatitis. Post-contrast CT scan showing localized fluid collections within the gland (arrows). Much of the normal gland parenchyma has been preserved.*

seen within the gland and the peripancreatic exudate is more extensive (Fig. 5.58). Phlegmon, consisting of inflammatory exudate, necrotic tissue and blood, is seen on CT as poorly defined, irregularly contoured, solid and fluid elements in the peripancreatic regions (Fig. 5.58). Like transient fluid collections, these are seen first within the lesser sac and in the anterior pararenal space, particularly on the left side. Fluid collections or phlegmon may extend inferiorly along the pararenal spaces, bilaterally continuing inferiorly along the psoas muscle border into the pelvis, and rarely into the thigh. Mesenteric, mesocolic, posterior pararenal space and perirenal space involvement occurs less commonly. Direct mediastinal extension and involvement of the liver and spleen also occur occasionally.

Focal or segmental pancreatitis demonstrates findings similar to acute pancreatitis but is localized to the involved area of the gland, usually the head.

Ultrasound examination of the pancreas may be normal in mild cases of pancreatitis and even occasionally in more severe forms. Its usefulness early in the evaluation of pancreatitis is primarily to exclude other causes of abdominal pain and to identify choledocholithiasis or cholelithiasis. The ultrasound findings are similar to those seen on CT, namely focal or diffuse glandular enlargement which is usually uniformly hypoechoic (Fig. 5.59). Peripancreatic phlegmonous changes result in loss of definition of the pancreatic edge and thickening of the peripancreatic fascial planes. Extrapancreatic fluid collections develop usually within 2–4 weeks after earliest clinical symptoms. They may be anechoic or septate and most resolve within weeks or months. Secondary findings include dilatation of the pancreatic duct, ascites and thickening of the gallbladder and bowel walls.

Figure 5.59 *Acute pancreatitis. Transverse ultrasound scan showing marked swelling of the gland, which contains multiple hypoechoic areas owing to necrosis (arrowed).*

Complications of pancreatitis and grading of severity

CT has been shown to be extremely accurate in grading the severity of acute pancreatitis by detecting the most frequent and important complications which include gland necrosis, pancreatic abscess, fluid collections (including pseudocyst) and vascular, gastrointestinal or biliary tract involvement. The clinical severity of pancreatitis is usually best assessed with Ranson's criteria. Poor correlation exists between CT and Ranson's criteria, probably because CT primarily grades local complications, whereas the Ranson classification evaluates systemic complications.

Figure 5.60 *Acute necrotizing pancreatitis. Contrast medium-enhanced CT scan showing areas of non-enhancing pancreatic parenchyma, with replacement of the pancreas by fluid and abnormal soft tissue.*

Figure 5.61 *Acute infection in necrotizing pancreatitis. CT scan showing multiple large pockets of gas within abnormal soft tissue (arrows) indicating infected necrosis.*

Pancreatic gland necrosis

Necrotizing pancreatitis is a severe form of acute pancreatitis, occurring in 8–15 per cent of patients, characterized by destruction of pancreatic parenchyma, peripancreatic tissues or both. Areas of pancreatic necrosis can be recognized on CT as areas of non-enhancing parenchyma after intravenous injection of a bolus of contrast medium (Fig. 5.60). Non-contrast CT cannot exclude pancreatic necrosis. Differentiating necrotizing from oedematous pancreatitis by ultrasound is not consistently possible. Pancreatic infection is a common complication, occurring in 40 per cent of patients, and is often responsible for the high mortality in these patients. It may be recognized by the appearance of gas bubbles within the necrotic tissue (Fig. 5.61).

Peripancreatic fluid collections

Peripancreatic fluid collections are common and usually develop early in the course of acute pancreatitis. They may be readily detected on ultrasound or CT. Many resolve spontaneously, usually within 6 weeks. Fluid collections which do not resolve within a few weeks tend to become encapsulated by fibrous connective tissue to form pseudocysts. Bacterial infection of a fluid collection will result in an abscess.

Pseudocysts

Pancreatic pseudocysts can be found virtually anywhere in the abdomen and pelvis, and have even been reported extending into the mediastinum, neck, scrotum, groin or lower extremities. They complicate acute pancreatitis in less than 10 per cent of patients and tend to occur in regions most likely to be affected by phlegmonous pancreatitis such as the lesser sac,

perisplenic region and transverse mesocolon. Up to 30 per cent resolve spontaneously, sometimes with spontaneous rupture into the pancreatic duct, stomach or peritoneal cavity. Spontaneous resolution of a cyst over 5 cm or multiple lesions is unlikely.

Signs of pseudocyst formation are seldom seen on plain film as calcification is very unusual. Most pseudocysts of the head and body of the pancreas are readily seen on ultrasound. The wall is smooth and well-defined, and the fluid can be entirely echo-free or have internal echoes or debris. The CT number of the fluid is usually close to 0 HU, but can be as high as 25–30 HU; the wall is usually thin and smooth (Fig. 5.62). When the cyst wall is irregular, thickened and its contents echogenic, the possibility of superimposed haemorrhage or infection should always be considered.

Figure 5.62 *Pseudocyst of the pancreas. Contrast-enhanced CT scan showing a septate fluid-filled pseudocyst of the pancreas (arrows).*

Figure 5.63 *Pancreatic abscess. CT scan showing pockets of air (arrows) within a thick-walled fluid collection within the body and tail of the pancreas due to infection of a pseudocyst.*

Overall, CT is better than ultrasound for depicting pseudocysts, especially those remote from the pancreas. Ultrasound often gives a better display of the internal architecture.

Pancreatic abscess

Pancreatic abscess is a localized collection of pus confined by a wall or rind of inflammatory tissue (Fig. 5.63). It can usually be differentiated easily from infected necrosis on CT, where the inflammatory tissue is not confined (Fig. 5.61). Like other fluid collections, abscesses may be confined to the pancreatic bed or extend beyond the organ, even into the pelvis. The most obvious sign of an abscess is air within the inflammatory mass. This, however, does not constitute absolute evidence of pancreatic abscess, as air within a fluid collection can be secondary to a fistula with the gastrointestinal lumen. Furthermore, a substantial proportion of pancreatic abscesses, probably the majority, do not contain gas.

Vascular complications

Vascular complications of acute pancreatitis include occlusion or thrombosis of the splenic vein or other regional veins, direct arterial erosion or pseudoaneurysm formation. Pseudoaneurysms most commonly arise from the splenic artery, followed by the gastroduodenal artery. On CT, the demonstration of a homogeneously, brightly enhancing structure within or adjacent to a pseudocyst, or contiguous with a vascular structure after injection of contrast medium, is highly suggestive of a pseudoaneurysm. Ultrasound also demonstrates pseudoaneurysms as hypoechoic structures within a larger cystic structure. Turbulent and pulsatile flow is seen on duplex and colour-flow Doppler imaging.

Gastrointestinal complications

Direct extension of inflammation from the pancreas can cause oedema, necrosis or perforation of the wall of the stomach or small bowel. Thrombosis of mesenteric vessels can cause similar changes. CT readily demonstrates these bowel wall changes. Pancreatico-enteric fistulae occur late in the course of pancreatitis, most commonly affecting the splenic flexure. These must be specifically suspected and sought with the use of gastrointestinal contrast studies. As many as 20 per cent of fistulae may not be discovered before surgery. ERCP does not opacify all fistulae. A fistula can be recognized on CT by the presence of oral contrast material or gas within a pancreatic phlegmon.

Common bile duct obstruction

Oedema in the head of the pancreas can cause transient compression of the common bile duct. This complication can be detected in about 6 per cent of patients with acute pancreatitis on ultrasound, CT or ERCP.

CHRONIC PANCREATITIS

Chronic pancreatitis can be considered to have two main morphological forms. The most common type is **chronic calcific pancreatitis**. Less common is **chronic obstructive pancreatitis** resulting from any non-calculous obstructive lesion of the pancreas. The hallmark of chronic calcific pancreatitis on any imaging study is the identification of calculi in the pancreas. **Pancreatic calcifications** develop in close association with progressive pancreatic dysfunction and usually develop five years after onset of chronic pancreatitis in alcoholic chronic pancreatitis. Pancreatic calculi are almost

Figure 5.64 *ERCP in a patient with chronic pancreatitis showing slight dilatation of the main pancreatic duct and impaired filling of the secondary ducts. Calcification of the pancreatic parenchyma (arrows) can also be seen.*

Figure 5.65 *ERCP in chronic pancreatitis showing marked 'beaded' dilatation of the main pancreatic duct, marked dilatation of several of the secondary ducts and non-filling of others.*

always intraductal; true parenchymal calcification is unusual and may occur after haemorrhage or necrosis (Fig. 5.64).

Demonstrating pancreatic calculi on abdominal radiography is the most cost-effective method for confirming chronic calcific pancreatitis as it will depict calculi in 90 per cent of patients when compared with CT.

The three main indications for ERCP in chronic pancreatitis are to establish a diagnosis, to assess pancreatic anatomy and to perform endoscopic therapy. As many as 30 per cent of patients with chronic pancreatitis have a normal pancreaticogram. The earliest identifiable changes are slight ectasia or clubbing of the side branches of the pancreatic duct. Side branch filling may be impaired. The main duct is usually minimally dilated and irregular (Fig. 5.64). Moderate chronic pancreatitis is characterized by dilatation, tortuosity and

stenosis within the main duct, with cystic dilatation and obstruction of branch ducts (Fig. 5.65). Marked chronic pancreatitis is present when both pancreatic duct and side branches are severely involved by dilatation, stenosis or obstruction. In most cases, the entire duct is involved and is usually beaded.

Signs on ultrasound include an enlarged main pancreatic duct (> 4 mm), gland atrophy, echogenic foci within the parenchyma and an irregular contour to the gland, particularly focal enlargement (Fig. 5.66). The diagnostic accuracy of ultrasound is reported to vary between 60 and 80 percent.

Pancreatic duct dilatation, parenchymal atrophy and pancreatic calcifications are the most common CT manifestations of chronic pancreatitis (Fig. 5.66). Fluid collections, focal pancreatic enlargement and biliary duct dilatation also occur. Focal enlargement, which occurs in about 30 per cent of cases of pancreatitis, can be difficult to distinguish from pancreatic malignancy unless calcification is present within the mass; calcifications are extremely uncommon in pancreatic adenocarcinoma. Cysts may also be found within the pancreas.

In the early stages of the disease, there is poor correlation between the radiological changes (as detected by ultrasound, CT and ERCP) and the degree of functional impairment. In the later stages, the correlation is good.

PANCREATIC TRAUMA

Following pancreatic trauma, CT may demonstrate diffuse focal swelling of the gland with or without

(a)

(b)

Figure 5.66 *Chronic pancreatitis. (a) CT scan showing marked dilatation of the pancreatic duct (arrows) with calculi within the duct (curved arrow). There is also marked atrophy of the pancreatic parenchyma. (b) Ultrasound scan on the same patient showing dilatation of the pancreatic duct (arrows) and parenchymal atrophy. An echogenic calculus can be seen within the duct (curved arrow).*

regional streaky inflammatory changes in the peripancreatic fat, anterior pararenal space, lesser sac or mesentery. A fracture may sometimes be identified. Trauma to the spleen, liver, gallbladder, bile ducts, duodenum and adrenal gland may be visible. Late sequelae of pancreatic trauma include pseudocysts, fistulae and abscesses. All of these findings can usually be demonstrated on CT. ERCP may be used on an emergency basis for the diagnosis of suspected pancreatic ductal rupture. It is more sensitive and specific for ductal rupture than combinations of CT, peritoneal lavage and serum amylase.

CONGENITAL ABNORMALITIES OF PANCREAS

A variety of congenital abnormalities of the pancreas can be demonstrated on imaging. CT may show the duodenum partially or completely encircled by an annular pancreas. An ERCP can be used to confirm the diagnosis by demonstrating a segment of pancreatic duct encircling the duodenum. Ectopic islands of pancreatic tissue are most commonly located in the wall of the stomach or duodenum. The diagnosis is usually made incidentally during barium examination, which shows a smooth, submucosal nodule. In patients with autosomal dominant adult polycystic disease of the kidney, cysts may be demonstrated in the pancreas on ultrasound or CT. In von Hippel–Lindau disease cystic pancreatic neoplasms may be seen in the pancreas.

CYSTIC FIBROSIS OF THE PANCREAS

The pathological changes of fibrosis, fatty replacement, calcification and cyst formation in the pancreatic ductules are all reflected as an increased echogenicity of the pancreas that is usually markedly increased for age on ultrasound. The usual CT picture is fatty replacement depicted as a normal pancreatic contour with decreased attenuation values in the range of fat. Pancreatic cysts are occasionally seen.

SPLEEN

IMAGING TECHNIQUES

ULTRASOUND

The normal echo pattern of the spleen is evenly distributed echoes, similar but slightly greater than the liver. The size and shape of the spleen, the position of the hilum and its relationship to adjacent organs (diaphragm, stomach, pancreas, left kidney) can all be identified. Often the splenic vein can be identified in the hilum.

Ultrasound is useful for detecting and characterizing focal lesions within the spleen as cystic or solid, and can be used to estimate splenic size and volume. Colour Doppler ultrasound is useful for demonstrating the splenic artery and vein; this can be helpful in differentiating vascular structures, such as normal vessels or aneurysms, from non-vascular structures, such as pancreatic pseudocysts. Rapid measurements of splenic volume can be made, which is useful when following splenic size.

CT SCANNING

Computed tomography is exquisite in its ability to demonstrate the size, shape and location of the normal spleen, and in demonstrating focal intrasplenic abnormalities. Technical artefacts may result from motion or unusual enhancement. The density of the spleen on CT is usually close to that of liver and has a normal range of 35–55 HU. The splenic hilum and its relations are well visualized. The posterior surface of the spleen abutting the pleural space is called the 'bare area' and has a constant relation to Gerota's fascia. The significant variation in the size, shape and position of the spleen is well shown on CT. Enhancement with intravenous contrast medium is generally indicated when looking for splenic disease and results in dense enhancement of the normal spleen within 2 minutes after injection.

MAGNETIC RESONANCE IMAGING

MRI can equal, if not surpass, other modalities in the detection of focal splenic lesions, provided rapid scanning techniques combined with compensation for respiratory and cardiac motion (with or without contrast agents) are used.

RADIONUCLIDE IMAGING

^{99m}Tc-sulphur or tin colloid scanning of the spleen for the detection of focal abnormalities has largely been replaced by cross-sectional imaging such as ultrasound, CT and MRI. Gallium citrate scanning may be helpful in investigating inflammatory conditions.

ANGIOGRAPHY

Selective catheterization and injection of contrast medium into the coeliac axis or splenic artery provides excellent visualization of the arteries, and delayed images show the splenic and portal veins. In many patients it is possible to show the main splenic artery and normal splenic and portal veins using **intravenous digital subtraction angiography. Splenoportography**, achieved by injecting contrast medium through a cannula or needle introduced percutaneously into the splenic pulp, has now become obsolete.

SPLENIC NEOPLASMS

BENIGN NEOPLASMS OF SPLEEN

Splenic haemangioma

Haemangiomas are the most common benign splenic neoplasms and have similar appearances to liver haemangiomas. On ultrasound, they are usually hyperechoic and calcification may cause bright echoes with acoustic shadowing. On CT, the lesion is hypodense before contrast and then, like liver haemangioma, 'fills in' after intravenous contrast medium (Fig. 5.67). In patients presenting acutely with rupture of a splenic haemangioma, CT may show perisplenic or intraperitoneal blood.

Hamartoma (splenoma, splenoadenoma, nodular hyperplasia of the spleen)

To date the ultrasound and CT appearances do not allow differentiation from haemangiomata.

MALIGNANT NEOPLASMS OF SPLEEN

Lymphoma

Splenic lymphoma is usually a manifestation of generalized lymphoma and is the most common splenic malignancy. Primary splenic lymphoma is rare and comprises

(a)

(b)

(c)

Figure 5.67 *Splenic haemangioma. (a) CT scan taken during intravenous injection of contrast medium showing a well-defined focal abnormality. (b) Scan taken after a delay of 3 minutes showing progressive enhancement of the margins of the lesion. (c) After 10 minutes further 'filling in' of the lesion is seen confirming the presence of a haemangioma.*

(a)

(b)

Figure 5.68 *Non-Hodgkin's lymphoma of the spleen. (a) A longitudinal ultrasound scan of the liver showing multiple large inhomogeneous areas of abnormal echogenicity (arrows). (b) CT scan on the same patient showing the same focal abnormalities owing to infiltration by non-Hodgkin's lymphoma.*

only 2 per cent of all lymphoma. Laparotomy with splenectomy reveals splenic involvement at presentation in 23–34 per cent of patients with Hodgkin's disease and 30–40 per cent of patients with non-Hodgkin's lymphoma. CT is the primary technique for diagnosing splenic lymphoma, evaluating the volume and extent of the tumour and monitoring response. However, CT is relatively insensitive for the detection of splenic involvement, partly because 45–70 per cent of splenic tumours manifest with either diffuse tumour infiltration or tumour foci well under a centimetre in size.

The ultrasound, CT or MRI appearance of splenic lymphoma includes homogeneous enlargement without a discrete mass, a solitary mass, multifocal lesions, and diffuse infiltration. A poor correlation exists between the size of the spleen and the presence of splenic lymphoma. Splenomegaly does not always indicate involvement and a normal-sized spleen does not exclude disease. The majority of focal lesions are hypoechoic on ultrasound and of decreased density on CT before and after intravenous injection of contrast medium (Fig. 5.68). Diffuse infiltration may be seen as diffusely low echogenicity on ultrasound and diffusely low attenuation on CT before injection of contrast medium, and irregular enhancement after contrast medium. Infarction of the spleen is not uncommon and wedge-shaped peripheral areas of low CT attenuation may, therefore, be seen.

Non-lymphatous tumours and metastases

The rare, primary, benign and malignant splenic tumours including angiosarcoma, lymphangioma, malignant fibrous histiocytoma, leiomyosarcoma and fibrosarcoma, all show a non-specific cystic, solid or complex mass.

Splenic metastases are found at autopsy in 7 per cent of patients with malignancy but are seen relatively uncommonly on imaging. They occur most frequently from the breast, lung, ovary, stomach, cutaneous melanoma and prostate. The ultrasound appearance of metastases varies greatly: they may be hypoechoic or hyperechoic. Cystic splenic metastases are seen typically in patients with melanoma, or primary tumours in the ovary, breast and endometrium (Fig. 5.69). Occasion-

Figure 5.69 *Cystic splenic deposits. Contrast medium-enhanced CT scan showing multiple cystic lesions in the spleen in patient with disseminated malignant melanoma.*

Figure 5.70 *Spontaneous rupture due to splenic deposit. Unenhanced CT scan showing high attenuation within the spleen owing to a spontaneous bleed in a patient with disseminated breast cancer. Removal of the spleen revealed the presence of a deposit within it.*

Figure 5.71 *Splenic abscess. CT scan performed after intravenous injection of contrast medium showing a large fluid-filled abscess with an air–fluid level anteriorly (arrows).*

ally splenic metastases may present with a spontaneous splenic haemorrhage (Fig. 5.70). No correlation exists between the ultrasound features of metastases and the type of primary tumour. Lesions are more commonly multifocal than solitary. On CT, metastases are typically areas of slightly decreased attenuation in relation to normal spleen.

INFECTIONS OF SPLEEN

BACTERIAL ABSCESS

The frequency of splenic abscess has recently increased because of a rising number of immunocompromised people. Complications such as rupture and subsequent subphrenic abscess and peritonitis may result from delayed diagnosis. CT is currently the diagnostic method of choice because of its high sensitivity (up to 96 per cent), non-invasiveness, applicability in unstable patients and value in allowing accurate localization of the lesion in relation to contiguous viscera. Bacterial abscess is frequently seen as a low-attenuation centre of fluid with peripheral contrast enhancement once a capsule has developed. The presence of gas within the fluid collection is diagnostic of abscess, although the majority of splenic abscesses do not contain air (Fig. 5.71). A splenic abscess may contain septa of various thicknesses. Ultrasonography may be technically difficult because of an ileus, overlying ribs and perisplenic fluid, but has the advantage that it can be performed at the bedside if necessary.

The ultrasound appearance depends on the stage of development. Initially there is an ill-defined mass of decreased echogenicity, which may develop into a complex lesion with septations, debris and border nodularity. When a capsule has developed, the lesion is well-defined with a thick hyperechoic rim.

FUNGAL ABSCESS

Fungal abscesses occur almost exclusively in immunocompromised individuals. Candida is the most frequent followed by Aspergillus and Cryptococcus. Because the lesions are often very small, fungal abscesses in neutropenic patients are not always detectable on imaging. On ultrasound they have a typical 'bulls-eye' appearance with bright central echogenic areas surrounded by a hyperechoic periphery (Fig. 5.72). On CT, typical lesions are smaller than 2 cm in diameter and are of relatively low attenuation (Fig. 5.72). Ring-like enhancement may be seen with contrast-enhanced CT on MR imaging. The appearance of *Pneumocystis carinii* infection can produce similar, multiple, small focal abnormalities early in the disease. With time, calcification may develop, often within a few months.

In patients with AIDS, the differential diagnosis of low-density lesions in the spleen includes fungal or mycobacterial infection, lymphoma or disseminated Kaposi's sarcoma.

SPLENIC TRAUMA

Splenic trauma may follow blunt or penetrating injuries and may be spontaneous or iatrogenic. In cases of blunt

(a)

(b)

Figure 5.72 *Fungal abscesses within the spleen. (a) Contrast-enhanced scan in a patient with leukaemia showing multiple minute low-density foci within the spleen (arrows) owing to candidal abscesses. (b) Longitudinal ultrasound of the spleen in the same patient showing multiple hypoechoic foci corresponding to the candidal abscesses (arrows).*

abdominal trauma, the spleen is the most commonly injured organ. Splenic injuries have been classified in a variety of ways, but a useful scheme is:

- contusion
- subcapsular haematoma
- parenchymal injury with small capsular tear
- rupture with haemoperitoneum

The need for imaging depends on the severity of the injury. Patients who are haemodynamically unstable are taken directly to laparotomy. Patients who are stable with suspected splenic injury should undergo CT as CT can be more than 95 per cent accurate in identifying splenic injury. If CT is done after peritoneal lavage, it will be unclear whether the intraperitoneal fluid is from the initial trauma or the lavage. Thus if CT is to be used, peritoneal lavage should be delayed or omitted. Furthermore, haemoperitoneum can be diagnosed radiologically and the severity and extent of other organ injuries assessed.

Plain film findings are necessary primarily to look for evidence of intraperitoneal or retroperitoneal air, pneumothorax and other injuries. When bleeding is

(a)

(b)

Figure 5.73 *Splenic trauma. (a) Precontrast CT scan showing high density soft tissue consistent with haematoma within the spleen, in the subcapsular region and in the extracapsular space (arrow). Ascites is also present around the liver. (b) After intravenous injection of contrast medium there is gross disruption of the splenic architecture with pools of contrast medium extravasating in the subcapsular haematoma (arrows). Non-enhancement of portions of the spleen is due to devascularization.*

confined to the parenchyma or subcapsular region, a plain film may show splenic enlargement with resultant displacement of the stomach. The presence of rib fracture(s), pleural effusion or severe gastric dilatation should raise the possibility of significant splenic injury.

On **CT**, subcapsular haematomas are seen as peripheral low density lesions that flatten the contour of the spleen. Lacerations produce low-density bands across the splenic substance. Lacerations tend to involve the lateral aspect of the spleen and are associated with free intraperitoneal fluid. Splenic rupture may be seen as fragmentation of three or more sections of devascularized (non-enhanced) spleen (Fig. 5.73).

Although CT has now become established as the primary means of evaluating splenic trauma in the stable patient, it is not a useful predictor of outcome after splenic trauma, presumably because it fails to quantify active haemorrhage as opposed to inactive, old blood. Nevertheless, part of its value lies in the fact that a normal CT scan virtually excludes significant splenic injury.

Figure 5.74 *Epitheloid ('true') cyst of the spleen. Longitudinal reconstruction of a contrast-enhanced CT scan showing a typically large epitheloid splenic cyst with scalloping of the splenic margin.*

SPLENIC CYSTS

Splenic cysts represent a heterogenous group of lesions and include cystic neoplasms, parasitic cysts, 'true' and 'false' cysts. True cysts, also called primary, epithelial, epidermoid or congenital cysts, contain an epithelial lining, and false or pseudocysts are without an epithelial lining. False cysts are probably post-traumatic in origin and may be haemorrhagic or serous.

Plain films may show a left upper quadrant mass with elevation of the left hemidiaphragm with left lower lobe atelectasis. Curvilinear or plaque-like calcification may be present on plain abdominal films, more commonly in post-traumatic than true cysts. Ultrasound shows the usual features of a cyst. If haemorrhagic, ultrasound may demonstrate layering of two fluids within the cyst. Trabeculation may be seen. True cysts are well seen on CT (Fig. 5.74) and the differential diagnosis includes echinococcal cysts (which are usually multiseptated), large solitary abscess, haematoma, cystic neoplasm or an intrasplenic pancreatic pseudocyst.

FURTHER READING

Dachman, A.H., Friedman, A.C. 1993: *Radiology of the spleen*. St Louis, MO: Mosby-Year Book Inc.

Friedman, A.C., Dachman, A.H. 1994: *Radiology of the liver, biliary tract and pancreas*. St Louis, MO: Mosby-Year Book Inc.

Gazelle, G.S., Saini, S., Mueller P.R. (eds) 1998: *Hepatobiliary and pancreatic radiology. Imaging and intervention*. New York, Stuttgart: Thième.

Ros, P.R. (ed.) 1998: Hepatic imaging: an overview. *Radiologic Clinics of North America* **36**: 237–46.

Adrenal glands

RODNEY H. REZNEK

IMAGING TECHNIQUES

COMPUTED TOMOGRAPHY

CT, because of its very high accuracy, has assumed the primary role in imaging the adrenal glands. A complete study of the adrenal gland involves narrow collimation (3 or 5 mm) scans through the adrenal gland both before and after intravenous injection of a bolus of contrast medium. Contrast medium will help to separate the adrenal glands from adjacent vessels and to assess the nature of an adrenal mass.

MAGNETIC RESONANCE IMAGING

Magnetic resonance imaging offers multiplanar imaging with better contrast resolution than CT or ultrasound and does not use ionizing radiation. It can now achieve spatial resolution close to that of CT. Imaging in the coronal and sagittal plane helps to determine invasion into adjacent structures by large mass lesions. Chemical shift imaging sequences can be performed to distinguish benign cortical adenomas from other adrenal mass lesions. Paramagnetic contrast agents can be administered intravenously to assess the vascularity of a lesion.

With continued development in hardware technology and imaging sequences, MRI may become the technology of choice in most cases of adrenal pathology.

ULTRASOUND

Ultrasound can demonstrate most adrenal masses over 2 cm, but has far lower accuracy than CT or MRI, especially in obese patients.

RADIOPHARMACEUTICALS

Radiolabelled analogues of cholesterol such as ^{75}Se-$^{6}\beta$-selenomethylnorcholesterol are used in the depiction and localization of adrenal cortical function. Appropriate imaging time intervals are dictated by the particular disease process under study and may require the addition of dexamethasone suppression studies of adrenal cortical function. Meta-iodobenzylguanidine (MIBG), an analogue of guanethidine, is concentrated in sympathoadrenal tissue. Studies with ^{131}I- and ^{123}I-MIBG take advantage of the ability to screen the whole body for sympathomedullary function. Imaging is performed 1–3 days following administration of the radiopharmaceuticals. Numerous drugs such as reserpine, tricyclic and antidepressants and others interfere with the uptake of iodocholesterol into the adrenal cortex and MIBG into the sympathoadrenergic tissues, and must be avoided.

VENOUS SAMPLING

Venous sampling is extremely accurate in the preoperative localization of the source of abnormal hormone secretion. It is, however, an invasive procedure that is technically difficult to perform and necessitates long fluoroscopy times and consequently entails high radiation exposures. The technique usually requires hospitalization. Because of these disadvantages and the availability of less invasive procedures, venous sampling is best reserved for equivocal cases. Nevertheless, adrenal venous sampling is still used and is extremely accurate in the preoperative evaluation of primary aldosteronism. Whole body venous sampling is used in defining the source of ACTH-dependent Cushing's syndrome, ectopic sources of catecholamine excess and abnormal function in virilization syndromes.

PERCUTANEOUS BIOPSY

The accuracy of percutaneous adrenal biopsy ranges from 80 to 90 per cent. Sonography can be used for imaging guidance if the adrenal mass and adjacent organs are sufficiently well demonstrated, but usually CT provides the best anatomical imaging for guidance. The most common complications are pneumothorax

and haemorrhage. The major risk is biopsy of an unsuspected phaeochromocytoma, as a catecholamine storm following biopsy can be a life-threatening complication and is fatal in 50 per cent of unsuspected phaeochromocytomas. The potential risk of this happening is high, since only 50 per cent of patients with phaeochromocytomas have paroxysmal hypertensive episodes and 14 per cent may have atypical or absent signs.

NORMAL RADIOLOGICAL ANATOMY

The adrenal glands are enclosed within the perinephric fascia and are usually surrounded by a sufficient amount of fat for identification on CT or MRI (Fig. 6.1). The right adrenal gland lies immediately posterior to the IVC, between the right crus of the diaphragm medially and the right lobe of the liver laterally. The left adrenal gland lies lateral to the aorta and the left crus of the diaphragm, anteromedial to the upper pole of the left kidney and posterior to the pancreas and splenic vessels. The adrenals normally extend over 2–4 cm in the craniocaudad direction. The shape of the adrenals can vary, depending on the orientation of the gland and the level of the image. The limbs of the adrenal gland have a uniform thickness and, on any cross-section, the normal thickness of these limbs, perpendicular to their long axes, does not exceed 4 mm, except at the apex of the gland where these limbs converge.

Demonstrating the normal adrenal glands and small adrenal lesions remains difficult on ultrasound, despite the introduction of high-resolution, real-time scanners.

(a)

(b)

Figure 6.1 *(a) T1-weighted MRI scan showing normal left adrenal gland (arrow). (b) T1-weighted MRI scan showing normal right adrenal gland (arrows) lying posterior to the inferior vena cava.*

These small organs are high in location, deep within the rib cage, adjacent to the vertebrae, and are thus easily obscured by bone shadow and by stomach and bowel gas on ultrasound.

ADRENAL CORTICAL HYPERFUNCTION

Adrenal cortical hyperfunction includes primary hyperaldosteronism, Cushing's syndrome and androgen-producing lesions of the adrenal.

CONN'S SYNDROME (PRIMARY HYPERALDOSTERONISM)

In 79 per cent of cases, a benign cortical adenoma will be responsible for primary hyperaldosteronism; in 20 per cent, the cause will be bilateral adrenal hyperplasia and very rarely an adrenocortical carcinoma will be responsible. As surgery should be considered for adenomas and bilateral hyperplasia is best treated medically, the distinction between these causes is extremely important. Imaging plays an important role in making this distinction.

Adrenal CT scanning is highly effective for the localization of small **adrenocortical adenomas**, which tend to be small, with an average size of approximately 1.6 cm, and of much lower density than the surrounding adrenal tissue (−18 HU to +13 HU), due to a high content of cytoplasmic lipid (Fig. 6.2a). These adenomas do not enhance significantly after intravenous injection of contrast medium and rarely calcify. As about 15–20 per cent of aldosteronomas are micronodules, measuring less than 1 cm, meticulous examination technique is required to detect them, including very narrow collimation and magnification. The sensitivity of CT for detecting these small adenomas has improved markedly in recent years and currently about 90 per cent of tumours will be detected. False-negative results arise when micronodules are missed. Conversely, CT cannot distinguish between aldosteronomas, macronodules in nodular hyperplasia and non-functioning adenomas, especially when the lesion is solitary. Nevertheless, false-positive results are infrequent, because the chance of a solitary adrenal mass in normal-sized glands, visualized by CT in the appropriate clinical and biochemical setting, being something other than an aldosteronoma, is extremely low. Similarly, although a macronodule in nodular hyperplasia can cause confusion, postural plasma aldosterone and 18-hydroxycorticosterone tests will provide an indication as to whether the patient has idiopathic hyperplasia or an adrenal adenoma.

Available data suggest that MRI is as sensitive and specific as CT in identifying adrenal adenomas in patients with hyperaldosteronism. Most adenomas appear slightly hypointense or isointense relative to the liver on T1-weighted images (Fig. 6.2b) and slightly hyperintense or isointense relative to hepatic parenchyma on T2 images. MRI has little advantage over CT in the evaluation of adrenal hyperplasia or in the identification of hyperfunctioning cortical adenomas, which are best evaluated with thinly collimated CT sections.

The adrenal gland can be functionally characterized in primary aldosteronism using adrenal scintigraphy

(a)   (b)

Figure 6.2 *Conn's tumour (a) CT scan after intravenous injection of contrast medium showing a small, low-density, non-enhancing mass in the right adrenal gland (arrow). (b) T1-weighted MRI scan showing the same small mass of low signal intensity (arrow).*

with a cholesterol-based radiopharmaceutical and dexamethasone suppression. This technique will distinguish between a unilateral adenoma and bilateral hyperplasia (Plate 4, opposite page 358). As with CT, the sensitivity of the technique is dependent partly on the size of the adenoma, and its accuracy compares unfavourably with that of CT. Because of this, and also because the procedure is time-consuming and expensive, it is seldom used as the initial investigation in patients with Conn's syndrome, except in cases considered equivocal on CT.

Venous sampling, when successful, is the most accurate means of localizing aldosteronomas. However, even in experienced hands, failure to catheterize the right adrenal vein occurs in 10–30 per cent of cases. In those cases successfully catheterized, a sensitivity approaching 100 per cent and a positive predictive value of 90 per cent has been achieved. However, complications of the procedure are not infrequent and include adrenal infarction, adrenal vein thrombosis or perforation and intra-adrenal haemorrhage. Hypotensive crises and adrenal insufficiency may result.

In most institutions, in practice, CT is considered sufficiently accurate for localizing cortical adenomas to proceed to surgery without any further investigation, especially when the CT appearance is clear-cut and correlates with all the biochemistry. Venous sampling is reserved for those cases in which:

- the adrenal glands appear normal on CT (as a micronodule may be undetected);
- there are bilateral nodules on CT scans that may be due to nodular hyperplasia or multiple adenomata;
- there is disagreement between the CT findings and the biochemistry.

CUSHING'S SYNDROME

Biochemical studies, including determination of plasma ACTH levels and response to high-dose dexamethasone suppression, are used to distinguish between Cushing's disease, ectopic ACTH-producing tumours and cortisol-producing adrenal neoplasms. While these tests are usually successful in making this distinction, difficulties in interpretation can arise. The purpose of imaging is to localize or exclude an adrenal mass and, when the biochemical tests point to an ectopic source of ACTH, to identify the source. In 75 per cent of cases, Cushing's syndrome results from an excess of ACTH production, of which about 80 per cent is due to a pituitary abnormality (Cushing's disease) and the remainder is due to an ectopic source. In 25 per cent of cases the syndrome is due to excess cortisol from an adrenal neoplasm, more commonly an adenoma than a carcinoma. **Adrenal cortical adenomas** resulting in Cushing's syndrome are usually over 2.0 cm and are thus readily

detected on any cross-sectional technique. On CT, these masses are of soft-tissue density, although occasionally they show lower density due to a high fat content. The mass may enhance after intravenous injection of contrast medium (Fig. 6.3).

Adenomas over 2 cm may well be demonstrated on ultrasound (Fig. 6.3). The ultrasound reflectivity of adenomas is low compared to the high reflectivity of the surrounding fat. A right adrenal mass typically compresses the inferior vena cava or displaces it forward, and may indent the inferior surface of the liver. Whilst all tumours are usually homogeneous, heterogeneous reflectivity due to focal areas of necrosis or haemorrhage may be seen in larger masses.

MRI also readily identifies functioning adrenal adenomas and, because of their relatively large size, identifies them with similar sensitivity to CT. As with adenomas in Conn's syndrome, functioning adenomas are usually of low signal intensity relative to the liver on T1-weighted images and isointense or hyperintense relative to the liver on T2-weighted images (Fig. 6.3).

On all imaging techniques, the contralateral gland appears normal but, rarely it may appear atrophic due to the suppression of ACTH.

Imaging with cholesterol-based radiopharmaceuticals is not usually performed except where the diagnosis is problematical. The usual pattern then is of unilateral activity in the functioning adenoma with virtual absence of uptake of the radiopharmaceutical in the contralateral gland.

Adrenal carcinomas account for 10–15% of cases of Cushing's syndrome (Fig. 6.4), almost always exceed 6 cm at the time of presentation and are readily detected on ultrasound, CT or MRI. Only about 15 per cent of carcinomas are over 6 cm in diameter. Ultrasound can be extremely useful in distinguishing between a primary adrenal or renal mass, because it is easy to scan in the longitudinal plane (Figs 6.4a,b), the optimal plane for making this distinction. On CT, adrenal tumours are usually heterogeneous with areas of high and low density, which enhance patchily after intravenous enhancement of contrast medium (Fig. 6.4c). On MRI they are also usually inhomogeneous on T1- and T2-weighted images, showing areas of low and high signal intensity on both sequences (Figs. 6.4d,e). Invasion of adjacent viscera such as the liver and venous structures is common. All three techniques can readily evaluate extension of thrombus into the inferior vena cava, although MRI most accurately predicts the true extent of the involvement of the entire inferior vena cava, including the intra- and infrahepatic portions. Direct involvement of the adjacent lymph nodes and extension into the liver and adjacent bones is equally well assessed on CT or MRI.

There is usually no uptake of cholesterol-based radiopharmaceutical by adrenal cortical carcinoma. Very rarely, a well differentiated carcinoma may show

(a)

(b)

(c)

(d)

Figure 6.3 *Functioning adrenal adenoma. (a) Longitudinal ultrasound scan showing a well-defined hypoechoic mass (arrows) easily separated from the upper pole of the right kidney. (b) CT scan after intravenous injection of contrast medium showing the right adrenal mass (arrow). (c) T1-weighted MRI scan showing the adrenal mass of low signal intensity (arrows). (d) Longitudinal T2-weighted MRI scan showing the adrenal mass of intermediate signal intensity.*

uptake, but in clinical practice, failure of uptake by a large adrenal mass in a patient with or without Cushing's disease is good evidence of a malignancy.

The differential diagnosis for an adrenal mass in a patient with Cushing's syndrome includes a functioning adenoma, a carcinoma, a metastasis from an ACTH-producing primary carcinoma elsewhere in the body, an incidental non-cortisol-producing adenoma, or even an ACTH-producing phaeochromocytoma.

The adrenals in ACTH-dependent Cushing's syndrome become hyperplastic pathologically. In about one third of patients, hyperplastic adrenal glands look normal on CT or MRI. In some, the gland appears smoothly enlarged, with preservation of the normal contours of the gland. When there is nodular hyperplasia pathologically, a nodular configuration may be seen together with the diffuse enlargement on CT or MRI. Multiple nodules of varying size are usually seen but infrequently one of the nodules becomes dominant, reaching up to 4–5 cm in size and can be misdiagnosed as a unilateral adenoma, especially if the biochemical findings are equivocal.

There is a rare cause of Cushing's syndrome – **primary, pigmented nodular cortical disease** – in which multiple small nodules demonstrated on imaging, produce cortisol autonomously in the absence of elevated ACTH levels. This condition is indistinguishable on CT or MRI from secondary nodular hyperplasia.

Figure 6.4 *Adrenal carcinoma. (a) Longitudinal ultrasound scan showing a large inhomogeneous right suprarenal mass (arrows). (b) Longitudinal ultrasound scan through the inferior vena cava showing tumour extending into the inferior vena cava (arrows) above the level of the entry of the middle hepatic vein (A). (c) CT scan after intravenous injection of contrast medium showing the right suprarenal mass extending into the inferior vena cava (arrows). (d) MRI axial T2-weighted image showing the suprarenal mass of mixed signal intensity extending into the inferior vena cava (arrows). (e) MRI longitudinal T1-weighted image showing thrombus within the IVC (arrows) extending above the level of the diaphragm into the right atrium.*

Primary macronodular hyperplasia is the rarest of the nodular adrenal syndromes associated with hypercortisolaemia. The adrenals are replaced by multiple large nodules that distort the normal adrenal shape. Occasionally on CT or MRI, the hyperplasia is diffuse.

ANDROGEN-PRODUCING TUMOURS

The role of imaging techniques in the evaluation of patients with virilism centres on the detection or exclusion of a tumour, or other surgically curable sources of

Figure 6.5 *Congenital adrenal hyperplasia. CT scan after intravenous injection of contrast medium showing massive bilateral adrenal enlargement (arrows).*

Figure 6.6 *Neuroblastoma. CT scan after intravenous injection of contrast medium showing a large inhomogeneous mass originating in the left adrenal, extending across the midline and encasing the splenic (arrow) and hepatic (curved arrow) arteries. Calcification is demonstrated (open arrows).*

androgen excess, in the adrenals, ovaries or testes. Androgen-producing tumours of the adrenals are rare; they are usually carcinomas, adenomas being less common. They usually exceed 2 cm in diameter and have the same characteristics described elsewhere for adenomas and carcinomas.

The commonest adrenal cause of excess androgens is **congenital adrenocortical hyperplasia,** usually the result of an inborn enzyme deficiency causing a partial block in adrenocortical steroids synthesis. The compensatory elevation of ACTH results in gross enlargement of the adrenals, easily recognizable on CT or MRI (Fig. 6.5). The adrenals, particularly when imaged in older patients, are likely to be so large as to simulate adrenal mass lesions.

CT has a limited role in the localization of extraadrenal sources of virilizing syndromes because of the ionizing radiation dose to the gonads of patients who are often young. MRI is the best technique to image both the adrenal glands and the ovaries.

NEUROBLASTOMA

Neuroblastoma is one of the most common tumours of childhood with 80 per cent occurring in children under 5 years of age and a third under 2 years; 50–80 per cent arise in the adrenal medulla, but the posterior mediastinum is the second most common site. Up to three quarters have metastases at the time of presentation.

Ultrasound almost always demonstrates a mass which must be distinguished from other causes of abdominal masses such as a nephroblastoma. Neuroblastomas are typically heterogeneous on ultrasound with areas of high reflectivity which represent calcification. The margins of the tumour are usually ill-defined. Neuroblastomas often cross the midline and encase the coeliac and superior mesenteric vessels. Ultrasound is usually the first investigation but is often limited in showing the exact extent of the mass. It is, however, particularly valuable in monitoring the response of the tumour to chemotherapy.

On CT, the tumour is recognized as an irregular, pararenal soft-tissue mass which is lobulated, but has no definable rim or pseudocapsule (Fig. 6.6). On noncontrast enhanced scans, the mass usually has a density lower than that of surrounding tissues. Intravenous administration of contrast medium accentuates this difference. Calcification within the tumour, which can be coarse, mottled, solid or ring-shaped, can be observed in almost 85 per cent of neuroblastomas on CT, whereas plain radiographs identify calcification in only 50 per cent of patients. Prevertebral extension across the midline, which occurs in up to 60 per cent of patients, is well demonstrated, as are encasement of the aorta and inferior vena cava, hepatic metastases and renal invasion.

On MRI, neuroblastoma has a low signal intensity relative to hepatic parenchyma on T1-weighted sequences, which increases relative to the liver on T2-weighting. Tumour heterogeneity is best demonstrated on T2-weighted sequences, and reflects calcification and necrosis. MRI is superior to CT in defining vascular encasement, hepatic metastases and particularly intraspinal extension through the intervertebral foramina, which occurs in 15 per cent of patients. MRI is thus currently the most accurate imaging method for staging the extent of the disease.

Neuroblastomas may also take up MIBG; in a small group of patients this can be shown to be more accurate than CT or MRI, usually by showing bony metastases.

GANGLIONEUROBLASTOMA AND GANGLIONEUROMA

Ganglioneuroblastoma is a malignant tumour comprised of both primitive and differentiated cells; it may be totally or partially encapsulated. Ganglioneuroma is a benign tumour that is well circumscribed and consists entirely of ganglion cells. Both appear as soft-tissue masses with flecks of calcification. Differentiation of the various types of ganglion tumours requires tissue sampling.

PHAEOCHROMOCYTOMA

Phaeochromocytoma (also termed adrenal paraganglionoma) is a catecholamine-producing tumour which arises from the paraganglion cells. These cells are derived from the neural crest in close association with the autonomic ganglion cells, and paraganglionomas may thus arise anywhere from the neck to the bladder; 98 per cent, however, originate in the abdomen and 90 percent arise in the adrenal medulla. Most extra-adrenal phaeochromocytomas arise in the paravertebral sympathetic ganglia, in the aortic bifurcation, and rarely in the bladder. Neuroectodermal disorders such as neurofibromatosis, tuberous sclerosis, von Hippel–Lindau syndrome or multiple endocrine neoplastic syndrome are associated with 10 per cent of phaeochromocytomas. Multiplicity and malignancy, each of which occur in about 10 per cent of cases, are more frequent when phaeochromocytomas occur in association with other diseases. Malignancy is also more frequent when the tumour is extra-adrenal. Tumours are more frequently non-functioning when extra-adrenal and when present as part of a systemic disorder. About 90 per cent of adrenal medullary phaeochromocytomas are functional, whereas only

(a)

(b)

(c)

Figure 6.7 *Phaeochromocytoma. (a) Longitudinal ultrasound scan showing an inhomogeneous right-sided suprarenal mass (arrows). (b) CT scan after intravenous injection of contrast medium showing enhancement of the periphery of the lesion (arrows) with central necrosis. A small phaeochromocytoma is seen on the contralateral side (open arrow). (c) Longitudinal T2-weighted MRI scan showing typical high signal intensity in bilobed suprarenal mass.*

50 per cent of sympathetic and 1 per cent of parasympathetic tumours are functional.

On **ultrasound scanning** phaeochromocytomas are typically well-defined, round or ovoid masses with uniform reflectivity (Fig. 6.7a). Large tumours frequently undergo necrosis or haemorrhage with loss of homogeneity. The accuracy of ultrasound for detecting phaeochromocytomas is less than CT, MRI or MIBG scintigraphy, particularly for detecting small masses in the left adrenal gland or ectopic masses in the retroperitoneum where the ultrasound beam can be obscured by bowel gas.

On **CT**, in sporadic cases of phaeochromocytomas, unassociated with any syndrome, over 90 per cent of masses will exceed 2 cm, with an average size of 5 cm. The lesions are often smaller when detected in patients with multiple endocrine abnormalities as they are often specifically sought. On unenhanced scans, these tumours are of similar density to surrounding soft-tissue structures. Calcification, usually speckled, occurs in about 12 per cent of tumours. The hallmark of phaeochromocytomas is intense enhancement after intravenous injection of a bolus of contrast medium. Not infrequently, the tumours undergo marked necrosis so that the mass may have a fluid-filled centre (Fig. 6.7b). Nevertheless, marked enhancement of a peripheral soft-tissue part of the mass can usually be shown. As intravenous injection of contrast medium can precipitate a hypertensive crisis in some patients, α-adrenergic blockade is routine prior to performing the CT. The overall accuracy of CT for detecting adrenal phaeochromocytomas is very high with sensitivities ranging from 93 to 100 per cent, and a positive predictive value exceeding 90 per cent. This exceeds the accuracy of CT for detecting extra-adrenal paraganglionomas.

Meta-iodobenzylguanidine (MIBG) is an analogue of noradrenaline used for sympathoadrenal imaging. Paraganglionomas, including phaeochromocytomas, are depicted as abnormal focal collections of activity. [123]I- or ^{131}I-MIBG scintigraphy is especially useful for the detection of ectopic phaeochromocytomas and also for detecting metastatic or locally recurrent disease because, unlike ultrasound, CT or MRI, it is inherently a whole body imaging technique. The sensitivity of MIBG scintigraphy for detecting functioning phaeochromocytomas is slightly less than 90 per cent; the specificity exceeds 90 per cent. A positive MIBG always requires correlation with CT or MRI.

CT and MRI are equally accurate for identifying adrenal phaeochromocytomas. The multiplanar capability of **MRI** gives it the advantage of being slightly more accurate than CT for detecting extra-adrenal phaeochromocytomas. On T1-weighted images, phaeochromocytomas show similar or slightly lower signal intensity than the liver, but most cases of phaeochromocytomas reported in the literature have been markedly hyperintense on T2-weighted images (Fig. 6.7c). This feature

gives MRI a higher specificity than CT for differentiating between cortical adenomas and phaeochromocytomas when the biochemistry is equivocal.

The choice of initial investigation in a patient suspected of having a phaeochromocytoma depends on several factors other than accuracy, as CT, MRI and MIBG scintigraphy are of roughly equal sensitivity. MIBG has the advantage of allowing assessment of the whole body, but is not universally available, is very expensive and, because of poor spatial resolution, always requires supplementary imaging. Also, in patients with associated syndromes, MIBG scintigraphy will not demonstrate other associated tumours such as renal cell carcinoma, islet-cell tumours, neurofibromas or the other tumours which comprise the various multiple endocrine neoplastic syndromes. In time, CT may be replaced by MRI as the predominant imaging modality for adrenal phaeochromocytomas as it has the advantages of non-ionizing radiation, improved specificity and multiplanar display.

NON-HYPERFUNCTIONING ABNORMALITIES

METASTASIS

Tumours of the lung, kidney, melanoma, breast and digestive tract are the most common primary sites to metastasize to the adrenal glands. The presence of an adrenal mass in a patient with a known malignancy does not necessarily indicate metastatic disease, as 40–50 per cent will turn out to be non-metastatic, representing adenomas rather than metastases.

On CT, metastases tend to be of soft-tissue density, inhomogeneous, with irregular margins; they enhance inhomogeneously after intravenous injection of contrast medium. They are more commonly unilateral than bilateral. On MRI, they are typically hypointense compared to the liver on T1-weighted imaging and relatively hyperintense on T2-weighted imaging. Features that favour malignancy include a size over 3 cm, poorly defined margins, heterogeneous internal architecture and no imaging evidence of fat contained within the mass.

ADENOMA

Incidental, silent adenomas with a diameter of 1–3 cm are detected in 0.6–1.0 per cent of upper abdominal CT examinations performed for indications other than for the detection of adrenal disease. On CT (Fig. 6.8a), they are characteristically round, well-defined in outline, homogeneous, without a perceptible wall, and usually are of low density, owing to relatively large amounts of

(a)

(b)

(c)

Figure 6.8 *Incidentally discovered adenoma. (a) Small, low-density, non-enhancing mass demonstrated in the left adrenal gland on a contrast-enhanced CT scan (arrow). (b) T1-weighted MRI image, showing the mass to be of low signal intensity (arrow). (c) T2-weighted MRI scan showing the mass to be of equal signal intensity to the liver (arrow).*

lipid. They enhance only minimally after intravenous injection of contrast medium. These criteria usually allow a confident distinction between a metastasis and an adenoma. Cholesterol-based scintigraphy usually shows increased uptake in an adenoma compared with a normal gland. Distorted, absent or reduced uptake on the suspect side suggests pathology such as a carcinoma, metastasis or other space-occupying lesion.

Most adenomas appear either slightly hypointense or isointense relative to the liver on MRI T1-weighted images and slightly hyperintense or isointense relative to the hepatic parenchyma on T2-weighted images (Figs 6.8b,c). As with adrenal metastasis, atypical adenomas exist that can be considerably hyperintense, relative to the liver on T2-weighted images.

CARCINOMA

About 60 per cent of adrenal carcinomas are non-functioning, the remainder can result in Cushing's syndrome, hyperaldosteronism, virilization or preco-

cious puberty. The characteristic features on imaging are described earlier in this chapter.

INFECTION

Tuberculosis of the adrenal glands has increased in frequency recently, particularly in immunocompromised patients. The appearance of the gland on CT varies with the stage of infection. Involvement is usually bilateral and, if active, the glands are enlarged and inhomogeneous in density. Punctate calcification is a feature (Fig. 6.9). After intravenous injection of contrast medium, numerous small, non-enhancing areas representing caseous necrosis can often be identified. Long-standing tuberculosis results in atrophic glands.

HAEMORRHAGE

Bilateral adrenal haemorrhage is usually associated with anticoagulant therapy (or other bleeding disorders) or

(a)   *(b)*

Figure 6.9 *Adrenal tuberculosis. (a) Precontrast CT scan showing bilateral adrenal masses (arrowed). Speckled calcification is demonstrated in the left adrenal mass. (b) Postcontrast CT scan showing multiple small focal non-enhancing areas within the enlarged adrenals corresponding to the caseating granulomata.*

with stress caused by surgery, burns and hypotension. Most cases of massive bilateral cortical haemorrhage in fulminant septicaemia occur in infants or children, but can occur in adults. On CT, the adrenals are usually bilaterally markedly enlarged and often mass-like (Fig. 6.10). If the adrenals are examined in the acute or subacute phase, the density of the enlarged adrenal is markedly increased and follow-up study shows a decrease in density. The increase in density of the centre of the gland is characteristic of adrenal haemorrhage.

Bilateral adrenal haemorrhage, owing to blunt abdominal trauma, is very unusual. It is usually unilateral, results from injury to the right side of the abdomen, and is associated with ipsilateral visceral injury. It is seen in only 3 per cent of children who have CT after blunt abdominal trauma.

Figure 6.10 *Adrenal haemorrhage. Precontrast CT scan showing bilateral adrenal enlargement in a patient who had recently undergone a splenectomy for hypersplenism due to myelofibrosis. High-density haemorrhage is seen within the enlarged right adrenal gland (arrow).*

CYSTS

On CT, ultrasound and MRI, adrenal cysts have the same characteristics as cysts seen elsewhere in the body: fluid density, a clearly defined margin, a thin wall, and on CT and MRI, no enhancement after intravenous injection of contrast medium (Fig. 6.11). On CT, small adenomata, when they show uniform low density of their content, may simulate a cyst on CT, but unlike cysts, small adenomata usually enhance after intravenous injection of contrast medium. Endothelial cysts account for 45 per cent of all adrenal cysts; the remainder being epithelial, parasitic or pseudocysts. They are almost always unilateral and detected incidentally. Pseudocysts are thought to represent the result of previous haemorrhage.

LYMPHOMA

Involvement of the adrenals in lymphoma is usually a part of widespread lymphoma, being detected in about 5 per cent of cases of non-Hodgkin's lymphoma. Primary lymphoma is extremely rare. On CT, secondary adrenal lymphoma usually appears as solid homogeneous masses of soft-tissue density which enhance slightly after intravenous injection of contrast medium (Fig. 6.12).

Figure 6.11 *Adrenal endothelial cyst. Coronal reconstruction on a spiral CT scan showing a benign right suprarenal cyst with calcification in the wall.*

Figure 6.12 *Adrenal lymphoma. Bilateral adrenal masses demonstrated in both adrenal glands owing to infiltration with high grade non-Hodgkin's lymphoma (arrows). A retroperitoneal mass caused by lymph node infiltration is also seen.*

MYELOLIPOMA

Myelolipoma is a rare benign neoplasm composed of fat and bone marrow elements in varying proportions, and is usually incidentally discovered in asymptomatic patients. Occasionally, spontaneous haemorrhage may cause pain. The diagnosis is based on the demonstration of fat within an adrenal mass on ultrasound, CT or MRI. However, the proportion of fat may vary and those with only a small amount of fat may be difficult to differentiate from other adrenal masses.

HYPOADRENALISM

Imaging in patients with hypoadrenalism can be useful in identifying treatable causes. The usual cause in

Western countries is primary idiopathic atrophy in which the adrenals appear extremely small and uncalcified, and may be difficult to identify. Calcification within small adrenals usually indicates tuberculosis, but can also be seen in amyloid, sarcoidosis, metastatic disease, haemochromatosis or fungal infections. In acute hypoadrenalism, CT can be useful in identifying haemorrhage.

INCIDENTAL ADRENAL MASS

With increased use of cross-sectional imaging, adrenal masses are found incidentally in 1–3 per cent of abdominal CT scans. The initial step in the assessment of an incidentally discovered adrenal mass is a biochemical evaluation as detection of a biochemical abnormality dictates further management. A unilateral non-hyperfunctioning adrenal mass seldom, if ever, represents a metastasis if there is no other clinical or radiological evidence of malignancy, and the differential diagnosis rests between adenoma and carcinoma. However, if there is a known underlying malignancy, then the diagnosis lies between an adenoma and metastasis.

Adrenal masses larger than 3 mm are malignant in 90–95 per cent of cases, and 78–87 per cent of lesions less than 3 cm are benign. Nevertheless, size alone is poor at discriminating between adenomas and non-adenomas. The demonstration of the benign nature of an adrenal mass is based on the presence of intracellular lipid lowering the attenuation value on CT. An attenuation value on CT of less than 10 HU on non-contrast-enhanced scans indicates a benign tumour. A much greater overlap between benign adenomas and other lesions is seen on contrast-enhanced scans.

More recently, MRI with chemical shift imaging has been used to characterize adrenal masses. Chemical shift relies on the phenomenon that, in a magnetic field, protons in water molecules spin at a slightly different frequency to protons in lipid molecules. By selecting the appropriate time to sample the signal, one can acquire an in-phase image where the signal is derived from the signal of water plus fat protons. On the out-of-phase image, the signal intensity is derived from the difference in signal from water and fat protons. Therefore, if a lesion contains intracellular lipid, there will be a loss of signal on the out-of-phase compared with the in-phase sequences (Fig. 6.13). This has been shown to have a specificity of 100 per cent for identifying large adenomas.

Cholesterol-based radiopharmaceuticals and positron-emission tomography with [18]fluorodeoxyglucose can also differentiate benign adenomas from metastasis. However, both techniques are infrequently used. Even with improved imaging and new techniques,

(a)   (b)

Figure 7.1 *Oblique plain film (a) showing calcification overlying right lower pole on AP film (b) is due to both a partial staghorn calculus (black arrow) and multiple gallstones (white arrow), which lie away from the kidney on the oblique film. (Reproduced with permission from W.R. Cattell, J.A.W. Webb and A.J.W. Hilson,* Clinical renal imaging, *published by John Wiley, Chichester, 1989.)*

INTRAVENOUS UROGRAPHY

Intravenous urography (IVU) gives an excellent rapid overview of urinary tract anatomy. It shows more detail of pelvicalyceal and ureteric anatomy than do the other imaging methods. It provides more limited information about the renal parenchyma and bladder than ultrasonography and computed tomography. Although production of the urogram depends on a functioning kidney which filters and concentrates the contrast medium, the functional information provided by urography is relatively limited.

INTRAVENOUS CONTRAST MEDIA

During the intravenous injection of contrast medium it is usual for the patient to feel a warm sensation and sometimes to notice a metallic taste or feel nauseated. None of these sensations constitute a 'contrast medium reaction'. Significant systemic side effects that constitute a 'reaction' occur in about 5 per cent with high osmolar contrast media and 1 per cent with the newer low osmolar agents. The majority of reactions involve bronchospasm, urticaria, angioneurotic oedema or hypotension. Only a very small proportion of patients develop cardiac arrhythmias or cardiac arrest. The mortality following intravenous contrast media is of the order of 1:50 000 for high osmolar and 1:250 000 for low osmolar agents. The mechanism of these reactions is as yet poorly understood but they do seem to have an 'allergic' basis and are treated with steroids as well as symptomatic measures. Patients who give a history of

previous contrast medium reaction or asthma should be given one of the low osmolar contrast media. Although the role of steroid premedication is controversial, the general consensus is that it should still be used as well. A suitable regime is prednisolone 20 mg tds for 48 hours, starting 24 hours before the contrast medium injection.

Although contrast media have no adverse effect on renal function in subjects with normal function, they can cause deterioration in function, usually temporary, in about 10 per cent of patients with impaired renal function. To reduce the risk, such patients should always be well hydrated before they are given contrast medium, and care should be taken not to exceed the recommended contrast medium dose limits.

FILMS OBTAINED AND NORMAL APPEARANCES

Immediate (1-minute) films

A film of the renal area immediately after contrast medium injection shows the renal parenchyma (nephrogram) at its best. On this film the following features should be checked:

- The **renal length** should be the same length as the first three and a half lumbar vertebrae and their intervening discs, and should be more than 11 cm.
- The **renal axis** should be such that the upper pole lies medial to the lower.
- The **renal outline** should be examined for scars or masses.

Figure 7.2 *IVU. Coned view of the kidneys with ureteric compression in place and good pelvicalyceal distension. (Reproduced with permission from W.R. Cattell, J.A.W. Webb and A.J.W. Hilson,* Clinical renal imaging, *published by John Wiley, Chichester, 1989.)*

Figure 7.3   *IVU. Full-length film showing normal pelvicalyceal systems, ureters and bladder. (Reproduced with permission from H.N. Whitfield, W.F. Hendry, R.S. Kirby and J.W. Duckett.* Textbook of genitourinary surgery, *published by Blackwell, Oxford, 1998.)*

5-minute renal film

Contrast medium should have entered the pelvicalyceal systems. If they appear normal, ureteric compression is usually applied with a tight band, which compresses the ureters as they cross the pelvic brim. This band is left in place for 5 minutes.

10-minute renal film

The pelvicalyceal systems should be fully distended on this 'pyelogram' film obtained with ureteric compression in place (Fig. 7.2). The film should be checked for:

- filling of all the calyces;
- filling defects in the pelvicalyceal system;
- contrast medium collections outside the pelvicalyceal system.

Full-length film

This is obtained following release of ureteric compression and shows the ureters and bladder filled with contrast medium (Fig. 7.3). A further full-length film is obtained after voiding to check bladder emptying and drainage of the upper tracts. These films should be checked for:

- ureteric position, filling defects, strictures or calculi (normal ureteric peristalsis often makes it difficult to see the whole ureter filled with contrast medium at any one time);
- bladder position and size, filling defects, wall thickness and emptying.

Additional films such as oblique views, or tomograms, may be obtained by the radiologist to clarify the appearances. The techniques of emergency and frusemide urography are described on pages 201 and 203 respectively.

ULTRASONOGRAPHY

Ultrasonography provides predominantly structural information about the kidneys and bladder. It does not visualize the normal ureter, which is obscured by overlying bowel, and in most instances does not show the normal pelvicalyceal system. However, it provides more detail about renal parenchymal structure and the perinephric space than the IVU and can characterize masses as cystic or solid. It also provides more information than urography about many intrinsic bladder abnormalities, such as tumours and calculi. Doppler techniques permit the detection of renal arterial and venous blood flow.

TECHNIQUE AND NORMAL APPEARANCES

Scans of the **kidneys** (Fig. 7.4) are obtained in the longitudinal and transverse axes of the kidney by scanning through the flanks, usually with the patient lying on their side. The kidney is seen as an ovoid structure on the longitudinal scans and appears round on the transverse scans. It shows a central cluster of echoes – the sinus echoes – produced predominantly by fat in the

Figure 7.4 *Normal renal ultrasound scans. (a) Longitudinal scan showing renal sinus echoes (arrowed); (b) transverse scan through hilum: note the sinus echoes extend to the renal margin (arrowed). (Reproduced with permission from R.W. Schrier and C.W. Gottschalk,* Diseases of the kidney, *5th edn, published by Little, Brown & Co., Boston MA, 1993.)*

renal sinus. On good quality parenchymal images, the pyramids are seen as triangular black structures arranged around the sinus, and surrounded by the more echogenic cortex. Renal length can be measured from the longitudinal scans. The examination must be done carefully to ensure that the distance between the upper and lower poles is measured, because oblique longitudinal measurements will underestimate length. A normal adult kidney measures 10–12 cm with 9 cm being the lower limit of normal. These measurements are less than the urographic measurements because the radiographic technique produces magnification.

The full **bladder** (Fig. 7.5) is seen as an ovoid, echo-free, fluid collection immediately superior to the pubic symphysis. The wall of the distended bladder should be less than 3 mm thick. From measurements of length, transverse and antero-posterior diameter, bladder volume before and after voiding can be estimated. A widely used formula is:

bladder volume =
0.7 × length × width × antero-posterior diameter.

COMPUTED TOMOGRAPHY

CT is used as a second-line investigation of the kidneys, ureters and bladder, giving predominantly anatomical information. Like ultrasonography it can characterize

Figure 7.5 *Bladder ultrasound. (a) Transverse scan: note seminal vesicles (arrowed); (b) longitudinal scan in another patient: note thick-walled bladder with sacculation (long arrow) and enlarged prostate (short arrow) at bladder base.*

(a)

(b)

(c)

Figure 7.6 *Normal renal CT scans. (a) Precontrast medium scan. Arrow indicates renal fascia. (b) Early post-contrast medium scar. Note cortex (short arrow) defined from medulla, and left renal vein (long arrow) with renal artery posterior to it. (c) Late post-contrast medium scan in another patient shows pelvicalyceal opacification.*

masses and show the perinephric space. It has the additional advantages of being a very sensitive detector of calculi, including 'lucent' calculi, of visualizing the ureter and retroperitoneum and of providing some limited functional information.

TECHNIQUES AND NORMAL FINDINGS

Kidneys and ureter

A full renal CT examination necessitates intravenous contrast medium. On the scans before contrast medium (Fig. 7.6a), the normal renal parenchyma is clearly outlined by the perinephric and sinus fat. The perinephric fascia is often seen. Scans immediately after intravenous contrast medium show the renal artery and vein with the renal pelvis lying posteriorly. Immediate scans show opacification of the renal cortex only (Fig. 7.6b). Subsequently, the medulla also opacifies giving a homogeneous nephrogram, and pelvicalyceal filling occurs by 2 to 3 minutes (Fig. 7.6c). The normal ureter can only be seen with certainty on postcontrast medium scans, but the water density of a dilated ureter can be seen without giving contrast medium.

Figure 7.7 *Normal bladder CT scan. The bladder wall (small arrows) is outlined by unopacified urine and perivesical fat, and the seminal vesicles (large arrow) lie posterior to the bladder.*

CT of bladder (Fig. 7.7)

The bladder is seen as a rounded water density structure clearly outlined by perivesical fat. On scans after contrast medium, the bladder opacifies and the dense

(a)

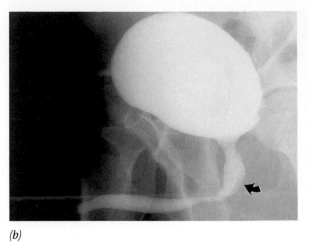

(b)

Figure 7.8 *(a) Normal male ascending urethrogram. Note smoothly tapered bulbar urethra (arrowed) and poor distension of posterior urethra superior to this. Rounded filling defects in the penile urethra are caused by air bubbles. (b) Normal male micturating cystogram. The posterior urethra is well distended and posteriorly is indented by the lucency of the verumontanum (arrowed). (Reproduced with permission from W.R. Cattell, J.A.W. Webb and A.J.W. Hilson,* Clinical renal imaging, *published by John Wiley, Chichester, 1989.)*

contrast medium often layers posteriorly. The seminal vesicles are seen as ovoid soft-tissue structures posterior to the bladder at its base, and inferior to the bladder base thc prostate appears as a rounded soft tissue density.

URETHROGRAPHY

Urethrography in the male is used to diagnose urethral stricture and to evaluate the **urethra** after trauma. Female urethrography is technically difficult. The only indication is to check for urethral diverticulum and this can usually be demonstrated more easily by micturating cystography or transvaginal ultrasonography.

In male urethrography the external meatus is occluded either by the nozzle of a specially designed clamp (e.g. Knutsson clamp) or by the balloon of a Foley catheter in the fossa navicularis. The penile and bulbar parts of the anterior urethra normally distend with the contrast medium to the level of the smoothly tapering proximal bulbar urethra (Fig. 7.8a). Since contrast medium is being injected against the external sphincter, there is usually incomplete distension of the posterior urethra. The bladder is usually filled after the anterior urethra has been visualized and a voiding study (micturating cystogram, see below) is then performed (Fig. 7.8b).

Recently, an **ultrasonographic technique** for urethrography has been described in which the urethra is distended by saline rather than contrast medium and longitudinal and transverse ultrasound images of the distended urethra are obtained. The advantage is that the periurethral tissues are visualized and may appear abnormal in inflammatory disease; the disadvantage is that only the anterior urethra is visualized.

MICTURATING CYSTOGRAPHY

This examination is performed alone relatively rarely in adults. It is not indicated in the routine evaluation of adult urinary tract infection. It may be performed following urethrography in the male to give a functional assessment of any obstructing lesion. It is also used in suspected bladder fistula, to check for vesico-ureteric reflux, and occasionally to look for tumour in a bladder diverticulum or for a urethral diverticulum in females. Cystography alone is used in the assessment of bladder trauma.

The **bladder** is catheterized and filled with contrast medium. Intermittent fluoroscopy is used to check for bladder leaks in suspected trauma or fistula and for vesicoureteric reflux. For a micturating study, the catheter is removed when the bladder is full and the patient voids in the erect oblique position. In the normal male micturating cystogram, the prostatic urethra distends fully (Fig. 7.8b). It is usually indented posteriorly by an ovoid filling defect, the verumontanum. The membranous urethra extends from the lower verumontanum to the upper bulbar urethra. The anterior urethra is also visualized but, in the absence of obstruction, is less well distended than with anterior urethrography. In the female, the short urethra distends fully and may have a variable shape, usually being either ovoid or tubular.

VIDEOURODYNAMICS

When functional bladder disturbance is suspected, e.g. bladder instability, neuropathic bladder or stress incontinence, videourodynamic evaluation is more helpful. Bladder and rectal pressure transducer lines are placed and bladder detrusor pressure is measured during bladder filling and emptying by subtracting rectal from bladder pressure. Video images of the bladder and urethra are also obtained so that both functional and anatomical assessment are performed.

NUCLEAR MEDICINE

Nuclear medicine studies are used to obtain information about renal function. There are two principal types of study; dynamic and static. In **dynamic studies**, radioactive tracers are attached to substances excreted by the kidneys so that serial images provide information about the excretion process. In a **static study**, the tracer is attached to a substance which is taken up and retained in functioning kidney tissue. Such uptake is proportional to renal function.

DYNAMIC STUDIES

The agents used for dynamic studies are ^{99m}Tc-labelled MAG-3 (mercaptoacetyl triglycine), which is excreted by glomerular filtration and tubular secretion, and ^{99m}Tc-labelled DTPA (diethylene triamine pentacetic acid), which is excreted by glomerular filtration only.

The hydrated patient is given an intravenous injection of the radioactive tracer and then lies on a couch above a gamma camera while data are collected. The information obtained may be presented as serial images that show the distribution of radioactivity in the patient. These images are viewed from the position of the gamma camera looking at the patient, so that the patient's right side is on the right side of the image. Alternatively, the information may be presented in the form of a plot of radioactivity over the kidney against time (renogram curve).

When the scintigram is studied, a series of phases may be appreciated (Fig. 7.9). The first 30 seconds represents the **perfusion or vascular phase** during which the tracer passes down the aorta into the kidney via the main renal artery. This is followed by the **uptake phase** in which the tracer enters the renal tubules and the activity of the renal parenchyma increases to a peak. There is then **parenchymal transit and clearance** as the tracer passes along the nephrons and enters the renal collecting system. In the **outflow phase** activity over the collecting system decreases as tracer passes to the bladder where a final **bladder phase** is seen. Bladder images before and after voiding are usually obtained.

Figure 7.9 ^{99m}Tc-labelled DTPA dynamic nuclear medicine scan images and renogram. The pelvicalyceal system in the left kidney is dilated but tracer clears rapidly after frusemide indicating that the kidney is not obstructed. (Reproduced by permission of Dr A.J.W. Hilson.)

A dynamic study may be used to evaluate:

- perfusion abnormalities, particularly renal artery stenosis;
- suspected obstruction (frusemide is often used to distinguish non-obstructed from obstructed dilated systems; if the pelvicalyceal system is dilated but not obstructed, tracer is rapidly washed out by frusemide) (Fig. 7.9);
- glomerular filtration rate (DTPA only);
- relative uptake of the two kidneys (divided renal function).

STATIC STUDIES

The usual agent for static renal scanning is ^{99m}Tc-labelled DMSA (dimercaptosuccinic acid). Approximately 30 per cent of the intravenously administered tracer is taken up and retained by the proximal tubular cells. Scans obtained 3 hours later can be used to estimate the relative function in each kidney. The images provide a sensitive method of detecting renal scars (Fig. 7.10) and are also helpful in showing whether bulges of the renal contour represent true masses or are 'pseudotumours' composed of normal functioning renal tissue, which simulate masses.

ANTEGRADE AND RETROGRADE PYELOGRAPHY

In both antegrade and retrograde pyelography, contrast medium is directly introduced into the kidney or ureter.

Figure 7.13 *Horseshoe kidney on IVU. Note the abnormal renal axes and medially pointing lower pole calyces (arrowed).*

Figure 7.14 *Bilateral ureteroceles on IVU. Note the typical 'cobra head' appearance and the mild ureteric hold-up caused by the right ureterocele (arrowed).*

appearances at IVU (Fig. 7.13) with the two kidneys lying lower than usual, their long axes paralleling the spine. The isthmus joining the lower poles opacifies if it contains functioning renal tissue. The renal pelves usually face anteriorly and the lower pole calyces point medially because there is associated malrotation. It may be more difficult to make the diagnosis with ultrasound since the isthmus can be difficult to visualize when overlain by bowel gas. CT is an excellent method of examining horseshoe kidneys, including the isthmus, and is helpful when the presence of abnormalities such as tumours or stones is suspected.

MEGACALYCES

Megacalyces is a congenital anomaly in which there is poor papillary development leading to non-obstructive dilatation of the calyces. The pelvis and ureter are normal, distinguishing the condition from obstructive or postobstructive dilatation.

URETEROCELE

A ureterocele is a dilated segment of the distal ureter which prolapses into the bladder at its insertion. The dilated contrast medium-filled ureter is surrounded by a lucent margin consisting of the ureteric wall and overlying prolapsed bladder wall. This gives rise to the 'cobra-head' appearance at urography (Fig. 7.14). Simple ureteroceles are common and of no pathologi-

cal significance. When the ureteric orifice is stenotic, ureteric obstruction and stone formation within the ureterocele may occur.

RETROCAVAL URETER

Retrocaval ureter occurs as a result of persistence of the right posterior cardinal vein during development of the inferior vena cava. This results in medial displacement of the right ureter which passes posteriorly to the inferior vena cava. The ureter may become obstructed at vena caval level, and may show a characteristic 'reversed J' appearance.

STONE DISEASE, RENAL CALCIFICATION

A distinction must be made between renal stones and renal calcification. **Stones** lie in the lumen of the urinary tract: calyx, pelvis, ureter, bladder or urethra. The great majority of urinary tract stones (approximately 90 per cent) appear opaque on plain films because they contain either calcium or cystine which is moderately radiopaque. So-called 'lucent' stones contain urate, xanthine or pure matrix and are readily detected by CT because of its high sensitivity to densities greater than that of soft tissue. They may also be

Figure 7.15 *Plain film showing right staghorn calculus.*

202), renal tubular acidosis or hyperparathyroidism. More rarely it occurs in a variety of hypercalcaemic states. **Focal renal parenchymal calcification** is seen in tuberculosis (Fig. 7.50, p. 216), some adenocarcinomas (Fig. 7.37, p. 210), infarcts, haematomas and in the papillae in some patients with papillary necrosis.

Plain films, if necessary supplemented by plain tomography, readily demonstrate renal calcification. With the appropriate combination of plain films it should be possible to establish whether calcification is in the kidneys or is only projected over them (Fig. 7.1, p. 190). In most instances, further localization of the calcification requires urography, although the nature of large calculi which fill the pelvicalyceal system (**staghorn calculi**) may be recognized on plain films alone (Fig. 7.15).

Plain films are only moderately sensitive and specific for the detection of opaque ureteric stones. Small stones may be missed because of underlying bone (transverse processes, sacrum), or overlying bowel, or because their density is relatively low. Calcifications in the bony pelvis caused by phleboliths and arterial calcification are relatively common. **Phleboliths** may be suspected if the calcifications are rounded with lucent centres and lie below the level of the ischial spines, but from plain films alone it is impossible to be sure that they are not ureteric.

Intravenous urography remains the investigation of choice in the diagnosis and further evaluation of most urinary tract stone disease. With urography, opaque renal calculi can be distinguished from renal parenchymal calcification. Lucent renal calculi are seen as filling

demonstrated with ultrasound where they show the characteristic features described below.

Diffuse calcification in the renal parenchyma is described as **nephrocalcinosis**. Nephrocalcinosis is commonly medullary in distribution and is usually associated with medullary sponge kidney (Fig. 7.21, p.

(a)

(b)

Figure 7.16 *(a) Plain film shows calcification adjacent to L4 (arrowed). (b) IVU shows calcification lies in left ureter, which is causing mild hold-up.*

(a)

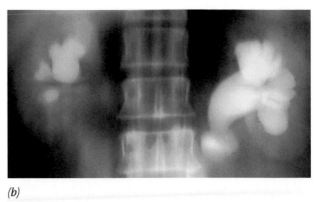
(b)

Figure 7.23 *IVU in chronic obstruction. (a) Film obtained immediately after contrast medium shows central negative pyelogram (arrowed). (b) Delayed film shows dilated calyces and pelvis in the position of the previous negative pyelogram. (Reproduced with permission from W.R. Cattell, J.A.W. Webb and A.J.W. Hilson,* Clinical renal imaging, *published by John Wiley, Chichester, 1989.)*

(a)

(b)

Figure 7.24 *(a) Frusemide IVU in left pelviureteric junction obstruction. Note slight fullness of the left pelvis. (b) 15 minutes after frusemide the left pelvicalyceal system has dilated further and the right has washed out. (Reproduced with permission from W.R. Cattell, J.A.W. Webb and A.J.W. Hilson,* Clinical renal imaging, *published by John Wiley, Chichester, 1989.)*

increase in size of the pelvis and calyces with no ureteric filling, and the patient develops loin pain, whereas with an extrarenal pelvis the contrast medium will have washed out of the pelvis by this time.

Ultrasonography is a sensitive method of detecting pelvicalyceal dilatation in chronic obstruction. The dilated pelvicalyceal system is seen as a group of communicating, rounded fluid collections centrally in the renal sinus, representing the dilated pelvis surrounded by dilated calyces (Fig. 7.25). The upper and lower few centimetres of a dilated ureter may also be seen. In long-standing obstruction, thinning of the renal parenchyma from obstructive atrophy will also be present.

(a) (b)

Figure 7.25 *Moderate pelvicalyceal dilatation (arrowed). Longitudinal (a) and transverse (b) renal ultrasound scans in renal obstruction. (Reproduced with permission from D. Cosgrove, H. Meire and K. Dewbury,* Clinical ultrasound, *published by Churchill Livingstone, Edinburgh, 1993.)*

Figure 7.26 *Mild pelvicalyceal dilatation. Longitudinal ultrasound scan in severe renal obstruction caused by retroperitoneal fibrosis (both kidneys appeared similar). (Reproduced with permission from D. Cosgrove, H. Meire and K. Dewbury,* Clinical ultrasound, *published by Churchill Livingstone, Edinburgh, 1993.)*

Figure 7.27 *CT scan in bilateral renal obstruction. Note bilateral pelvicalyceal dilatation, parenchymal thinning on the left and the periaortic soft-tissue mass (arrowed) of retroperitoneal fibrosis.*

Since minor dilatation can be associated with severe obstruction (Fig. 7.26), in a setting where obstruction is suspected, any degree of dilatation must be taken seriously and investigated further. This will, however, lead to a significant number of false-positive diagnoses. Ultrasound is more limited in this regard than IVU which, by virtue of its ability to show the ureter and to demonstrate drainage of the upper tracts, is associated with less false-positive diagnoses of obstruction.

On precontrast **CT scans** (Fig. 7.27) the dilated pelvicalyceal system of an obstructed kidney can be detected as a water-density central structure surrounded laterally by dilated calyces. At CT a dilated intrarenal pelvis can be distinguished from an extrarenal pelvis, which is a normal variant. The intrarenal pelvis is defined as that part of the pelvis lying lateral to a line joining the hilar lips, the convexities of the parenchyma

which border the renal sinus. Renal parenchymal thinning will be seen in long-standing obstruction. CT has the additional advantage over ultrasound that the water density of urine in a dilated ureter can be traced through the retroperitoneum to the level of the obstruction. Scans after contrast medium will show delayed filling of the dilated pelvicalyceal system and ureter which eventually opacify to the level of the obstruction.

MAG-3 or **DTPA scintigraphy** of an obstructed kidney shows delayed clearance of the parenchyma and delayed outflow from the collecting system. On the renogram, renal activity either rises to a plateau or keeps rising. A dilated extrarenal pelvis alone without obstruction may be associated with delayed outflow from the collecting system, but parenchymal clearance should be normal. **Frusemide renography** is very helpful. If frusemide is given after the postvoiding

Figure 7.28 *⁹⁹ᵐTc-labelled DTPA dynamic nuclear medicine scan images and renogram in a patient with a dilated, obstructed right pelvicalyceal system. Note that the obstructed system does not wash out after frusemide. (Reproduced by permission of Dr A.J.W. Hilson.)*

(a) *(b)*

Figure 7.29 *Antegrade pyelogram in partial ureteric obstruction caused by a urate calculus. (a) Nephrostomy catheter in the pelvicalyceal system; (b) lucent filling defect (arrowed) in the distal ureter.*

image is obtained, a subsequent image shows washout of a baggy, non-obstructed, extrarenal pelvis, but increase in size and retained activity in true pelvi-ureteric junction obstruction (Fig. 7.28).

CAUSE OF OBSTRUCTION

Intravenous urography often shows the level and the cause of obstruction. Extrinsic ureteric obstruction is associated with smooth ureteric tapering, while an intrinsic lesion produces a filling defect in the lumen of the ureter.

When pelvicalyceal dilatation is shown by **ultrasound**, possible causes should be sought by examining the retroperitoneum and pelvis. It may be difficult to show by ultrasound retroperitoneal causes of obstruction but ultrasound can detect pelvis masses or the enlarged bladder of chronic retention. Where ultrasound shows pelvicalyceal dilatation in suspected obstruction, but not the cause of obstruction, either antegrade pyelography or CT is likely to be helpful.

Like urography, **antegrade pyelography** can usually distinguish intrinsic from extrinsic causes of obstruction (Fig. 7.29), but lesions of the ureteric wall such as transitional cell tumours may appear either intrinsic or extrinsic in origin. When polypoid they produce a filling defect and, if they lie in the wall, they produce smooth tapering, which mimics an extrinsic obstruction. Antegrade pyelography is a usual preliminary to percutaneous drainage of the kidney.

CT is an excellent method for demonstrating masses such as enlarged nodes, tumours or retroperitoneal fibrosis causing extrinsic ureteric obstruction (Fig. 7.27).

Figure 7.30 *Retrograde pyelogram. Note lucent filling defect (arrowed) of transitional cell carcinoma in the lower ureter. (Reproduced with permission from W.R. Cattell, J.A.W. Webb and A.J.W. Hilson,* Clinical renal imaging, *published by John Wiley, Chichester, 1989.)*

It can also distinguish stones (Fig. 7.18, p. 000), because of their high density, from other intraluminal filling defects such as transitional cell tumours or blood clots.

Retrograde pyelography is occasionally used to outline the lower end of an obstructed ureter if pelvicalyceal dilatation is mild and antegrade pyelography is likely to be difficult (Fig. 7.30). One of the reasons that the antegrade route is generally preferred is that the retrograde technique carries a risk of introducing infection into the obstructed system.

RENAL MASSES AND TUMOURS

A renal 'mass' detected by imaging most commonly represents a simple cyst, but a wide differential diagnosis must be considered, including benign and malignant tumours, inflammatory masses, pseudotumours, obstructed calyces, haematoma and aneurysm. Masses and tumours can be classified into:

- Cysts
  - simple
  - complicated
    - ▶ septate
    - ▶ haemorrhagic
    - ▶ infected
- Tumours
  - benign
    - ▶ adenoma
    - ▶ angiomyolipoma
  - malignant: primary
    - ▶ adenocarcinoma
    - ▶ Wilms' tumour
    - ▶ invasive transitional cell tumour
  - malignant: secondary
    - ▶ metastasis
    - ▶ lymphoma
- Inflammatory
  - abscess
  - focal acute pyelonephritis
- Pseudotumour
  - hypertrophied column of Bertin
  - compensatory hypertrophy, e.g. in a scarred kidney in reflux nephropathy
- Obstructed calyces
  - obstructed upper pole moiety of duplex kidney
  - obstructed calyx, e.g. TB, stone, transitional cell tumour
- Haematoma
- Aneurysm, arteriovenous malformation

SIMPLE CYSTS

Simple renal cysts are common, occurring in more than 50 per cent of individuals aged over 50. They may be

Figure 7.31 *Simple renal cysts. Tomogram from IVU shows two typical cysts (large arrows) in the upper kidney. Note the lucent masses are well defined and have 'beaks' (small arrows) at their margins. (Reproduced with permission from H.N. Whitfield, H.F. Hendry, R.S. Kirby and J.W. Duckett,* Textbook of genitourinary surgery, *published by Blackwell, Oxford, 1998.)*

multiple. With the widespread use of ultrasound and CT, simple cysts are now frequently detected.

At **IVU** a simple cyst is seen as a mass lesion which typically is lucent with a clear rounded margin. If the cyst protrudes from the kidney, smooth beaks of renal parenchyma are seen at its margins, and the part protruding from the kidney should not have a detectable wall (Fig. 7.31). If the cyst lies centrally in the

Figure 7.32 *Simple renal cyst on ultrasonograph. Note the band of increased through-transmission of sound (arrowed) posterior to the cyst (white arrow). (Reproduced with permission from R.W. Schrier and C.W. Gottschalk,* Diseases of the kidney, *5th edn, published by Little, Brown, W., Boston, MA, 1993.)*

(a)

(b)

Figure 7.33 *Simple renal cyst on CT. Round water-density mass (arrowed) (a) with no enhancement after contrast medium (b). (Reproduced with permission from W.R. Cattell, J.A.W. Webb and A.J.W. Hilson,* Clinical renal imaging, *published by John Wiley, Chichester, 1989.)*

kidney it may cause smooth displacement or compression of the pelvicalyceal system. However, the urographic criteria for diagnosing that a mass is cystic rather than solid are only correct in about 50 per cent of cases. Detection of a renal mass always necessitates further investigation by ultrasound, even if the mass has features suggestive of a cyst at IVU.

Ultrasonography shows a renal cyst as a rounded echo-free mass with a sharply defined back wall and increased through transmission of sound, seen as a white band posterior to the cyst (Fig. 7.32). If these criteria are strictly observed, the ultrasound diagnosis of

a benign cyst is correct in over 95 per cent of cases, and the majority require no further investigation.

CT shows a renal cyst as a rounded, well-defined, homogeneous mass of water density, which has a smooth interface with the adjacent renal parenchyma, no detectable wall, and no enhancement after intravenous contrast medium (Fig. 7.33). If these criteria are strictly observed, the CT diagnosis of a simple cyst is virtually certain.

MRI shows a renal cyst as a rounded, well-defined, homogeneous mass of lower signal intensity than adjacent normal parenchyma on T1-weighted images

(a)

(b)

Figure 7.34 *Simple renal cyst on MR. (a) T1-weighted axial image after gadolinium. Note the low signal intensity of the cyst (arrowed), which has not enhanced, and the corticomedullary differentiation in the normal enhanced kidney. (b) T2-weighted axial image shows high signal intensity in the cyst.*

Figure 7.35 *Septate renal cyst (large arrows) on ultrasound scan. Note the central septum (small arrows). (Reproduced with permission from R.W. Schrier and C.W. Gottschalk, Diseases of the kidney, 5th edn, published by Little, Brown & Co., Boston MA, 1993.)*

Figure 7.36 *Renal adenocarcinoma (arrowed) with peripheral and central calcification shows patchy opacification on IVU.*

with no enhancement after gadolinium. On T2-weighted images the cyst is of high intensity compared to normal parenchyma (Fig. 7.34).

ATYPICAL CYSTS

A number of features may lead to a cyst being classed as atypical of ultrasound or CT:

- calcification: some simple cysts have a pencil-thin rim of calcification in their wall, but such calcification may also occur in adenocarcinoma;
- septation (Fig. 7.35);
- echoes within the cyst at ultrasound;
- increased density or enhancement at CT.

These appearances raise the possibility of a variety of conditions including haemorrhagic cyst, infected cyst or abscess, necrotic tumour or haematoma. Further investigation is always indicated to confirm or exclude tumour. If the ultrasound features are atypical, CT or cyst puncture is performed. CT is preferred if the cyst is multilocate or there are multiple cysts. If the CT features are atypical, ultrasound or cyst puncture may be helpful.

RENAL ADENOCARCINOMA (RENAL CELL CARCINOMA)

A proportion of renal adenocarcinomas calcify and typically the calcification is central and irregular. Peripheral calcification, however, does occur in adenocarcinoma and **any calcified renal mass should be considered malignant until proved otherwise.**

On **urography** the tumour usually opacifies in an irregular manner (Fig. 7.36) and is poorly defined from adjacent renal parenchyma. If it has a definable wall, the wall is thicker than 1 mm. If the tumour lies centrally within the kidney it may displace and compress the pelvicalyceal system and possibly invade it, producing irregular filling defects.

Renal adenocarcinoma is seen at **ultrasound** as a solid mass, typically slightly hypoechoic to adjacent renal parenchyma and commonly inhomogeneous (Fig. 7.37). It may, however, have similar or increased echogenicity compared to the parenchyma. If the tumour necroses it may show increased through-transmission of sound indicating the presence of fluid, but the fluid contains echoes and the wall is thickened. If the mass contains calcifications, bright echoes with associated acoustic shadowing are seen.

Renal adenocarcinoma typically has attenuation values close to or less than adjacent renal parenchyma on **CT** before contrast medium, and may contain calcification. After contrast medium the mass enhances and has an irregular interface with renal parenchyma (Fig. 7.38). If it is necrotic and partly fluid-containing, the wall is thickened. The CT diagnosis of renal adenocarcinoma is sufficiently accurate that preoperative biopsy is not usually performed.

The most common pattern of renal adenocarcinoma on **MRI** is a mass of reduced signal intensity on T1-weighted images which enhances after gadolinium and shows inhomogeneous higher signal intensity than normal kidney, but less than fluid on T2-weighted images.

Staging of renal adenocarcinoma

Currently **CT** is considered the best staging method for renal adenocarcinoma. It can define whether the tumour breaches the capsule or the renal fascia, show venous

(a)   *(b)*

Figure 7.37 *Renal adenocarcinoma. (a) Solid upper pole mass (arrowed) on longitudinal ultrasound scan. (b) Tumour extension (large white arrow) into the vena cava (small arrows indicate caval walls) seen on longitudinal ultrasound scan (open arrow indicates left lobe of liver).*

Figure 7.38 *Renal adenocarcinoma in same patient shown in Fig. 7.37. CT scan after contrast medium shows inhomogeneously enhancing renal mass (solid arrow). There is tumour extension into an enlarged left renal vein (small arrows) and the vena cava (open arrow).*

Figure 7.39 *Renal adenocarcinoma in same patient shown in Fig. 7.37. Coronal T1-weighted MR scan shows tumour extension into left renal vein (short arrows) and vena cava (long arrow).*

extension and para-aortic lymphadenopathy, and detect liver metastases. Venous extension initially involves the renal vein and then may extend up the vena cava (Fig. 7.38) to the right atrium. The affected veins expand and the filling defect produced by the tumour can be defined on the scans obtained after contrast medium.

Ultrasound is also useful in detecting venous extension and can show tumour in the right renal vein, terminal portion of the left renal vein and vena cava (Fig. 7.37b). It is particularly helpful in defining the relation of the upper end of the tumour to the diaphragm. Its limitations relate to the fact that bowel

gas commonly obscures the proximal left renal vein and the infrahepatic vena cava. Liver metastases are well detected but perinephric extension is assessed less well than with CT.

Magnetic resonance imaging is particularly successful at defining venous extension of tumour which can be imaged in the coronal plane (Fig. 7.39). It can also demonstrate perinephric, nodal and liver involvement.

Angiography is no longer used in the diagnosis of renal adenocarcinoma but may occasionally be requested to demonstrate arterial anatomy if partial nephrectomy is planned.

Figure 7.40 *Renal angiomyolipoma. CT scan shows fat density in mass (arrowed).*

Figure 7.41 *Transitional cell carcinoma of the left upper pole calyces on IVU. Note the multiple small lucent filling defects (arrowed). (Reproduced with permission from H.N. Whitfield, W.F. Hendry, R.S. Kirby and J.W. Duckett,* Textbook of genitourinary surgery, *published by Blackwell, Oxford, 1998.)*

ANGIOMYOLIPOMA

Angiomyolipoma is a benign tumour which contains fat. Solitary angiomyolipomas typically occur in middle-aged females and present with haemorrhage. Multiple angiomyolipomas occur in tuberous sclerosis. Small angiomyolipomas are frequently detected incidentally on ultrasound, where they are seen as small, well-defined masses with markedly increased echogenicity, similar to that of sinus fat. While the tumour may be suspected from this sonographic appearance, the diagnostic test is CT which shows fat density within the mass (Fig. 7.40). Diagnosis may be difficult if haemorrhage obscures the fat.

LYMPHOMA AND METASTASES

If solid renal masses are multiple and occur in a patient with a known primary tumour or with para-aortic lymphadenopathy, metastases or lymphoma should be considered. The imaging appearances may be indistinguishable from renal adenocarcinoma and, if either metastases or lymphoma are suspected, biopsy is appropriate.

WILMS' TUMOUR

Wilms' tumour is predominantly a tumour of childhood but can occur in young adults. The diagnosis may be suggested by the patient's age, and by the appearance of the tumour which is typically large and contains areas of haemorrhage and necrosis.

TUMOURS OF THE COLLECTING SYSTEM AND URETER

The majority of tumours arising in the collecting system and ureter are transitional cell tumours. Squamous cell carcinomas are less common and are associated with stones or chronic infection. The tumours arise in the mucosa and urography is the best method to show them because it depicts detailed pelvicalyceal and ureteric anatomy.

Calcium salts may encrust the surface of transitional cell tumours and rarely will be seen as faint stippled calcification on the plain film. On **intravenous urography** the tumours are seen as either polypoid or plaque-like filling defects in the pelvicalyceal system and ureter, and may be multiple (Fig. 7.41). With growth they narrow the lumen and can produce obstruction of a calyx, the pelviureteric junction or the ureter (Fig. 7.30, p. 206). The ureteric stricture may be indistinguishable from that produced by an extrinsic mass. Renal transitional cell tumours may invade the renal parenchyma to produce a renal mass; differentiation from renal adenocarcinoma invading the pelvicalyceal system is then difficult.

Ultrasonography only detects large renal transitional cell tumours. Typically they are seen as hypoechoic solid masses centrally in the sinus displacing the normal bright echoes of the sinus.

Computed tomography also shows larger transitional cell tumours as masses of soft-tissue density or as thickening of the wall of the pelvis or ureter. CT is particularly helpful in the differential diagnosis of 'lucent' filling defects in the pelvicalyceal system, allowing calculi with their high CT density to be separated from tumour and blood clot.

RENAL CYSTIC DISEASE

Simple cysts are often multiple and their features are described on p. 207. Multiple simple cysts may distort

Table 7.1 *Summary of the typical features of renal cystic disease.*

Type	Heredity	Laterality	Kidney size	Cyst size	Cyst number	Liver	Renal adenocarcinoma risk
1. Multiple simple cysts	Not inherited	Uni- or bilateral	Normal	Variable mm to 8–10 cm	Countable	Not involved	Normal
2. Autosomal dominant polycystic kidney disease	Dominant	Bilateral	Large	Variable mm to 8–10 cm	Not countable	Cysts in 30%	Normal
3. Autosomal recessive polycystic kidney disease	Recessive	Bilateral	Large	Very small mm or less	Not countable	Liver fibrosis Liver cysts	Normal
4. Medullary sponge kidney	Not inherited	Uni- or bilateral	Normal or large	Few mm	Depends on severity	Not involved	Normal
5. Medullary cystic disease	Recessive or dominant (see text)	Bilateral	Small	mm to 2.0 cm	Not countable (too small)	Not involved	Normal
6. Multicystic dysplastic kidney	Not inherited	Unilateral	Large: neonates Small: adults	mm to several cm	Countable 'bunch of grapes'	Not involved	Normal
7. Acquired cystic disease	Not inherited	Bilateral	Small	0.5–2.0 cm	Countable	Not involved	Increased

Reproduced by permission from W.R. Cattell, J.A.W. Webb and A.J.W. Hilson, *Clinical Renal Imaging*, published by John Wiley, Chichester, 1989.

renal anatomy but renal size is usually normal; normal parenchyma can be seen, and the cysts are few enough to be counted.

Multiple renal cysts also occur in a variety of other conditions, some inherited, some sporadic and some acquired. There is considerable overlap in the imaging appearances of these conditions. Diagnosis involves a consideration both of the imaging features (renal size, whether involvement is uni- or bilateral, size and number of cysts, evidence of involvement of other organs, such as the liver), and of the clinical features (family history, renal function, and whether the patient has had dialysis) (Table 7.1). In some of these conditions, particularly autosomal dominant polycystic kidney disease, the genetic abnormality is known and identification of the abnormal chromosome permits a specific diagnosis.

AUTOSOMAL DOMINANT POLYCYSTIC KIDNEY DISEASE (ADULT POLYCYSTIC KIDNEY DISEASE)

Autosomal dominant polycystic kidney disease is always bilateral, although involvement may be asymmetric.

Ultrasonography is the diagnostic method of choice. In the established disease, the kidneys are enlarged. There is loss of the normal corticomedullary differentiation and of the normal pattern of sinus and parenchyma, because the whole kidney is replaced by multiple cysts of varying sizes, too numerous to count (Fig. 7.42). This latter feature distinguishes the condition from multiple simple cysts.

Urography shows enlarged kidneys with lobulated outlines and multiple mass lesions. These produce rounded lucencies in the nephrogram with stretching and compression of the pelvicalyceal systems. Since these appearances can also be produced by multiple solid masses, ultrasound is necessary to confirm the diagnosis.

Computed tomography also shows enlarged kidneys replaced by multiple cysts of varying sizes (Fig. 7.43).

About one third of patients have liver cysts and 10 per cent have pancreatic cysts detectable by ultrasound

Figure 7.42 *Autosomal dominant polycystic kidney disease. Longitudinal ultrasound scan shows enlarged kidney (calipers mark poles) with normal internal structure replaced by multiple cysts.*

Figure 7.43 *Autosomal dominant polycystic kidney disease. CT scan with contrast medium enhancement shows enlarged kidneys containing multiple cysts.*

or CT. There may be haemorrhage into the renal cysts or they may become infected. Ultrasound or CT often then detect atypical features: contained echoes or increased density. Autosomal dominant polycystic kidney disease is not associated with an increased risk of renal malignancy.

Early disease may be detected before clinical presentation. Ultrasound is the method of choice for screening the relatives of affected individuals at age 18–20. In the early stages of the disease renal size is normal and a few small cysts only may be present.

AUTOSOMAL RECESSIVE POLYCYSTIC KIDNEY DISEASE (INFANTILE POLYCYSTIC KIDNEY DISEASE)

Autosomal recessive polycystic kidney disease is a rare inherited condition in which both the kidneys and the liver show cysts and fibrosis. The younger the presentation, the more severely the kidneys are affected, while liver involvement occurs in later childhood. Renal involvement is always bilateral and results in renal enlargement. At **ultrasonography** the cysts are commonly too small to be seen and the renal parenchyma shows diffuse increase in echogenicity caused by the walls of the multiple tiny cysts. Occasionally small discrete cysts are seen. **Urography** shows enlarged kidneys with a dense nephrogram, which persists for up to 24 hours and appears streaky because of contrast medium in dilated tubules.

MULTICYSTIC DYSPLASTIC KIDNEY

Multicystic dysplastic kidney is a sporadic condition in

(a)

(b)

(c)

Figure 7.44 *Renal adenocarcinoma in acquired cystic disease in a patient who had had haemodialysis for 10 years. (a) Renal ultrasound shows multiple small cysts but no solid masses (both kidneys appeared similar). (b) Enhanced CT shows typical multiple cysts with (c) an enhancing 2 cm solid mass (arrowed) at the left lower pole.*

which the kidney fails to develop normally and consists of a collection of non-functioning cysts and primitive tissues. In neonatal life, a large abdominal mass containing multiple cysts at ultrasound is the typical appearance. In older children and adults the dysplastic kidney is small. It may show curvilinear calcification peripherally. Faint enhancement only may be seen at urography with no pelvicalyceal filling. Ultrasound shows a collection of non-communicating cysts of varying sizes. If retrograde ureterography is performed, an atretic ureter may be shown. The contralateral kidney is usually hypertrophied and has an increased incidence of other congenital anomalies, especially pelviureteric junction obstruction.

ACQUIRED CYSTIC DISEASE

Acquired cystic disease occurs in many patients on long-term dialysis. The shrunken end-stage kidneys develop multiple, usually small cysts which may be detected by ultrasound or CT. Complications include haemorrhage into the cysts, which may lead to cyst rupture, and an increased incidence of malignancy. While ultrasound can reliably detect the cysts, CT is a better method to search for solid tumours in these shrunken abnormal kidneys (Fig. 7.44).

RARE CYSTIC CONDITIONS

Medullary cystic disease occurs in an autosomal recessive type which presents in childhood (**juvenile nephronophthisis**) and an autosomal dominant type, which presents in early adult life. Patients present with salt wasting, growth retardation and renal failure. The kidneys are usually small and small medullary cysts may be demonstrable with ultrasound or CT.

Tuberous sclerosis is associated with multiple renal angiomyolipomas and cysts. In some patients the cysts are very numerous, replacing normal renal structure and, on imaging, the condition is indistinguishable from autosomal dominant polycystic kidney disease.

In **von Hippel–Lindau disease** the kidneys contain multiple cysts. Typical simple cysts arise from the distal tubules and do not have malignant potential. In von Hippel–Lindau disease cysts also arise from the proximal tubules and adenocarcinoma can develop within them. Renal adenocarcinoma is a significant cause of death in these patients and regular renal imaging (usually with MR or CT) is used to detect malignant tumours early.

UPPER URINARY TRACT INFECTION

ACUTE URINARY TRACT INFECTION

The diagnosis of acute urinary tract infection depends on the demonstration of significant bacteriuria, usually

Figure 7.45 *Acute pyelonephritis. Enhanced CT shows wedge- and band-shaped areas of reduced enhancement in the right kidney.*

in association with typical clinical features. **The great majority of patients with acute urinary tract infection do not require imaging.**

Occasionally, if renal pain is severe, ureteric colic may be suspected and an IVU may be performed. In acute pyelonephritis the IVU may be normal. In about 25 per cent of patients there may be swelling of the kidney, reduced nephrogram density and poor filling of the pelvicalyceal system, which is compressed by the swollen parenchyma.

Imaging is indicated if the patient fails to respond normally to antibiotic treatment and if obstruction or focal sepsis is suspected. **Ultrasonography** is usually chosen and in acute pyelonephritis images may be normal or show diffuse or focal renal swelling. If **computed tomography** is performed, patients with severe pyelonephritis may show renal swelling on the precontrast medium scans. After **intravenous contrast** medium, these patients may show a distinctive pattern of enhancement with streaky and wedge-shaped areas of reduced enhancement within the parenchyma (Fig. 7.45).

FOCAL ACUTE SEPSIS: RENAL AND PERINEPHRIC ABSCESS, PYONEPHROSIS

Renal abscess is seen at IVU as a mass with no specific features unless it contains air. Both on ultrasound and CT, a renal abscess may be seen as a simple fluid collection, or may show a thickened wall (Fig. 7.46); on ultrasound there may be contained echoes, which may layer; on CT there may be increased density of the contents. Air will be readily detected by CT and may be suspected on ultrasound if bright echoes with associated acoustic shadows are seen. Either ultrasound or CT may be used to guide needle puncture of an abscess for diagnostic purposes or for drainage.

Figure 7.46 *Left renal abscess (arrowed). CT scan after contrast medium shows its thickened enhancing wall. (Reproduced with permission from W.R. Cattell,* Infections of the kidney and urinary tract, *published by Oxford University Press, Oxford, 1996.)*

Figure 7.47 *Right perinephric abscess on CT scan. A lateral renal abscess has spread into the perinephric (large arrow) and paranephric (small arrow) spaces. (Reproduced with permission from W.R. Cattell,* Infections of the kidney and urinary tract, *published by Oxford University Press, Oxford, 1996.)*

Perinephric abscesses are most often secondary to rupture of an obstructed infected collecting system, but can also arise from rupture of an intrarenal abscess. On plain films the psoas and renal outlines may be lost, and at urography displacement of the kidney superiorly and anteriorly may be noted.

Ultrasound shows a fluid collection predominantly postero-inferior to the kidney, which may appear simple or show contained echoes or features suggestive of air. Computed tomography provides an excellent demonstration of the extent of perinephric abscesses (Fig. 7.47) which may appear of water or increased density and may contain air. Either ultrasound or CT can be used to guide percutaneous drainage of a perinephric abscess.

In **pyonephrosis** an obstructed infected pelvicalyceal system may show features identical to a simple dilated collecting system or may show air or other findings indicating a complex fluid collection. At ultrasound, there may be contained echoes, which may layer (Fig. 7.48), and at CT increased density may be shown. Usually no contrast medium excretion into the pelvicalyceal system is seen at CT.

Figure 7.48 *Pyonephrosis. Longitudinal ultrasound scan of kidney shows dilated pelvicalyceal system with echoes layering posteriorly (arrowed). (Reproduced with permission from W.R. Cattell,* Infections of the kidney and urinary tract, *published by Oxford University Press, Oxford, 1996.)*

CHRONIC SEPSIS: XANTHOGRANULOMATOUS PYELONEPHRITIS

Some patients with obstruction and infection develop the unusual chronic inflammatory condition of xanthogranulomatous pyelonephritis. This is characterized by macrophages which ingest fat ('foamy macrophages') within the chronic inflammatory tissue. The whole kidney is usually affected. Typically the renal pelvis is contracted, and contains a calculus. The ultra-sonographic and CT findings are similar to those in the pyonephrosis, and there is commonly extension of the inflammatory process into the perinephric space or psoas muscle. The affected kidney enhances poorly after intravenous contrast medium and there is no pelvicalyceal filling. Despite the pathological findings, fat density is not detected at CT.

RECURRENT URINARY TRACT INFECTION

In patients with proven recurrent urinary tract infection, further imaging investigation may be warranted to check whether there are associated complicating factors

(a)

Figure 7.49 *Bilateral reflux nephropathy. Small left kidney (poles indicated by arrows) with diffuse calyceal blunting and irregularly scarred right kidney with multiple blunt calyces. (Reproduced with permission from W.R. Cattell, J.A.W. Webb and A.J.W. Hilson,* Clinical renal imaging, *published by John Wiley, Chichester, 1989.)*

that increase the risk of renal damage (such as stones, obstruction, reflux or papillary necrosis), or whether there are factors likely to predispose to relapse or reinfection (such as stasis, scars or poor bladder emptying). Whilst some of these conditions may be detectable by ultrasound and plain films, the best investigation in the majority of instances is intravenous urography because of the detailed anatomical information it provides.

REFLUX NEPHROPATHY

The term reflux nephropathy is applied to the late sequelae of reflux of infected urine into the kidney, usually in early childhood. Occasionally it may develop later in life. The diagnosis usually requires urography. Typically the condition is focal and has a predominantly polar patchy distribution with areas of thinned parenchyma (scars) overlying blunted calyces (Fig. 7.49). Scarring at the poles is frequently associated with a smooth renal outline. The affected kidney often grows poorly and renal asymmetry is common. More rarely the condition is diffuse with generalized parenchymal loss and calyceal blunting, an appearance indistinguishable from the appearances following obstruction.

TUBERCULOSIS

Tuberculosis in the urinary tract is usually multifocal.

Urography is the best method to show the changes especially in early disease where detailed pelvicalyceal anatomy needs to be shown.

(b)

Figure 7.50 *Right renal and ureteric tuberculosis. (a) Plain film shows calcification (arrowed) at both upper poles. (b) IVU shows no calyceal filling at the right upper pole and dilatation of the remaining right pelvicalyceal system and ureter to the level of a ureteric stricture at the pelvic brim.*

Calcification is frequent. In the kidney it may be focal and speckled (Fig. 7.50) or more widespread and hazy. Late in the disease the whole pelvicalyceal system and ureter may be calcified: so-called tuberculous autonephrectomy. Calcification also occurs in the ureter, bladder, vas, seminal vesicles and prostate.

The earliest renal change is papillary with destruction of the papillary margins leading to poor definition of the calyces. Contrast medium density in the affected pelvicalyceal system is often poor. With progression, cavities develop that communicate with the pelvicalyceal system. Healing occurs with fibrosis, and this causes stenosis of the calyceal infundibula with delayed or non-filling of dilated calyces proximal to the stenoses (Fig. 7.50). Pelviureteric junction obstruction may also develop by the same mechanism, and eventually the pelvicalyceal system filled with caseous material may calcify.

The ureters may develop smooth or irregular strictures. These may occur during treatment and a limited urogram is usually performed after the patient has been on chemotherapy for 3 months to check for ureteric strictures.

Ultrasound can show the calcification and pelvicalyceal dilatation associated with advanced disease but the appearances are usually non-specific. **Computed tomography** can also show the changes of advanced disease, particularly calcification, pelvicalyceal dilatation, ureteric strictures and extrarenal spread, but is less sensitive than urography in the detection of early renal and ureteric tuberculosis.

TRAUMA

RENAL TRAUMA

Most renal trauma is due to blunt injury. Less commonly, injuries are penetrating or iatrogenic, for example following percutaneous nephrolithotomy or renal biopsy.

Plain films may show fractures of the lower ribs or transverse processes of the lumbar vertebrae. The renal and psoas outlines may no longer be seen if there is perinephric bleeding, and if the haematoma is large it may displace bowel.

Urography is usually performed first in localized blunt loin trauma in order to show:

- that the injured kidney is perfused, as evidenced by contrast medium excretion. (If there is injury to the renal pedicle, there will be no contrast medium excretion, and urgent intervention is then indicated.)
- any abnormality in the uninjured kidney which may affect decisions about nephrectomy, if conservative management is unsuccessful.

These questions can be answered with a relatively limited IVU (Fig. 7.51). To define the renal injury fully, a more detailed study with tomography is necessary. This will show abnormalities in the nephrogram, either local or diffuse reduction of the nephrogram or a wedge-shaped defect if there is laceration. The pelvicalyceal system may be compressed by haematoma and oedema, or may be disrupted with leak of contrast medium (Fig. 7.51). Clot in the pelvicalyceal system produces lucent filling defects.

Figure 7.51 *Left renal trauma. IVU shows contrast medium extravasation (arrowed) from left pelvicalyceal system. (Reproduced with permission from W.R. Cattell, J.A.W. Webb and A.J.W. Hilson,* Clinical renal imaging, *published by John Wiley, Chichester, 1989.)*

Computed tomography is used when the injury is more severe, when injury to multiple organs is suspected, or if there has been a penetrating injury. On the scans before contrast medium, high-density haematoma may be seen in the pelvicalyceal system, parenchyma or perinephric space. Following contrast medium, rapid sequence scans allow the renal vessels to be visualized. On the nephrogram phase lacerations can be detected as nephrogram defects. Contrast leak from the pelvicalyceal system will be shown and an excellent assessment of the size and extent of the perinephric haematoma can be made (Fig. 7.52). If there is injury to the renal artery resulting in occlusion, the renal artery shows abrupt cut-off and there is no renal excretion of contrast medium; however, there may be perfusion of a rim of cortex peripherally from collateral and capsular vessels.

Figure 7.52 *Right renal trauma. CT scan with contrast medium enhancement shows large perinephric haematoma (arrowed) and disruption of the anterior renal parenchyma. (By permission of Dr S.E. Mirvis and Dr K. Shanmuganathan.)*

Figure 7.53 *Renal laceration (large arrow) and perinephric haematoma (small arrows) seen on longitudinal ultrasound scan. (Reproduced with permission from W.R. Cattell, J.A.W. Webb and A.J.W. Hilson,* Clinical renal imaging, *published by John Wiley, Chichester, 1989.)*

Ultrasound may be used to assess the size of perinephric and intrarenal haematoma (Fig. 7.53). The use of ultrasonography is in part limited by the necessity to move the patient to obtain a good examination. This may not be practicable in severely injured patients. Initially haematomas have the same appearance as fluid, but with the development of clot, echoes appear within the fluid collection making it more difficult to visualize. Doppler ultrasound may be used to assess renal perfusion.

Angiography is no longer used in the diagnosis of renal injury, but may be employed if treatment of haemorrhage by embolization is planned.

Scintigraphy may be used to demonstrate renal perfusion and excretion but gives less anatomical information than the other methods.

Late effect of renal injury

When renal injury is managed conservatively the end result is often parenchymal loss with a relatively normal underlying pelvicalyceal system, appearances indistinguishable from a renal infarct.

URETERIC TRAUMA

The ureter is mobile and relatively rarely damaged by blunt injury. It may be injured by penetrating or iatrogenic trauma, for example during bowel or gynaecological surgery.

Intravenous urography is the best method to show injury. Contrast medium leakage from the ureter may be seen, or there may be obstruction if there has been transection or ligation of the ureter. Following gynaecological surgery, there may be a ureterovaginal fistula with contrast medium entering the vagina (Fig. 7.54).

Figure 7.54 *Left ureterovaginal fistula following hysterectomy. IVU shows contrast medium leak from left ureter (small arrow) and contrast medium in the vagina (large arrow).*

RENAL PARENCHYMAL DISEASE

The diagnosis of most renal parenchymal disease is dependent on biopsy, but imaging can provide some information. Urography, ultrasound and CT may show parenchymal swelling in acute parenchymal disease and parenchymal thinning (focal or diffuse) in chronic parenchymal disease.

Urography is the best method to diagnose **papillary necrosis** and **reflux nephropathy** (p. 216). Papillary necrosis occurs in patients with interstitial nephritis secondary to diabetes mellitus, analgesic abuse, non-steroidal anti-inflammatory drug ingestion and sickle cell disease or trait. Typically, involvement is patchy and bilateral. Usually the **plain film** is normal but there may be central spotty or peripheral linear papillary calcification. Necrosis may occur centrally in the papillae and communicate with the calyx ('egg in a cup') or may occur peripherally, resulting in tracks and horns of contrast medium extending out from the calyceal fornices (Fig. 7.55). If these surround the papilla, sloughing occurs, with the papilla seen as a lucent filling defect in a blunted calyx. The parenchyma overlying the abnormal calyces is normal until late in the disease, when papillary sloughing results in a shrunken kidney which typically has a 'wavy' irregular outline.

Figure 7.55 *Papillary necrosis. Multiple papillary contrast pools ('egg in a cup') (arrowed) in a man with ankylosing spondylitis who had taken analgesics over many years. Note the typical vertebral fusion.*

On **ultrasound** normal parenchyma has reflectivity similar to or less than the adjacent liver and spleen. When parenchymal reflectivity is greater than that of the adjacent organs, parenchymal disease is usually present (Fig. 7.56). Problems with using this as a method of identifying renal parenchymal disease are its low sensitivity, dependence on normal reflectivity of the liver and spleen, and the fact that it gives no indication of the type of parenchymal disease. As a result, the observation of altered parenchymal reflectivity rarely affects clinical management and certainly does not obviate renal biopsy.

Computed tomography shows an abnormal enhancement pattern after intravenous contrast medium in patients with acute pyelonephritis (Fig. 7.45, p. 214).

Figure 7.56 *Renal parenchymal disease in sickle cell trait. Longitudinal ultrasound scan shows renal parenchymal reflectivity is markedly increased compared to adjacent normal liver.*

Angiography can demonstrate the typical 2–3 mm microaneurysms of polyarteritis nodosa in the arcuate and interlobar arteries. There is often also arterial narrowing and focal parenchymal loss with scarring.

RENAL HYPERTENSION

Over 90 per cent of adult patients with hypertension have primary, or essential, hypertension. In a minority of adults, hypertension is secondary to renal disease, renovascular disease, endocrine disease or aortic coarctation. The younger the patient, the more likely that hypertension is secondary.

Clues that the hypertension is secondary to renal disease may be obtained from the history, especially if there has been glomerulonephritis, childhood urinary tract infection, or if there is a family history of cystic disease. Raised serum urea and creatinine, proteinuria or haematuria also raise the possibility of underlying renal disease. Such patients warrant renal imaging. **Ultrasonography** can be used to measure renal size and parenchymal thickness, to exclude renal obstruction and to detect evidence of autosomal dominant polycystic kidney disease. Ultrasonography may detect renal scars but, to diagnose reflux nephropathy, urography is necessary to show the typical associated calyceal blunting (Fig. 7.49, p. 216).

RENOVASCULAR HYPERTENSION

Renovascular hypertension may be defined as hypertension caused by reduced renal perfusion, which in the majority of cases is caused by **renal artery stenosis** (RAS). However, not all RAS causes hypertension, and true renovascular hypertension can only be identified when the blood pressure reverts to normal following correction of the RAS by surgery or angioplasty. It is estimated that less than 5 per cent of hypertensives have renovascular hypertension.

When renal artery stenosis results in reduced renal perfusion pressure, the juxtaglomerular apparatus releases renin, which catalyses the conversion of angiotensinogen to angiotensin I. Angiotensin-converting enzyme (ACE) then catalyzes the conversion of angiotensin I to the active angiotensin II. Angiotensin II causes hypertension both by stimulating the release of aldosterone and by causing generalized vasoconstriction, and is also involved in the autoregulation of glomerular filtration rate (GFR) by causing vasoconstriction of the efferent arterioles.

Imaging

Intravenous urography may provide indirect evidence of renal artery stenosis. The typical findings are a small,

(a)

(b)

Figure 7.57 *Left renal artery stenosis on IVU. (a) 5-minute film shows small smooth left kidney with delayed pelvicalyceal filling. (b) 10-minute film shows increased pelvicalyceal density on the affected side. (Reproduced by permission from W.R. Cattell, J.A.W. Webb and A.J.W. Hilson,* Clinical renal imaging, *published by John Wiley, Chichester, 1989.)*

smooth kidney, with delayed pelvicalyceal filling with contrast medium, and increased contrast medium density in the pelvicalyceal system on the affected side (Fig. 7.57). There may also be indentation of the pelvicalyceal system by arterial collaterals. To detect delayed pelvicalyceal filling on the affected side, a 'rapid sequence' IVU is necessary with films obtained at 1 minute intervals following contrast medium injection. However, this method is no longer routinely practised as it is not sufficiently sensitive to be used as a screening method for renovascular hypertension.

Typical findings on **renography** in renal artery stenosis are a slow upslope of the arterial curve, reduced uptake on the affected side and prolonged transit through the kidney. These signs, however, have not proved sufficiently reliable to detect renal artery stenosis. The **captopril renogram** is a much more sensitive test and relies on the fact that captopril (an ACE inhibitor) blocks the autoregulatory effect of angiotensin II on the GFR. Following a baseline renogram, oral captopril is given and the renogram is repeated 60–90 minutes later. In the presence of RAS, captopril causes decreased uptake and reduced parenchymal clearance in the affected kidney.

Ultrasonography of the renal arteries is technically demanding because of their relatively deep position, and in many subjects bowel gas obscures part or all of their course. If the arteries are visualized, Doppler may be used to search for features suggestive of RAS. Within the stenotic segment there may be increased flow velocity

(a)

(b)

Figure 7.58 *Angioplasty for atheromatous renal artery stenosis. Digital subtraction aortograms show typical proximal atheromatous left renal artery stenosis (a) before (arrowed) and (b) after angioplasty. (Reproduced by permission of Dr J.E. Dacie.)*

Figure 7.59 *Medial hyperplasia of the right renal artery. Typical 'string of beads' appearance on a selective arteriogram. (Reproduced by permission from W.R. Cattell, J.A.W. Webb and A.J.W. Hilson,* Clinical renal imaging, *published by John Wiley, Chichester, 1989.)*

(a)

(b)

Figure 7.60 *Spiral CT of atheromatous left renal artery stenosis. (a) Original CT image. (b) Axial maximum intensity projection reconstruction showing proximal stenosis (arrowed) typical of atheroma. (Reproduced by permission of Dr C. Engelke.)*

(> 150 cm/s) or absent flow, and distal to the stenosis there may be turbulent flow and spectral broadening. The technical difficulties in examining the main renal arteries led to the study of Doppler arterial waveforms within the kidney that looked for a prolonged acceleration time (pulsus tardus) and decreased peak systolic velocity (pulsus parvus). These indirect indicators are, however, usually only positive when the stenosis is greater than 75 per cent.

Angiography visualizes the renal arteries directly and provides the gold standard for RAS diagnosis. Approximately two thirds of patients have atheromatous renal artery stenosis, which affects the proximal one third of the renal artery, often causing an eccentric or ostial stenosis (Fig. 7.58). The remaining one third of RAS is accounted for by fibromuscular hyperplasia, which typically affects younger patients and involves the distal two thirds of the renal artery, or is segmental. The commonest form of the condition is medial fibroplasia, in which the stenotic segments are interposed between areas where there is medial weakening, giving rise to the 'string of beads' appearance (Fig. 7.59).

When RAS is detected in a hypertensive patient, angioplasty may be undertaken (Fig. 7.58). A stent is often placed following dilatation of atheromatous stenosis. Results both for immediate technical success and long-term cure are better with fibromuscular dysplasia than with atheromatous stenoses. Ostial stenoses are particularly difficult to dilate.

Spiral CT provides a relatively non-invasive method for detecting renal artery stenosis. Data acquired from the volume containing the renal arteries are processed and reconstructed to produce images of the renal arteries. The method reliably demonstrates RAS (Fig. 7.60) but does necessitate irradiation and intravenous contrast medium.

MR angiography with gadolinium contrast medium enhancement during breathholding provides high resolution images of the renal arteries. It has excellent accuracy (> 90 per cent) in identifying RAS (Fig. 7.61) and can show segmental arteries. MR techniques can also be used to quantify renal blood flow. The gadolinium contrast agents used have lower potential for nephrotoxicity than iodinated media.

Diagnosis of renovascular hypertension

To **screen** for renovascular hypertension, captopril renography appears to be the best method. Doppler ultrasound is technically too difficult and IVU is not sensitive enough to be suitable. Availability and cost are likely to limit the use of MR angiography for screening for some time to come.

Rather than screening all hypertensives, many clinicians prefer to **select** patients at high risk of RAS and image their renal arteries directly. Criteria which are widely used are:

- hypertension which is difficult to control with drugs
- young patients (< 30 years)

(a)

(b)

Figure 7.61 *MR of atheromatous right renal artery stenosis. (a) Contrast enhanced MR angiogram. (b) Corresponding midstream aortogram. The stenosis is arrowed. (Reproduced by permission of Dr S.C. Rankin.)*

ultrasound. **Antegrade or retrograde pyelography** may also be helpful (p. 207).

Ultrasound may detect changes indicative of chronic nonobstructive parenchymal disease: small kidneys with thinned parenchyma, which may show increased reflectivity. Parenchymal thickness is generally considered normal if it is 2 cm or more, with 1.5 cm indicating moderate parenchymal thinning and 1 cm or less indicating marked thinning.

If either significant renal asymmetry or renal scarring are shown at ultrasound, a renovascular cause for renal failure is possible, and **angiography** or **spiral CT** or **MR angiography** should be considered. If there is renal artery stenosis, angioplasty may prevent further deterioration in function. Ultrasound can also detect autosomal dominant polycystic kidney disease (Fig. 7.42, p. 212) when this is the cause of renal failure.

Where renal size is normal or increased on ultrasound, and there is no pelvicalyceal dilatation, and no evidence of a prerenal cause for renal failure, renal parenchymal disease is likely. There may be increased parenchymal reflectivity (Fig. 7.56, p. 219). Ultrasound guided renal biopsy will usually provide the diagnosis.

- malignant hypertension
- patients whose renal function deteriorates on captopril.

Traditionally, such patients had renal angiography. CT angiography and, in the future, MR angiography are likely to become the methods of choice, with more invasive traditional angiography being reserved for patients in whom angioplasty is planned.

RENAL FAILURE

The main roles of imaging in a patient presenting with impaired renal function are the detection of renal obstruction and measurement of the kidneys, since normal or large kidneys indicate acute renal failure, and small kidneys indicate chronic irreversible failure.

Ultrasound is the best initial imaging method since it is a sensitive detector of pelvicalyceal dilatation in renal obstruction and can also measure the kidneys accurately. Ultrasound should always be combined with plain films to detect calculi. Since mild pelvicalyceal dilatation may occur in severe functional obstruction (Fig. 7.26, p. 205), any pelvicalyceal visualization must be evaluated further. This approach is associated with false-positive diagnoses, because of the variety of nonobstructive conditions that are associated with pelvicalyceal dilatation. **CT** is helpful in identifying many of the ultrasound false positives, and in showing the cause of obstruction when this cannot be demonstrated with

HAEMATURIA

Haematuria, both macroscopic and microscopic, necessitates urinary tract imaging. Particular concerns include renal adenocarcinoma, transitional cell carcinoma of the bladder, pelvicalyceal system and ureter and calculus disease. Other imaging diagnoses which may be made include renal infarction, papillary necrosis and tuberculosis.

Traditionally, **intravenous urography** has been used as the method of choice to evaluate the kidneys and ureters for causes of haematuria, with cystoscopy being used to check the bladder because of the recognized poor sensitivity of urography in detecting bladder carcinoma. Many still consider that IVU combined with cystoscopy remain the best initial investigations in haematuria.

Ultrasound is a more sensitive detector of renal adenocarcinoma and bladder carcinoma than urography, and has been recommended, combined with plain films, as the first imaging method of choice in haematuria. If this path is followed, the limitations of ultrasound in diagnosing calculi and the fact that detailed pelvicalyceal and ureteric anatomy are not shown must be borne in mind.

Where the ultrasonographic examination is negative and no cause for haematuria has been found, **IVU** is essential in order that many important causes of haematuria do not go undetected. Conversely, if IVU and cystoscopy are negative, ultrasonography or CT should be used to check for renal masses not detected by IVU.

FURTHER READING

Dunnick, N.R. (ed.) 1996: Advances in uroradiology I & II. *Radiologic Clinics of North America* **34**, (5 & 6).

Dunnick, N.R., Sandler, C.M., Amis, S., Newhouse, J. (eds) 1996: *Textbook of uroradiology* (2nd edition). Philadelphia, PA: Lippincott-Raven.

Pollack, H.M., McClennan, B.L. (eds) 2000: *Clinical urography* (2nd edition). Philadelphia, PA: W.B. Saunders.

Webb, J.A.W. 1997: Imaging in haematuria. *Clinical Radiology* **52**, 167–71.

Webb, J.A.W. (ed.) 2000: Imaging in urology. *British Journal of Urology Supplement*, **86** (Supp 1).

8

Lower urinary tract and male genital tract

JUDITH A.W. WEBB

BLADDER

TRAUMA

Severe bladder trauma produces bladder rupture. This may be intraperitoneal, if the bladder is full at the time of injury, or extraperitoneal, usually in association with pelvic fracture. Lesser injury produces contusion without rupture and may be associated with bladder displacement by pelvic haematoma.

To image bladder trauma adequately, cystography is necessary. If there is possible urethral trauma, urethrography must be performed first (p. 194) before catheterization of the bladder for cystography. The bladder must be well distended to visualize rupture. Intraperitoneal rupture is seen as contrast medium outlining bowel loops and spreading into the flanks (Fig. 8.1a). In extraperitoneal rupture there is streaky extravasation into the perivesical tissues (Fig. 8.1b). The two may coexist.

CT can detect extravasation and shows its distribution very accurately. However, if intravenous contrast medium alone is used to distend the bladder, CT appears to be less sensitive than cystography. If CT is to be relied on to detect bladder rupture, the bladder should be distended with contrast medium installed through a catheter (CT cystography).

NEOPLASM

The majority of bladder carcinoma is transitional cell in type. Squamous cell carcinoma is infrequent and associated with calculus and chronic infection. Adenocarcinoma is rare and arises in urachal remnants at the bladder fundus.

Calcification on the surface of the bladder tumour may be seen on **plain films**. On urography, the tumour may produce a polypoid or flattened filling defect (Fig. 8.2) or local bladder wall thickening. Oblique and postmicturition views may help to show whether an apparent filling defect is truly within the lumen rather than being caused by overlying bowel. **Urography is relatively insensitive in the detection of bladder cancer.**

(a)

(b)

Figure 8.1 *Cystograms in bladder trauma. (a) Intraperitoneal rupture. The extravasated contrast medium (arrowed) outlines bowel and has a smooth lower margin. (b) Extraperitoneal rupture with associated pelvic fracture (short arrow). Contrast medium is tracking irregularly into the perivesical tissues (long arrow). (Reproduced by permission of Dr S.M. Goldman, in J.J. McCort and R.E. Mindelzun (eds),* Trauma radiology, *published by Churchill Livingstone, Edinburgh, London, 1990.)*

Even quite large tumours may be missed when the bladder is full of contrast medium. The postmicturation bladder film may be helpful in detecting smaller masses.

At **ultrasonography**, bladder tumours are seen as solid masses protruding into the urine-filled bladder (Fig. 8.3) or as localized bladder wall thickening. Ultrasound is more sensitive in the detection of bladder cancer than IVU.

Relatively small amounts of calcification on the tumour surface can be detected at **computed tomography**. The soft tissue density mass of the tumour may be outlined either by non-opacified water density urine (Fig. 8.4) or by contrast medium within the bladder. CT is used to stage bladder cancer. It can demonstrate extension into the perivesical fat and involvement of the adjacent structures – uterus, prostate, seminal vesicles and bowel – and can show whether there is a clear plane of separation betweem the tumour and the pelvic side wall (Fig. 8.4). CT can also detect pelvic and retroperitoneal nodal metastases. It is not able to show the depth of extension of the tumour within the muscle of the bladder wall.

Figure 8.2 *Bladder carcinoma. IVU shows irregular left bladder mass (arrowed) causing ureteric obstruction.*

Figure 8.3 *Bladder carcinoma. Ultrasound shows solid tumour mass (arrowed) on the posterior right bladder wall.*

Figure 8.4 *Bladder carcinoma. CT shows posterior bladder tumour (black arrow). Note the clear plane between bladder and seminal vesicle. The white arrow indicates the left seminal vesicle.*

On **magnetic resonance imaging**, bladder cancer is isointense with the bladder wall on T1-weighted images. The mass or wall thickening stands out well against the low signal intensity urine and the high signal intensity perivesical fat (Fig. 8.5a, 8.5b). On T2-weighted images the tumour usually has higher signal intensity than the wall (Fig. 8.5c). The degree of muscle infiltration can be assessed more accurately with T2-weighted MRI than with CT. The coronal and sagittal planes (Fig. 8.5b) are particularly helpful in demonstrating basal and fundal tumours. MRI, like CT, can demonstrate perivesical spread and lymph node involvement.

INFECTION

Bladder infection produces bladder wall thickening of non-specific appearance which can be demonstrated by IVU, ultrasound or CT. Calcification in the thickened

(a)

(b)

Figure 8.5 *Bladder carcinoma. Axial (a) and sagittal (b) images show the tumour (arrowed) on T1-weighted MR images. Sagittal image clearly depicts involvement of the bladder base. (c) T2-weighted axial MR scan shows increased signal intensity in the tumour (arrowed). (By kind permission of Dr J. Husband.)*

(c)

Figure 8.6 *Bladder calculus (white arrow) on longitudinal ultrasound scan. Note the acoustic shadow (black arrows).*

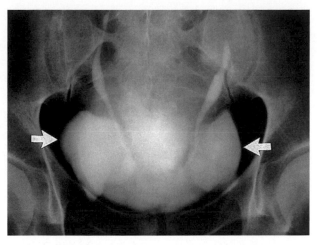

Figure 8.7 *Bladder diverticula. IVU shows bilateral diverticula (arrowed) causing medial deviation of the lower ureters.*

bladder wall suggests tuberculosis or schistosomiasis, both of which produce a contracted bladder in their later stages.

CALCULI AND FILLING DEFECTS

Bladder calculi should be detected on plain films if they are opaque, but on the **plain films** alone the location of pelvic calcifications may be uncertain.

Urography, with oblique or lateral views if necessary, demonstrates whether pelvic calcifications lie within the bladder. Bladder stones are well seen at ultrasound as mobile echogenic foci with associated acoustic shadows (Fig. 8.6). **Ultrasound** is more sensitive for the detection of small bladder stones than is IVU. On **CT** bladder calculi appear as high density mobile opacities within the bladder lumen.

A variety of other bladder filling defects are seen at urography and may need to be distinguished from calculi. Possible causes of a bladder filling defect are:

- calculus
  - lucent
  - opaque
- tumour
- blood clot
- sloughed papilla
- fungal ball
- foreign body
- ureterocoele
- enlarged prostate.

Lucent filling defects produced by tumour and blood clot may be indistinguishable, especially if clot is adher-

ent to the bladder wall. These two entities also appear identical on sonography. The clinical setting may suggest the possibility of a fungal ball or sloughed papilla. A ureterocoele usually has a characteristic appearance (Chapter 7, p. 198). Prostatic enlargement is usually smooth and basal, producing elevation of the bladder base (see Fig. 8.16, p. 231), but a basal bladder carcinoma may be indistinguishable. Overlying bowel gas can usually be distinguished from a bladder abnormality with oblique films. The lucent bowel gas usually does not overlie the bladder in all positions of the patient.

DIVERTICULA

Most bladder diverticula develop secondary to bladder outflow obstruction; rarely, diverticula are congenital. In bladder outflow obstruction there is also bladder wall thickening and often evidence of prostatic enlargement. Most diverticula fill at urography (Fig. 8.7) and cystography. Their size is variable and if large they may cause displacement of the ureter or bladder. Diverticula may enlarge after voiding. Filling defects within them raise the possibility of calculus or tumour and ultrasound or CT may be used to differentiate these.

FISTULAE

Fistulae from bladder to bowel are usually secondary to diverticulitis or carcinoma of the colon; more rarely they may occur in other inflammatory disease, e.g. Crohn's disease, or after trauma or pelvic radiotherapy.

Figure 8.8 *Rectovesical fistula following radiotherapy for carcinoma of cervix. Lateral film shows contrast medium has entered the rectum (large arrow) through a fistula (small arrow) at the bladder fundus.*

Figure 8.9 *Neuropathic bladder seen on IVU in patient with spina bifida. Note bladder wall thickening, multiple diverticula and contrast medium entering the urethra (arrowed).*

Fistulae may be suspected if air is seen in the bladder on plain films or at CT. Air in the bladder can however also result from previous instrumentation including bladder catheterization or from infection with gas-forming organisms.

Demonstration of fistulae may be difficult and **cystography** is more likely to show the fistula than urography or barium studies (Fig. 8.8). **CT** is also helpful in detecting fistulae and shows air in the bladder, focal thickening of the bladder wall and adjacent adherent thickened bowel. As with cystography, contrast medium extravasation through the fistula is more difficult to demonstrate.

Fistulae from bladder to vagina usually result from radical pelvic surgery and/or radiotherapy for malignancy and less commonly from obstetric injury. They are usually relatively easy to demonstrate at cystography. Lateral views are helpful to show contrast medium in the vagina.

NEUROPATHIC BLADDER

Full assessment of bladder dysfunction in neuropathic bladder requires videourodynamics. Either IVU or cystography may demonstrate anatomic abnormality. Spinal cord lesions above the parasympathetic outflow cause detrusor hyperreflexia and detrusor–sphincter dyssynergia. These are associated with bladder wall thickening and trabeculation (Fig. 8.9) and in severe cases with an elongated bladder shape, the so-called 'Christmas tree' or 'pine cone' appearance. There may be secondary dilatation of the ureters and pelvicalyceal systems caused by obstruction at bladder wall level

and/or by vesicoureteric reflux. **Bladder calculi** are relatively common. Pelvic nerve injury is associated with an atonic bladder which is very large and has a smooth outline. Because of the low intravesical pressure, an atonic bladder may not be associated with dilatation of the pelvicalyceal systems and ureters.

URINARY DIVERSION

Ileal loop diversion may be assessed on an IVU but, to show the anatomy in full, **ileal loopography** is required, a procedure in which a Foley catheter is placed in the

Figure 8.10 *Normal ileal loopogram. Arrow indicates ileal loop.*

ileal loop with the balloon inflated just deep to the abdominal wall in order to occlude the stoma. Contrast medium injected to distend the loop normally refluxes freely into both ureters (Fig. 8.10). Failure to show reflux suggests obstruction at the uretero-ileal insertion. Other late complications such as ileal loop stenoses may also be demonstrated.

A variety of continent urinary diversions (e.g. Kock pouch, Mainz pouch) are now also undertaken, and their anatomy can be demonstrated directly by contrast medium injection through a catheter placed in the pouch.

URETHRA: MALE

TRAUMA

In any male patient where urethral trauma is possible, urethrography should be performed before bladder catheterization is attempted, as such attempts may further damage a partially ruptured urethra. **Anterior urethral trauma** is usually secondary to a straddle injury, and contrast medium extravasates below the level of the membranous urethra into the soft tissues of the penis and scrotum (Fig. 8.11). **Posterior urethral trauma** is usually associated with pelvic fracture. The commonest pattern is a tear through the membranous urethra and urogenital diaphragm involving the prostatic and bulbar urethra (i.e. a combined anterior and posterior urethral injury). Contrast medium extravasation occurs both above and below the urogenital diaphragm. If the rupture is incomplete, some contrast medium may enter the bladder at urethrography (Fig.

Figure 8.11 *Anterior urethral trauma. Urethrogram shows contrast medium (arrowed) tracking into the penile, scrotal and inguinal soft tissues. (By kind permission of Dr S.M. Goldman.)*

Figure 8.12 *Posterior urethral trauma. Urethrogram shows contrast medium extravasation (white arrow) from the posterior urethra, tracking into the perivesical tissues (short black arrow) around the bladder base (long black arrow). (By kind permission of Dr S.M. Goldman.)*

8.12). Less commonly, there is stretching of the posterior urethra without rupture or rupture of the posterior urethra alone (Fig. 8.12).

STRICTURE

Stricture of the anterior urethra is usually either post-inflammatory (penile and bulbar urethra), post-traumatic (straddle injury to the bulbar urethra) or iatrogenic (at the penoscrotal junction following catheterization or other instrumentation). Posterior urethral strictures are less common: they follow external trauma or may be iatrogenic, especially after transurethral prostate resection.

Anterior urethral stricture is demonstrated at ascending urethrography as a narrowed segment (Fig. 8.13a). In inflammatory stricture this may be irregular and may involve a long segment which fails to distend normally. With inflammatory stricture there may also be filling of Littre's glands, seen as small contrast medium pools alongside the penile urethra, and of Cowper's glands alongside the proximal bulbar urethra. A voiding study shows dilatation of the urethra to the level of the stricture (Fig. 8.13b). Where obstruction is marked, there may be filling of prostatic glands with contrast medium.

URETHRA: FEMALE

The short female urethra is injured much less frequently than the male urethra. **Urethral diverticula** are

(a)

(b)

Figure 8.13 *Urethral stricture in a male. (a) Tight stricture of the bulbar urethra (arrowed) on ascending urethrogram. (b) Micturating cystography shows dilatation of the urethra to the level of the stricture (arrowed). (Reproduced with permission from H.N. Whitfield, W.F. Hendry, R.S. Kirby and J.W. Duckett,* Textbook of genitourinary surgery, *published by Blackwell, Oxford, 1998.)*

relatively uncommon. Many can be demonstrated as a small contrast medium pool inferior to the bladder on a postmicturition bladder film at IVU. The majority will be shown as a contrast medium pool posterior to the urethra at micturating cystography (Fig. 8.14). An alter-native method of showing a diverticulum is by trans-vaginal ultrasonography. Female urethrography is cumbersome and unpleasant for the patient because of the difficulties in obtaining occlusion of the external meatus, and is now rarely used.

Figure 8.14 *Urethral diverticulum in a female. Biloculate diverticulum (arrowed) fills at micturating cystography.*

PROSTATE

NORMAL ANATOMY

Conventional urography and micturating cystography may show indirect evidence of prostatic enlargement, for example by bladder displacement or urethral compression. The prostate is directly visualized by ultrasound, used either transabdominally, scanning through the full bladder, or transrectally. With **transrectal ultrasound**, a high frequency transducer provides high resolution images, usually in the longitu-dinal and transverse planes. The zonal anatomy of the prostate and the seminal vesicles is seen (Fig. 8.15). The transition and central zones are usually not separable and appear of reduced echogenicity compared to the peripheral zone, which occupies the posterolateral gland and gland apex.

CT provides relatively limited information about the prostate which is seen as a homogeneous rounded soft-tissue density structure inferior to the bladder base.

MRI shows homogeneous signal intensity in the gland on T1-weighted images, but on T2-weighted images the high signal intensity peripheral zone can be identified separately from the lower intensity central and transition zones (Fig. 8.19, p. 232).

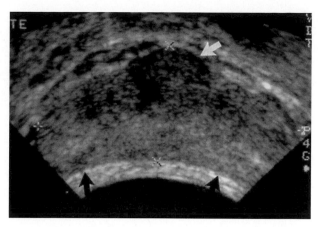

(a)   *(b)*

Figure 8.15 *Normal axial transrectal ultrasound scans. (a) Seminal vesicles (arrowed) lying posterior to the bladder base. (b) Periurethral hypoechoic transition zone (white arrow) and posterolateral peripheral zone (black arrows) on a scan inferior to (a).*

BENIGN PROSTATIC HYPERTROPHY

At **urography** the enlarged prostate of benign prostatic hypertrophy elevates the bladder base, commonly with a smooth lucent filling defect protruding into the bladder base (Fig. 8.16). Secondary effects of bladder outflow obstruction may be seen, with bladder wall thickening, trabeculation, diverticula, elevation of the distal ureters (so-called 'fish-hooking') and, in some patients, secondary pelvicalyceal and ureteric dilatation. Bladder emptying is usually impaired.

On **transabdominal sonography**, the soft tissue mass of the enlarged prostate is seen protruding into the bladder base (Fig. 7.5b, p. 192). On **transrectal ultra-** sound it can be appreciated that the enlargement involves the central transition zone; this is globular in shape, of inhomogeneous reduced echogenicity and it may contain defined adenomatous nodules (Fig. 8.17). The enlarged transition zone compresses the higher echogenicity peripheral zone. Prostate volume can be calculated from measurements of the prostate in three planes.

CARCINOMA

Approximately 70 per cent of prostate cancer affects the peripheral zone. The classic **sonographic** finding in early prostate cancer is a nodule of reduced echogenicity in

Figure 8.16 *Benign prostatic hypertrophy. Enlarged prostate produces a lucent filling defect (arrowed) at the bladder base and elevation of trigone causes 'fishhooking' of the distal ureters.*

Figure 8.17 *Benign prostatic hypertrophy. Axial transrectal ultrasound scan shows the enlarged hypoechoic transition zone (white arrows). Note the calcification (small black arrow) in the 'surgical capsule' between transition and peripheral zones in the right lobe of prostate.*

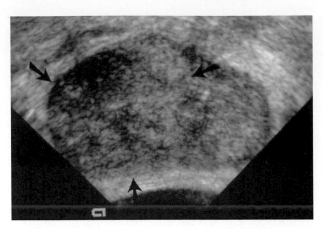

Figure 8.18 *Prostatic carcinoma. Irregular hypoechoic mass (arrowed) occupying the right peripheral and transition zones.*

the peripheral gland. It should, however, be appreciated that hypoechoic nodules in the peripheral zone are often inflammatory rather than malignant. Also, about 25 per cent of tumours have similar echogenicity to normal prostate. As the tumour grows, it spreads into the central and transition zones (Fig. 8.18). The minority of tumours that arise in the central and transition zones are much more difficult to detect with ultrasound, because most patients have some abnormality in this region caused by benign prostatic hypertrophy. Thus **transrectal ultrasound** of the prostate is associated with false-negative and false-positive scans for cancer.

The best assessment in suspected prostate cancer involves combining the findings at digital rectal exami-nation, transrectal ultrasound and the serum prostate specific antigen level. If any of these three methods raises the possibility of cancer, prostate biopsy can be performed either transperineally or transrectally using ultrasound guidance. The transrectal route is currently favoured because of the simplicity of obtaining multi-ple specimens and the ease with which guided biopsies of small abnormalities can be taken. It has the potential disadvantage of sepsis and antibiotic cover for transrec-tal prostate biopsy is, therefore, mandatory. Transrectal ultrasound may also be used for local staging of cancer, to see whether the gland capsule is intact and whether there is evidence of spread into the seminal vesicles.

On T2-weighted **MRI**, cancer in the peripheral zone is seen as an area of decreased signal within the high signal background of the normal peripheral gland (Fig. 8.19). T1-weighted images are best for assessing spread into the periprostatic fat, which is clearly seen as bright signal surrounding the lower signal intensity prostate. The major role of MRI in prostate cancer is for staging rather than detecting tumour. The use of endorectal coils to increase image resolution shows promise of being a more sensitive method than ultrasound in assessing capsular and seminal vesicle involvement.

Either MRI or CT may be used to assess whether there is spread into the perivesical fat or to lymph nodes.

PROSTATITIS

The findings on transrectal ultrasonography in prosta-titis are non-specific. There may be abnormality in the

(a)

(b)

Figure 8.19 *Prostatic carcinoma. Axial magnetic resonance images. (a) T1-weighted image where tumour is difficult to detect. Bright signal of periprostatic fat outlines the gland clearly with no evidence of tumour spread. (b) T2-weighted image shows tumour (arrowed) as an area of reduced signal highlighted against the bright signal of the remaining peripheral zone. (By kind permission of Dr J. Husband.)*

central or peripheral gland, and the latter may be indistinguishable from carcinoma. Prostatic abscess may be diagnosed as a fluid collection by transrectal ultrasound, CT or MRI. Ultrasound may be used to guide transperineal drainage of an abscess.

SCROTUM

NORMAL ANATOMY

Ultrasonography is the most commonly used scrotal imaging method. The testis appears as an ovoid, clearly defined structure of homogeneous echogenicity with a linear band of increased echogenicity, the mediastinum testis, at one side of its long axis. The epididymis is seen as a separate elongated structure paralleling the testis and tapering from the head towards the tail which lies inferiorly. Doppler sonography can be used to detect blood flow in the epididymis and testis.

Scintigraphy is used to demonstrate testicular perfusion. ^{99m}Tc-labelled DTPA is used and dynamic and static images are usually obtained in suspected torsion to check whether there is normal testicular perfusion.

MRI is a secondary scrotal imaging method. Preliminary evaluation indicates that coronal T2-weighted images provide excellent depiction of scrotal anatomy. The wider field of view compared to ultrasound is helpful and MRI has been recommended as useful in patients in whom ultrasound does not give a clear diagnosis.

CT has no role in imaging normally sited testes. It is an important technique, however, in checking for retroperitoneal node enlargement in patients with testicular malignancy, and may be used to search for an undescended testis (p. 235).

INFECTION

In epididymitis the epididymis enlarges and often shows reduced echogenicity on ultrasound (Fig. 8.20). Enlargement may particularly affect the tail. If the inflammatory process spreads to the testis, the testis also may enlarge and become inhomogeneous. If the testicular abnormality is inflammatory it should resolve with antibiotic treatment. Resolution should always be checked with ultrasound because of the possibility that the abnormality could represent a testicular tumour. In epididymitis and orchitis there may be an associated hydrocoele and scrotal skin thickening. In primary orchitis ultrasound shows an enlarged testis which is usually of reduced echogenicity. Rarely, inflammation in either the epididymis or the testis may progress to abscess formation which then shows central fluid contents.

TESTICULAR TUMOURS

Tumours of the testes are seen on ultrasound as intratesticular masses of reduced echogenicity. Seminoma is typically fairly homogeneous (Fig. 8.21), whereas teratomas and embryonal cell tumours are often inhomogeneous with cystic areas or calcifications. Differentiation of these appearances from a focal inflammatory process or infarct is not possible on ultrasound appearances alone. MRI may be helpful in delineating complex tumour masses (Fig. 8.22).

Figure 8.20 *Epididymitis. Longitudinal ultrasound of testis shows the enlarged hypoechoic epididymis (broad arrow) alongside the normal testis (long arrow).*

Figure 8.21 *Seminoma. Hypoechoic 2 cm solid mass (arrowed) seen at the upper pole of the testis on a longitudinal ultrasound scan.*

Figure 8.22 *Coronal T2-weighted image of the scrotum shows a low signal lymphomatous mass (M) arising in the right epididymis and infiltrating the right testis (short arrow). There is also a high signal hydrocoele (long arrow). (Reproduced by permission of Dr R.F. Mattrey and W.B. Saunders, in R.R. Edelman, J.R. Hesselink, J. Newhouse and D.J. Sartoris (eds),* Clinical magnetic resonance imaging, *published by W.B. Saunders, London, 1990.)*

CYSTS AND FLUID-CONTAINING ABNORMALITIES

Benign testicular cysts are relatively common but should be carefully evaluated to check that they do not represent the cystic component of a tumour.

Epididymal cysts are common in any part of the epididymis (Fig. 8.23).

Spermatocoeles usually occur in the epididymal head and may be multiloculate.

Hydrocoele is readily detected by ultrasound as fluid surrounding the testis (Fig. 8.24). The underlying testis and epididymis may be difficult to palpate and ultrasound is helpful to check for underlying testicular neoplasm.

Varicocoele is seen as a collection of dilated veins adjacent to the testis, which become more prominent when the patient stands or performs a Valsalva manoeuvre. Interventional radiological techniques may now be used to embolize the internal spermatic vein in patients with infertility and varicocoele.

TESTICULAR TORSION

Testicular torsion cannot be diagnosed by ultrasound imaging alone, because there is swelling of the testis and epididymis indistinguishable from the appearances in epididymitis or epididymo-orchitis. **Doppler** evaluation may be helpful by showing reduced epididymal and testicular blood flow compared to the normal side and

Figure 8.23 *Epididymal cysts. Transverse ultrasound scan through the upper testis shows two cysts (arrowed) in the epididymis lateral to the testis.*

Figure 8.24 *Hydrocoele. Large fluid collection surrounds a normal testis (arrowed) on a longitudinal ultrasound scan.*

scintigraphy may also show decreased perfusion. Since torsion may be intermittent and since neither method is infallible, early surgical exploration is vital if there is a strong clinical suspicion of torsion, even if Doppler ultrasound studies or scintigraphy do not confirm the diagnosis. Early studies with **MRI** indicate that it may provide helpful diagnostic information in torsion, especially subacute torsion (Fig. 8.25).

TRAUMA

Ultrasound is used following testicular trauma to check for testicular rupture. This may be seen as an interrup-

Figure 8.25 *Coronal proton density-weighted image of the scrotum in subacute left torsion. The thickened cord (black arrows) and knot (white arrow) are seen. There is a high signal haematocoele (h). (Reproduced by permission from Trambert, M.A., Mattrey, R.F., Levine, D. and Berthoty, D.P., Radiology 1990; 175: 53–56.)*

Figure 8.26 *Cavernosogram. Contrast medium in the corpora cavernosa (white arrow) with drainage into the pelvic veins (black arrow) indicating a venous leak.*

tion in the testicular contour or as a localized area of abnormal echogenicity within the testis caused by haemorrhage. Haemorrhage may also occur into the peritesticular tissues producing a haematocele. This has the same distribution as a hydrocele and shows contained echoes when blood clot develops.

UNDESCENDED TESTIS

The role of imaging in diagnosing the position of an undescended testis is controversial, and many consider that exploratory surgery is the best way to find an impalpable testis. When the undescended testis lies in the inguinal region, it can be readily shown by ultrasound. Identification of the mediastinum testis provides a helpful marker that the structure imaged is the testis and not an enlarged lymph node. Both CT and MRI have been used with moderate success to search for intra-abdominal undescended testes.

PENIS

There are relatively few indications for imaging the soft-tissue structures of the penis. In suspected **Peyronie's disease** ultrasound may be used to check for fibrous plaques, which may contain calcification. They are seen

as plaques of increased echogenicity surrounding the corpora cavernosa in whole or in part.

In **impotence**, if a problem with either arterial inflow into or venous leak from the corpora cavernosa is suspected, penile **Doppler ultrasound** studies following intracavernosal injection of prostaglandin (Alprostadil) may be undertaken. In a normal subject there should be increased systolic inflow in the cavernosal arteries following prostaglandin, followed by cessation of venous flow with a decrease to zero in diastolic velocity in the cavernosal arteries when an erection develops. If systolic velocity does not increase normally, arterial inflow is impaired. **Internal pudendal angiography** may be

Figure 8.27 *Longitudinal transrectal ultrasound scan showing a dilated ejaculatory duct (black arrow) which is obstructed just above the verumontanum. White arrow indicates bladder base and open white arrow periurethral hypoechoic area.*

carried out if the patient is a candidate for vascular surgery or angioplasty. If the diastolic velocity does not decrease normally, a venous leak from the corpora cavernosa may be suspected and this can be demonstrated by **cavernosography** in which contrast medium is infused into the corpora cavernosa (Fig. 8.26).

MALE INFERTILITY

Imaging may be used to investigate the patency of the genital tract as a part of the investigation of infertility.

Vasography may be used to outline the ductal system. The vas is cannulated at surgery and contrast medium is injected to outline the vas, seminal vesicle and ejaculatory duct. Contrast medium should flow freely into the posterior urethra.

Transrectal ultrasonography may be used to visualize the ejaculatory ducts as they traverse the prostate. Obstructed ducts appear dilated (Fig. 8.27) and the obstructing lesion, a calculus or Müllerian duct cyst for example, may sometimes be demonstrated.

FURTHER READING

Dunnick, N.R. (ed.) 1996: Advances in uroradiology I & II. *Radiologic Clinics of North America* **34** (5 & 6).

Dunnick, N.R., Sandler, C.M., Amis, S., Newhouse, J. (eds) 1996: *Textbook of uroradiology* (2nd edition). Philadelphia: Lippincott-Raven.

Hricak, H., Hamm, B., Kim, B. 1995: *Imaging of the scrotum*. New York: Raven Press.

Jafri, S.Z.H., Diokno, A.C., Amendola, M.A. (eds) 1998: *Lower genitourinary radiology*. New York: Springer-Verlag.

Pollack, H.M., McClennan, B.L. (eds) 2000: *Clinical urography* (2nd edition). London: W.B. Saunders.

Rifkin, M.D. 1997: *Ultrasound of the prostate* (2nd edition). Philadelphia: Lippincott-Raven.

Webb, J.A.W. (ed.) 2000: Imaging in urology. *British Journal of Urology Supplement* **86** (Suppl 1).

9

Female pelvis

JANE M. HAWNAUR

For most of the 100 years since X-rays were discovered by Wilhelm Röntgen, radiological diagnosis of pelvic conditions has relied on the plain film supplemented by X-ray contrast techniques such as intravenous urography, barium enema, hysterosalpingography, angiography and lymphangiography. Ultrasound and X-ray computed tomographic techniques, introduced in the 1970s, were technically refined and complemented by magnetic resonance imaging in the 1980s and 1990s. Modern pelvic imaging is largely based on these cross-sectional techniques, which are capable of demonstrating pelvic pathology and providing detailed anatomical information non-invasively.

RADIOLOGICAL ANATOMY AND TECHNIQUES

RADIOGRAPHIC PROTECTION

Radiological techniques employed in the investigation of the female patient with symptoms referable to the urinary tract, bowel or pelvic musculoskeletal system are similar to those in males, with the proviso that techniques using ionizing radiation should only be used with full awareness of radiation protection guidelines. X-rays and radionuclides should not be used if the patient has missed a menstrual period and could be pregnant. The '10-day rule', where X-irradiation for non-urgent diagnostic purposed is only carried out in the 10 days following the onset of menstruation, contin-

ues to be applied in some centres to examinations such as pelvic CT or barium enema studies that involve direct irradiation of the female reproductive organs. Both the clinician and radiologist have a duty to protect the patient and unborn child from unnecessary X-irradiation with a consequently greater emphasis on the application of imaging techniques employing non-ionizing radiation in females of child-bearing age.

PLAIN RADIOGRAPHY

The bladder and uterus can be identified on a supine abdominopelvic radiograph as soft-tissue density masses outlined by relatively lucent pelvic fat. Bone metastases from female reproductive tract cancers are unusual except in advanced disease, but are relatively common from breast and bronchial carcinomas. Radiodense foreign bodies or devices such as tubal ligation clips or intrauterine contraceptive devices can be seen. Calcified thrombotic nodules in the pelvic veins (phleboliths) are common and more linear calcification may be visible in the pelvic arteries, especially in patients with renal failure or diabetes. Characteristic calcification in uterine leiomyomata (fibroids) or the combination of fat and teeth in an ovarian dermoid occasionally allow a specific diagnosis to be made from the plain radiograph (Figs 9.1, 9.2). More typically, however, imaging with ultrasound, CT, MRI or contrast radiography is required to reach a diagnosis.

Figure 9.1 *Supine radiograph showing typical coarse calcification in a large uterine fibroid tumour.*

Figure 9.2 *Supine radiograph showing well-formed teeth in the pelvis, characteristic of a dermoid tumour arising in the ovary (large arrow). The adjacent round opacity has the typical appearance of a phlebolith (small arrow).*

CONTRAST RADIOGRAPHY

Barium examination of the large or small bowel remains the best method for localizing adhesions, strictures and fistulae caused by pelvic inflammatory or malignant disease, and for demonstrating mucosal lesions. Large pelvic masses may present with altered bowel habit; a barium enema then helps to exclude colonic carcinoma and evaluate the effect of the pelvic mass on the large bowel (Fig. 9.3).

Intravenous urography can demonstrate ureteric obstruction from a pelvic mass or malignant infiltration, and is indicated for demonstration of iatrogenic damage to the ureters following surgery.

ANGIOGRAPHY AND LYMPHANGIOGRAPHY

Pelvic arteriography is now rarely performed except in the investigation of pelvic haemorrhage. Pelvic venography is undertaken to assess iliac vein compression or thrombosis. Demonstration of lymph node metastases by lymphangiography has largely been superseded by CT and MRI.

HYSTEROSALPINGOGRAPHY

Hysterosalpingography is often performed as part of the investigation of recurrent miscarriage or infertility, since it enables the shape of the uterine cavity and the morphology and patency of the fallopian tubes to be assessed. The examination is contraindicated in pregnancy or if there is active pelvic infection or iodine sensitivity. Hysterosalpingography is carried out within 10 days of last menstrual period, to prevent irradiation of an early conception, but after menstruation has stopped, to reduce potential diagnostic error caused by blood clots in the uterine cavity. After the patient has been told about the nature of the procedure, a warmed speculum is inserted to identify the cervix, which is swabbed with a mild antiseptic solution. A wide variety of devices is available for performing hysterosalpingography. Catheters secured by a balloon in the uterine cavity may obscure the lower part of the uterine cavity; images of this area should be obtained with the balloon deflated at the end of the examination. Vacuum cup devices allow complete visualization of the uterine cavity and traction on the uterus without the use of a tenaculum to grip the cervix. Once the chosen cannula is in place, the speculum is removed and water-soluble iodinated contrast medium at room temperature is introduced by slow hand injection, 5–10 ml over 1 minute. Radiographic exposures are made as contrast medium fills the uterine cavity, delineates the fallopian tubes and spills into the peritoneal cavity. Any tubal spasm can be relieved by smooth muscle relaxants or turning the patient prone and injecting more contrast medium. The normal triangular shape of the uterine cavity is altered in congenital uterine anomalies, or if there are endometrial polyps, submucosal fibroids or synechiae (Asherman's syndrome). Abnormal morphol-

(a)   *(b)*

Figure 9.3 *(a) Supine radiograph taken at the end of the barium enema examination in an elderly woman complaining of altered bowel habit and pelvic fullness. The colon is displaced by a large abdominopelvic mass. (b) Ultrasound scan of the right iliac fossa shows the mass to be solid with multiple cystic areas (arrows): features consistent with ovarian carcinoma.*

ogy (Fig. 9.7b, p. 243) or obstruction of the fallopian tubes can be diagnosed and the presence of peritubal adhesions can be inferred, if contrast medium remains loculated in the peritoneal cavity (Fig. 9.4). Hysterosalpingography can have a therapeutic effect in infertility, presumably caused by contrast medium dislodging debris previously blocking the tube and preventing fertilization.

ULTRASOUND

Techniques

Transabdominal ultrasound is the imaging method for primary assessment of the uterus and related structures. Its application in pregnancy and obstetric complications is discussed in Chapter 10. In the non-pregnant patient, a full bladder is vital for successful scanning, pushing the uterus upwards from behind the pubic symphysis, displacing small bowel and behaving as an acoustic window, improving transmission of the ultrasound beam. The transducers used are of relatively low frequency (2.5–4.0 MHz) resulting in relatively poor spatial resolution. Visualization of pelvic structures may be limited in obese patients.

Transvaginal ultrasound is used to monitor infertility treatment and to assess early pregnancy and its

Figure 9.4 *Hysterosalpingogram performed in the investigation of infertility. The uterine cavity is of normal outline and the proximal tubes are of normal calibre. Saccular dilatation of the distal fallopian tubes with lack of peritoneal spill indicates bilateral hydrosalpinges.*

complications. It is the preferred technique for assessing pelvic inflammatory or malignant conditions, especially when the patient is obese or cannot achieve adequate bladder filling. With a transvaginal probe, the transducer is closer to the region of interest, there is less beam attenuation in superficial soft tissues and a higher ultrasound frequency (5–7.5 MHz) can be employed, increasing sensitivity and spatial resolution in the image. High-resolution ultrasound may also be performed by a transrectal route to assess local tumour spread in patients with carcinoma of the cervix.

Doppler ultrasound can provide useful additional information about vascular changes associated with physiological and pathological pelvic conditions. Ovarian vascularity fluctuates during the menstrual cycle, low resistance to flow occurring in the presence of a functioning corpus luteum. Postmenopausal ovaries are relatively hypovascular, and the demonstration of abnormal vascularity by Doppler ultrasound examination is suggestive of a neoplastic process causing new vessel formation.

Sonohysterosalpingography

Ultrasound can be used to evaluate tubal patency: transvaginal ultrasound is performed while saline or contrast medium is injected via a thin cannula through the cervical canal. When saline alone is used, only the proximal portion of the tube is visible, and patency is inferred when fluid accumulates in the peritoneal cavity. Echogenic ultrasound contrast agents containing stabilized microbubbles allow the full length of the fallopian tube to be visualized, especially when colour Doppler is used, which increases the sensitivity of ultrasound to detection of flow.

Normal ultrasound anatomy

In the reproductive period, the normal uterus measures about 7.5 × 5.0 × 2.5 cm, but is smaller in the prepubertal, postmenopausal or hypo-oestrogenized woman. Normal uterine stroma returns low-level, uniform echoes and the position of the endometrial and endocervical canals is indicated by linear echogenic stripes, representing the interfaces between mucus and mucosa. The ovaries normally lie in the ovarian fossae with their long axes parallel to the internal iliac vessels and ureters posteriorly. Ovarian volume ranges from 4–10 cm^3 depending on hormonal status. Ovarian follicles appear as spherical echolucencies within the ovary and may reach a size of 2.5 cm in normal cycles. Normal fallopian tubes are not visible. A small amount of fluid in the pouch of Douglas is a normal finding, frequently seen at ovulation.

When ultrasound is used to assess women with menstrual problems, abnormal bleeding or pelvic pain, awareness of the cyclic changes in the endometrium and ovaries is invaluable to correlate the ultrasound findings with the patient's symptoms and hormonal status (Table 9.1).

COMPUTED TOMOGRAPHY

Technique

CT is a second line investigation for pelvic disease in the female, particularly for patients of child-bearing age. It is often used for staging pelvic malignancy when, particularly in patients destined for radiotherapy, radiation protection considerations become irrelevant (Fig. 9.5). In young women with benign disease CT should be reserved for patients with complex bowel-related, traumatic or osseous pathology, in whom more basic radiographic or ultrasound techniques have not provided sufficient information for management decisions to be made. The technique involves a high radiation dose to the pelvic organs (around 25 mGy), with direct irradiation of the ovaries. Sections 10 mm thick are obtained from the pelvic brim to perineum. Opacification of the large and small bowel with oral contrast medium is important when pelvic soft-tissue masses or fluid collections are sought. Moderate distension of the bladder helps to improve demonstration of the bladder wall and lifts the uterus into a more vertical position. A tampon can be used to identify the

Table 9.1 *Ultrasound appearances of endometrium and ovaries in a normal menstrual cycle.*

Days (approx)	Endometrium	Ovaries
1–5	Menstrual phase Initially 10–15 mm thick, hyperechoic, +/– fluid, later thin bright echo < 3 mm	Early follicular phase Immature follicles < 10 mm
6–13	Proliferative phase Thickens to ~7 mm, increasing reflectivity from basal layer	Follicular phase Dominant follicle enlarges and secretes oestrogen
~14	Peri-ovulatory Trilaminar hyperechoic outer layer, hypoechoic centre, midline bright echo	Ovulation when follicle is 18–25 mm Ovum + fluid released Follicle collapses
15–28	Secretory phase Thickens to ~15 mm, echogenic with posterior acoustic enhancement	Luteal phase Corpus luteum forms and secretes progesterone

Figure 9.5 *CT of pelvis. Axial CT section obtained for radiotherapy treatment planning in carcinoma of the cervix. Uterus (U), muscle (M), vessels (V) and ovaries (O) have similar soft-tissue density, although follicles in the ovaries are visible because of lower density fluid content.*

position of the vagina in relation to the urethra and rectum. Repeated scanning after intravenous iodinated contrast medium may be necessary to identify the ureters, distinguish pelvic vessels from enlarged lymph nodes and assess the vascularity of any pelvic mass demonstrated.

Normal CT anatomy

The **cervix** is visualized as an ovoid soft-tissue density structure, which should not exceed 3 cm in diameter. The endocervical canal is not usually identifiable unless it contains gas, and the interface between cervix and vaginal fornix is usually unclear. Similar soft-tissue densities and partial volume effects between the uterus, bladder and rectum make the vesicouterine recess and the pouch of Douglas difficult to assess on CT. The orientation of the **body of the uterus** depends on the degree of filling of the urinary bladder and rectal distension. Consequently, axial CT sections are usually oblique in relation to the long axis of the uterus, so that measurements of the normal uterus or uterine masses are unreliable. The structure of the uterus is better shown after intravenous contrast medium, when the vascular endometrium enhances, leaving the uterine cavity visible as a relatively hypodense T-shaped structure. The **broad ligament** can sometimes be identified as a triangular density extending to the pelvic side wall. It encloses a layer of fibrous, vascular and fatty tissue lying lateral to the uterus, called the parametrium. The **round ligament** may be visible as a tubular density extending from the uterine fundus towards the inguinal canal, but the parametrial vessels require enhancement with contrast for their identification within the parametrial soft tissues. The **ovaries** lie between the internal

and external iliac arteries in the ovarian fossae, and have a density similar to other soft-tissue structures such as bowel, blood vessels and muscle (Fig. 9.5). Their identification can be helped by opacification of the ureters, which run posterior to the ovaries. The **ureter** also has an important relationship to the cervix, running 1–2 cm lateral to the cervix before entering the bladder trigone anterior to the uterus.

MAGNETIC RESONANCE IMAGING

Technique

MRI uses non-ionizing radiation and has no known side effects at diagnostic field strengths, provided that patients with ferromagnetic or electromagnetic implants are excluded. Image contrast can be manipulated extensively by altering sequence parameters, but in the pelvis the soft-tissue contrast of a combination of T1-weighted and T2-weighted spin-echo sequences is usually adequate for characterization of many tissues and is superior to that of ultrasound or CT. Sequences that suppress the signal from fat can also be useful in the pelvis. Bowel preparation with oral contrast material is not generally required, although agents which increase or decrease the signal intensity of the bowel lumen are commercially available. If obtrusive, gut peristalsis can be reduced with a short-acting smooth muscle relaxant given immediately before scanning. There are few specific indications for using intravenous paramagnetic MR contrast media in the female pelvis. Their administration is usually reserved for assessment of malignant disease, particularly if satisfactory T2-weighted sequences cannot be obtained.

Normal MRI anatomy

In the reproductive period, the **uterus** has distinctive zonal anatomy on T2-weighted MR images (Fig. 9.6a). The **myometrium** shows a medium intensity signal, separated from hyperintense **endometrium** by a band of low signal, representing the compact inner third of the myometrium. The cervical fibromuscular stroma is low in signal intensity. The **ovaries** show a low to medium signal on T1-weighted sequences, similar to that of adjacent vessels or bowel. Ovarian stroma has a medium to high signal intensity on T2-weighted sequences and the very high signal in developing follicles allows identification of the ovaries in the majority of women with normal ovarian function (Fig. 9.6b).

INFERTILITY

Infertility is defined as the inability to conceive after 12 months or more of unprotected sexual intercourse. It

(a)

(b)

Figure 9.6 *(a) Sagittal T2-weighted MRI scan demonstrates tumour (T) in the posterior cervical lip as medium signal density replacing the low signal of normal stroma. The zonal anatomy of the uterus is well shown, the outer two thirds of myometrium (M) having medium signal intensity separated from hyperintense endometrium by a band of low signal representing the 'junctional' zone of myometrium. (b) MRI of pelvis as in Fig. 9.5. A T2-weighted MRI scan obtained at a similar level shows high signal from urine in the bladder (B) and fluid in ovarian follicles (F), medium signal from cervical tumour (T) and low signal from normal cervix (C), vaginal wall (W) and flowing blood (V).*

affects about 15 per cent of couples, and in about half of these, infertility is partly or wholly caused by a problem in the female partner. Imaging can help to diagnose the cause, for example, ovulatory or endocrine dysfunction or structural abnormalities preventing fertilization and implantation of the ovum.

Ultrasound provides a useful preliminary non-invasive assessment, confirming the presence of a normal adult uterus and ovaries. If the ultrasound appearance of the ovaries and endometrium correlates with the phase of the menstrual cycle, a normal ovulatory cycle can be inferred (Table 9.1). Impending ovulation is assumed when a dominant follicle measuring 18–25 mm is present, in which the mature oocyte and surrounding granulosa cells (cumulus oophorus) may be visible. Signs indicative of ovulation include the collapse and disappearance of a dominant follicle in the second half of the cycle, identification of a corpus luteum, and development of a thick and echogenic luteal endometrium. Adnexal or uterine masses associated with subfertility can be identified. For example, submucosal fibroids can interfere with implantation, and intramural fibroids may obstruct the fallopian tube or cervical canal. MRI may help to localize a fibroid more accurately, especially if myomectomy is being considered to conserve uterine function. Other specific conditions associated with subfertility, identifiable on imaging, include polycystic ovarian syndrome, congenital uterine anomalies, endometriosis and pelvic inflammatory disease, which may be associated with hydrosalpinges (see below). In addition to ultrasound, hysterosalpin-

gography is often requested to assess the morphology of the uterine cavity and the patency of the fallopian tubes.

ASSISTED CONCEPTION

Patients with ovulatory dysfunction may be treated by clomiphene citrate or human menopausal gonadotropin to stimulate follicular development. Patients usually undergo serial transvaginal ultrasound to monitor the development of follicles and identify when a follicle is mature. Ovulation occurs, or the ovum can be retrieved, when a follicle attains a diameter of 20–25 mm. Transvaginal ultrasound is used to assess the receptivity of the endometrium to a gamete, in combination with measurements of serum oestradiol. It is also used to guide aspiration of ova from ovarian follicles, and the subsequent introduction of embryos fertilized *in vitro* into the fallopian tube or uterine cavity by transvaginal catheter, i.e. gamete intrafallopian transfer (GIFT).

Ovarian hyperstimulation syndrome is a complication of ovulation induction characterized by persistence of multiple physiological ovarian cysts after stimulation with gonadotropins. Painful ovarian enlargement owing to cyst formation and stromal oedema may be accompanied by ascites, pleural effusions, electrolyte imbalances and thromboembolism and can be life-threatening. Transvaginal ultrasound is used to detect early signs of hyperstimulation, so that management of the cycle can be modified to reduce the risk of the complication occurring.

IMAGING IN GYNAECOLOGY

Ultrasound is the most frequently requested imaging technique for assessing the patient with gynaecological symptoms, or confirming and identifying the cause of abnormal findings on clinical examination, for example, uterine enlargement caused by fibroids, or a palpable mass in the adnexae caused by an ovarian cyst or an hydrosalpinx. The premenopausal woman is often most concerned about the possible effect of gynaecological problems on her ability to have children whilst, in the postmenopausal woman, presentation with abnormal bleeding, pelvic pain or swelling raises anxieties about malignant disease.

CONGENITAL ANOMALIES

Duplication anomalies of the uterus and vagina are due to abnormal fusion of the Müllerian ducts in utero. Congenital maldevelopment of the genital tract occurs in about 0.5 per cent of women and may be associated with an increased incidence of spontaneous abortion. There are seven categories of congenital abnormality:

- Type I: hypoplasia or aplasia of vagina, cervix, uterine body or fallopian tubes, singly or in combination;
- Type II: unicornuate uterus: failure of one Müllerian duct to develop, often associated with ipsilateral renal agenesis;
- Type III: uterus didelphys: there are two separate uterine horns, each with its own cervix and upper vagina;
- Type IV: bicornuate uterus: there are two separate uterine horns, a single cervix and vagina;
- Type V: septate uterus: the uterine fundus is intact but the endometrial cavities are divided by a septum which may extend to involve the cervix and vagina;
- Type VI: arcuate uterus: the uterine cavity is indented at the fundus but the outer fundal contour is convex;
- Type VII: diethylstilboestrol-associated deformity: the uterus has a small T-shaped cavity and a short cervix; there is an association with clear cell carcinoma of the vagina.

Congenital uterine anomalies are often suspected initially on ultrasound or hysterosalpingography, but both methods have their limitations (Fig. 9.7). For example, a unicornuate uterus may be mistaken for a small, laterally situated uterus on ultrasound whilst, on hysterosalpingography, one horn of a bicornuate uterus may be rudimentary and non-communicating, appearing similar to a unicornuate uterus. Magnetic resonance imaging is the preferred method for detailed assessment and classification of complex anomalies.

(a)

(b)

Figure 9.7 *Congenital uterine anomalies. (a) Transabdominal ultrasound scan of the pelvis showing the two divergent horns of a uterus didelphys in transverse section. There was an associated absence of the left kidney. (b) Hysterosalpingography showing partial division of the uterine cavity due to congenital bicornuate uterus. The fallopian tubes are normal and there is peritoneal spill of contrast.*

Haemato(metro)colpos secondary to vaginal occlusion or imperforate hymen can present with a pelvic mass in an amenorrhoeic teenager.

INFLAMMATORY CONDITIONS

PELVIC INFLAMMATORY DISEASE

Sexually transmitted organisms are often responsible for pelvic inflammatory disease but adnexal inflammation may also be secondary to diverticulitis, appendicitis or

Figure 9.8 *Transverse pelvic ultrasound scan in a woman suspected of having pelvic inflammatory disease. There is a large fluid collection posterior to the uterus (U) secondary to appendicitis.*

inflammatory bowel disease (Fig. 9.8). If an abdominal radiograph is performed, findings suggestive of pelvic inflammatory disease include obliteration of pelvic fat planes, local ileus and the presence of an intrauterine contraceptive device. Ultrasound, however, is the imaging investigation of first choice. The uterus may appear slightly swollen and hypoechoic with ill-defined margins and a prominent endometrial echo. There may be an inflammatory adnexal mass or ancillary signs of pelvic inflammatory disease, such as free intraperitoneal fluid, loss of tissue interfaces or mild hydronephrosis. Normal pelvic ultrasound does not exclude the diagnosis. Once a clinical diagnosis of pelvic inflammatory disease is made, response of any inflammatory mass to conservative treatment with antibiotics can be monitored by ultrasound.

HYDROSALPINX

In acute salpingitis, the fallopian tubes may be visible on ultrasound as dilated tubular structures in the adnexae. In chronic pelvic inflammatory disease, hydrosalpinx is caused by secretions trapped in the tubal lumen by peritubal adhesions. Hysterosalpingography shows fusiform tubal dilatation with prolonged retention of contrast medium and no peritoneal spill (Fig. 9.4, p. 239). Demonstration of mucosal folds and continuity with the uterine cornua on ultrasound helps to differentiate hydrosalpinx from other cystic adnexal masses. Echogenic contents or layering of debris suggest the presence of

blood or pus within the fallopian tubes. Haematosalpinx may occur in ruptured ectopic pregnancy.

TUBO-OVARIAN ABSCESS

Acute salpingitis may be complicated by abscess formation, when pus from the fimbriated end of the fallopian tube becomes loculated between the tube and the adjacent ovary. The resultant tubo-ovarian abscess may involve adjacent bowel or bladder and, if rupture occurs, may be life-threatening.

Ultrasound demonstration of an irregular thick-walled cystic adnexal mass is not specific and may also occur in ectopic pregnancy, haemorrhagic or infected ovarian cyst, ovarian torsion, etc. Radio-nuclide scanning using gallium 67-citrate or indium 111-labelled leucocytes can be used to confirm the presence of infection and localize an abscess. CT and MRI are less commonly used, but may show a complex cystic mass incorporating the ovary, containing fluid of proteinaceous or haemorrhagic nature, and a thickened irregular wall enhancing after contrast.

ENDOMETRITIS

Endometritis is a common cause of fever in the puerperium especially after caesarian section or prolonged rupture of the membranes. Ultrasound demonstrates echogenic mterial within the endometrial canal in more advanced cases with fluid or gas in a distended endometrial cavity. The differential diagnosis includes retained products of conception and malignancy.

PYOMETRIUM

Impaired drainage of the uterine cavity associated with cervical or endometrial carcinoma, previous uterine surgery, radiotherapy, benign tumours (such as fibroids) or inflammatory processes, may underlie the formation of a pyometrium (pus-filled endometrial cavity) or haematometrium (blood-filled). The presence of a dilated endometrial cavity can be confirmed by any cross-sectional imaging technique, but characterization of the contents is most accurate on ultrasound or MRI (Fig. 9.9).

BENIGN UTERINE TUMOURS

UTERINE FIBROIDS

Uterine fibroid tumours (leiomyomata) are common in women aged over 30 years. Submucosal or intramural

(a)

(b)

Figure 9.9 *(a) Sagittal T2-weighted MRI scan in an elderly woman with uterine cancer and canal stenosis showing distension of the endometrial cavity by hyperintense material. (b) A postcontrast T1-weighted MRI scan helps to identify the intrauterine masses as part fluid (F) with a non-enhancing mass, possibly blood clot in the obstructed uterine canal. Lack of enhancement effectively excludes viable tumour.*

tumours often cause heavy menstrual blood loss and anaemia. Subserosal fibroids may be asymptomatic until so bulky as to cause pressure symptoms. Pedunculated fibroids may also arise from the cervix or broad ligament. In about 30 per cent of cases, the compact fibromuscular stroma of a fibroid becomes affected by haemorrhagic, mucinous or myxomatous degeneration. Sarcomatous degeneration is rare but cannot be distinguished from benign degeneration by diagnostic imaging methods.

In the UK, troublesome fibroids are often managed by hysterectomy in women who have completed their family. The surgical approaches to uterine leiomyomas with conservation of the uterus are hysteroscopic myomectomy for submucosal tumours or transabdominal myomectomy for intramural and serosal tumours.

MRI is the most accurate method for precise localization for planning such conservative surgery, but often fibroids can be equally well demonstrated by either **ultrasound** or MRI. On MRI, uncomplicated fibroids are well-circumscribed low signal intensity masses within the myometrium (Fig. 9.10). Degeneration of all types causes an increase in signal intensity, especially on T2-weighted sequences.

On ultrasound, fibroids appear as solid iso- or hypoechoic masses compared with normal myometrium (Fig. 9.11). Degeneration may produce cystic spaces or fluid-debris levels on ultrasound, and calcific foci produce areas of echogenicity with acoustic

Figure 9.10 *Sagittal T2-weighted MR scan through the uterus showing multiple low signal intensity intramural and submucosal fibroids.*

shadowing. The density of a simple fibroid is similar to that of normal myometrium on CT, but morphological distortion and the presence of coarse calcification within the mass suggest the diagnosis (see Fig. 9.20, p.

Figure 9.11 *Transabdominal ultrasound of the uterine body in longitudinal section, showing intramural fibroids (between cursors).*

Figure 9.12 *Sagittal T2-weighted MR scan through the uterine body showing myometrial thickening due to diffuse adenomyosis. Hyperintense intramural foci (arrows) are typical for adenomyosis. The widening of the endometrial cavity is due to endometrial hyperplasia.*

251). Degenerative changes cause increased tissue heterogeneity, with the appearance of hypodense areas or intralesional gas. Tumour margins may become more visible after bolus contrast administration.

ADENOMYOSIS

In adenomyosis, portions of the basal layer of the endometrium are ectopically deep within the myometrium, exciting reactive hyperplasia of the surrounding muscle. The condition may be asymptomatic, but dysmenorrhoea is common. Diffuse adenomyosis causes enlargement of the uterus whereas focal adenomyosis is difficult to distinguish from fibroids on CT and ultrasound. On T2-weighted MRI scans, diffuse adenomyosis results in uterine enlargement with thickening and loss of definition of the junctional zone extending into the outer myometrium (Fig. 9.12). Focal adenomyosis appears as a low signal mass on T2-weighted sequences, similar to a fibroid, but with a more ovoid shape and less well-defined margins.

MALIGNANT UTERINE TUMOURS

ENDOMETRIAL CARCINOMA

Endometrial cancer is typically a well-differentiated adenocarcinoma with a slow rate of progression, manifesting with postmenopausal bleeding. At presentation, 75 per cent of women have tumour confined to the endometrium (stage IA) for whom the 5-year survival rate is 80 per cent following total hysterectomy. The International Federation of Obstetrics and Gynaecology (FIGO) committee recommends staging by total

abdominal hysterectomy, bilateral salpingo-oophorectomy and lymphadenectomy, a counsel that is not achievable in all cases. Preoperative imaging may be helpful in assessing the depth of myometrial invasion, the presence or absence of cervical involvement and lymphadenopathy in patients in whom clinical examination is difficult or full staging laparotomy is inappropriate.

Transabdominal ultrasound can demonstrate uterine enlargement but does not adequately assess depth of myometrial invasion or lymph node enlargement. **Transvaginal ultrasound** gives a better assessment of the uterus but is insufficient to assess extrauterine spread.

On **CT** with intravenous contrast enhancement, a large endometrial carcinoma may be visible as a hypodense mass deforming the uterus, often with eccentric spread within the myometrium and low density areas representing avascular tumour necrosis or retained secretions within the endometrial cavity.

Endometrial carcinoma is more easily shown by **MRI**, although early cancers may be difficult to detect because of similarity in signal intensity to endometrium on T2-weighted sequences. When tumours become large enough to distend or distort the uterine cavity, differentiation from benign tumour or blood clot may require intravenous paramagnetic contrast administration. Intravenous contrast also increases the accuracy of staging and allows assessment of the volume of viable tumour, since necrotic tumour, blood clot or other

Figure 9.13 *Sagittal T2-weighted MR scan in a postmenopausal woman showing expansion of the endometrial cavity by a large tumour of heterogeneous signal intensity.*

Figure 9.14 *Sagittal T2-weighted MR scan of an endocervical carcinoma. Hyperintense tumour is surrounded by low signal cervical stroma, i.e. it is confined to the cervix.*

debris do not enhance (Fig. 9.9, p. 245). When tumour invades the myometrium, there is loss of the normal low signal intensity of the junctional zone, although this may ordinarily be indistinct in post-menopausal women (Fig. 9.13). Tumour invading less than half the myometrial depth is given a stage of IB, and greater than half, stage IC. Accuracy of staging of endometrial carcinoma by MRI is about 80 per cent.

UTERINE SARCOMA

Leiomyosarcoma accounts for less than 1 per cent of uterine malignancy. Although malignant transformation of uterine fibroids may occur, most leiomyosarcomas arise *de novo*. No imaging technique can reliably differentiate between benign degenerative fibroids and sarcoma.

CERVICAL CARCINOMA

In 60–70 per cent of cases, cervical carcinoma is squamous in histological type, developing in the squamocolumnar junction, and potentially detectable in the preinvasive stages by the cervical smear population screening programme.

Adenocarcinomas tend to arise deeper in the endocervical canal and may remain occult until advanced (Fig. 9.14). Diagnostic imaging is only appropriate in invasive cancer, the spatial resolution of currently available radiological techniques being insufficient to identify microinvasive disease. Clinical staging of invasive carcinoma of the cervix is inaccurate, particularly in women with disease extending beyond the uterus. Demonstration of lymph node enlargement by cross-sectional imaging may also modify treatment pathways, although no imaging method can reliably differentiate reactive from metastatic nodal enlargement. Although both ultrasound and CT have applications in cervical cancer staging, MRI is the most consistently useful modality in all tumour stages and is as accurate as contrast-enhanced CT for assessing lymph node status. It is the most suitable imaging method for staging women with carcinoma of the cervix during pregnancy (Fig. 9.15).

Transabdominal ultrasound does not contribute to staging the primary cervical tumour, but can show urinary tract obstruction, ascites or hepatic metastases in advanced disease. **Transrectal ultrasound** can demonstrate cervical enlargement and parametrial extension but, because of a limited range of view, cannot evaluate the full extent of bulky tumours or screen the relevant lymph node regions.

On unenhanced **CT**, the density of cervical carcinoma is similar to normal cervix, but carcinoma can be inferred when there is eccentric enlargement of the cervix. An irregular or ill-defined interface with the parametrial soft tissues implies parametrial invasion, although a similar appearance may be seen following pelvic inflammatory disease or surgery. Obliteration of pelvic fat planes is well demonstrated by CT, enabling diagnosis of tumour

(a)   (b)

Figure 9.19 *Transaxial MR scans in a patient with bilateral endometriomas. (a) T1-weighted sequence showing high signal intensity. (b) T2-weighted sequence showing intermediate signal caused by the presence of chronic haemorrhage.*

Doppler ultrasound may be minimal. The diagnostic advantages of CT or MRI over ultrasound have not been determined and these techniques are not appropriate unless immediatley available in the emergency situation.

OTHER ADNEXAL MASSES

Cysts of the broad ligament are usually derived from embryonic remnants and can reach a massive size. They can be complicated by infection, haemorrhage, torsion or rupture presenting as a surgical emergency. On imaging, broad ligament cysts are difficult to distinguish from ovarian or other adnexal cysts.

Peritoneal inclusion cysts occur in patients with pelvic adhesions from previous surgery or pelvic inflammatory disease. Fluid is trapped between thickened and adherent peritoneum and may be visualized on ultrasound as a cystic adnexal mass distorting the ovary.

On all imaging modalities, a **lymphocoele** is a unilocular thin-walled cyst on the pelvic side wall, containing watery or proteinaceous fluid.

ENDOMETRIOSIS

Functioning endometrial cells may implant on the ovary, broad ligament, uterine serosa or in the pouch of Douglas. The endometriotic tissue undergoes cyclical growth and bleeding in response to hormonal stimula-

tion, forming haemorrhagic 'chocolate cysts'. Rupture causes intense serosal irritation and adhesions. Imaging techniques are generally unable to show small implants but may demonstrate secondary effects related to inflammation and scarring. Endometriotic adhesions can distort pelvic anatomy and cause conditions such as rectal tethering, hydrosalpinx and small bowel obstruction. Large implants are more likely to be detectable by ultrasound, CT or MRI.

Endometriotic cysts, or endometriomas, have variable morphology on imaging and can mimic other lesions that have a complex mixed cystic/solid appearance such as tubo-ovarian abscess, infected or haemorrhagic cysts and ovarian malignancy. The most characteristic appearance is multiloculated thin-walled cysts with ill-defined margins. On **ultrasound**, internal echoes reflect the presence of blood products in the cyst fluid (Fig. 9.17). Endometriomas usually have increased density on **CT** and high signal intensity on **MRI** owing to their haemorrhagic content. Signal intensity may vary in different parts of the cyst, especially on T2-weighted sequences, because of various stages of degradation of blood products; a low signal rim due to haemosiderin-laden macrophages or fibrosis may be visualized at the periphery of chronic endometriomas (Fig. 9.19). The cysts often have angulated margins or show evidence of tethering. Implants occurring in unusual locations, such as on bowel serosa or the liver, are best investigated using ultrasound or CT scanning with full bowel preparation. MRI has a higher sensitivity and specificity than ultrasound or CT for the diagnosis of endometrioma. The definitive technique for staging endometriosis is, however, laparoscopy, at which the severity of endometriosis and the extent of pelvic adhesions is scored. Once diagnosed, the response of endometriomas to hormonal therapy can be assessed using ultrasound or MRI.

BENIGN OVARIAN TUMOURS

Tumours arising from the surface epithelium of the ovary include serous, mucinous, endometrioid, clear cell, Brenner and undifferentiated types, and account for 60 per cent of ovarian tumours (Fig. 9.20). Cellular differentiation into benign and malignant types is not always clear-cut, up to one third being classified as borderline malignancy on histological examination. The classification of ovarian masses by imaging is also imperfect. Benign tumours often have the appearance of simple cysts, while malignant tumours are more heterogeneous complex masses with a higher proportion of solid tissue. Any solid or complex pelvic mass demonstrated by imaging is therefore regarded with suspicion. Unfortunately, certain benign ovarian tumours, such as fibromas and granulosa cell tumours (derived from ovarian stroma) and Brenner tumours, are characteristically solid. Ovarian malignancy is also more likely to be associated with ascites.

OVARIAN CYSTADENOMA

Serous cystadenomas account for 30 per cent of benign ovarian neoplasms and are usually thin-walled unilocular or multilocular cysts, often bilateral, measuring 5–10 cm in diameter, with watery or minimally haemorrhagic contents. Fine calcification may occur in the cyst wall. Mucinous cystadenomas constitute 20 per cent of benign ovarian tumours and are usually larger in size, more frequently multilocular and less often bilateral compared with the serous type. The wall is generally diffusely thickened and the cyst contents are mucinous. Cyst leakage into the peritoneal cavity can

(a)

(b)

Figure 9.21 *(a) Ultrasound scan, performed to assess an asymptomatic pelvic mass in a 21-year-old woman, demonstrates a uniformly echogenic mass arising centrally in the pelvis. A specific diagnosis could not be made from the ultrasound scan. (b) CT scan in the same patient shows a mass containing proteinaceous fluid (20 HU) with a fat–fluid level (vertical arrow) anteriorly and rim calcification (horizontal arrow). These features are typical of an ovarian dermoid cyst.*

Figure 9.20 *Contrast-enhanced CT scan showing a cystic mass in the right adnexa, with poor definition and frond-like soft-tissue density posteriorly (straight arrow). A benign clear cell ovarian tumour was resected. Calcification is present in a uterine fibroid (curved arrow).*

(a)

(b)

Figure 9.22 *(a) Sagittal T2-weighted MRI scan in a 66-year-old woman with an ulcerating mass in the posterior vaginal fornix, thought clinically to be cervical in origin. In addition to tumour (T) in the pouch of Douglas invading the vagina and rectum, multiple complex cystic tumours (C) are present, consistent with ovarian carcinoma. Apart from a small fibroid in the anterior myometrium, the uterus is normal. (b) Coronal T1-weighted MRI scan demonstrates a cystic ovarian tumour (T) on the left, and right pelvic lymphadenopathy (arrow).*

result in pseudomyxoma peritonei, with large gelatinous masses which may contain amorphous calcification filling the abdominal cavity.

OVARIAN DERMOIDS

Cystic ovarian teratomas, or dermoid tumours, account for 20 per cent of ovarian tumours, and may be bilateral. Dermoid ovarian tumours classically contain a complex mixture of tissues in a multicompartmental, part cystic and part solid adnexal mass. The presence of fat, bone or teeth within the mass is characteristic (*see* Fig. 9.2, p. 238).

Other possible constituents include proteinaceous or serous cysts, soft-tissue septa or nodules and rim calcification, which altogether may result in a complex and bizarre appearance on diagnostic imaging. Fat has a speckled hyperechoic appearance on ultrasound, a negative attenuation value on CT and a high signal intensity on both T1- and T2-weighted MR sequences (Fig. 9.21). Fat–fluid levels may be apparent on all imaging methods. On MRI, the chemical shift artefact which occurs at interfaces between lipid and water, or reduction in lesional signal on fat-suppression sequences may be useful corroborative evidence of the presence of fat within the tumour.

Calcification is identified as echo-bright areas with acoustic shadowing on ultrasound and as very high attenuation tissue on CT. MRI is relatively insensitive to calci-

fication and will not identify fine mural calcification or focal calcification but can identify teeth and bone tissue if well-developed. Soft-tissue fronds, mural nodules and septa can be identified by all techniques. Differentiation between benign and malignant teratomas (2 per cent of total), which also contain a mixture of mesodermal elements, is imprecise by all imaging techniques.

MALIGNANT OVARIAN TUMOURS

Ovarian cancer is a disease of postmenopausal women predominantly, most of whom present with advanced disease. After clinical examination, which may demonstrate a pelvic mass, ultrasound is the imaging investigation of first choice (*see* Fig. 9.3b, p. 239).

In postmenopausal women the ovaries are atrophic, measuring around 1–2 cm in maximum diameter, and can be difficult to visualize on ultrasound. Any solid or cystic ovarian enlargement has to be regarded as malignant until proven otherwise, and requires follow-up. A simple cyst of less than 4 cm in diameter in a postmenopausal woman is unlikely to be malignant and can be followed by ultrasound. Larger cysts, especially those with a wall thickness of more than 3 mm, solid nodules, multiple irregular septa, prominent papillary excrescences or echogenic cyst contents, are more likely to be malignant. Benign cysts complicated by haemorrhage or infection can have an

Figure 9.23 *CT scan showing complex cystic masses arising from the pelvis in a ptient with bilateral ovarian serous cystadenocarcinoma.*

Figure 9.24 *Contrast-enhanced CT in a patient with advanced ovarian cancer. An 'omental cake' of metastatic ovarian tumour is present (arrows). The contrast-filled ureters can be seen posteriorly lying on the psoas major muscles (arrowheads).*

identical ultrasound appearance and although ultrasound demonstration of ascites or peritoneal masses favours underlying malignancy, the specific diagnosis may ultimately require laparoscopy.

Similarly, CT or MRI may confirm the clinical suspicion of an ovarian tumour with comparable features, but they do not provide a more specific diagnosis than ultrasound (Figs 9.22, 9.23). Transvaginal ultrasound with colour flow Doppler has a higher sensitivity and specificity, tumour neovascularization being associated with a low impedance to blood flow through the ovarian vascular bed.

Treatment of ovarian carcinoma is usually total hysterectomy, bilateral salpingo-oophorectomy and infracolic omentectomy, at which time formal laparoscopic staging is performed. Preoperative imaging can assist the surgeon when planning surgery and may help postoperatively to assess the volume of residual disease and its subsequent response to chemotherapy. CT is particularly able to demonstrate peritoneal and omental tumour, hepatic metastases and lymphadenopathy (Fig. 9.24). Although MRI can stage the primary tumour and assess lymphadenopathy, it is less capable of demonstrating bowel and peritoneal involvement.

OVARIAN CYSTADENOCARCINOMA

Two thirds of ovarian cancers arise in the surface epithelium, producing serous or mucinous cystadenocarcinoma, endometrioid carcinoma, or more unusually, clear cell, Brenner, or undifferentiated types of carcinoma. **Serous cystadenocarcinoma** accounts for 40 per cent of malignant ovarian tumours. Tumour cysts tend to be larger than 10 cm in diameter, with variable solid components, and are bilateral in 50 per cent (Fig. 9.23).

On CT and MRI, malignant soft-tissue nodules enhance after intravenous contrast medium. Psammomatous or dystrophic calcification may be apparent. Focal papillary projections disrupting the normally smooth outer margin indicate capsular invasion, associated with seeding of tumour cells into the peritoneal cavity.

Mucinous cystadenocarcinomas comprise 5–20 per cent of malignant ovarian tumours; they are multicystic tumours containing mucinous material, haemorrhage, necrotic and solid tumour, and are bilateral in 15–25 per cent. The rarer **endometrioid tumour** is a complex cystic or solid mass on imaging, affecting one or both ovaries or the fallopian tubes and spreading intraperitoneally.

OTHER OVARIAN MALIGNANCIES

Malignant neoplasms may also arise from germ cell, sex cord stromal or mesenchymal cell lines in the ovary. These often appear on imaging as a solid soft-tissue mass, with or without lymphadenopathy. The ovaries are favoured sites of metastasis from primary gastrointestinal or breast adenocarcinoma producing so-called **Krukenberg tumours**, identical on imaging to primary ovarian carcinoma.

VAGINA AND VULVA

The vagina and external genitalia are readily accessible to clinical examination, and diagnostic imaging

Figure 9.25 *T1-weighted MRI scan performed to stage carcinoma of the vulva in a 63-year-old woman. The primary tumour (T) was shown on other images to involve the anus, vagina, urethra and pubis. Bilateral pelvic lymphadenopathy is present (arrows).*

techniques are only used to assess deep invasion of vaginal or vulvar carcinoma and the presence of pelvic lymphadenopathy (Fig. 9.25). Imaging may also help to confirm the presence of fistulae.

TREATED PELVIC MALIGNANCY

Tumour recurrence

After hysterectomy for uterine malignancy, tumour recurrence usually occurs initially in the vaginal stump or on the pelvic side wall, with subsequent spread to the pelvic viscera and lymph nodes. Suitability for further treatment, e.g. pelvic exenteration, depends on the extent of local involvement and the absence of systemic dissemination. Pelvic imaging by CT or MRI can be very useful to demonstrate tumour extent, particularly when clinical pelvic examination is hindered by postoperative changes.

Postoperative changes

Postoperative changes can be easily demonstrated by cross-sectional imaging, with MRI being the most sensitive to inflammatory changes following surgery. This sensitivity and the lymph node enlargement, which may follow even relatively localized surgery, hinders the ability of all imaging methods to assess residual tumour in the first few weeks after operation.

Imaging is thus best delayed for a minimum of 6 weeks postoperatively, unless base-line scans are available for comparison or there is a case for urgent scanning. Over the period between 6 weeks and 3 months after uncomplicated surgery, vascular granulation tissue matures into a relatively avascular fibrous scar. Haematoma and oedema also tend to resolve. Three months after radical hysterectomy, CT should demonstrate the vaginal stump as a thin soft-tissue

(a)

(b)

Figure 9.26 *Axial T1-weighted MRI scans (a) pre- and (b) post-gadolinium-DTPA in a patient with dysuria and bilateral hydronephrosis on ultrasound. Diffuse thickening of the bladder wall and rectum, enhancing after contrast, is secondary to inflammation rather than tumour recurrence. The patient received radical radiotherapy for cervical carcinoma 4 years previously.*

structure, the uterine bed being filled with fatty tissue containing only thin dense strands of fibrous scar.

The presence of nodular soft-tissue densities at the operative site or on the pelvic wall indicates tumour recurrence, especially if associated with enlargement of pelvic lymph nodes. Central low density from necrosis may be apparent within recurrent tumour, but demonstration of a predominantly cystic mass with ring enhancement is more suggestive of abscess or organizing haematoma. If abnormal soft tissue is demonstrated on postoperative pelvic MRI, absence of high signal on T2-weighted sequences or lack of enhancement on T1-weighted sequences makes recurrent tumour very unlikely, although microscopic foci of tumour within scar or scirrhous cancers are causes of error. On CT, fibrous tissue tends to be more dense than other soft tissues but the differentiation is often unclear.

Postradiotherapy changes

Symptomatic acute cystitis and proctitis are frequent in women receiving intracavitary radiotherapy. Chronic radiation complications are less common and may involve the colon or small bowel, producing strictures or fistulae, or may involve the bladder or distal ureters, resulting in upper renal tract obstruction. The presence of hydronephrosis can be quickly ascertained by ultrasound, but the level and nature of the obstruction is best investigated by CT or MRI (Fig. 9.26).

Barium studies remain the most sensitive investigation for demonstrating bowel complications such as strictures, adhesions and fistulae. Asymptomatic thickening of bowel or bladder wall is a frequent incidental finding in patients imaged after radical pelvic radiotherapy. Changes are often diffuse, symmetrical and with little change on sequential scans, findings that help to differentiate postradiation inflammation from recurrent tumour. However, both diseases may present with a discrete enhancing pelvic mass on MRI and CT. Differential diagnosis may require image-guided biopsy or sequential scanning to assess change.

FURTHER READING

Brown, D.L., Doubilet, P.M., Miller, F.H. *et al.* 1998: Benign and malignant ovarian masses: selection of the most discriminating gray-scale and Doppler sonographic features. *Radiology* **208**, 103–10.

Callan, P.W. (ed.) 1994: *Ultrasonography in obstetrics and gynecology*. Philadelphia, Pennsylvania: W.B. Saunders.

Collins, J.I., Woodward, P.J. 1995: Radiological evaluation of infertility. *Seminars in Ultrasound, CT and MR* **16**, 304–16.

Fleischer, A.C., Javitt, M.C., Jeffrey, R.B. Jr, Jones, H.W. (eds) 1997: *Clinical gynecological imaging*. Philadelphia, Pennsylvania: Lippincott-Raven Publishers.

Forstner, R., Hricak, H., White, S. 1995: CT and MRI of ovarian cancer. *Abdominal Imaging* **20**, 2–8.

Fried, A.M., Kenney, C.M. III, Stigers, K.B., Kacki, M.H., Buckley, S.L. 1996: Benign pelvic masses: sonographic spectrum. *RadioGraphics* **16**, 321–34.

Hricak, H., Yu, K.K. 1996: Radiology in invasive cervical cancer. *American Journal of Roentgenology* **167**, 1101.

Langer, J.E., Jacobs, J.E. 1966: High resolution computed tomography of the female pelvis: spectrum of normal appearances. *Seminars in Roentgenology* **31**, 267–78.

Levine, D. 1998: Gynaecological ultrasound. *Clinical Radiology* **53**, 1–9.

Lipson, S.A., Hricak, H. 1996: MR imaging of the female pelvis. *Radiologic Clinics of North America* **34**, 1157–82.

Mayer, D.P., Shipilov, V. 1995: Ultrasonography and magnetic resonance imaging of uterine fibroids. *Obstetric and Gynecology Clinics of North America* **22**, 667–725.

Outwater, E.K., Siegelman, E.S., Van Deerlin, V. 1998: Adenomyosis: current concepts and imaging considerations. *American Journal of Roentgenology* **170**, 437–41.

Thurmond, A.S., Jones, M.K., Cohen, D.J. 1996: *Gynecologic, obstetric and breast radiology. A text/atlas of imaging in women*. Cambridge, Massachusetts: Blackwell Science Ltd.

Urban, B.A., Fishman, E.K. 1995: Spiral CT of the female pelvis: clinical applications. *Abdominal Imaging* **20**, 9–14.

Woodward, P.J., Wagner, B.J., Farley, T.E. 1993: MR imaging in the evaluation of female infertility. *RadioGraphics* **13**, 293–310.

10

Obstetrics

PETER TWINING

In no other area of medicine has a single imaging modality had a greater impact on patient management than ultrasound in obstetrics and gynaecology. The introduction of ultrasound has truly revolutionized the practice of obstetrics and gynaecology, which is facilitated by the compact high resolution real-time ultrasound machines currently available.

Obstetric ultrasound basically falls into three main types of scans carried out in each of the three trimesters of pregnancy.

First trimester scans are carried out to date the pregnancy accurately, exclude pregnancy complications, confirm fetal viability and diagnose multiple gestation. Major fetal anomalies may also be detected, particularly around 12 weeks' gestation, using the transvaginal probe. Nuchal translucency scanning has also recently been introduced, which can be used to detect both chromosomal disease and also certain fetal anomalies.

Mid trimester scans are carried out to detect fetal abnormalities and to assess placental position. In the UK all women are offered a routine fetal anomaly scan at 18–20 weeks' gestation.

Third trimester scans are carried out to assess fetal growth and well-being, and placental position can also be reassessed. Fetal growth can be assessed by carrying out fetal measurements, and fetal well-being may be assessed using umbilical artery Doppler waveforms and biophysical profiles.

Using ultrasound the fetus can be comprehensively assessed from conception right through to term.

FIRST TRIMESTER SCANNING

NORMAL APPEARANCES

Scanning in the first trimester is begun transabdominally, but a transvaginal scan is almost invariably performed until 10 weeks gestation, as so much more information is gained by scanning transvaginally; it also obviates the need for the patient to have a full bladder. Pregnancy can be confirmed with the transvaginal probe as early as 4½ weeks after the first day of the woman's last menstrual period (LMP). At this stage a gestational sac will be present but no fetal pole or fetal heart beat. Scanning the ovaries will also reveal a corpus luteal cyst.

At 5 weeks' gestation, a yolk sac should be seen and a fetal pole may also be visible adjacent to the yolk sac (Fig. 10.1). The yolk sac is seen as a echodense structure, often with a transonic centre in the gestation sac (Fig. 10.2).

Figure 10.1 *Transvaginal scan of a 5-week pregnancy showing a gestational sac with a yolk sac (arrow). Adjacent to the yolk sac is a developing fetal pole. At this stage of gestation the fetal heart beat may not be present.*

Figure 10.3 *Transvaginal scan of an 8-week pregnancy. The calipers are measuring the crown-rump length of 20 mm, which equates with just over 8 weeks' gestation. The yolk sac is also clearly seen adjacent to the fetus (arrow).*

Figure 10.2 *Transvaginal scan of a 6½-week pregnancy showing the yolk sac (curved arrow), the amniotic sac (straight arrows) and the fetal pole (open arrow).*

Figure 10.4 *Transabdominal scan of a normal 12-week pregnancy. The arrows indicate the nuchal translucency, which is the thin trace of fluid occurring on the back of the fetal head (H). (B, fetal body.)*

A 6 weeks, a fetal heartbeat should be demonstrated within the fetal pole. A crown rump measurement can be carried out (the longest distance from one end of the fetal pole to the other) and this measurement can be used to date the pregnancy.

From 7 weeks onwards there should be a distinct fetus, amniotic sac, yolk sac and trophoblastic tissue which will subsequently become the placenta (Fig. 10.3).

From 8 weeks the fetus has a distinct head and trunk, and limb buds may be visible. Fetal development continues, so that by 12 weeks' gestation major fetal anomalies may be diagnosed and the nuchal translucency measurement can be carried out (Fig. 10.4). At this stage of pregnancy evaluating the fetus for anomalies should be carried out with the transvaginal probe.

Besides evaluating the fetus, abnormalities of the uterus and ovaries may be demonstrated. Congenital abnormalities of the uterus such as a bicornuate uterus

Figure 10.5 *Transabdominal scan through a fibroid associated with a 20-week pregnancy. The fibroid shows central cystic degeneration.*

Figure 10.6 *Transvaginal scan of an ectopic pregnancy. The ectopic gestational sac is adjacent to the left ovary and is clearly seen to be separate from the uterus.*

may be present, when the fetus may develop in one horn of the uterus.

Leiomyomas (fibroids) are present in 1 per cent of pregnant patients, and may be responsible for the uterus being larger than expected for the gestational age. Leiomyomas usually arise in the body or fundus of the uterus but when situated lower in the uterus they may obstruct labour. Fibroids may increase in size under the normal influences of pregnancy and occasionally undergo cystic degeneration (Fig. 10.5).

Corpus luteum cysts may be seen in the ovaries but they frequently involute as the pregnancy progresses.

EARLY PREGNANCY COMPLICATIONS

Early pregnancy complications occur commonly and are extremely distressing to the woman concerned. Ideally these patients should be assessed in dedicated units with highly trained and sympathetic personnel with access to ultrasound machines with transvaginal probes. These patients need to be seen and counselled in a sensitive and private setting, and any further treatment carried out as soon as possible.

ECTOPIC PREGNANCY

Ectopic pregnancy has an incidence of about 1.4 per cent of all pregnancies and this has increased in recent years with the introduction of *in vitro* fertilization techniques. There is also a higher risk if there has been previous tubal surgery, pelvic inflammatory disease (PID) or a previous ectopic pregnancy. Clinically

ectopic pregnancy should always be suspected in any woman with vaginal bleeding and/or pelvic pain and a positive pregnancy test.

Ultrasound scanning using the transvaginal approach is used to confirm an intrauterine pregnancy, which should be possible to demonstrate from 5 weeks' gestation. The presence of an intrauterine pregnancy virtually excludes an ectopic pregnancy. However, there is a small risk (1:7000) of both an intrauterine and an ectopic pregnancy occurring at the same time. It is therefore prudent, even if an intrauterine pregnancy is seen, to assess both adnexal regions for other pathology.

An ectopic pregnancy should always be suspected if there is no intrauterine gestation sac in the presence of a positive pregnancy test. Positive signs of an ectopic pregnancy include a decidual cast within the uterus and an adnexal mass separate from the ovary. There may be a corpus luteum cyst or haemorrhagic fluid containing low level echoes in the pouch of Douglas (Fig. 10.6). On rare occasions a fetal pole and heart beat may be seen within the adnexal mass.

Difficulties in diagnosis can arise when there is fluid within the endometrial cavity (pseudosac), which may be confused with a true gestational sac. Fluid within the cavity is usually centrally located, whereas a gestation sac is eccentrically positioned. The gestation sac may also have a yolk sac present and a ring of trophoblastic tissue around it. Haemorrhage around a gestation sac might also create difficulties in diagnosis, but careful assessment of the uterus will reveal the presence of a gestational sac if there is a viable pregnancy. It should be remembered, however, that in up to 20 per cent of cases there will be no positive signs of ectopic pregnancy on scanning.

Abdominal pregnancy, resulting from the implantation of the embryo on the omental or mesenteric surface, can be difficult to diagnose on ultrasound, and MRI may be useful to show the pregnancy outside the uterus.

NON-VIABLE PREGNANCY

Non-viable pregnancy includes conditions such as incomplete abortion, blighted ovum and intrauterine fetal death, and missed abortion. Patients usually present with vaginal bleeding, and estimation of human choronic gonadotrophin (HCG) may reveal low values for that particular gestational age. Clinically it is often difficult to differentiate the varying early pregnancy complications and so ultrasound is useful in assessing non-viable pregnancy.

Incomplete abortion

The patient usually presents with heavy vaginal bleeding and pain following a positive pregnancy test.

Scanning the uterus reveals a variable picture depending on the amount of trophoblastic tissue and blood within the uterine cavity. Essentially there is usually a combination of fluid (blood) and tissue showing increased echogenicity (trophoblastic tissue) within the uterus cavity with no gestation sac or fetal pole present.

Blighted ovum

A blighted ovum is thought to occur when there is early death of the fetus and so a gestational sac but no fetal pole is present. The mean gestational sac diameter increases with gestational age and increases in a linear fashion from early pregnancy by approximately 1 mm/day. The absence of a fetal pole within a gestational sac of mean diameter of 2 cm or greater indicates a blighted ovum and thus a non-viable pregnancy (Fig. 10.7).

If there is any doubt or the dates indicating gestational age do not match the size of the gestation sac, then a repeat scan 1 week later is performed to reassess the pregnancy. If a viable pregnancy is present then the

Figure 10.8 *Intrauterine fetal death. Transvaginal scan of a 10-week pregnancy showing an irregular gestational sac. There is a fetal pole (F) measuring 12 mm in length, but no fetal heart beat was detected.*

mean gestational sac diameter will have increased significantly over this period.

The Joint Standing Committee of the Royal College of Obstetricians and Gynaecologists and Royal College of Radiologists have issued guidelines for the assessment of early pregnancy complications.

Intrauterine fetal death

Intrauterine fetal death can be diagnosed if a gestational sac is present with a yolk sac and fetal pole, but there is no fetal heart motion seen. Fetuses with crown rump length (CRL) measurements of over 6 mm should always demonstrate fetal heart motion and so, if fetal heart motion is absent in a fetus of this size and over, then an intrauterine fetal death can be diagnosed (Fig. 10.8). When the CRL measurement is less than 6 mm and fetal heart motion is not seen, a repeat scan after 1 or 2 weeks is indicated to reassess viability.

Missed abortion

A missed abortion may be unsuspected or follow an episode of light bleeding. A scan may show either a gestation sac greater than 2 cm in diameter with no fetal pole, or a fetal pole greater than 6 mm in length with no fetal heart beat.

MULTIPLE GESTATION

Twin pregnancies have an incidence of 1:80 live births. Multiple gestation, however, is increasing owing to

Figure 10.7 *Blighted ovum. A transabdominal scan through a 10-week pregnancy. A gestational sac measuring 2.7 cm in diameter is seen. There is no fetal pole and so the pregnancy is non-viable.*

Figure 10.12 *Lateral ventricles. Transverse section through the fetal head of an 18-week fetus showing the lateral ventricles (arrows). The echogenic choroid (C) is seen to lie within the posterior horn of the lateral ventricle.*

Figure 10.13 *Placenta praevia. Scan at 20 weeks' gestation showing the placenta completely covering the lower part of the uterus. (B, bladder; P, placenta; F, fetus.)*

types of minor and major abnormalities can be detected and some of the more important will be discussed. The detection of fetal anomalies, however, requires careful training and meticulous attention to detail. The fetus needs to be assessed in a systematic way so that organ systems are not missed. In addition if one fetal anomaly is detected, then the fetus must be carefully searched for other abnormalities. The presence of multiple abnormalities carries a poor prognosis and often indicates chromosomal disease or a genetic syndrome.

An indication of fetal abnormality is **polyhydramnios**, since this is due to fetal anomaly in 20 per cent of cases. Polyhydramnios is defined as twice the volume of amniotic fluid expected for the period of gestation; the diagnosis is often made by a visual estimate of the amount of fluid or by finding a pool of liquor deeper than 8 cm.

SPINE

The antenatal ultrasound diagnosis of **spina bifida** is based on the demonstration of a number of ultrasound signs within the fetal head, which provide the clue to the diagnosis. There are three important ultrasound findings in the head and these include the lemon-shaped head, banana-shaped cerebellum and ventriculomegaly (Fig. 10.14). When these signs are present there is a very high likelihood of an **open spina bifida**. Assessing the spine may reveal a cystic component

(a)

(b)

Figure 10.14 *(a) Spina bifida. Transverse section through the fetal head showing the pointed appearance of the frontal bones (lemon head). (b) Transverse section through the fetal head showing the 'banana cerebellum' (arrows).*

Figure 10.15 *Spina bifida. Sagittal section through the fetal spine showing a lumbar sacral meningomyelocele (arrows).*

Figure 10.17 *Hydrocephalus. Transverse section through the fetal head showing quite marked dilatation of the lateral ventricles (V), caused by aqueduct stenosis.*

Figure 10.16 *Spina bifida. Transverse section through the lower spine showing the skin defect over the neural tube defect (arrows). Note that the posterior elements of the spine are widely separated.*

caused by a meningomyelocele or a soft-tissue defect over the spine (Fig. 10.15). In addition, on transverse scanning, there will be separation of the central processes of the neural arch to produce a 'V'- or 'U'-shaped appearance to the spine (Fig. 10.16). The outcome of a fetus with spina bifida depends on the level of the defect, with small sacral lesions having the best outcome and large thoracolumbar defects the worst prognosis. **Closed lesions** (i.e. the defect is covered by soft tissue or skin) have a better outcome than open defects (no soft tissue or skin over the lesion).

HEAD

Hydrocephalus is usually caused by an obstruction at some point within the ventricular system. In the fetus

the commonest causes are aqueduct stenosis (obstruction at the aqueduct of Sylvius) (Fig. 10.17), spina bifida and Dandy–Walker syndrome (obstruction of the exit foramina in the posterior fossa). Obstruction of the ventricular system causes dilatation of the lateral ventricles and also of the third ventricle. These signs are useful in differentiating hydrocephalus from other causes of ventriculomegaly, such as agenesis of the corpus callosum, where the third ventricle is usually of normal size. The outcome of fetuses with hydrocephalus depends on the presence of any other abnormalities. Rapidly progressing hydrocephalus will have a poorer outcome than static ventriculomegaly.

Anencephaly may be diagnosed after 14 weeks by the absence of a visible skull vault, though echoes from the skull base and face may be seen. The fetal body is usually well formed and moves actively. In **microcephaly** there is a small skull containing small brain.

The choroid plexuses are echogenic structures lying within the lateral ventricles. **Cysts in the choroid plexus** are a fairly common occurrence but usually these cysts are of no clinical significance, normally resolving by 24 weeks' gestation (Fig. 10.18). However, there is an association with chromosomal abnormalities, notably trisomy 18 but, if no other abnormality is defected on ultrasound, fetal karyotyping is not normally advised.

CARDIAC DEFECTS

Many cardiac abnormalities can be diagnosed *in utero*; however, the overall detection rate for cardiac defects is

Figure 10.18 *Choroid plexus cyst. Transverse section through the fetal head showing a cyst within the choroid plexus (arrow).*

Figure 10.20 *Ventricular septal defect. Four-chamber view through the fetal thorax showing a large VSD (arrow).*

only 30 per cent using the routine four-chamber view at mid trimester scanning. On the normal four-chamber view (Fig. 10.19) the following observations should be made:

- The heart occupies approximately a third of the thorax.
- There are two atria of approximately the same size.
- There are two ventricles of approximately equal size and thickness and contractility.

Figure 10.19 *Transverse section through the fetal thorax showing a normal four chamber view. (RV, right ventricle; LV, left ventricle; RA, right atrium; LA, left atrium.)*

- The atrial and ventricular septa meet the atrioventricular valves to form an offset cross.
- Two opening atrioventricular valves seen.

The commonest cardiac abnormality is the **ventricular septal defect**; however, this is also one of the most difficult to detect (Fig. 10.20). A less common defect is the atrioventricular septal defect (AVSD) and in this condition the central portion of the heart is missing, associated with both ventricular and atrial septal defects. When an AVSD is seen prenatally it carries a 30 per cent risk of the baby having Down's syndrome.

Other common cardiac anomalies detected *in utero* include hypoplastic left heart syndrome, pulmonary atresia and outflow tract problems, such as transposition of the great arteries and truncus arteriosus. In these two latter conditions the standard four-chamber view will usually be normal.

GASTROINTESTINAL TRACT

Diaphragmatic hernia is an uncommon anomaly, which occurs when there is a defect in the diaphragm, usually on the left side, and which allows herniation of abdominal contents into the thorax. This produces mediastinal shift away from the defect, and the stomach is often seen displacing the heart to the right on transverse scanning through the thorax (Fig. 10.21).

The condition is usually diagnosed at the mid trimester scan; however, herniation can be delayed until the third trimester. The outcome is variable, but approximately 50 per cent of prenatally diagnosed cases

Figure 10.21 *Diaphragmatic hernia. Transverse section through the fetal thorax showing the stomach (S) within the thorax, displacing the heart (H) to the right.*

will survive. Poor prognostic factors include an early diagnosis, the presence of other anomalies and the development of polyhydramnios.

The two most common **abdominal wall defects** are omphalocele and gastroschisis, which can both be treated surgically in the neonatal period.

In **omphalocele** there is herniation of bowel and occasionally other abdominal organs, through a large central abdominal defect. The bowel is always surrounded by a membrane into which the cord inserts. Omphaloceles are often associated with other fetal abnormalities, particularly cardiac anomalies, and there is a high association with chromosomal disease.

Gastroschisis is a different form of abdominal wall defect, as there is no membrane surrounding the bowel, which floats freely in the amniotic fluid (Fig. 10.22). In addition the umbilical cord inserts normally and the defect is always on the right side of the cord insertion. There is also a very low incidence of associated anomalies and chromosomal disease.

Duodenal atresia can be recognized by the presence of two round cystic structures in the upper abdomen representing the distended stomach and duodenum in the 'double bubble' appearance. Duodenal atresia is associated with Down's syndrome.

Oesophageal atresia cannot be directly demonstrated, but is associated with polyhydramnios.

URINARY TRACT

The two most common form of renal anomalies seen are hydronephrosis and multicystic kidney.

Hydronephrosis is usually secondary to a pelvi-ureteric junction obstruction (Fig. 10.23). The best means of assessing the degree of dilatation of the renal collecting system is to measure the anteroposterior renal pelvic diameter. It is now well established that a renal pelvic diameter greater than 1 cm requires full postnatal investigation when a high incidence of significant renal pathology will be detected. Renal pelvic diameters between 0.5 and 1 cm have a debatable significance, but can indicate vesicoureteric reflux in a small number of cases. Renal pelvic diameters below 5 mm are normal.

Figure 10.22 *Gastroschisis. Multiple loops of small bowel are seen to be floating freely within the amniotic fluid adjacent to the fetal abdomen (A).*

Figure 10.23 *Hydronephrosis. Coronal section through the fetus showing a hydronephrotic kidney (H). The renal pelvis is dilated and the appearances are due to a pelviureteric junction obstruction. (S, spine.)*

Figure 10.24 *Multicystic kidney. Coronal section through the fetal abdomen showing a multicystic kidney (C, cysts). A normal contralateral kidney (K) is also seen. Ao = aorta.*

Multicystic kidney is caused by obstruction to the kidney at a very early stage of development producing a dysplastic kidney containing multiple cysts of varying sizes (Fig. 10.24), which may be difficult to differentiate from hydronephrosis. The affected kidney is usually non-functioning and, if the condition is unilateral, the outcome is good.

The kidneys contribute significantly to the volume of the amniotic fluid, so profound oligohydramnios should raise the possibility of bilateral renal disease, which can cause death in the neonatal period from pulmonary hypoplasia. Severe oligohydramnios is seen with bilateral multicystic kidneys, infantile polycystic kidneys and renal agenesis, where there is absence of both kidneys and the bladder.

Infantile polycystic kidney disease is always bilateral with cysts in both kidneys, which vary in size from microscopic to several millimetres. The size of the cysts determine the ultrasound appearances but tend to produce echogenic kidneys which may be enlarged.

Bladder outlet obstruction can cause bilateral hydronephrosis, and the most common causes are posterior urethral valves or urethral atresia. As well as hydronephrosis, there are hydroureters and a dilated thick walled bladder. The outcome is variable and, with posterior urethral valves, depends on the degree of obstruction, as the back pressure affects the development of the kidneys. In urethral atresia the outlook is poor. Intrauterine intervention may be performed by insertion of a catheter to drain the bladder into the amniotic cavity, to relieve the obstruction.

SKELETON

Skeletal abnormalities that can be recognized by ultrasound are absence of a complete limb or part of a limb, shortening of the long bones giving rise to dwarfism, and defective mineralization and/or fracture. Lethal skeletal dysplasias are often associated with polyhydramnios, and other abnormalities may be present as well.

TUMOURS

These are rare, with the commonest being **cystic hygroma**, which is an abnormality of lymphatics, resulting in cystic swellings around the fetal neck. There is an association with Turner's syndrome.

When **sacrococcygeal teratoma** is diagnosed *in utero*, it is invariably benign. It is a solid, cystic or complex structure, and may contain calcification.

HYDROPS FETALIS

Hydrops refers to an increase in total body water, where there is oedema from either ascites, pleural or pericardial effusions. In the past hydrops was due to the presence of anti-D Rhesus antibodies, but following the programme of prophylaxis this condition is now much less common. There are many non-immune causes of hydrops including haematological conditions, such as thalassaemia; cardiovascular disorders, such as dysrhythmias and hypoplastic left heart syndrome; liver causes, such as hepatitis; and peritonitis, chromosomal abnormalities and infections, for example, from cytomegalic virus.

THIRD TRIMESTER SCANNING

Scans are carried out in the third trimester to assess fetal growth and well-being.

Fetal growth is best assessed by the abdominal circumference measurement (Fig. 10.25), as the first sign of growth retardation may be lack of growth of the fetal body. The abdominal circumference can then be correlated with the head circumference measurement, which is more accurate than the BPD in the third trimester because it compensates for any degree of head flattening, which commonly occurs in the third trimester.

INTRAUTERINE GROWTH RETARDATION

Intrauterine growth retardation or restriction is diagnosed when fetal measurements are below the fifth centile for gestation, or if there has been a lack of growth or reduced growth on serial scans over a period

Figure 10.25 *Abdominal circumference measurement. On this section where the measurement should be taken, the fetal stomach (S), and the intra-abdominal portion of the umbilical vein (arrows), should be seen.*

of time. Growth scans should be carried out at 2-weekly intervals at least to demonstrate a significant change in growth.

Historically growth retardation has been classified into two types – symmetrical and asymmetrical. In **symmetrical growth retardation**, both the head and abdominal measurements are reduced whereas, in the **asymmetrical type**, head growth is maintained at relatively normal values, but the abdominal measurements are reduced. It is generally accepted that symmetrical growth retardation is often caused by intrinsic fetal pathology, such as chromosomal disease, fetal infection and certain genetic syndromes, whereas asymmetrical growth retardation is usually a result of uteroplacental insufficiency.

Growth retardation can be suspected by reduced fundal height measurements or the maternal abdomen appearing small for dates. Measurements of the fetus can then confirm the diagnosis. Once a diagnosis has been made, a search for the cause of the growth retardation should be carried out. The commonest maternal causes are: uteroplacental insufficiency, maternal hypertension, smoking and autoimmune disorders, such as systemic lupus erythematosis. The common fetal causes are: chromosomal disease, viral infections, such as cytomegalovirus and toxoplasmosis, and rare genetic syndromes.

Where the cause of the growth retardation is maternal, the fetus is anatomically normal and may show an asymmetrical growth picture and reduced liquor volume. In fetal causes of growth retardation, there may well be fetal abnormalities present; the type of growth retardation may be symmetrical and liquor volume may

be normal or increased. Where infection is suspected, a TORCH screen can be carried out to look for toxoplasmosis, rubella, cytomegalovirus, herpes simplex or other infections.

Growth-retarded fetuses require careful monitoring during the remainder of pregnancy with 2-weekly growth measurements and regular Doppler ultrasound carried out.

UMBILICAL ARTERY DOPPLER ULTRASOUND

Within the umbilical cord there are two umbilical arteries and one umbilical vein. Doppler ultrasound of the umbilical artery is extremely useful for monitoring fetuses with growth retardation. In normal pregnancy the placental resistance is low and, as a large proportion of the fetal cardiac output flows through the placenta, there is a high diastolic flow shown by the flow velocity waveform from the umbilical artery (Fig. 10.26). Placental resistance to blood flow indicates a poor fetal outcome, and is shown by a reduced diastolic flow; if there is absent or even reversed diastolic flow, then more severe resistance is present.

Figure 10.26 *Normal umbilical artery Doppler flow velocity waveform. The arrows indicate the period of diastolic flow.*

In severe growth retardation the fetus will redistribute its circulation to maintain a normal blood supply to important organs such as heart, brain and adrenals, but reduce the blood supply to other body organs. This is classically demonstrated in the asymmetrical type of growth retardation, where head growth is normal because cerebral blood flow is maintained. Abdominal growth is reduced because blood through the liver is bypassed – flow is increased through the ductus venosus, and so liver growth and subsequently the abdominal circumference measurement are reduced. Liquor volume falls because renal perfusion is also reduced to improve blood flow to other organs. At this stage umbilical artery Doppler waveforms are abnormal and may show absent end diastolic flow or reversed diastolic flow (Fig. 10.27).

Normal umbilical artery Doppler waveforms are reassuring in the presence of growth retardation, but

(a)

(b)

Figure 10.27 *(a) Umbilical artery trace showing absent end diastolic flow. (b) Umbilical artery trace showing reversed end diastolic flow, which indicates severe fetal compromise.*

should be repeated on at least a weekly basis with 2-weekly growth measurements. The presence of absent end diastolic flow requires intensive monitoring with regular Doppler, biophysical profiles and cardiotacography (CTG). The majority of babies with absent end diastolic flow and growth retardation will require delivery by caesarean section, the timing of which can usually be planned, depending on the rate of fetal growth, the degree of oligohydramnios, the result of the biophysical profiles and the stage of fetal viability. Fetuses demonstrating reversed end diastolic flow are severely compromised and usually require immediate delivery by caesarean section if the fetus is viable.

BIOPHYSICAL PROFILES

As well as umbilical artery Doppler ultrasound, biophysical profiles, which use five indices to indicate fetal health, can be performed in the at-risk fetus (Table 10.1). The assessment may need to be performed over a 30-minute period.

DIABETES

Diabetic pregnancies can be complicated by growth retardation. However, another common problem is **macrosomia** where the fetus becomes significantly larger than expected for dates. In diabetic pregnancies, therefore, regular growth measurements are indicated to detect such complications.

PLACENTA

The placenta can easily be recognized at 8 weeks' gestation, and is seen as a well-defined structure lining the inner wall of a portion of the uterus. The surface of the placenta, the chorionic plate, appears as a line of bright echoes. Changes are seen in the texture of the placenta during the course of pregnancy, but these changes, even when calcification or placental lakes are present, are not thought to be of clinical significance.

At mid trimester the placenta is often low in position but, owing to the differential rate of growth of the uterus (the lower segment grows more than the rest of the uterus) the placenta is carried away from the cervical os towards the fundus as the pregnancy progresses. Only those placentas that actually cover the os at mid trimester are likely to become a placenta praevia in later pregnancy.

The two common causes of **antepartum haemorrhage** are placenta praevia and placental abruption.

PLACENTA PRAEVIA

A placenta praevia is a placenta lying wholly or partially in the lower uterine segment. The degree of placenta praevia can be identified by the placenta encroaching onto the lower uterine segment, reaching or covering the internal os (Fig. 10.28). Although the internal os cannot always be identified as such, the position of the cervix can be inferred from the position of other structures. Errors can occur identifying a low-lying placenta if the placenta is located posteriorly, because it then becomes more difficult to identify the lower uterine segment. Anteriorly the bladder is an important landmark for the lower uterine segment. The fetal head

Table 10.1 *Biophysical profiles*

Variable	Normal (2)	Abnormal (0)
Fetal breathing movements	> 1 episode of 30 s duration	No episode in 30 min
Body movements	≥ 3 discrete body/limb movement in 30 min	≤ 2 movements
Fetal tone	≥ 1 episode of active flexion and extension of limbs; opening and closing of hand	Absent fetal movement; slow extension; partial flexion
Reactive fetal heart rate	≥ 2 accelerations of ≥ 15 beats/min lasting 15 s associated with fetal movement	< 2 accelerations in 30 min
Amniotic fluid volume	At least 1 pocket of amniotic fluid, at least 1 cm in 2 perpendicular planes	No amniotic fluid pockets > 1 cm

A score of 0–2 is given to each variable. A total score of 8–10 is regarded as normal, 6 as equivocal, ≤ 4 abnormal.

Figure 10.28 *Placenta praevia. Sagittal scan in third trimester showing the placenta completely covering the lower segment of the uterus. (B, bladder; F, fetus; P, placenta.)*

may obscure the margin of the placenta making its localization difficult.

If a placenta praevia is found on a third trimester scan, serial scans are performed, because the position of the placenta is an important factor in determining the mode of delivery.

PLACENTAL ABRUPTION

Placental abruption, which is also known as **accidental haemorrhage**, is haemorrhage from premature separation of the placenta. Most cases do not involve trauma and occur spontaneously. In the majority of cases no specific cause can be found. The haemorrhage may be concealed when the extravasated blood remains entirely within the uterus or revealed when the blood appears at the vulva.

The diagnosis is made on clinical grounds and, in the acute stage, ultrasound has a limited role, but it may be helpful in excluding placenta praevia and confirming that the fetus is still alive. It may be difficult on ultrasound to differentiate between a retroplacental

haematoma and normal intravascular blood, and the haematoma may be misdiagnosed as a thick placenta. As the haematoma matures its echo pattern may change and so becomes easier to recognize.

COMPLICATIONS OF PREGNANCY

TROPHOBLASTIC DISEASE

Hydatidiform mole occurs in 1 in 1500 pregnancies, although commoner in certain parts of the world such as South East Asia. The embryo dies but fails to abort normally, and the chorionic villi proliferate to form multiple grape-like vesicles distending the uterine cavity. A partial mole contains fetal parts, and in invasive mole there is penetration of uterine muscle by trophoblastic elements. Very rarely a mole may coexist with a living pregnancy.

Choriocarcinoma arises from malignant transformation of hydatidiform mole or from retained placenta after normal pregnancy or abortion. Signs include vaginal bleeding, high levels of beta human chorionic gonadotrophin, and uterine enlargement greater than expected for the stage of pregnancy. On ultrasound, a complex multicystic/solid mass fills the uterine cavity and multiple theca lutein ovarian cysts may be seen (Fig. 10.29). Ultrasound cannot distinguish between complete hydatidiform mole, invasive forms and choriocarcinoma. Choriocarcinoma metastasises via the bloodstream to give haemorrhagic and necrotic metastases in the lung, kidney and brain.

OVARIAN VEIN THROMBOSIS

Ovarian vein thrombosis may occur postpartum from sudden reduction in flow and venous stasis in the ovarian vein (usually the right). Symptoms and signs resemble those of appendicitis, patients often presenting with fever, pain and a tender, tubular mass in the

Figure 10.29 *Ultrasound scan in a pregnant woman with abnormal vaginal bleeding. The uterus is larger than expected for a 10-week pregnancy and contains no viable fetus, but is enlarged by a mass containing cystic and solid elements (arrows). A complete hydatidiform mole was subsequently evacuated.*

Figure 10.31 *Sagittal MRI scan giving a pelvic AP inlet measurement of 11.1 cm and an AP outlet of 12.3 cm.*

APPENDICITIS

Approximately 1 in 1500 pregnancies are complicated by appendicitis, the diagnosis of which is made more difficult by the high prevalence of nausea, vomiting and leucocytosis in normal pregnancies and the migration of the appendix towards the right iliac crest as the uterus enlarges. The decision to perform a laparotomy is made on clinical grounds and should not be unduly deferred to await imaging studies. Fetal loss is high if appendiceal perforation occurs. In the stable patient, ultrasound examination may be able to identify the inflamed appendix, or show other causes of a similar clinical picture, such as biliary colic, ovarian lesions or urinary tract disease (Fig. 10.30).

Figure 10.30 *Right iliac fossa ultrasound showing a thick-walled fusiform mass containing debris, which was tender and contiguous with the caecal pole, indicating an inflamed appendix mass rather than a mass of adnexal origin.*

PELVIMETRY

Pelvimetry is a technique used to determine the dimensions of the pelvis. It is used infrequently nowadays because of the increased use of caesarean section in difficult labour; the pelvic measurements following a difficult labour give little indication of the outcome in future pregnancies, and pelvimetry cannot predict the outcome of vaginal breech delivery.

From an erect lateral radiograph the anteroposterior measurements of the pelvic inlet and outlet can be made. The transverse diameter of the inlet and bispinous diameter can be measured from a supine anteroposterior film. These measurements are of limited use as they are made from bone to bone surfaces and make no allowance for the all important thickness

iliac fossa. On ultrasound, the thrombosed vein can be appreciated as a tender mass with internal echoes and no flow, and on CT or MR the enlarged ovarian vein can be followed proximally in the retroperitoneum to renal level.

Deep vein thrombosis in the legs can be readily diagnosed with ultrasound.

of soft tissues. Because of the radiation hazard to both mother and fetus from plain film radiographs and CT, other methods have been introduced. Measurements can be made by MRI (Fig. 10.31) which involves no ionizing radiation.

FURTHER READING

Chudleigh, P., Pearce, J.M. 1992: *Obstetric ultrasound* (2nd edition). Edinburgh: Churchill Livingstone.

Fleischer, A.L., Kurjak, A., Granberg, S. 1997: *Ultrasound and the endometrium. Progress in obstetrical and gynaecological sonography*. New York: Parthenon Publishing Group.

Fleischer, A.C., Romero, R., Manning, F.H., Jeanty, P., Everette, J.A. 1991: *The principles and practice of ultrasonography in obstetrics and gynaecology* (4th edition). London: Prentice Hall Inc.

James, D.K., Steer, P.J., Weiner, C.P., Gomik, B. (eds). 1999: *High risk pregnancy*. London: W.B. Saunders.

Kurjak, A. 1992: *An atlas of ultrasonography in obstetrics and gynaecology*. London: Parthenon Publishing Group.

Kurjak, A. 1994: *Ultrasound and the ovary. Progress in obstetrics and gynaecological sonography*. New York: Parthenon Publishing Group.

Osmers, R., Kurjak, A. 1997: *Ultrasound and the uterus. Progress in obstetrical and gynaecological ultrasound*. New York: Parthenon Publishing Group.

Snijders, R.J.M., Nicolaides, K.H. 1996: *Ultrasound markers for fetal chromosome defects*. London: Parthenon Publishing Group.

Twining, P., McHugo, J., Pilling, D.W. (eds). 1999: *A text book of fetal abnormalities*. London: Churchill Livingstone.

11

Interventional radiology

ANTHONY F. WATKINSON, ANDREAS ADAM

Interventional radiology has made a significant contribution to the management of many diseases. Technological advances are continuing to increase the success rate and minimize the complication rate of many procedures. In some instances, such as the control of haemorrhage, interventional radiology can replace conventional surgical methods, whereas in other situations it is a useful adjunct to surgery. The increasing complexity and sophistication of both surgery and interventional radiology demand careful joint planning for the choice of the optimum method of treatment.

DILATATION OF BENIGN AND MALIGNANT LOWER OESOPHAGEAL STRICTURES

In patients with dysphagia the underlying cause must be investigated and fully evaluated. Benign causes of obstruction include achalasia or strictures secondary to reflux oesophagitis, postsurgical narrowing, radiation fibrosis, Crohn's disease, postvariceal sclerotherapy and caustic ingestion. Malignant obstruction in the lower third of the oesophagus is most likely to be due to squamous cell carcinoma or adenocarcinoma.

The dilatation of oesophageal lesions is not a new phenomenon: bougienage with whalebone dates back many centuries. Until recently, the treatment of benign lower oesophageal obstruction was by open surgical bypass or by unguided, transorally placed, soft mercury-weighted or rigid metal dilators. More recently, fluoroscopically guided dilatation using balloon catheters has been employed.

Balloon dilatation has the advantage of providing a controlled radial dilating force without producing the high longitudinal shear forces associated with bougie dilatation that are thought to predispose to oesophageal rupture. In addition the balloon inflation and oesophageal dilatation can be viewed in real time, the severity of the waist seen in the balloon indicating the degree of success.

Recent advances in **self-expanding metallic stent technology** has meant that malignant dysphagia can be treated effectively, with minimal hospital stay and a rapid return to a normal environment. These stents can create a normal-sized oesophageal lumen with some transmission of peristaltic waves and, in many instances, patients can resume a near normal diet. In addition, the newer stents have a variety of plastic covers to prevent tumour ingrowth. This design is also useful for dealing with oesophageal perforation or fistula formation.

ACHALASIA

Pneumatic dilatation is the initial treatment of choice for achalasia, with surgical myotomy being reserved for failure after several attempts of balloon dilatation. The aim is to purposely overdilate and traumatize the lower oesophagus

(a)

(b)

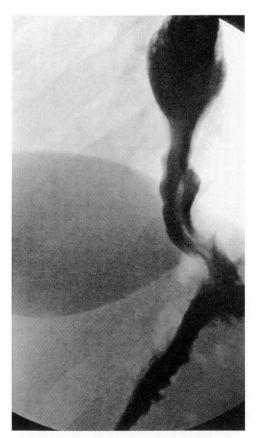

(c)

Figure 11.1 *Balloon dilatation of achalasia. (a) Barium swallow demonstrating dilated oesophagus above a smooth tight stricture (arrows) in the lower oesophagus, typical of achalasia. (b) Dilatation of the lower oesophageal stricture using a 35 mm balloon. The balloon has been partially inflated with dilute contrast medium. Note the central waisting (arrows) at the site of the stricture. (c) Barium swallow after the procedure demonstrates satisfactory dilatation of the stricture.*

in the region of the sphincter, and cause sufficient tissue injury with rupture of the muscle layers, to eliminate the functional obstruction that exists in achalasia. The improvement in symptoms is immediate, the risks are low and the morbidity minimal when compared with surgery. Most cases can be performed with light intravenous sedation; however, general anaesthesia may be required in children or in patients unable to cooperate.

An initial contrast study is required to confirm the diagnosis, identify the level of obstruction and assess the amount of food residue in the dilated oesophagus (Fig. 11.1a). If significant food residue is identified, endoscopic washout prior to the procedure minimizes the risk of aspiration. Patients should receive antibiotic cover as bacteraemia is common during the dilatation. Light intravenous analgesia and sedation are used. Local anaesthetic, e.g. lignocaine, is applied to the oropharynx and a catheter introduced and passed into the stomach over a guidewire under fluoroscopic guidance. This ensures that the stricture is traversed with minimal trauma and that the risk of perforation is minimized.

The catheter is then withdrawn and successively larger diameter balloons used. In most cases the oesophagus is initially dilated to 20 mm progressing in 5 mm increments to a maximum diameter of 35 mm (Fig. 11.1b). At each stage it is hoped to achieve absence of waisting of the balloon. The procedure is terminated if the patient experiences significant pain or if there is blood on the balloon following withdrawal. Long-term symptomatic improvement is usually observed if dilatation of 30 mm or greater is achieved.

The radiographic result on a postdilatation contrast study (Fig. 11.1c) has been shown to correlate well with symptomatic relief. Overall, approximately 85–90 per cent of patients are symptom free at 4–24 months.

BENIGN OESOPHAGEAL STRICTURES

There are many causes of benign strictures, the most common being reflux oesophagitis and postsurgical narrowing. A lumen of less than 12 mm almost always results in dysphagia and, if the lumen is greater than 20 mm, the vast majority of patients will be asymptomatic. Consequently, dilatation to a diameter of 20 mm is usually enough to relieve symptoms and enable the patient to eat a normal diet.

The technique is the same as for achalasia with the introduction of a balloon over a guidewire under fluoroscopic guidance. The initial balloon may be as small as 6 mm, the end-point of the procedure being full dilatation of a 20 mm balloon with no residual waist. The procedure is terminated if the patient experiences significant pain or there is marked blood staining of the balloon. Even the tightest strictures can be traversed with a guidewire and subsequently dilated. Postradiation strictures tend to be more rigid and may require initial dilatation with small, high-pressure balloons before larger balloons are used.

MALIGNANT OESOPHAGEAL STRICTURES

Patients with lower oesophageal malignancy should be rigorously investigated and, if there is no evidence of metastatic disease or extensive local spread, offered surgical resection as a curative procedure. If the lesion is unresectable but the patient has few oesophageal symptoms, palliative radiotherapy or chemotherapy may be appropriate.

Patients with unresectable disease and symptoms of dysphagia, owing to partial or complete oesophageal obstruction, are a difficult group. They have a limited life expectancy and therefore treatment should be minimally invasive, with the aim of returning patients to their home environment with good swallowing as quickly as possible. Surgery in these advanced cases now plays a minor role. **Laser therapy**, to reduce tumour volume within the oesophageal lumen and maintain patency, has been used extensively but requires numerous retreatments and also runs the risk of perforation.

The endoscopic placement of rigid plastic tubes, such as Celestin or Atkinson tubes, is gradually being superseded by self-expanding **metal stents**. Advantages include a wide lumen (up to 25 mm) and some flexibility, which allows movement with peristalsis and thus near normal swallowing. Some of these stents are covered with plastic, minimizing tumour ingrowth and also sealing any associated perforation or fistulae. Covered metallic stents are now the treatment of choice in such cases. They relieve symptoms rapidly and the patient can return to a normal environment and tolerate a near normal diet. If the fistulae is too high to achieve a seal a tracheal stent may also be required. Early problems with migration at the gastro-oesophageal junction have been resolved with the development of conical stents (Fig. 11.2a,b). Reflux has been a problem in low stents and recent developments to control this include the use of a stent with an anti-reflux valve.

A contrast swallow demonstrates the level of obstruction and any associated fistulae (Fig. 11.3a). Local anaesthesia to the oropharynx and intravenous analgesia and

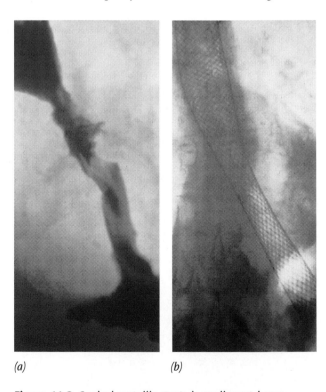

(a)   *(b)*

Figure 11.2 *Conical metallic stents in malignant lower oesophageal obstruction. (a) Contrast swallow demonstrating a malignant stricture in the lower oesophagus extending to the gastro-oesophageal junction. (b) Following placement of a conical self-expanding stent to minimize migration with the lower end in the gastric fundus.*

(a)   *(b)*

Figure 11.3 *Metallic stents in malignant oesophageal obstruction. (a) A contrast swallow demonstrating a malignant stricture in the lower oesophagus with evidence of fistulation (arrows). (b) A contrast swallow after placement of a self-expanding plastic-covered metal stent. There is rapid, free flow through the stent with no evidence of leakage. (Reproduced with permission from A.F. Watkinson et al. in* Radiology, *1995,* **195***, 821–827, published by the Radiological Society of North America.)*

sedation are used. The stricture is traversed with a catheter and guidewire under fluoroscopic guidance. It is virtually always possible to traverse the stricture with the aid of hydrophilic guidewires. Serial balloon dilatation to a maximum diameter of 15 mm is performed under fluoroscopic guidance. In the presence of fistulae or perforation the dilatation is limited to 10 mm. The self-expanding metallic stent is then introduced over a guidewire and deployed across the stricture. If the postcontrast swallow (Fig. 11.3b) is satisfactory the patient can resume a near normal diet immediately.

MANAGEMENT OF ENTERIC STRICTURES

Traditionally, gastrointestinal strictures have been treated with surgical resection or bypass. Although surgical treat-

ment is generally associated with a high success rate, it can be associated with significant morbidity and mortality, particularly in debilitated patients with multisystem disease. The radiological management of enteric strictures was first described in 1981 and since then many cases have been reported which document the ease of fluoroscopically guided **balloon dilatation** at many different sites along the gastrointestinal tract. This technique combines a high success rate with minimal morbidity. Any stricture that can be reached with a balloon catheter can be treated with balloon dilatation, and it is worth trying this method before resorting to surgery. Self-expanding metallic stents are now used routinely in malignant disease, and in benign cases in rare instances.

Local anaesthesia is required at the mouth, anus or stoma site, and intravenous analgesia and sedation may be helpful in certain circumstances. Extra long guidewires and catheters are required; otherwise the equipment is standard. Access to the gastric outlet or small bowel is via the mouth or an indwelling gastrostomy, if present. Progress through the small bowel requires gently curved catheters and soft guidewires. Rectal intubation is performed in the left lateral position and, with a combination of soft guidewires and gentle catheters, it is usually possible to reach the stricture site. Injection of water-soluble contrast agents will help to confirm the stricture location and define its contours and length. During manipulation in the upper gastrointestinal tract in patients with gastric stasis and in all manipulations in the lower gastrointestinal tract, mucosal disruption and bleeding can occur, which may lead to bacteraemia. Antibiotic cover in these patients is therefore advisable. Relatively few studies of gastric, small bowel and large bowel stricture dilatations and stent insertions have been published. However, sufficient information and experience have been obtained to identify factors which influence success, failure and complications.

GASTRIC OUTLET STRICTURES

Pyloric or antral scarring is usually the result of long-standing peptic disease, but occasionally results from ingestion of strongly acidic or caustic substances, or as a complication of pyloric surgery. Surgically created gastroenterostomies and surgical procedures that involve restriction of gastric volume or jejunal bypass for the treatment of morbid obesity are other settings which may lead to gastric outlet obstruction. In these settings balloon dilatation is appropriate. However, if malignancy, either gastric, duodenal or pancreatic, is the cause of gastric outlet obstruction, primary stent insertion is appropriate.

PYLORIC STRICTURES

Pyloric canal or antral strictures are traversed using the catheter guidewire technique. Access is usually peroral although transgastric dilatation can be performed. In benign disease the goal of pyloric dilatation is to achieve full expansion of a 15 mm balloon, as this will usually relieve obstructive symptoms. Some pyloric strictures are very resistant and may require sequential dilatation.

Technically, the most difficult part of any gastrointestinal stricture dilatation is the intubation of the stricture itself. Once this has been crossed, exchange for the balloon catheter and expansion of the balloon are straightforward in comparison. In cases where intubation is unsuccessful (usually < 10 per cent) a combined endoscopic approach may help. Strictures following surgical gastroenterostomy can also be balloon dilated although the stricture is often extremely difficult to locate. Preprocedure review of available imaging studies, particularly barium studies and CT scans, can be invaluable in choosing the optimum patient orientation and which initial catheters and guidewires to use. Once located, however, the technique is identical with balloon dilatation to 15 mm, usually with good results

and with symptomatic relief in approximately 70 per cent of patients over a 2-year period. Poor results appear to correlate with eccentric lesions and where a kink in the bowel exists rather than a true stricture. If balloon dilatation fails, metallic stent insertion can be used as a surgical alternative.

Patients who have strictures following morbid obesity can also be treated although the varied post-surgical anatomy can present a challenge. In general, the channel remaining after restrictive gastroplasty should not be dilated to more than 12 mm.

In malignant obstruction of the gastric outlet or duodenum there is increasing usage of self-expanding stents for palliation; thus surgical bypass with its associated morbidity and mortality is avoided. Stents up to 22 mm in diameter are now available on 10 Fr introducer systems. The technique is the same as for balloon dilatation using a catheter guidewire technique either perorally, transgastrically or rarely transhepatically (Fig. 11.4).

(b)

(a)

(c)

Figure 11.4 *Self-expanding metallic stents in gastric outlet obstruction. (a) Barium meal demonstrating significant gastric distension and stasis with concentric narrowing of the second part of the duodenum from carcinoma of the pancreas. (b) CT scan in the same patient demonstrating a markedly distended stomach with food residue and an inhomogeneous soft-tissue mass in the region of the head of the pancreas. A tiny area of increased attenuation in the centre of this soft-tissue mass represents retained contrast in the narrowed duodenal lumen from the previous barium meal. (c) Self-expanding metallic stent placement. A guidewire has been advanced through the obstruction from a peroral approach and a stent released following introduction of the device over the wire. The intrinsic expansile force of the stent will enable full expansion to 22mm over 24–48 hours.*

COLORECTAL STRICTURES

The technique in reaching, cannulating and dilating strictures of the lower gastrointestinal tract is the same as for upper gastrointestinal strictures whether via the anus or via a stoma. If the stricture is at some distance from the entry site, a combined endoscopic and fluoroscopic approach is often successful. Benign strictures can be **balloon dilated** using standard catheter-guidewire technique. In general larger balloon sizes are required in the lower gastrointestinal tract with dimensions up to 40 mm being required in some instances to achieve a normal faecal stream.

There has been significant interest and progress in recent years in the management of malignant colorectal strictures with expandable **metallic stents**. The devices have been used in both acute and chronic malignant colorectal obstruction. In patients who present acutely, placement of a stent can stabilize an extremely

sick patient and enable appropriate staging to be performed. If surgery is appropriate, then a resection and primary colorectal anastomosis can be performed electively within a few days. If curative surgery is not appropriate then the stent can remain *in situ* and provide effective palliation. This management strategy avoids operating on extremely debilitated patients and also prevents a two-stage procedure with intermittent colostomy. In patients with colorectal malignancy with metastatic disease who present with change of bowel habit, again stent placement can provide effective palliation (Fig. 11.5).

If the stricture can be reached and traversed with a catheter and guidewire, then it can be stented in most instances. Access with fluoroscopy alone is usually successful for strictures to the descending colon, although this becomes increasingly difficult for more proximal strictures. For lesions in the ascending and transverse colon, endoscopic assistance can be

(a)

(b)

(c)

Figure 11.5 *Self-expanding metallic stents in colorectal obstruction. (a) Barium enema demonstrating apple core stricture in the mid sigmoid from carcinoma. (b) Radiograph taken immediately following stent placement demonstrating considerable waisting at the stricture site. (c) Radiograph at 24 hours showing good stent position and reasonable expansion, although some persistent waisting at the stricture site persists. Multiple sclerotic bony metastases can be seen throughout the bony pelvis.*

extremely helpful. Antibiotic cover is usually required. Balloon dilatation pre- and post-stent insertion is not advised because of the risk of perforation. Newer stent designs have recently been introduced on 10–12 Fr introducer systems with diameters of 30 mm post-deployment. The complications relating to the procedure include perforation and stent migration.

There is increasing evidence in the literature to demonstrate this is a cost-effective and efficacious technique in managing colorectal malignancy in both acute and chronic cases.

PERCUTANEOUS MANAGEMENT OF GASTROINTESTINAL FISTULAE

Fistulae vary in complexity from a single track to multiple tracks with associated abscesses. In general, the simpler types are more likely to heal with conservative therapy, whilst those associated with abscesses require intervention. Upper gastrointestinal fistulae are divided into low output and high output. Those with outputs of ≤ 200 ml/24 h are defined as high output. Traditionally the volume of output has been inversely related to the likelihood of spontaneous closure without intervention. However, the recent aggressive use of total parenteral nutrition and pharmacological agents has made this distinction less valid. The location of the fistula along the gastrointestinal tract and the underlying aetiology are more important prognostic factors.

Abdominal surgery is the most common cause of gastrointestinal fistulae. Inadvertent enterostomy and leaking anastomoses are the major subgroups of surgically related fistula. Other causes include penetrating trauma, inflammatory diseases such as ulcers, diverticulitis, radiation enteritis and Crohn's disease as well as neoplasm.

The management of persisting fistula is to occlude the tract and prevent leakage as considerable fluid and electrolyte loss can occur. Also the bowel contents can be irritating, leading to skin ulceration. Sepsis and malnutrition frequently complicate management.

All patients presenting with gastrointestinal fistulae should be evaluated with cross-sectional imaging, preferably CT scanning and contrast medium fistulography. The primary purpose of cross-sectional imaging is to detect abdominal abscesses associated with fistula, which will need to be drained before healing can occur. Also, the underlying disease process may be identified, e.g. bowel wall thickening in Crohn's disease or a pericolic abscess associated with diverticulitis. If a soft-tissue mass suggestive of an abscess is seen, injection of dilute contrast medium along the fistulous tract whilst the patient is in the CT scanner, and re-imaging at this level, will demonstrate communication of the fistula

with the abscess. If this is the case, then contrast medium will outline the abscess cavity, which can be drained, in most instances, under fluoroscopic guidance. If no contrast medium enters the abscess, then a separate puncture to localize the abscess should be done under CT guidance.

The purpose of fistulography is to determine the site of origin of the fistula, to establish whether there is distal obstruction and to show any abscess communicating with the tract. If there is neither, then conservative management has a reasonable chance of success. Conservative management focuses on decreasing fistula output whilst treating infection, malnutrition and skin breakdown.

Enterocutaneous fistulae that are complicated by associated abscesses, fistulae that are discovered after initial drainage of abscesses, and simple fistulae not responding to conservative measures are all amenable to percutaneous therapy. The goals are:

- to place a tube or tubes precisely, which will divert the bowel contents away from the site of the defect in the bowel wall;
- to drain thoroughly associated abscess collections.

CANNULATION OF ENTEROCUTANEOUS FISTULAE

An initial fistulogram is performed to define clearly the relationship between a sinus tract, the hole in the bowel and any abscesses. Subsequent cannulation of the sinus track is made with extreme caution to avoid dissection of the friable, often tortuous, pathways. Once the catheter has reached the lumen of the bowel, additional contrast is injected to evaluate the bowel distal to the fistula.

DIVERSION OF ENTERIC CONTENTS

Control of the effluent from the bowel can be achieved by placing a catheter just inside the bowel lumen, thus diverting the bowel contents before they leak into the subcutaneous tissues. This is particularly advantageous when the leaking fluid is irritating, such as from duodenal fistulae containing both hydrochloric acid and pancreatic enzymes. Alternatively, if the fistula is smaller, a drainage catheter can be positioned just outside the hole in the bowel to collect the contents as they leak, and divert them from the subcutaneous tissues. Once the associated abscesses are resolved, all that then remains is a single fistula tract drain. When the volume of drainage falls below 100 ml/24 h, the tube is positioned several centimetres from the bowel wall. When drainage finally ceases, a sinogram is performed to confirm closure of the fistula and the tube is removed incrementally.

DRAINAGE OF ASSOCIATED ABSCESSES

The second major focus of percutaneous therapy of enteric fistulae is drainage of associated abscesses. This may require multiple drainage tubes. The general principle is the same as for abscesses (see p. 288) not associated with fistula; however, a combination of fistula and abscess or abscesses tends to require more aggressive and longer term drainage. Once the fistula is controlled, the abscesses will heal with tube drainage. As with any drainage tubes, the drains must be kept patent by frequent flushing, typically with 10–20 ml saline three times daily. Repositioning and replacement are done in conjunction with repeat sinograms that monitor progress and direct optimal catheter position. When the sinogram demonstrates resolution of the abscess cavities, the drainage tubes are backed out incrementally and removed.

Gastrointestinal fistulae related to pancreatic inflammatory disease are particularly challenging, with abnormal communications to the pancreatic duct and biliary tree. They most commonly occur after pancreatic surgery or drainage of pancreatic abscesses. Catheter diversion of both pancreatic and biliary output is sometimes necessary to allow healing. Prolonged healing is routinely required in this setting. However, the principles applied are the same as for other gastroenteric fistulae, with the initial focus being resolution of the abscesses followed by closure of any fistulae.

RESULTS

Before the aggressive use of total parenteral nutrition, the spontaneous closure rate of gastroenteric fistulae was reported to be as low as 25 per cent. Parenteral nutrition has doubled this closure rate, but about 50 per cent of fistulae will require intervention. Complete closure can be achieved in approximately 60–80 per cent with the use of percutaneous techniques. The success rate depends on a number of factors.

- It was previously thought that low output fistulae resolved in a higher proportion of cases; however, with aggressive use of total parenteral nutrition and pharmacological manipulation of the effluent, the initial output volume appears to be less important.
- Location appears to be important. Gastric and proximal duodenal fistulae are very difficult to treat percutaneously, with approximately 75 per cent eventually requiring surgery. Distal duodenal and other small bowel fistulae tend to close on average between 60–80 per cent of the time.
- If the underlying bowel at the site of the fistula is diseased, the likelihood of cure is small. Crohn's disease is a good example: a spontaneous fistula to bowel involved by Crohn's will close with percuta-

neous drainage in only 20 per cent of cases. However, if the fistula occurs postoperatively following removal of a diseased segment of Crohn's disease then it will close in approximately 80 per cent of cases with percutaneous management.
- The success rate of percutaneous management of colonic fistulae is dependent on the underlying disease. Fistulae secondary to diverticulitis or appendicitis appear to respond well to tube drainage. However, in cases secondary to abnormal segments of bowel affected by radiation enteritis or colitis, successful closure with percutaneous management is unlikely.

PERCUTANEOUS GASTROSTOMY AND GASTROJEJUNOSTOMY

Patients unable to maintain nutrition with oral intake require either enteral or parenteral feeding. The most common indications are inability to swallow following cerebrovascular accident or upper gastrointestinal malignancy. Other indications include chronic neurological disorders (multiple sclerosis, senile dementia, Alzheimer's and Parkinson's disease), severe burns, chronic pancreatitis, Crohn's disease and radiation enteritis. Enteral feeding is preferable, if possible, as it is more physiological and cost-effective. This form of feeding has traditionally been via surgical gastrostomy or nasogastric feeding tube. Surgical gastrostomy has the disadvantage of high cost with a higher morbidity and mortality. Long-term nasogastric tube feeding is cheap but poorly tolerated and can lead to gastro-oesophageal reflux, peptic oesophagitis and stricture formation.

Recent advances for placement of **gastrostomy feeding tubes** using endoscopy and fluoroscopy with the Seldinger technique have rendered surgical gastrostomy almost obsolete. The choice between endoscopic and fluoroscopic placement depends on local expertise, although the fluoroscopically guided method does have several advantages: apart from reduced cost, there is a decreased risk of wound infection and aspiration. In addition, the fluoroscopic placement of a gastrojejunostomy tube, in patients who require jejunal infusional feeding, is a relatively simple extension of the basic technique. Although endoscopic placement of the catheter into the jejunum is possible, the procedure is more tedious to perform and catheters are difficult to exchange. The complications associated with endoscopic placement have been as high as 80 per cent with catheter dysfunction in more than 50 per cent. The decision to perform gastrostomy or gastrojejunostomy depends on the underlying pathology and the general condition of the patient. If the patient is ambulatory and can tolerate a single large feed two to three times daily, without risk of reflux, a gastrostomy tube is indicated. In addition, a small group of patients with advanced abdominopelvic malignancy requires gastrostomy tube placement for palliative bowel decompression. If the patient is bed-bound with a decreased level of consciousness, a gastrojejunostomy tube with a slow infusion feed is placed to reduce the risk of reflux.

TECHNIQUE

An abdominal ultrasound scan is performed prior to the procedure to map out the position and so avoid puncture of the left lobe of the liver. Following placement of a nasogastric tube the stomach is inflated with carbon dioxide or air in order to increase the size of the stomach and make it an easier target. It also causes the anterior wall to lie subcutaneously just beneath the abdominal wall. If passage of a nasogastric tube is not possible, direct percutaneous puncture of the collapsed gastric antrum is possible (with ultrasound or CT guidance) with direct inflation of the stomach with carbon dioxide down the needle lumen.

Anteroposterior and lateral fluoroscopy is then performed to ensure that the stomach lies subcutaneously with no interposing small bowel and that the transverse colon has been deflected inferiorly. The procedure is performed under local anaesthesia, intravenous analgesia and sedation.

Under fluoroscopic guidance an appropriate puncture site is selected overlying the body of the stomach near the antrum clear of the liver and transverse colon. A 22-gauge fine bore needle is introduced such that the tip lies within the insufflated stomach angled towards the fundus for a gastrostomy tube or the pylorus for a gastrojejunostomy tube. If a gastrostomy is required, various guidewires and dilators are used coaxially and a 12F loop catheter is positioned with its retention loop in the stomach.

If a gastrojejunostomy is required, a catheter-guidewire combination is manipulated across the pylorus into the duodenum and onward beyond the ligament of Treitz; the catheter is then removed leaving the guidewire in place. A 12F gastrojejunostomy catheter can then be introduced over the guidewire such that the tip is in the jejunum and the retention loop lies in the stomach (Fig. 11.6). There is a variety of catheters on the market but most have 20 side holes in the last 15 cm. The catheter can be left *in situ* for up to 6 months before exchange is required.

The technique has a success rate which approaches 100 per cent with low morbidity (5–8 per cent) and mortality (< 1 per cent). Minor complications include wound infection and tube dislodgement. The main major complication is peritonitis, which some authors have attempted to minimize by performing gastropexy. Others argue that the incidence of gastric leakage and

(a)

(b)

Figure 11.6 *Gastrojejunostomy tube insertion. (a) and (b) A 12F gastrojejunostomy tube is seen with the retention loop in the stomach and the tip of the tube beyond the ligament of Treitz. (Reproduced with permission from A.F. Watkinson et al. in* European Radiology, *1995,* **5,** *13–18, published by Springer Verlag, Berlin.)*

peritonitis is no higher with the percutaneous endoscopic approach and no higher than following surgical gastrostomy. With careful selection of patients for gastrostomy and gastrojejunostomy tubes, the incidence of chronic aspiration is extremely low.

PERCUTANEOUS MANAGEMENT OF BENIGN AND MALIGNANT BILIARY STRICTURES

In patients with obstructive jaundice good imaging is required with CT or ultrasound to identify the level of obstruction and the cause. It still may not be possible to make a diagnosis and direct cholangiography is often required. The least invasive approach is via endoscopy; however, this is not always successful, does not always demonstrate the intrahepatic radicles completely and depends on local expertise. Percutaneous transhepatic cholangiography provides excellent delineation of the intra- and extrahepatic biliary tree and is the initiating step in percutaneous access and treatment of biliary strictures.

Good clotting function is essential with a platelet count of more than 80 000 and a prothrombin time of no more than 4 seconds greater than control. All patients should receive prophylactic broad-spectrum antibiotic therapy during the procedure. The initial diagnostic study is carried out using a 22-gauge needle from a right intercostal approach. Although easier to perform if the intrahepatic biliary tree is dilated, it is still successful in most instances if the biliary tree is only minimally dilated; however, more needle passes may be required. Once a duct has been punctured it is impor-

tant to aspirate bile, so that contrast can be introduced in equal aliquots and not further distend the biliary tree, which would increase the risk of endotoxic shock or cholangitis. Good images are then obtained (Fig. 11.7) which, when combined with the clinical history, ultrasound or CT, should indicate the diagnosis, though a fine-needle aspiration biopsy may be necessary for final confirmation.

If a decision is made to proceed to drainage, a suitable duct for access is selected. This should have a direct line of approach toward the common hepatic duct. In most instances a peripheral duct on the right is chosen in both benign and malignant disease. Initial puncture is once again performed with a 22-gauge needle, and access to the intrahepatic ducts is obtained using the Seldinger technique. Further manipulation in the biliary tree is performed with specially designed catheters and guidewires. Teflon-coated hydrophilic guidewires are particularly useful for traversing even the tightest strictures.

BENIGN BILIARY STRICTURES

About 95 per cent of biliary strictures are postoperative secondary to surgery. Other causes include sclerosing cholangitis and chronic pancreatitis (Fig. 11.8), or are secondary to biliary calculi. Postoperative strictures usually occur at the site of a hepaticojejunostomy following bile duct excision (Fig. 11.9a) or at the site of insertion of the cystic duct postcholecystectomy. Recurrent strictures cause intermittent bouts of cholangitis associated with pain and jaundice. The traditional method of treatment is surgical repair; however, the

Figure 11.7 *Percutaneous transhepatic cholangiography (PTC). There is a tight stricture (arrows) of the common hepatic duct caused by cholangiocarcinoma, with intrahepatic biliary dilatation above the stricture. If it is decided to proceed to percutaneous drainage, a second puncture should be performed via a suitable duct (curved arrow).*

Figure 11.8 *Benign biliary stricture. PTC demonstrating a smooth tapered stricture of the lower common bile duct secondary to pancreatitis (straight arrows). Note the catheter is entering the biliary tree via a duct providing good access for percutaneous intervention (curved arrows).*

(a)

(b)

(c)

Figure 11.9 *Dilatation of benign biliary stricture. (a) PTC demonstrating complete obstruction of the common hepatic duct (arrow) after construction of a hepaticojejunostomy. (b) The obstructed hepaticojejunostomy has been traversed and a balloon dilatation catheter introduced along the percutaneous tract. This has been inflated (arrows) across the strictured segment. (c) A cholangiogram performed via a percutaneous catheter with the tip in the left main hepatic duct. The hepaticojejunostomy is now widely patent (arrow) and the catheter can be removed. (Reproduced with permission from A.F. Watkinson and A. Adam (1996)* Interventional radiology: a practical guide, *published by Radcliffe Medical Press, Oxford.)*

recurrence rate is 10–40 per cent with an operative mortality of 2–4 per cent. Balloon dilatation through a percutaneous tract was first described in 1978 and since then has become a well-established technique.

Technique

If the stricture can be traversed using standard catheter-guidewire techniques then a balloon catheter can be introduced coaxially over the guidewire after catheter withdrawal. Subsequent balloon inflation can then be performed to dilate the stricture (Fig. 11.9). This is usually performed using 8–10 mm balloon catheters, which can be inflated to at least 12 atm (1216 kPa). If biliary sepsis is present, balloon dilatation should not be performed until this has settled during a period of external drainage and antibiotic therapy. After balloon dilatation an access catheter is sometimes left in place to facilitate repeat dilatation should early recurrence occur. The catheter is removed following check cholangiography 3–4 weeks later, provided the patient is asymptomatic and the anastomosis fully patent (Fig. 11.9).

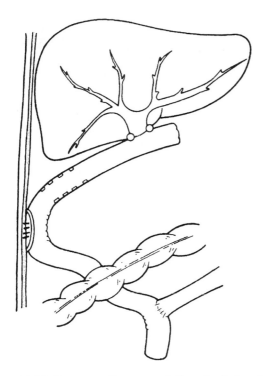

Figure 11.10 *Diagrammatic representation of a Hutson loop. An end-to-side hepaticojejunostomy has been constructed and the jejunal loop attached to the abdominal wall with a radiopaque metal ring marker to facilitate future percutaneous access. (Adapted from A.F. Watkinson and A. Adam (1996)* Interventional radiology: a practical guide, *published by Radcliffe Medical Press, Oxford.)*

Figure 11.11 *Malignant biliary stricture. PTC demonstrating a markedly dilated intra- and extrahepatic biliary tree. There is an irregular stricture in the lower common bile duct secondary to carcinoma of the pancreas (white arrows). The ideal duct for percutaneous access has been punctured (black arrows).*

Results

The success rate is approximately 80 per cent after 30 months. The results of balloon dilatation are, however, poor in patients with sclerosing cholangitis.

Good surgical practice demands that all patients undergoing hepaticojejunostomy should have a Hutson loop formed (Fig. 11.10). This should be marked with a radiopaque circular ring to facilitate repeated percutaneous access for stricture dilatation in the event of future problems.

Expandable metal stents should be used only as a last resort in benign disease when strictures are resistant to balloon dilatation or if the patients are unfit for surgery.

MALIGNANT BILIARY STRICTURES

Biliary drainage is usually a palliative procedure in patients with biliary tract obstruction owing to unresectable malignancy. The most common neoplasm producing extrahepatic biliary obstruction is carcinoma of the pancreas, which, if inoperable, has a mean survival time of approximately 6 months. Percutaneous relief of this obstruction is an accepted mode of treatment; however, the recent advances in endoscopically placed stents have meant the role of percutaneous drainage in pancreatic carcinoma is usually limited to endoscopic failures. The choice of treatment varies according to local expertise.

Primary bile duct tumours are more difficult to manage endoscopically, particularly when located at the hilum of the liver (**Klatskin tumours**) or extending into the intrahepatic ducts. In non-surgical candidates these lesions are readily treated by percutaneous techniques. Transhepatic biliary drainage may also provide palliation for patients with metastases or other tumours at the hilum of the liver. However, in patients with multiple peripheral intrahepatic metastases associated with biliary tract obstruction, drainage should be avoided as it is generally ineffective in relieving jaundice. Usually, it is sufficient to drain only one side of the obstructed biliary tree as drainage of 30 per cent or greater of the liver parenchyma will relieve the obstructive symptoms.

The initial technique is identical to the approach in benign biliary strictures with diagnostic cholangiography as the initial step. The anatomy of the biliary tree and the level of obstruction determine the choice of appropriate duct for drainage (Fig. 11.11). Biliary drainage on the left side may be necessary in cases of

(a) *(b)*

Figure 11.12 *Malignant biliary stricture. (a) A self-expanding metallic stent has been positioned across a malignant stricture in the lower common bile duct secondary to carcinoma of the head of the pancreas. The narrowing (arrows) of the stent represents the site of the stricture. A safety catheter has been left within the stent. (b) A cholangiogram via the safety catheter 24 hours after stent placement demonstrates free flow into the duodenum with a satisfactory radiological result. The safety catheter can now be withdrawn. (Reproduced with permission from A.F. Watkinson and A. Adam (1996)* Interventional radiology: a practical guide, *published by Radcliffe Medical Press, Oxford.)*

extensive tumour invasion, via an anterior subcostal approach. A combination of specifically designed catheters and hydrophilic guidewires ensures that even the tightest strictures can usually be traversed; if not, a period of external drainage for two to three days usually opens up the stricture to allow the guidewire through. The stricture is then dilated with a balloon catheter prior to stent placement.

Choice of endoprosthesis: plastic or metal?

Plastic endoprostheses require a percutaneous tract of 12F or greater with associated increased morbidity and patient discomfort. The recent introduction of self-expanding metallic endoprostheses means that a smaller percutaneous tract is sufficient and that the stent can often be inserted at one sitting without a period of external drainage. The disadvantage of cost is overcome by a reduced reintervention rate because of the decreased rate of occlusion of metallic stents compared with conventional devices. This factor is important in the treatment of cholangiocarcinoma, which grows

more slowly than pancreatic lesions and, with adequate decompression, patients can achieve a 1-year survival of approximately 50 per cent. Metallic stents are thus the treatment of choice for percutaneous palliation of inoperable biliary strictures.

Metallic endoprostheses, which are self-expanding, are introduced over a guidewire across the predilated stricture. Once the stent has been released across the stricture a small safety catheter can be left within the stent (Fig. 11.12a) so that a cholangiogram can be performed the following day to check patency of the endoprosthesis prior to removal of the catheter (Fig. 11.12b).

Stent occlusion is usually the result of bile encrustation, tumour ingrowth or overgrowth. The problem of bile encrustation is reduced by the use of metallic stents. Early promise that the use of covered stents would help solve the problem of tumour occlusion has not been realised and studies have not shown improved patency. Tumour growth above or below the endoprosthesis can be reduced by the placement of long stents extending from the intrahepatic radicles to the duodenum just beyond the ampulla of Vater.

(a)

(b)

Figure 11.13 *Percutaneous removal of common hepatic duct calculi. (a) PTC demonstrates a large intraluminal filling defect (arrows) in the common hepatic duct. (b) A basket introduced coaxially (arrows) has captured the calculus; this can now be fragmented and pushed into the duodenum or removed percutaneously.*

The perfect biliary stent would be a removable endoprosthesis that is safe to insert along a narrow tract associated with a low rate of complications, in particular recurrent jaundice, cholangitis and stent occlusion. Metallic stents have gone a long way to solving some of these problems; however, new developments are awaited to further improve the design and reduce the initial cost.

MANAGEMENT OF PROBLEMATIC BILIARY TRACT CALCULI

Stones in the common bile duct are found in approximately 10 per cent of patients undergoing cholecystectomy, rising to over 30 per cent in those over 80 years of age. Since the advent of endoscopic sphincterotomy in 1974, the approach to treating common bile duct calculi has changed fundamentally. The overall success rate of endoscopic sphincterotomy in clearing these stones is 85–90 per cent with a lower morbidity and mortality than surgery. This procedure is therefore the technique of choice in the majority of cases for removal of common bile duct calculi. An exception is in patients who have a T-tube *in situ*; here, percutaneous removal under fluoroscopic guidance, with a steerable catheter and basket (as popularized by Burhenne who performed this technique on the Shah of Iran in 1979), has a high success rate with very low morbidity. The disadvantage is that the T-tube tract must be left to mature for 5–6 weeks. T-tubes are not usually left in place after laparoscopic cholecystectomy; any retained stones are usually removed postoperatively via an endoscopic sphincterotomy.

Problematical biliary calculi are ductal or intrahepatic stones that are not amenable to treatment with endoscopic sphincterotomy or removal via a T-tube tract using basket techniques. Patients with these stones usually have one of the following:

- **Inaccessible biliary tree**. Because of altered anatomy, secondary to either gastric surgery or the presence of a duodenal diverticulum, it may not be possible to cannulate the ampulla of Vater.
- **Bile duct stricture**. With bile stasis, calculi often form proximal to strictures and even with endoscopic papillotomy and dilatation the calculi are often difficult to clear.
- **Large and impacted stones**. Stones larger than 1.5 cm in diameter are often difficult to remove and can become impacted. Intrahepatic stones can be remote from the ampulla and difficult to reach with the basket.

TECHNIQUE OF PERCUTANEOUS BILIARY STONE REMOVAL

Percutaneous cholangiography, as described on page 281, is performed through the right or left intrahepatic bile ducts depending on the location of the stones. If the stones are in the extrahepatic biliary tree then a relatively horizontal approach to the right main duct allows access to the common bile duct. Once drainage has been performed, the tract is allowed to mature for 1–2 days, in order to enable sheath systems of up to 18F to be introduced with minimal discomfort (Fig. 11.13a,b). With a percutaneous access route, various methods can be used to fragment, flush and dissolve the stones. **Direct fragmentation** with baskets (Fig. 11.13b) and **electrohydraulic lithotripsy** are the most commonly used techniques. Stone fragments are usually removed by antegrade passage through the ampulla, although retrograde removal through the larger sheaths is possible. A prior endoscopic or transhepatic sphincterotomy or balloon dilatation of the ampulla is usually required (Fig. 11.14a–c). **Chemical dissolution** has not been widely adopted and is unlikely to become so, because only cholesterol-containing stones are amenable; dissolution may take a prolonged period and the agents used (methyl *tert*-butyl ether [MTBE] and mono-octanoin) have potentially significant side effects and complications.

An alternative method for stone removal is the combined **radiological endoscopic approach**. The initial percutaneous puncture is performed as previously described and, following access to the biliary tree with a standard catheter-guidewire technique, a guidewire is manipulated into the duodenum (or jejunum if the patient has had a Roux loop formed). An experienced endoscopist can then locate the wire and use this to guide retrograde access to the ampulla of Vater and common bile duct, thus overcoming the problems of abnormal anatomy.

If endoscopic cannulation of the ampulla is possible, but the stones are too large or too many for removal even after sphincterotomy and basket fragmentation, then alternative techniques are necessary. These include chemical dissolution through a nasobiliary tube, extracorporeal shockwave lithotripsy and intracorporeal lithotripsy devices introduced via the endoscope.

INTERVENTIONAL RADIOLOGY OF THE GALLBLADDER

Interventional radiology and surgery of the gallbladder have gone through dramatic changes in recent years and, although the overwhelming success of laparoscopic techniques now means that the radiologist no longer offers alternatives to elective surgery, gallbladder puncture and catheterization techniques remain useful in the management of complicated gallbladder disease.

FINE NEEDLE ASPIRATION

Fine needle aspiration of the gallbladder is a relatively safe procedure and is usually performed under ultrasound guidance via the transhepatic or transperitoneal approach. The aspirate can be sent for cytology and culture; however, patients are often on intravenous antibiotics and the infective agent can only be determined in approximately 60 per cent of cases. Consequently, the decision to proceed to percutaneous drainage is often made on clinical grounds rather than from the bacteriological results.

PERCUTANEOUS CHOLECYSTOSTOMY

The current indications for performing percutaneous cholecystostomy are:

- decompression and drainage in acute cholecystitis and empyema;
- to develop an access tract for stone removal (which may follow the above);
- access for biliary drainage.

Technique when treating acute cholecystitis and empyema

Percutaneous cholecystostomy is usually performed under local analgesia with intravenous sedation. Anaesthetic assistance may, however, be requested as these patients are frequently unfit for major surgery. The traditional approach has been the transhepatic route under ultrasound guidance. The aim is to puncture the bare area of the liver and thus minimize the risk of bile leak into the peritoneal cavity. The incidence of peritonitis via the transperitoneal approach appears to be no different and, therefore, either method is acceptable. The gallbladder can be punctured directly with a sheathed needle or a fine-needle introduction set, the aim being to leave a self-retaining catheter, with a locking loop at the tip, within the gallbladder lumen. The single-stick technique is frequently used in patients with an empyema and profound sepsis, as the gallbladder is usually distended in an immediately subcutaneous position. Recovery in such circumstances can be dramatic, and catheter drainage can be performed for 2–3 weeks prior to definitive cholecystectomy. The technique does not preclude laparoscopic cholecystectomy. If the cholecystitis is secondary to malignant obstruction of the biliary tree, then long-term drainage can be carried out with repeated catheter exchange, although, if possible, internal drainage via an endopros-

(a)

(b)

(c)

Figure 11.14 *Percutaneous sphincteroplasty of the ampulla of Vater. (a) PTC demonstrates obstruction of the lower end of the common bile duct, with a curved meniscus (arrows), caused by an impacted common duct calculus. (b) A balloon catheter has been introduced percutaneously and inflated across the ampulla of Vater (arrow) to perform sphincteroplasty. (c) A cholangiogram after sphincteroplasty demonstrates free flow into the duodenum. The calculus has passed spontaneously through the dilated ampulla of Vater. (Reproduced with permission from A.F. Watkinson and A. Adam (1996)* Interventional radiology: a practical guide, *published by Radcliffe Medical Press, Oxford.)*

thesis should be used following recovery from the initial episode.

There is increasing evidence to support performing percutaneous cholecystostomy in patients in intensive therapy units who are septic without traceable cause. Culture of the bile is usually unhelpful in diagnosing bile infection, because these patients are usually receiving a wide range of antibiotics. The ultrasound features of acalculous cholecystitis are thickening of the gallbladder wall and pericholecystic fluid. Sludge, a non-specific finding, is usually present within the bile. Approximately half the patients in this clinicoradiological setting will improve following percutaneous cholecystostomy.

STONE EXTRACTION AND DISSOLUTION

The traditional technique for treatment of gallstones has been open cholecystectomy since Langenbeck first performed the operation in 1884. In the 1980s, prior to the introduction of laparoscopic cholecystectomy, there was great interest and development in the fields of lithotripsy and various mechanical devices to crush and fragment the stones if a percutaneous tract existed. Nowadays, the combination of **laparoscopic surgery** and **endoscopic sphincterotomy** manages the vast majority of gallbladder and common duct calculi, but there is still a small group of patients who require alternative methods of treatment for a variety of reasons.

Patients who have had percutaneous cholecystostomy performed for acute cholecystitis secondary to gallstones can have these removed percutaneously when the acute episode has settled. The tract is left to mature for 4–6 weeks and then dilated up to 12–14F gauge. The stones can then be extracted with a variety of baskets or forceps. Alternatively rotary lithotrite devices can be introduced to emulsify the stones. For very large or impacted stones it may be necessary to deal with these stones using a rigid nephroscope via the original tract dilated to 28–30F under general anaesthesia.

If a percutaneous catheter is in the gallbladder lumen, and the gallstones consist predominantly of cholesterol, they can be successfully dissolved using methyl *tert*-butyl ether or mono-octanoin via manual instillation. This technique has proved to be unpopular because of the toxicity of the dissolution agents, the time involved to carry out the procedure and the high stone recurrence rate, as residual calcium carbonate fragments act as future nidi for gallstone formation. Extracorporeal shockwave lithotripsy is still appropriate in patients who decide they do not want surgery, either laparoscopic or open. Modern units can usually fragment most gallstones of a size up to 3 cm, although more than one session may be required. This technique is carried out under local anaesthesia on an out-patient basis, and the patient is usually started on oral ursodeoxycholic acid as a dissolution agent. If the gallbladder is functioning and the cystic duct is patent (assessed on ultrasound pre- and post-fatty meal), clearance of stones will be achieved in greater than 70 per cent of cases at 1 year. However, if the gallbladder is left *in situ*, there is a significant risk of stone recurrence.

If there is no contraindication to surgery, and the patient gives informed consent, the best treatment for symptomatic gallstones is laparoscopic cholecystectomy by an experienced surgeon.

BILIARY DRAINAGE

In the acute setting in a jaundiced, septic patient with a distended gallbladder, a rapid percutaneous cholecystostomy under ultrasound guidance (which can be performed at the bedside) can dramatically improve the patient's condition. More formal assessment of the biliary tree with subsequent intervention can be delayed until more clinically appropriate.

PERCUTANEOUS ABDOMINAL BIOPSY AND ABSCESS DRAINAGE

IMAGE-GUIDED BIOPSY

Percutaneous biopsy can provide information about the presence, nature and extent of intra-abdominal disease, and almost any radiologically detected abnormality is technically amenable to needle biopsy or aspiration.

Patients with a prothrombin time over 4–5 seconds above control or a platelet count less than 80 000/ml should have these parameters corrected, if possible prior to biopsy. Patients who have severe, uncorrectable coagulopathies and require liver biopsy should be considered for a percutaneous biopsy with plugging of the tract or biopsy via the transvenous route (transjugular or transfemoral). If there is gross ascites, this should be drained prior to biopsy.

Antibiotic prophylaxis should be considered in immunocompromised patients or if there is a high probability of traversing a contaminated field (e.g. transcolonic biopsy). All patients should have an intravenous line inserted prior to the procedure in case analgesia or resuscitation is required. Most percutaneous biopsies can be performed on an out-patient basis. Patients should be observed for at least 2 hours afterwards and, if vital signs remain stable, they can be discharged.

Choice of needle

The choice of needle type and size often depends on personal preference and the suspected underlying pathology. In patients with suspected malignancy, immediate cytological analysis of a cellular aspirate obtained through a fine needle (19 gauge or smaller) is often sufficient to make the diagnosis. If after two or three passes a diagnostic specimen has not been obtained a core biopsy is taken with an 18-gauge cutting needle (manual or spring-loaded) and sent for histological examination. In patients with benign parenchymal disease affecting the liver or kidney, where architectural information is important, an 18-gauge core biopsy with a cutting needle is usually required. If larger needles are used the complication rate appears to increase.

Choice of imaging modality

Generally the shortest route from the skin to the lesion is chosen, providing no vital structures (e.g. the spleen

Figure 11.15 *Fluoroscopically-guided percutaneous biopsy. Bilateral indwelling biliary internal–external drainage catheters have been positioned across a stricture at the confluence of the right and left main hepatic ducts (arrow). A 21-gauge needle has been introduced percutaneously, under fluoroscopic guidance, to biopsy the hilar lesion.*

or lung) are interposed. The size and location of the lesion combined with operator preference determine the optimum imaging modality. When the target is visible on conventional radiography, fluoroscopy is suitable for biopsy guidance. In the abdomen, a contrast examination is often needed (e.g. bile duct stricture with an indwelling biliary stent [Fig. 11.15]).

Most biopsies, however, are performed using CT or ultrasound guidance. Targets affected by respiratory motion are often biopsied more readily using ultrasound because real time imaging can be used. Similarly,

because of the multiple scan planes possible with ultrasound, angled approaches (e.g. craniocaudal angulation) are easier. Other advantages include low cost, rapid scan time and no radiation dose. CT should be used for small lesions, especially in areas that cannot be imaged satisfactorily with ultrasound, such as masses in the retroperitoneum (Fig. 11.16a,b) or bone. CT is also useful for biopsying partially necrotic lesions, when intravenous contrast enhancement allows targeting of the viable part of the tumour.

Results and complications

Overall accuracy rates of most percutaneous abdominal biopsies exceed 80 per cent. False-negative biopsies may be due to an off-target biopsy or sampling of the necrotic or fibrous portion of a tumour (e.g. pancreatic carcinoma) or the reactive hyperplasia accompanying many tumours. Thus, a negative biopsy should be repeated when there is strong clinical suspicion of malignancy. Complication rates from percutaneous abdominal biopsy are extremely low (< 1.5 per cent), especially when fine gauge needles are used (smaller than 19 gauge). If peripheral liver lesions are biopsied, it is important to traverse normal parenchyma first as the normal tissue will help to tamponade any haemorrhage.

IMAGE-GUIDED DRAINAGE

Percutaneous drainage has replaced surgery as the treatment of choice for most intra-abdominal abscesses and collections. Almost any intra-abdominal fluid collection demonstrated by either CT or ultrasound may be considered for drainage. This not only includes simple, unilocular fluid collections but also more

(a)

(b)

Figure 11.16 *CT-guided biopsy. (a) A CT scan at the level of the mid abdomen demonstrating a 2 cm mass on the lateral limb of the left adrenal gland (arrows). (b) A prone CT scan in the same patient demonstrating a needle with its tip in the adrenal lesion. Note how CT guidance has enabled puncture of the lung to be avoided.*

complicated collections such as necrotic tumour, haematomas and phlegmonous masses. Percutaneous drainage may not always totally eradicate these complex collections; however, the procedure allows improvement in the patient's general state of health so that definitive surgical drainage and debridement can be performed.

There are few contraindications to percutaneous drainage and most are relative. Any clotting abnormality should be corrected and the access route should avoid bowel or lung. A retroperitoneal, as opposed to a transperitoneal, approach is preferable to reduce the risk of intraperitoneal spillage of infected material. Except for simple cysts and loculated ascites, an intravenous line is mandatory and patients not already receiving antibiotics should be given broad-spectrum cover before and after percutaneous drainage.

Choice of imaging modality

The image guidance techniques are the same as for percutaneous biopsy. Percutaneous drainage of intra-abdominal collections is most often performed using **ultrasound guidance**; however, CT either alone or with fluoroscopy can also be used. Ultrasound is particularly useful in the drainage of superficial collections and those requiring an angled approach (e.g. subphrenic, high hepatic and splenic abscesses). Deep abdominal and pelvic collections are poorly visualized by ultrasound, and CT guidance is preferred. However, CT-guided drainage is not real time and the guidewire, tract dilators and drainage catheter are inserted by feel alone. Therefore, extra care is required to avoid misplacement of the catheter, and combination with fluoroscopy can be helpful in difficult cases.

Technique

The CT and ultrasound appearances of intra-abdominal fluid collections cannot reliably differentiate between abscess, sterile collections and organizing haematomas. When the decision to drain a collection depends on its nature or the presence of infection, diagnostic fine needle aspiration may be performed before drainage (Fig. 11.17). If the fluid is not obviously purulent, immediate microscopy should be performed. Biochemical analysis may also help to characterize the fluid (e.g. identification of a bile leak after a cholecystectomy or injury to the pancreas after splenectomy).

Subsequent catheter insertion uses the Seldinger guidewire exchange technique or a single-step trocar drainage catheter system, depending on personal preference. The trocar technique is more appropriate for large, superficial collections when there is little risk of misdirection. The pigtail catheter should end up in a coiled position within the abscess cavity. Multiple adjacent abscess cavities may require several drainage catheters for adequate treatment. The choice of catheter

Figure 11.17 *CT-guided aspiration. A needle is seen within a right paracolic collection for diagnostic aspiration.*

depends on the viscosity of the fluid. The catheter should be large enough for steady drainage and usually 8–10F is adequate for bilomas and loculated ascites. If the material aspirated is thick or particulate, larger bore catheters, 12–18F in diameter, are required. The cavity should be evacuated as completely as possible; however, aspiration should be stopped if the patient experiences sudden pain or the aspirate becomes bloody. Sudden decompression of large collections may be extremely uncomfortable and can precipitate haemorrhage from the abscess wall. Gentle irrigation with saline may help to decrease the viscosity of the contents and encourage drainage.

Good care following catheter placement is essential. Regular saline irrigation (10–20 ml three times daily) is important to maintain patency during the postdrainage days. The patient's condition usually improves noticeably within 24–48 hours after successful drainage. Failure to improve usually means drainage is inadequate, the collection is loculated or the catheter sideholes are incorrectly positioned. Repositioning of the catheter may be required. Continued drainage of 50 ml/day or more several days after the procedure often suggests a fistulous communication (e.g. with bowel, bile duct or pancreas), which can be confirmed by a contrast study. As long as the normal internal flow is unobstructed, these fistulae will close, although drainage may continue for 4–6 weeks or more. The catheter should not be removed until drainage has ceased and ultrasound or CT and a contrast study through the catheter confirm that the cavity has been obliterated.

Results and complications

With good technique and meticulous catheter care the overall success rate should be approximately 80 per cent and approach 100 per cent for unilocular collections. Success rates are lower for patients with complex collections (multiloculations, inflammatory masses and enteric or biliary fistula). The major complications include sepsis, haemorrhage and injury to adjacent structures. Minor complications include skin infection, catheter blockage and displacement. Careful planning of the approach to the collection should minimize the risk of inadvertent puncture of bowel, vascular structures and pleura.

PANCREATIC COLLECTIONS

The radiological management of pancreatic collections deserves special mention and depends on the type of collection.

Pseudocysts

Pseudocysts are walled-off collections of pancreatic secretions within or adjacent to the pancreas. They most commonly occur in the lesser sac region and usually form 4–6 weeks after acute pancreatitis. Although pseudocysts frequently resolve spontaneously, those over 5 cm in diameter often require intervention. Endoscopic retrograde pancreatography may be useful prior to drainage to demonstrate any communication with the duct system. Drainage in patients with pseudocysts with persisting communication with the duct system is less successful and usually takes longer. In these cases a transgastric approach is advised (see below). An uninfected pseudocyst with no communication to the duct system should be drained electively

when the wall has become well-defined and acute pancreatitic inflammation has subsided (usually at least 4 weeks after the acute episode). Earlier drainage may be contemplated if the patient's symptoms (abdominal pain and upper gastrointestinal obstruction) are worsening or the pseudocyst is enlarging. Infected pseudocysts should be drained more urgently. The reported success rate of percutaneous pseudocyst drainage ranges between 60 and 90 per cent.

Technique

A transgastric approach is attempted after the stomach has been distended with air. Puncture of the cyst is through the anterior abdominal wall and the anterior and posterior walls of the stomach. The procedure is best performed under CT guidance, although fluoroscopy or ultrasound may be used. Drainage via a direct percutaneous approach is acceptable, if the transgastric route is not feasible, but there is at least a theoretical risk of development of a persistent cutaneous pancreatic fistula.

The catheter is removed after CT once catheter contrast medium injection has confirmed complete resolution of the collection with no residual loculated areas, and drainage volumes have decreased to below 10 ml/day. Persistent drainage suggests communication with a pancreatic duct and in this case the catheter should be left in place until an established tract has formed between the cyst and the stomach. Alternatively a double pigtail stent may be used to establish communication between the pseudocyst and stomach to ensure internal drainage. The stent may be removed endoscopically later.

(a)

(b)

Figure 11.18 *Percutaneous pancreatic abscess drainage. (a) Contrast-enhanced CT scan demonstrating a large pancreatic collection of relatively low attenuation, surrounding the origin of the coeliac axis (the hepatic and splenic arteries are marked with curved arrows). The collection is of higher attenuation than water and is consistent with pus. (b) A 12F catheter has been inserted into the collection and, after 72 hours, a repeat CT scan shows considerable resolution. The catheter is seen coiled within the pancreatic bed (arrows).*

Pancreatic phlegmon, abscess and necrosis

The success rate of percutaneous drainage of pancreatic phlegmon, abscesses and necrosis is less successful than for other intra-abdominal abscesses. Contrast-enhanced CT should be performed (Fig. 11.18a). If a definite fluid collection is identified, with an attenuation value higher than simple fluid and consistent with pus, then percutaneous drainage, as previously described, should be performed with large bore catheters (Fig. 11.18b). Even if the abscess does not resolve this can serve as an interim measure to improve the condition of a critically ill patient before surgical debridement and drainage. However, if the CT scan reveals an enlarged, oedematous pancreas with areas of non-perfusion consistent with necrosis but no identifiable collection, percutaneous drainage will probably be of no value and intervention, when required, should be primarily surgical.

LIVER BIOPSY IN PATIENTS WITH ABNORMAL COAGULATION

Percutaneous liver biopsy is an established procedure with a very low morbidity and mortality in patients with normal coagulation. Image-guidance with ultrasound or CT is advised, even in the presence of diffuse disease, as there is a risk of pneumothorax, puncture of the bowel and damage to large vascular structures within the liver parenchyma. In many patients with diffuse liver disease, such as cirrhosis or widespread malignant infiltration, there are abnormalities of blood coagulation, which significantly increase the risk of bleeding after a biopsy. This can be minimized by performing percutaneous biopsy with subsequent **plugging** of the tract or the use of a **transvenous approach** via the femoral or jugular veins.

In patients with abnormal clotting (prothrombin time 4–5 seconds greater than control or a platelet count < 80 000/ml) every effort should be made to correct the abnormality with vitamin K, fresh frozen plasma or platelet transfusions. If the clotting abnormalities cannot be corrected, then the biopsy technique must be modified.

In patients with a moderate coagulopathy with an INR (International Normalized Ratio) of 1.4–2.0, or a platelet count of 50 000–80 000/ml, plugging of a percutaneous tract is a safe procedure with good results and minimal complications. However, in patients with an INR > 2.0 or a platelet count of < 50 000 the percutaneous approach is not advised as, although tract plugging can occlude the bleeding site in the liver, small subcutaneous or subcapsular veins cannot be occluded and can cause catastrophic haemorrhage. A transvenous approach is advised in patients with an INR > 2.0 or a platelet count < 50 000 that will not correct with vitamin K, fresh frozen plasma or platelet transfusions.

PLUGGED LIVER BIOPSY

There are various versions of this technique but the basic principle is biopsy through a sheath followed by embolization of the tract with steel coils or particulate material. The appropriate needle is usually of the 'Trucut' type which consistently produces satisfactory specimens.

Technique

An intravenous line is established and the patient given platelets or coagulation factors as required. The biopsy is performed under fluoroscopic guidance. Preliminary screening helps to identify the position of the liver and any adjacent bowel gas. The needle is introduced inside a covering sheath in the mid-axillary line parallel to the table top. The biopsy is taken and the needle withdrawn. Contrast medium is injected to demonstrate the point of communication between the tract and the vessel responsible for the bleeding, usually a hepatic or portal vein branch. The embolic material is deposited within the tract, adjacent to the bleeding vessel. The sheath is then withdrawn and more embolic material deposited within the tract (Fig. 11.19). Particular care is taken to place a coil close to the liver capsule to prevent extracapsular leakage.

Various modifications of this technique have been described using differing needles and embolic agents, including gelfoam and other haemostatic agents,

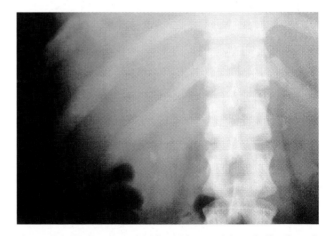

Figure 11.19 *Percutaneous liver biopsy with embolization of the tract. Steel coils can be seen in the right upper quadrant following embolization of the biopsy track. (Reproduced with permission from A.F. Watkinson and A. Adam in* Seminars in Interventional Radiology *1994,* **11***(3), 254–266, published by Thieme Medical Publishers, NY.)*

depending on personal preference. The use of a covering plastic sheath, rather than direct deposition of embolic material through the needle cannula minimizes damage to the liver capsule during respiratory movement of the liver. We prefer steel coils because other haemostatic agents are not suitable for stopping massive bleeding, as may occur from a transected artery or large portal vein radicle. In addition the embolic fragments may be swept out of the tract by the force of blood flow.

TRANSJUGULAR LIVER BIOPSY

This form of biopsy is performed within the liver parenchyma via the hepatic veins thus avoiding external bleeding. The procedure is performed under fluoroscopic guidance with an intravenous line in place and a pulse oximeter monitoring oxygen saturation. In the supine position the internal jugular vein is punctured and a sheath positioned in the right or middle hepatic vein. The 7Fr Quick Core biopsy needle is then advanced until it lies at the tip of the sheath (Fig. 11.20), the inner stylet advanced into the liver substance and the outer sheath advanced to obtain a core sample.

Complications

The main complication is perforation of the liver capsule leading to intraperitoneal bleeding. Capsular perforation is seen in approximately 3.9 per cent of

Figure 11.20 *Transjugular liver biopsy. A biopsy needle is seen positioned in the middle hepatic vein (arrows). This can now be advanced into the liver parenchyma to acquire a biopsy specimen.*

patients, but usually there are no clinical sequelae, significant intraperitoneal haemorrhage occurring in only 0.35 per cent of patients. The mortality rate is approximately 0.13 per cent. Other complications mostly relate to the puncture site and access route. These include haematoma, puncture of the carotid artery, transient hoarseness, Horner's syndrome, cardiac arrhythmias, pneumothorax and interference with indwelling central lines. In addition patients often find the procedure frightening because of the proximity of such a large needle to the face.

Results

It is possible to pass the needle into the liver in 90 per cent of cases, but the success rate is lower in patients with small livers or when the diaphragm has been elevated by ascites. The Quick Core needle has replaced the former suction needle technique and has shown to be safe and provide samples in > 90 per cent of cases.

EMBOLIZATION OF THE LIVER, PANCREAS, SPLEEN AND GASTROINTESTINAL TRACT

Embolization or, more precisely, transcatheter vascular occlusion therapy of visceral structures makes a significant contribution to the treatment of abdominal inflammatory disease, blunt or iatrogenic abdominal trauma and both benign and malignant tumours. It may have a curative role for a variety of conditions, such as intractable bleeding or vascular malformations, or may have a palliative role in the alleviation of symptoms caused by malignant disease.

Before visceral artery intervention, it is important to perform coeliac and superior mesenteric arteriography to identify the abnormality and to demonstrate any variants of vascular anatomy. Some lesions need to be treated by superselective catheterization with the catheter tip as peripheral as possible; others should be treated more centrally.

No single embolic material is suitable for all purposes and in each clinical situation certain substances are more appropriate than others (as discussed in Chapter 25, p. 636).

LIVER

Embolization is indicated in a variety of benign and malignant conditions. Pre-existing occlusion of the portal vein is a contraindication to embolization of the hepatic artery, unless it is performed at a subsegmental level to avoid major parenchymal loss. Sepsis and decreased liver function from any cause are relative contraindications.

Indications

Benign disease

In general, haemorrhage from blunt abdominal trauma is managed either conservatively or surgically in the first instance. The main indication for embolization is the identification of a circumscribed intrahepatic vascular lesion:

- a pseudoaneurysm, not accessible to surgery and causing significant blood loss;
- haemorrhage following a liver biopsy, when the bleeding site is usually focal;
- the relatively rare arteriovenous malformation that causes pain or has led to right heart failure;
- on occasion, benign liver tumours, such as ruptured adenomas, that may cause life-threatening haemorrhage, or giant haemangiomas to reduce the volume of the lesion and the risk of haemorrhage.

Malignant disease

Unresectable liver tumours, especially hepatocellular carcinoma, represent the most frequent indication for liver embolization. The procedure is usually performed for palliation of abdominal pain and ascites; however, in some patients with unresectable tumours in the liver, chemoembolization may prolong life expectancy.

More recently embolization of portal venous branches has been performed in patients with extensive malignancy occupying either the left or right lobe of the liver in whom the contralateral lobe (the non-tumour affected lobe) represents less than 30 per cent of the total liver parenchyma. This is thought to represent the minimum residual liver volume required for adequate hepatic function post surgery. Embolization of the portal vein supplying the lobe with tumour load allows for hypertrophy of the contralateral lobe over 30 per cent within a few weeks, such that safer curative surgery can be performed.

(a)

(b)

Figure 11.21 Embolization of hepatic artery–bile duct fistula following percutaneous biopsy. (a) A coeliac axis arteriogram demonstrates a focal bleeding site in the right lobe of the liver (arrow). (b) The catheter has been advanced selectively within the right hepatic artery. A delayed phase arteriogram demonstrates opacification of the intra- and extrahepatic biliary tree and flow into the duodenum. (c) Selective embolization of the arteriobiliary fistula with a steel coil (arrows) has effectively sealed the leak.

(c)

(a)

(b)

Figure 11.22 *Chemo-embolization of hepatocellular carcinoma. (a) A CT arterioportogram (CTAP) following selective catheterization of the superior mesenteric artery. This demonstrates a large non-enhancing lesion in the right lobe of the liver, with several small satellite nodules, consistent with hepatocellular carcinoma. (b) A delayed CT scan at 72 hours after selective chemoperfusion with cis-platinum and lipiodol followed by particulate embolization of the feeding artery.*

The effectiveness of therapeutic embolization for **palliation for malignant disease** depends partly on the histological characteristics of the tumour. Colorectal primary neoplasms are the most frequent source of liver metastases; such deposits usually cause no symptoms and therapeutic embolization is unnecessary in most patients. Hypervascular metastases from malignant endocrine pancreatic or other intestinal tumours (apudomas) may produce clinical symptoms early in the course of the disease. For example, carcinoid syndrome is characterized by episodes of flushing, vomiting and diarrhoea. In addition hypervascular liver metastases tend to be more painful than colorectal metastases and embolization may provide useful palliation.

Technique

Pseudoaneurysms should be treated as selectively as possible; steel microcoils are preferred with a microembolization catheter introduced coaxially and advanced to the site of the pseudoaneurysm, ideally within the neck of the lesion. If this is not possible then the coil should be positioned in the feeding vessel as close to the lesion as possible. The same technique is used to occlude a focal bleeding site following trauma or percutaneous liver biopsy (Fig. 11.21a–c). If the source of bleeding or a pseudoaneurysm can be reached subselectively then the success rate is near 100 per cent and the complication rate is very low.

Embolization of **benign liver tumours** also requires a subsegmental approach and a coaxial catheter technique. In giant haemangioma or bleeding adenoma without evidence of arteriovenous shunting, peripheral embolization with non-resorbable particulate matter is

most appropriate. In arteriovenous malformations a different approach is necessary: whilst embolization at a subsegmental level is still required, special attention must be paid to arteriovenous shunts. The safest and quickest method is to deploy coils in the feeder artery because particulate matter may reach the pulmonary circulation via arteriovenous shunts.

Focal malignant lesions (Fig. 11.22a), fed by distinct subsegmental arteries, may be treated using selective chemoperfusion with *cis*-platinum, epirubicin or I^{131}, often combined with lipiodol as a CT contrast agent, followed by occlusion of the feeding artery with particulate matter. Within a period of 24–72 hours a CT scan will establish the extent of tumour embolization, which is reflected in the lipiodol distribution around the tumour (Fig. 11.22b). A CT examination at 1 month demonstrates the effectiveness of the embolization and, if unsatisfactory, the procedure can be repeated. Primary occlusion of the hepatic artery should be avoided in order to maintain access for further embolization procedures. Various percutaneous techniques, such as injection of alcohol or laser photocoagulation under ultrasound guidance, are also being used in an attempt to reduce tumour volume, treat symptoms and improve survival. However, it remains to be seen which combination will achieve these aims most effectively.

In patients with **metastatic deposits** the approach is slightly different. The metastases most suitable for embolization are hypervascular lesions, such as those arising from neuroendocrine tumours or renal carcinoma. The hypervascularity of the deposit is used to flow-direct the embolization material, which makes subsegmental positioning of the catheter unnecessary. The tip of the catheter can be placed in either the right or left hepatic arteries, and non-resorbable material infused until peripheral stasis occurs. Embolization tends to be effective in relieving severe clinical symptoms and improving survival in patients with hypervascular endocrine tumours. In patients with colorectal carcinoma the procedure usually results in relief of symptoms but does not prolong survival in most cases.

Complications

The most common complication is vascular damage caused by catheter introduction, which may cause severe vasospasm, intimal tears or dissection. The incidence of this type of complication has decreased since the introduction of coaxial catheters. Reflux and inadvertent transport of embolic material to inappropriate areas is a dangerous complication, which may occur with any embolic substance. When coils lodge elsewhere in the liver, there are usually no serious clinical sequelae because of the presence of a good collateral supply in most instances. When liquid embolization substances are used, the danger from reflux is much more significant, particularly when the reflux occurs into the cystic and gastroduodenal arteries. Therefore, whenever substances are injected that are toxic to mucosa, the catheter tip must be well beyond the origins of these arterial branches.

PANCREAS

In general, the indications for embolization of the pancreas are less frequent and less well defined than those for liver embolization. Also the multiple arterial supply of the pancreas may reduce the effectiveness of therapeutic embolization.

Embolization in benign disease is usually employed in the control of haemorrhage from pseudoaneurysms caused by chronic pancreatitis. The technical success rate of embolization of pseudoaneurysms approaches 100 per cent but the clinical success depends on the initial condition of the patient. Patients may die when the time gap between the onset of symptoms and treatment is too long and multiorgan failure develops; 30-day mortality often approaches 20 per cent.

Embolotherapy has no role in the palliation of the commonest forms of carcinoma, but in recurrent hypervascular tumours, such as malignant apudomas (carcinoid tumours, gastrinomas), superselective embolization may have a role in the management of intractable pain or other severe tumour-related symptoms. The success rate in the embolization of recurrent endocrine tumours is high, with clinical regression of the tumour being observed in most cases.

Technique and complications

Most false aneurysms have a number of feeding vessels and the technique is aimed at direct occlusion of the aneurysm with coaxial superselective catheters and microcoils. If the false aneurysm cannot be reached, all feeding vessels should be occluded with coils. In recurrent pancreatic apudomas it is best to use particulate material in order to preserve access for repeat embolization.

When steel coils in the pancreas are being used, complications are uncommon because of the multiple arterial supply. An exception is misdirection of the coils down the main trunk of the superior mesenteric artery with subsequent bowel necrosis. Particulate matter may backflow after overembolization.

SPLEEN

Elucidation of the role of the spleen in the immune response has increased the interest in splenic salvage for patients who have suffered blunt abdominal trauma. The outcome of conservative treatment in patients who have splenic damage demonstrated on CT is poor, approximately 70 per cent having recurrent or persistent bleeding requiring delayed laparotomy. However, in certain cases timely therapeutic embolization of the splenic artery can obviate the need for splenectomy.

Haemodynamically unstable patients who have suffered blunt abdominal trauma should have diagnostic peritoneal lavage and, if this is positive, the patient should undergo exploratory laparotomy. If the patient is haemodynamically stable, but diagnostic peritoneal lavage is positive, CT should be performed. If damage to the spleen is seen, the patient should be further evaluated with arteriography and, if extravasation of contrast material is seen, embolization of the proximal splenic artery can be carried out with steel coils; these can be delivered by coaxial catheters in the proximal splenic artery. Embolization of specific bleeding intrasplenic arteries prior to main splenic artery occlusion should only be attempted when it is safe and technically possible to advance the catheter into the spleen. Experience is currently limited. As interest increases, the technique may become more widely adopted. In haemodynamically stable patients with evidence of contrast extravasation on CT and angiography, splenic salvage and avoidance of laparotomy is achieved in over 95 per cent of cases.

Complications specific to splenic embolization are the theoretical risks of infarction from incorrect coil positioning, or perforation of the damaged splenic capsule from catheter manipulation within the splenic substance.

GASTROINTESTINAL TRACT

Indications

The indications for gastrointestinal embolization depend on the section of bowel affected by the disease and on the feasibility of surgical or endoscopic methods of management. Hence embolization procedures in the stomach or rectum are rare whilst embolotherapy is performed more frequently for duodenal, small bowel and proximal large bowel lesions. Attention to technical detail is vital for the achievement of satisfactory results and avoidance of complications. Capillary embolization should be avoided because of the risk of bowel gangrene, but delivery of emboli into large, proximal vessels is ineffective.

A frequent problem is the difficulty of demonstrating the source of bleeding. Direct angiographic visualization of intestinal haemorrhage requires a substantial rate of blood loss at the time of the procedure (> 1–2 ml/min). Unfortunately, by the time most patients are brought to the angiographic table, the bleeding has either stopped or fallen below the level necessary for angiographic visualization.

In patients with **gastric haemorrhage**, embolization is only indicated if both endoscopy and an aggressive haemostatic drug regimen have failed to control active bleeding. Indications include:

- inoperable tumours;
- bleeding caused by chemotherapeutic agents, particularly in lymphoma;
- anastomotic bleeding after gastric surgery, particularly in septic patients;
- ruptured pseudoaneurysms.

Duodenal embolization, too, is only considered as second-line therapy after failure of endoscopy. The incidence of acute bleeding from duodenal ulcers has decreased with the advent of effective medication for the treatment of early ulcer disease. Consequently, the commonest source of duodenal haemorrhage is a pseudoaneurysm of the gastroduodenal arteries or one of its major branches. These can occur as a result of atherosclerotic disease or as a rare, late complication of pancreatitis. Duodenal haemorrhage may also occur following gastrectomy or papillotomy.

Small or large bowel embolization is a rare procedure performed in carefully selected cases. There is a significant risk of infarction (in contrast to embolization in the liver, stomach or duodenum) because of the end-artery character of the vascular supply to the bowel. For satisfactory results a careful embolization technique, involving superselective catheterization combined with a detailed knowledge of the arterial supply of the bowel, is required. Colonoscopy of the large bowel should always precede angiography and attempted embolization in order to identify the bleeding site and arrest haemorrhage. If a bleeding site is identified which is not correctable at endoscopy then surgery is the treatment of choice in most instances. If several unsuccessful attempts have been made to localize the source at open surgery, or patients are not fit for general anaesthesia or have objections to surgery,

embolization may be considered. Indications include vascular malformations, telangiectasia, postanastomotic haemorrhage and bleeding diverticula.

Technical success is defined as complete occlusion of the lesion and no recanalization during the 30-day post-treatment period; when the lesion can be selectively accessed, success should approach 100 per cent. However, the clinical results are often influenced by the generally poor state of the patient at the time of the procedure; the outcome is often determined by renal or multiorgan failure if the patient has experienced prolonged periods of hypotension.

Technique and complications

The femoral artery approach is most commonly used with selective catheterization of the appropriate mesenteric vessel. The approach to the lesion should be as superselective as possible. The main limitation of the technique is difficulty of access to the bleeding site in certain instances; for example, the left gastric artery is often technically demanding to cannulate. When gastric or duodenal embolization is performed, coils are the embolic material of choice, although particulate matter is used in certain cases. Considerable caution should be exercised in small and large bowel embolization if bowel necrosis is to be avoided. Coils are the preferred embolic material and should be placed as close to the lesion as possible. Particulate or liquid embolic agents are not usually employed as they can occlude capillaries and lead to bowel necrosis. Mere reduction of flow by the insertion of a few coils combined with correction of any coagulation defects may be clinically sufficient. The exception is mesenteric telangiectasia where complete obstruction of the feeding vessels often requires a combination of coils and particulate material.

The main risk of embolization of gastrointestinal lesions is bowel necrosis from occlusion of the superior or inferior mesenteric arteries or their branches. There is, however, increasing usage of embolization in the lower gastrointestinal tract in the management of acute gastrointestinal haemorrhage, possibly due to improved technique and availability of smaller microcatheters enabling much more selective catheterization. The use of coils rather than particulate matter or liquid agents is often sufficient to reduce the bleeding significantly but not compromise the immediate adjacent bowel. Pancreatitis can also result from ischaemia secondary to embolic infarction.

TREATMENT OF PRIMARY LIVER TUMOURS AND METASTASES

Hepatic resection is the mainstay in the curative management of primary and secondary hepatic malignancies. It offers the only proven chance for cure of both primary and certain metastatic liver tumours. Actuarial survivals achieved in patients undergoing resection for hepatocellular carcinoma range from 55 to 80 per cent at 1 year and 25 to 50 per cent at 5 years. Similar outcomes have been achieved with the resection of colorectal hepatic metastases.

Although surgical resection has significantly improved survival in operated candidates, only a minority of patients are surgical candidates because of tumour volume, lesion location, extrahepatic metastases or, in the case of hepatoma, limited hepatic functional reserve secondary to associated cirrhosis.

PERCUTANEOUS LIVER TUMOUR ABLATION

Percutaneous techniques of local tumour ablation may be categorized into three major groups:

- injectables (ethanol, acetic acid, hot saline);
- heating (radiofrequency, electrocautery, interstitial laser therapy, microwave coagulation therapy, and high intensity focus ultrasound);
- freezing (cryotherapy).

Of these the most widely used are percutaneous ethanol injection for hepatocellular carcinoma and thermal ablation methods for hepatic metastases.

Percutaneous ethanol injection therapy

Percutaneous ethanol injection therapy (PEIT) was first described in 1983. Since that time PEIT has been used extensively for treatment of unresectable hepatocellular carcinoma. There is no absolute limitation to the size or number of lesions treated. However, as tumour size increases, homogeneity of ethanol diffusion diminishes at the periphery, increasing the probability that residual viable tumour cells will persist at the margin of the lesion following therapy. The limitation of diffusion radius and homogeneity is particularly relevant to metastases that have a firmer consistency than hepatocellular carcinoma, making them more resistant to ethanol diffusion at any size. The frequent need for multiple treatment sessions per lesion, and the limited injection volume tolerated in a single session, place practical limitation on the number of lesions treated. For these reasons, as well as the documented greater effectiveness of PEIT for solitary tumours 3 cm or less in diameter, many authors have restricted PEIT to nodular lesions 3 cm or less in diameter and three or fewer in number. Others have used PEIT for tumour nodules up to 5 cm in size and up to four in number. Techniques such as insertion of multiple needles into different parts of large lesions, and single-session, high-dose therapy under general anaesthesia, have been used

to overcome these limitations and extend the applicability of PEIT to lesions as large as 9 cm, patients with as many as five nodular lesions, and even infiltrating neoplasms.

Thermal ablation

Lesional heating techniques such as radiofrequency (RF) ablation and interstitial laser photocoagulation (ILP) affect tumour necrosis from the effects of hyperthermia. RF electrodes or laser fibres are inserted into the tumour under ultrasound, CT or MRI guidance. They generate intralesional heat by local hyperthermia, which has been shown to cause almost immediate coagulation necrosis at temperatures of 60°C or greater, and to have a preferential cytotoxic effect on tumour cells at temperatures between 41° and 45°C. The time required to achieve a cytotoxic effect at these lower temperatures ranges from 15 minutes at 45° to 240 minutes at 41°, with the time doubling for each degree drop in temperature.

Radiofrequency waves induce ionic agitation, which results in frictional heat production within the tissue. The size and shape of the necrotic lesion produced by RF has been shown to be a function of the probe gauge, length of the exposed probe tip, temperature along the exposed electrode, and duration of therapy. Lesion diameter increases with local temperature up to 90° and reaches a maximum of 1.6 cm for a single probe. Strategies aimed at increasing the volume of tissue coagulation include the use of multiprobe electrodes and saline enhancement. The procedure is well tolerated and causes either no or only slight and transient elevations of liver function tests. Serious complications are rare, and consist mainly of intraperitoneal haemorrhage and liver abscess formation.

Interstitial laser photocoagulation (ILP) produces thermal coagulation by conversion of absorbed light energy into heat. Conduction and convection of heat extends the cytotoxic effect beyond the 8 mm of light penetration into surrounding tissues, reaching a plateau of 16 mm in diameter at 2 W and 600 J. With a 1 × 4 coupler to achieve simultaneous activation of four fibres placed 1.5 cm apart, it is possible to create a single coalescent necrotic lesion measuring approximately 3 × 3 × 3 cm in most cases.

The follow-up of patients after all forms of percutaneous tumour ablation includes a combination of imaging, tumour marker assay and selected use of fine needle aspiration biopsy. It is useful to follow serial levels of alpha-fetoprotein or carcinoembryonic antigen, in the case of hepatocellular carcinoma or metastatic disease respectively, only when the serum levels of these markers are elevated prior to the initiation of therapy. The immediate goal of imaging is to assess whether complete necrosis has been achieved. Ultrasound does not usually provide useful information, as the echogenicity of fibrosis and neoplastic tissue overlap. Contrast enhanced MRI and contrast enhanced CT are capable of demonstrating remaining viable tumour requiring treatment. However, in difficult cases, PET scanning may provide additional information.

Better methods of imaging guidance and more sophisticated equipment are likely to increase the importance of percutaneous tumour ablation in the future.

TRANSJUGULAR INTRAHEPATIC PORTOSYSTEMIC SHUNT (TIPS)

The percutaneous creation of a communication between the portal and hepatic venous systems for the relief of portal hypertension was first attempted in patients with the use of repeated balloon dilatation in the early 1980s. However, it was not until the introduction of expandable metal stents that the problem of progressive shunt occlusion was resolved. The first successful procedure was performed by Richter in Germany in 1988 and since then the technique has become well established worldwide. As clinical and technical experience has increased, the clinical indications have become better defined. However, longer term follow-up, particularly on stent occlusion, and reintervention rates will help to outline a treatment strategy accurately. The advantages of TIPS include:

- avoidance of open surgery that may be difficult because of the large varices;
- an entirely intrahepatic shunt (avoiding adhesions, which may interfere with subsequent liver transplantation);
- ability to measure and adjust the degree of shunting.

INDICATIONS

Current indications for TIPS include:

- chronically recurring variceal bleeding despite continuing sclerotherapy or endoscopic banding;
- recurring variceal bleeding and severe ulcerative or erosive disease from repeat sclerotherpy;
- repeat bleeding episodes from major gastric varices inaccessible for sclerotherapy or endoscopic banding;
- recurring variceal bleeding from occluded surgical shunts;
- intractable ascites;
- Budd–Chiari syndrome.

Patients may be considered for TIPS because the risks associated with surgery are unacceptable in certain cases. For this particular subset of patients no therapeutic choice other than TIPS exists. For patients fit for surgery with Child's stage A or B liver disease, the traditional surgical option has been a distal splenorenal shunt. In this group of patients TIPS competes with surgery and more information is required on outcome (patency rates, encephalopathy, morbidity and mortality) to decide on appropriate treatment strategies.

One area where TIPS has emerged as the treatment of choice is in patients already enrolled on a liver transplantation programme who are at high risk of bleeding. In these patients the shunt relieves the portal hypertension leaving the main vascular structures untouched. It is not clear yet whether TIPS is indicated in intractable ascites. Early results indicate a role in rapid-onset ascites with a high portosystemic gradient. However, in patients with a long history of cirrhosis, small liver and only a moderate portosystemic pressure gradient, TIPS may precipitate rapid liver failure from deprivation of portal blood nutrition.

CONTRAINDICATIONS

Absolute contraindications include:

- right heart failure or other cardiopulmonary factors contributing to substantial elevation of right ventricular pressure;
- presence of pulmonary or ascitic sepsis;
- significant acute liver failure not attributable to active bleeding;
- presence of extensive malignancy (hepatocellular carcinoma or metastatic disease) compressing or infiltrating the hepatic vessels or liver parenchyma in the proposed shunt tract.

Relative contraindications include portal vein occlusion or a peripheral, small hepatocellular carcinoma in a patient unfit for surgical resection.

TECHNIQUE

The procedure is performed on the patient in a supine position, with a fluoroscopic machine. Intravenous access is obtained and analgesia and sedation administered via this route. ECG and pulse oximetry are mandatory. Usually, acutely bleeding patients in whom medical treatment has failed to control variceal haemorrhage present in a poor or critical clinical state, resulting from substantial blood loss and coagulopathy, often with hepatic encephalopathy. Consequently anaesthetic assistance is required to maintain clinical stability.

The internal jugular vein is punctured with a standard Seldinger technique and a 9F catheter positioned in the proximal right or middle hepatic vein. The hepatic vein

(a)

(b)

Figure 11.23 *Transjugular intrahepatic portosystemic shunt (TIPS). (a) A catheter (curved arrows) has been introduced through the liver parenchyma from the middle hepatic vein into the portal vein. A venogram demonstrates the portal vein (straight arrows) and its tributaries (b). A self-expanding metal stent (arrows) has created a shunt between the left branch of the portal vein and the hepatic venous system. Embolization coils (curved arrows) have been used to occlude gastric varices. (Reproduced with permission from A.F. Watkinson and A. Adam (1996)* Interventional radiology: a practical guide, *published by Radcliffe Medical Press, Oxford.)*

pressure is then recorded. A modified Colapinto needle is introduced through the catheter and, under ultrasound guidance, it is advanced into one of the main portal branches. The correct position can be confirmed by a direct portal venogram through the puncture needle (Fig. 11.23a). As experience is gained, it is possible to puncture the portal branches without ultrasound guidance. The portal vein pressure is then recorded. With the use of standard catheter-guidewire-angioplasty techniques, the track is then predilated to a diameter of 8–10 mm and an expandable metallic stent positioned to create the portosystemic shunt (Fig. 11.23b). The stent diameter is chosen to reduce the portosystemic gradient to within 10–15 mmHg. This lowers the gradient sufficiently to reduce variceal bleeding but does not create a high-volume shunt with subsequent increase in the incidence of postprocedural encephalopathy. If bleeding gastric varices are present they can be embolized with steel coils prior to catheter withdrawal.

RESULTS AND COMPLICATIONS

The technical success rates of TIPS is over 90 per cent and the average procedure time is between 1 and 2 hours. Procedural mortality is uncommon (1–4 per cent) and usually relates to inadvertent puncture of the extracapsular portal vein or septic complications. Postprocedural morbidity includes puncture site haematomas, transient elevation of liver enzymes and complications related to the sedatives used.

The clinical success after 30 days is over 90 per cent with rebleeding occurring in less than 10 per cent of

patients. Hepatic encephalopathy can occur after the procedure and is highest in patients where the gradient is reduced to less than 10 mmHg. In many patients with hepatic encephalopathy prior to shunting, the symptoms do not seem to worsen after the procedure, probably because the hepatic encephalopathy is caused by severe acute bleeding and significant intestinal protein uptake, which decreases once the shunt is established. The most common late complication is shunt occlusion, usually owing to intimal hyperplasia. This appears to be more common than initially thought with reintervention rates (involving balloon dilatation or second stent insertion) approaching 50 per cent in patients surviving ≥ 12 months.

As currently performed, TIPS is a safe, non-invasive and efficient method for the treatment of variceal haemorrhage. It is particularly indicated in patients awaiting liver transplantation both in the emergency stage and also possibly at an earlier stage of the underlying liver disease. If transplantation is performed within 6–12 months, then the problems of late shunt occlusion and intimal hyperplasia should not happen. Further research is required to investigate haemodynamically significant intimal hyperplasia which appears to be responsible for late shunt occlusion, rebleeding and reintervention rates.

RENAL INTERVENTION

The specialty of urology has undergone many changes in recent years with advances in minimally invasive therapy in the treatment of diseases of the kidney, ureter, bladder and prostate. The application of the Seldinger technique to percutaneous catheterization of the renal pelvis has enabled techniques such as percutaneous nephrostomy, percutaneous nephrolithotomy, antegrade ureteric stent placement and ureteric balloon dilatation to be performed without resorting to open surgery.

PERCUTANEOUS NEPHROSTOMY

Percutaneous nephrostomy can be both diagnostic and therapeutic. Diagnostic indications include:

- accurate delineation of the anatomy of the collecting system in cases of filling defects or outflow obstruction (in most cases this is combined with a drainage procedure);
- aspiration of urine for microscopy, culture and sensitivity;
- evaluation of suspicious lesions in the urinary tract with cytology of brush biopsy specimens;
- a Whitaker test to quantify the significance of pelvi-ureteric or ureteric obstruction.

Therapeutic indications include:

- relief of urinary tract obstruction that may be secondary to calculus, stricture, tumour or pyonephrosis;
- percutaneous nephrolithotomy in patients not suitable for lithotripsy;
- urinary diversion in patients with fistula;
- abscess drainage and relief of urinoma.

Technique and results

Patient preparation is extremely important to minimize the risk of sepsis and haemorrhage. A complete blood count, coagulation profile, serum electrolytes and urine culture are mandatory. Intravenous access is established and the procedure is performed with the patient in the prone position, with appropriate antibiotic cover, analgesia and sedation. An initial ultrasound examination determines the location and depth of the kidney as well as the degree of hydronephrosis.

The preferred entry site is just medial to the posterior axillary line inferior to the twelfth rib. Under ultrasound guidance a fine needle is guided into an appropriate renal calyx. In most circumstances the preferred angle of approach is via a posterior middle calyx as this gives a direct line of access to the renal pelvis and ureter. If the procedure is the initiating step for percutaneous nephrolithotomy then the needle should be directed towards the stone-containing calyx or the posterior calyx nearest to the stone. Aspiration of

Figure 11.24 *Bilateral nephrostomies are seen inserted via the lower pole calyx on both sides. Nephrostograms demonstrate bilateral hydronephrosis and hydroureter to the level of the vesicoureteric junctions. Obstruction is caused by extensive carcinoma of the cervix.*

urine confirms that the needle is within the collecting system and a catheter can be introduced coaxially. Instillation of dilute contrast delineates the anatomy of the collecting system often giving information on the level and cause of obstruction (Fig. 11.24).

The refinement of interventional guidewires and catheters ensures that an appropriate nephrostomy catheter (usually 8 or 10F) with a self-locking loop can then be introduced with the minimum of trauma and discomfort. The self-locking catheters have reduced the risk of catheter dislodgement; however, the catheter should still be firmly attached to the skin with sutures or one of the many available specific devices. The technique, with ultrasound guidance, should ideally gain access to the collecting system after a single pass, thus minimizing the incidence of haemorrhage and septic shock from urinary leakage into the renal substance and renal vessels. If long-term drainage is required, the catheter should be exchanged every two to three months. However, long-term drainage is best achieved by a double-J pigtail stent inserted antegradely thus dispensing with the need for an external catheter (see below).

If the procedure is the initiating step for percutaneous nephrolithotomy, the puncture is directly onto the calculus. The tract is then sequentially dilated to an appropriate diameter (usually 24–28F) and the largest

(a)   *(b)*

Figure 11.25 *Embolization of a false aneurysm of a segmental renal artery. (a) Digital subtraction arteriography of a lower pole artery of the right kidney after percutaneous liver biopsy. This demonstrates a large false aneurysm (arrows). (b) The feeding artery has been embolized with steel coils occluding the aneurysmal sac. (We are grateful to Dr J .Reidy for donating these illustrations.) (Reproduced with permission from A.F. Watkinson and A. Adam in* Seminars in interventional radiology *1994,* **11***(3), 254–66, published by Thieme Medical Publishers, NY.)*

diameter sheath left *in situ* for endoscopic access and forceps removal of the stone. A safety wire is usually left in the upper ureter in case of sheath dislodgement.

If there is more than a mild hydronephrosis, the technical success of the procedure approaches 100 per cent. If the pelvicalyceal system is not dilated, then the correct positioning of a nephrostomy can be extremely difficult, with success being directly proportional to experience. This problem can occur if there is a leak of the renal pelvis or ureter decompressing into the retroperitoneum, or in acute calculous obstruction of the collecting system where the system has not had time to dilate. There is normally good renal function in these instances and an intravenous pyelogram usually helps to delineate the pelvicalyceal system to assist successful puncture.

Complications

The incidence of complications is low compared to open surgical nephrostomy, which has a perioperative mortality rate as high as 10 per cent and a morbidity

rate of over 30 per cent. Minor complications include catheter dislodgement or occlusion. The introduction of self-locking catheters has reduced dislodgement; however, ward staff must be made aware of this technical modification and asked not to attempt removal of the catheter. Catheter occlusion can lead to hydronephrosis, pyonephrosis, septicaemia and urinoma. If signs of obstruction are present a new catheter should be inserted. This is usually a straight-forward procedure with the placement of a guidewire down the mature tract.

Clinically significant haemorrhage occurs in 1–2 per cent of cases and can lead to massive intrarenal bleeding with haematuria as well as expanding pararenal haematomas. Usually the haematuria decreases after 1–2 days and the nephrostomy can be kept patent with frequent saline flushes. If the haematuria continues or there is a significant drop in the haemoglobin, then arteriography is advised. If a bleeding point, arteriovenous fistula or false aneurysm is identified then it should be embolized with coils, as selectively as possible (Fig. 11.25).

The incidence of septic complications varies in the range 1–2 per cent. These are potentially fatal and every precaution should be taken to minimize their occurrence including antibiotic cover and minimal catheter-guidewire manipulation. Urinomas and infected perirenal haematomas usually resolve with appropriate antibiotic cover and a functioning nephrostomy.

ANTEGRADE STENT PLACEMENT

If double-J pigtail stent insertion is required to relieve ureteric obstruction, the initial approach should be retrogradely via cystoscopy. Only when unsuccessful, or if the patient already has an indwelling nephrostomy, should the stent be positioned antegradely.

Indications

Antegrade stent placement allows urine to flow from the pelvicalyceal system to the bladder in ureteric obstruction or perforation, thus obviating the need for long-term nephrostomy. It is indicated in a number of clinical situations including:

- relief of ureteric obstruction secondary to calculi, which can be due to a single large obstructing calculus or postextracorporeal shock wave lithotripsy with many small fragments;
- healing of ureteric perforations or rupture;
- relief of ureteric obstruction secondary to benign or malignant strictures; in both instances associated balloon dilatation assists in passage of the stent. In benign disease stenting is temporary, but in malignant disease it is usually permanent; if necessary stent change can be performed retrogradely at 3–4 monthly intervals.

Technique

In most instances a percutaneous nephrostomy tube is already *in situ*. If not, one should be inserted as described above. An initial nephrostogram is used to define the anatomy and level of obstruction or leakage. The nephrostomy tube, if present, is then withdrawn over a guidewire and the guidewire with specially shaped catheters is manipulated into the ureter, advanced to the level of obstruction and, if possible, pushed through the strictured segment into the bladder. Most strictures can be traversed with the aid of low-friction, hydrophilic guidewires. If it is not possible to traverse the stricture during the initial session, a period of external drainage, via a nephrostomy, usually allows reduction of oedema and passage of a guidewire. The hydrophilic guidewire is then exchanged for a stiff exchange wire and a protective peel-away sheath inserted through the renal parenchyma into the ureter;

Figure 11.26 *Ureteric dilatation. A guidewire and balloon catheter are seen traversing the right ureter, with the tip of the guidewire in a partially filled bladder. The balloon is partially inflated showing waisting (arrows) at the site of a tight ureteric stricture.*

Figure 11.27 *Antegrade ureteric stent placement. Bilateral double-J pigtail stents have been positioned satisfactorily with the upper ends in the pelvicalyceal systems and the lower ends in the bladder. A safety nephrostomy catheter is seen within the left collecting system.*

(a)

(b)

(c)

Figure 11.28 *Renal stent placement. (a) Magnetic resonance angiography with gadolinium demonstrating bilateral renal artery stenosis confirmed on (b) digital subtraction angiography (DSA). (c) DSA following bilateral renal artery stent placement showing a satisfactory technical result.*

this prevents buckling at the level of the kidney, allows easy introduction of a balloon catheter to dilate the stricture (Fig. 11.26) and aids insertion of the double-J pigtail stent (Fig. 11.27). It is important to choose the correct length of stent to ensure that the upper and lower pigtails are in the renal pelvis and bladder respectively.

Results

The technical success rate exceeds 95 per cent and the complications are the same as for percutaneous nephrostomy, with the added risk of ureteric perforation during balloon dilatation or passage of the guidewire. If this occurs, then the patient should be given antibiotics and placed on external drainage via a nephrostomy; antibiotics should be given until healing occurs. The stent will eventually occlude from encrustation and should be replaced via the retrograde approach every 3–4 months or earlier if required.

RENAL ARTERY ANGIOPLASTY AND STENT PLACEMENT

As equipment and techniques have advanced, interest in the use of angioplasty for the treatment of renovascular hypertension and improvement, or maintenance, of renal function has increased. Non-invasive imaging using ultrasound, CT and magnetic resonance angiography (Fig. 11.28a) have made significant advances in the assessment of renal artery stenosis; however, confirmation of the significance of renal artery narrowing is most effectively performed during intra-arterial angiography (Fig. 11.28b). Lesions that are resistant to balloon dilatation, such as ostial stenoses, are increasingly an indication for primary placement of metallic endoprostheses (Fig. 11.28c).

Indications

Indications for angioplasty include:

- renovascular hypertension (blood pressure (> 140/95), from either atherosclerosis or fibromuscular dysplasia, which is poorly controlled on medical therapy and where a lesion is seen on arteriography;
- impaired or deteriorating renal function with a proven lesion on arteriography;
- renal transplant arterial stenosis.

Technique and results

The femoral approach is used preferentially for both native and transplant kidneys. In patients with severe atherosclerosis, with associated abdominal aortic aneurysms or atheromatous pelvic vessels, a brachial approach may be necessary. Abdominal aortography prior to cannulation of the renal artery confirms the presence of the lesion (Fig. 11.28b). The renal artery is engaged with a catheter specially shaped to cannulate the orifice, and 5000 units of heparin are given intra-arterially. The lesion is then traversed gently with a hydrophilic guidewire and the catheter advanced. A stiff guidewire is introduced enabling the catheter to be withdrawn and the angioplasty balloon to be introduced over the wire to straddle the lesion. On balloon inflation a waist will appear at the site of the lesion; this disappears at full distension of the balloon. A postangioplasty flush aortogram will show if the procedure has been technically successful. If the lesion does not dilate or recurs with a short time period, then a metal stent may be indicated. Balloon-expandable endoprostheses are preferable, as accurate placement is easier to achieve with these than with self-expandable devices (Fig. 11.28c).

Renal angioplasty has a technical success rate of approximately 90 per cent. Patients with hypertension from fibromuscular disease show improvement of their hypertension in 80–90 per cent of cases. In patients with unilateral atherosclerotic stenoses away from the renal ostium, there is usually an improvement in only 60–70 per cent of cases. Ostial stenoses are difficult to treat; they result from large atheromatous plaques in the aorta, which partially occlude the origin of the renal artery. In these patients primary success from angioplasty may be as low as 20–30 per cent and primary **metallic stenting** is increasingly being used (Fig. 11.28c). Angioplasty in patients with deteriorating renal function is less successful with improvement or stabilization of biochemistry in approximately 50 per cent of cases.

Complications

The complications of the procedure can threaten the viability of the kidney and a vascular surgeon should be aware of all renal angioplasty and stent cases so that intervention can be undertaken if required. The most common complication, occurring in approximately 5 per cent of cases, is deteriorating renal function. Occlu-

sion of the renal artery, which can occur from thrombosis or a dissection flap, has an incidence of approximately 3–4 per cent. If a clot occludes the artery, thrombolysis using tissue plasminogen activator may recanalize the vessel. However, if the dissection flap is significant, a metallic stent may be required to re-establish patency of the vessel. The renal artery ruptures in approximately 1 per cent of cases, in which case the angioplasty balloon should be re-advanced, over a guidewire, across the ruptured segment and reinflated. The vascular surgeon should then be contacted urgently. Prompt action can minimize the blood loss, thus decreasing the warm ischaemic time preventing loss of the kidney.

FURTHER READING

Adam, A., Gibson, R.N. (eds). 1994: *Interventional radiology of the hepatobiliary system and gastrointestinal tract*. London: Edward Arnold.

Casteneda-Wilkins, W.R. (ed.). 1997: *Interventional radiology* (3rd edition). Philadelphia, PA: Williams and Wilkins.

Livraghi, T., Solbiati, L. 1993: Percutaneous ethanol injection in liver cancer: methods and results. *Seminars in Interventional Radiology* **10**(2), 69–77.

Mainar, A., Ariza, M.A., Tejero, E. *et al*. 1999: Acute colorectal obstruction: treatment with self-expandable metallic stents before scheduled surgery – results of a multicentre study. *Radiology* **210**(1), 65–71.

Pinson, N.M., Tisnado, J., Cho, S.R. (eds). 1989: *Emergency interventional radiology*. Boston, MA: Little Brown & Co.

Steger, A., Lees, W.R., Shrovon, P., Walmsley, K., Brown, S.G. 1992: Multiple-fibre low-power interstitial laser hyperthermia: studies in normal liver. *British Journal of Surgery* **79**, 139–45.

Watkinson, A.F. Adam, A. 1994: Complications of abdominal and retroperitoneal biopsy. *Seminars in Interventional Radiology* **11**(3), 254–66.

Watkinson, A.F., Adam, A. (eds). 1996: *Interventional radiology: a practical guide*. Oxford: Radcliffe Medical Press.

Watkinson, A.F., Adam, A. 1996: The role of self-expanding metallic endoprostheses in esophageal strictures. *Seminars in Interventional Radiology* **13**, 17–26.

Watkinson, A.F., Adam, A. 1997: Esophageal stents. In Adam, A., Mueller, P., Dondelinger, R. (eds). *Textbook of metallic stents*. Oxford: Isis Medical Media, pp. 87–105.

Watkinson, A.F., Adam, A. 1997: The percutaneous management of malignant biliary tract obstruction. In Rossi, P. (ed.) *Biliary tract radiology*. New York, NY: Springer Verlag, pp. 343–65.

Watson, D., Wallace, S., Jackson, J. *et al*. 1997: Interventional radiology. In Grainger, R., Allison, D. (eds). *Textbook of radiology* (3rd edition). Edinburgh: Churchill Livingstone. 2483–551.

Skeletal trauma

SARAH BURNETT, ASIF SAIFUDDIN

Rather than give an exhaustive description of all fractures, we provide general principles of skeletal trauma, followed by a section devoted to specific fractures. We attempt to illustrate these principles with examples of classic fractures. (Spinal trauma is covered in Chapter 14).

A radiograph is not the most important aspect of the evaluation of a case of trauma. A carefully performed physical examination and the taking of a precise history to determine the mechanism of injury should precede any decision to image. It is essential to understand the common patterns of injury and their associations. Successful treatment starts with an accurate diagnosis, and a radiograph must be well performed and accurately interpreted. Therefore, the patient should be stabilized and possible fractures splinted in order to reduce morbidity and ease patient handling. Radiographs should, where possible, be performed in two projections and include the bone ends. Most fractures are readily identified on the plain film, but subtle evidence may be overlooked and serious injuries may even exist in the absence of radiographic findings. A search for specific signs on the film will be more accurate than a general viewing and soft-tissue clues can point to the site of injury. Direct searching will lead to easier recognition, confident interpretation and a correct diagnosis.

The location, nature and number of fractures is dependent on the age of the individual and the nature and severity of trauma. The skeleton is weak when immature, increases in strength in adulthood, and is again weakened by age and underlying disease, both local and systemic. Hence the same mechanism of injury will produce different fractures at different ages. For example, the fall on an outstretched hand in a child may produce a greenstick fracture of the radius, in an adult a fractured scaphoid, and in an elderly or osteopenic patient a Colles' fracture.

CLASSIFICATION OF FRACTURES

Fractures are described and classified by the extent, direction, position, number of fracture lines and integrity of the overlying skin. In a long bone, the precise position within the bone should be described.

A **complete** fracture implies discontinuity between two or more fragments of bone. Where part of the cortex remains intact the fracture is described as **incomplete**. The latter is more common in children, where the cortex bends, and is termed a **greenstick** fracture. If the overlying skin is intact the fracture is **closed**; if there is a skin breach then it is **open** or **compound**. This may occasionally be identified radiologically by bone protruding through the skin, or the presence of air in the adjacent soft tissues on the immediate postinjury film.

Direction is determined in relation to the long axis of the bone, and the location is stated in terms of its anatomical relationship. The shafts of long bones are conventionally divided into thirds. **Transverse** fractures may occur because of a direct blow, but are uncommon and are likely to be pathological. **Oblique** fractures result from a compressive force, with or without angulation, and are very common. A **spiral** fracture results from torque around the shaft of a long bone, and is usually associated with some compression, resulting in the ends of the fracture being more obliquely orientated. **Vertical** fractures occur from vertical loading and are rare but may occur as a component of a comminuted fracture. A **comminuted** fracture refers to more than two fragments. **Avulsion** fractures occur when a fragment of bone is pulled away from its origin by a ligament or tendon, and is defined by the site of insertion. Sharpey's fibres are sufficiently strong that the bone may yield before the soft tissue, particularly in children. Avulsion injury results from an indirectly applied force and is often a marker for more serious soft-tissue injury.

A fracture involving the end of the bone often extends into the joint or is limited to the joint surface, in which case it is termed an **intra-articular** fracture. It can be oblique, resulting from excessive angulation, and oblique views may be necessary to demonstrate this extension. A comminuted intra-articular fracture becomes impacted, and an **osteochondral** fracture results when shearing or rotational forces are applied. The osteochondral fragment is often entirely cartilaginous and cannot therefore be identified on plain films. It can subsequently cause problems as a loose body and, if radiolucent, can be identified with MRI. Injury may involve the joint capsule, internal structure, ligaments or tendons, without bony abnormality.

Displacement of one bone relative to the apposing bone at a joint is termed dislocation, subluxation or diastasis, and is defined by the movement of the distal bone relative to the proximal. **Dislocation** is defined as complete loss of continuity at a joint surface, while **subluxation** is partial loss of continuity. **Diastasis** is displacement of bone in relation to the apposing bone in a normally minimally mobile joint. This separation may involve either a fibrous or cartilaginous joint and is sometimes associated with fracture of one of the involved bones.

Stress fractures happen in otherwise normal bone due to repeated activities. There is usually no history of an acute injury and X-rays may be normal initially. A radionuclide bone scan (Fig. 12.1) may, however, be positive at this stage, and may reveal an occult contralateral fracture. At 10 days to 3 weeks a transverse or oblique radiolucency can be identified on the plain films. Other changes include a periosteal reaction (Fig. 12.2) and endosteal sclerosis, and the differential diagnosis includes an osteoid osteoma, osteomalacia, Paget's disease, osteomyelitis or a malignant neoplasm. A history of repeated physical activity and occurrence in a characteristic site should lead to the correct diagnosis. It is important to diagnose a stress fracture, as

Figure 12.1 *⁹⁹ᵐTc-MDP bone scan. A stress fracture is indicated by the area of increased uptake in the distal right tibia.*

continued athletic activity can result in conversion to a frank fracture. If clinical suspicion remains high and the plain film or bone scan findings are confusing, then a CT may demonstrate the characteristic linear appearance of the fracture line.

Stress fractures are particularly common in runners; occurring in the second or third metatarsals; the so-called **march** fracture is the most common stress fracture (Fig. 12.2). It is undisplaced and not visible until 7–10 days when early callus formation or periosteal reaction is seen. In the distal fibula a stress fracture will occur 3–7 cm from the tip of the fibula and, rarely, fractures of the junction of the pubis and ischium can be seen in female marathon runners. Horizontal stress fractures of the navicula and vertical stress fractures of the calcaneum are seen in joggers. Another common site for a stress fracture is the proximal tibial shaft; in runners, gymnasts and dancers, they occur in the posterior or anterior cortex and can be seen as a dense periosteal reaction.

An **insufficiency** fracture is the result of normal activity in a weakened bone, commonly from osteoporosis or osteomalacia, or in the elderly. It can also be the result of trivial trauma. Common sites are the tibia, fibula, femoral neck, sacrum (Fig. 12.3), and again march fractures are seen.

Figure 12.2 *AP view of the metatarsal. The curved arrows indicate a localized area of fluffy periosteal reaction around a march fracture in the third toe metatarsal.*

Figure 12.3 *CT scan of sacrum. An insufficiency fracture is present in the right sacral ala of this elderly woman. The open arrow demonstrates an area of sacroiliac joint diastasis posteriorly and the closed arrow shows the position where the fracture breaches the anterior sacral cortex.*

Insufficiency fractures occur characteristically in the sacrum owing to osteoporosis, and are usually vertical. They are seen as a dense line, parallel to the sacroiliac joint. They are difficult to see and thus frequently missed, although they are readily evident on bone scan or CT. Insufficiency fractures of the pubic rami are also common. In the presence of marked osteoporosis, the fracture line may expand and resemble infection or neoplasm. Pubic rami fractures may mimic the clinical findings of a fractured neck of femur.

In the ribs, insufficiency fractures may result from coughing. These may, on occasion, produce confusion on bone scans performed for the evaluation of diffuse metastatic disease, but with insufficiency fractures, like conventional traumatic rib fractures, the hot spots characteristically occur in a vertical line running across several ribs.

A **pathological** fracture is a fracture occurring at a site of abnormal bone. It can be due to either a focal or generalized process, e.g. rheumatoid arthritis. Both lytic and sclerotic bone abnormalities can fracture; distorted trabecular anatomy will weaken even dense bone. Outside the spine, the most common cause of a pathological fracture is a metastasis (Fig. 12.4), and clues to the presence of an underlying lesion are thinning of the cortex, expansion, bone destruction and the presence of a transverse fracture line. Common primary sites for metastases are breast, responsible for more than half of all metastatic pathological fractures, prostate, lung,

(a)   *(b)*

Figure 12.4 *(a) AP view of right hip. A transverse fracture is seen of the proximal femoral shaft. There is some ill-defined lucency in the proximal fragment but the suspicious nature of the fracture cannot be identified with certainty. (b) Three months later, following internal fixation, a large lytic lesion is now evident at the site of the previous fracture. The patient had a primary renal carcinoma.*

kidney and thyroid, and the proximal axial skeleton is predominantly affected. The most frequent primary bone lesion to produce a pathological fracture is myeloma. The presence of a pathological fracture does not imply that a neoplastic process is malignant, as fractures occur from many benign lesions.

Other causes of pathological fracture include osteoporosis, osteomalacia, neuropathy, Paget's disease and osteogenesis imperfecta.

SIGNS OF FRACTURE

A fracture is a discontinuity in bone. On X-rays this is shown as an **abnormal line of radiolucency**, the width of which is dependent on the degree of displacement. The clarity of the line is dependent on the alignment of the beam, and therefore two views in orthogonal planes (at 90° to each other) are mandatory, whenever practical. Most commonly these views will be anteroposterior and lateral; 90 per cent of fractures are identified on both views, while 5 per cent will be visible on one view alone, and a further 5 per cent only identified on special views or further imaging techniques. A fracture may also be evidenced by **irregularity of the cortex** or an angular projection or distortion in the flare of the metaphysis, for example the torus fracture (p. 310) in children. An abnormal line of radiopacity may be seen where fracture fragments over-ride each other. There may be disruption of certain anatomical lines or angles, as described in more detail later in this chapter.

The **soft tissues** may provide clues to the presence of a fracture. Oedema or haemorrhage can lead to displacement or effacement of fascial planes or the presence of an effusion. These lucent lines are due to the fat in normal fascial planes. In the chest, a pleural effusion, pneumothorax or lung contusion can result from a rib fracture; indeed exclusion of these complications is the main purpose of performing a chest film in cases of suspected rib fracture. Free intraperitoneal air or fluid may result from perforation of a viscus by a fracture fragment. When there has been an intra-articular fracture medullary fat can enter the joint creating a fat–fluid level seen on a horizontal beam X-ray; the finding of such a lipohaemarthrosis should lead to renewed vigour in searching the film for a fracture (Fig. 12.5).

NORMAL VARIANTS MIMICKING FRACTURE

A number of normal variants and radiographic phenomena can occur that may mimic a fracture. The lucent component of a joint may be projected through an adjacent bone and look like a fracture site. The **'Mach' effect** occurs where two bones overlap, a line of

Figure 12.5 *Horizontal beam film of knee. Although the tibial plateau fracture is not identifiable on this lateral film, the fat–fluid level in the suprapatellar pouch is clearly seen (arrow).*

lucency closely parallels the periphery of the cortex of one of the bones. It is seen commonly in the ankle and the wrist and may be mistaken for an undisplaced fracture. Further views, possibly including an oblique view, should confirm or refute the presence of genuine pathology.

Unfused ossicles and **apophyses** are seen in many sites, classically around the foot and ankle; for example, the os trigonum is often seen posterior to the talus, the os peroneum by the cuboid, and the os tibiale externum adjacent to the navicula. These may be confused with fracture fragments but are more rounded, have a distinct cortical margin and may often be symmetrical. They occur in characteristic positions and are therefore readily recognizable. Serious clinical confusion arises when the diagnosis of a fracture has important clinical consequences, such as the os odontoideum, an unfused ossicle at the tip of the odontoid peg. A further site that may cause confusion with a fracture is the unfused apophysis at the base of the fifth metatarsal (Fig. 12.6); the apophysis shows a vertical plane of cleavage, whilst a fracture line is horizontal. The patella and sesamoid bones may be bipartite or multipartite. If doubt persists, a reference text of normal variants should be consulted.

(a)

(b)

Figure 12.6 *(a) AP view of base of fifth toe metatarsal in an adult. The unfused apophysis at the base of the fifth metatarsal shows a vertical line of cleavage (curved arrows). (b) The same view in a different patient. The Jones' fracture (p. 328) of the base of the fifth metatarsal demonstrates the fracture line in a horizontal plane (arrow).*

SPECIAL CONSIDERATIONS IN CHILDREN

The young, although accident-prone, are both more agile and more flexible and therefore less likely to injure themselves. The forces generated in an accident are not as great because children and infants weigh less and their shorter stature reduces leverage. The skeleton of the young individual is less brittle because it contains a higher percentage of water. Also the periosteum is thicker and more elastic; therefore, it is more likely to remain attached to the fragments and act as a hinge, which helps considerably in both the reduction and stabilization of the fracture. Non-union is rare.

Complete fractures are the most common fractures seen in children but several types of incomplete fractures are also seen.

The classic **greenstick** fracture is an incomplete transverse fracture of one cortex (Fig. 12.7). There may be a longitudinal component; the opposite cortex remains bent or bowed but is intact. It most commonly occurs in the radius, ulna and clavicle. In hyperextension injuries of the fingers, greenstick fracture may occur at the diametaphysis of the proximal phalanx, and these fractures are often overlooked in the emergency situation.

A **torus** fracture is a buckling of the cortex due to compression perpendicular to the long axis (Fig. 12.8); the buckling is subtle and may be missed. They occur at metaphyses, which normally should be gently flared. Even minor changes, if they correspond to the site of tenderness, should be viewed with suspicion. Impaction at the fracture site may produce a fine line of increased density. **Bowing** fractures are due to a series of microfractures leading to curvature of the affected bone, usually a slender long bone. As the associated clues to the presence of a fracture are usually absent, this entity may be overlooked unless the observer is aware of its existence. It is most common in the radius or ulna, followed by the fibula. In paired bones, both may be bowed, or one actually fractured. Callus will develop subsequently and a permanent, worsening deformity may result; this may also interfere with the correct alignment of an associated fracture. Successful treatment may depend on converting the bowing into a complete fracture.

SALTER–HARRIS FRACTURES

The **epiphyseal complex** (epiphysis, physis or growth plate and metaphysis) is involved in 6–15 per cent of

Figure 12.7 *Lateral film of the wrist in a child showing the buckled dorsal cortex of both the radius (arrow) and ulna (open arrow).*

Figure 12.8 *AP film of the wrist in a child showing a concentric buckling of the cortex of the distal radius (arrows).*

fractures of the long bones in a child. Growth disturbances such as deformities and shortening commonly result as the integrity of the complex is responsible for normal growth and contour.

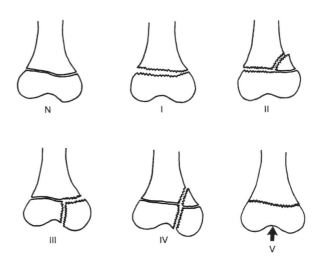

Figure 12.9 *Salter–Harris classification. N = Normal appearance of epiphyseal complex; I = the physis is widened; II = a fragment from the metaphysis accompanies the displaced epiphysis; III = only a fragment of the epiphysis is detached; IV = the fracture extends across the metaphysis, physis and epiphysis; V = the arrow denotes the direction of force; the physis is compressed between the epiphysis and metaphysis.*

TYPE I

Epiphyseal separation was first described by Poland in 1898, and can be thought of as the analogue of dislocation or ligamentous injury in the adult. There is no involvement of the metaphysis or epiphyseal ossification centre. It is relatively uncommon and is seen at a younger age. The only plain film evidence is displacement of the ossification centre, or a residual widening of the physis if there has been spontaneous reduction (Figs 12.9 I and 12.10). An identical injury occurs at an apophysis, where there is a bony projection for musculotendinous insertion. Violent contraction of the muscle may thus avulse the apophysis. The prognosis is generally favourable unless callus forms across the growth plate anchoring the epiphysis to the metaphysis leading to a cessation of growth.

TYPE II

Type II is the most common type, accounting for 75 per cent of Salter–Harris fractures. A fragment from the metaphysis accompanies the displaced epiphysis; thus a triangular fragment of metaphysis may be identified, and oblique views may aid detection (Figs 12.9 II and 12.11). The prognosis is favourable.

Figure 12.10 *AP view of the ankle in a child with a Salter–Harris Type I fracture. The entire tibial epiphysis has been displaced laterally (closed arrow). Note also the fracture through the distal fibular shaft (open arrow).*

Figure 12.12 *AP view of the ankle in a child with a Salter–Harris Type III fracture through the lateral aspect of the tibial growth plate (large arrow) and through the middle part of the epiphysis (long arrow)*

Figure 12.11 *AP view of the ankle in a child with a Salter–Harris Type II fracture showing widening of the lateral aspect of the physis (arrow) in association with an obliquely placed fracture line through the metaphysis (curved open arrow).*

TYPE III

An intra-articular shearing force results in a fracture line running vertically through the epiphysis and growth plate and then turning horizontally, through the growth plate, to the periphery. On the X-rays a portion of the epiphysis is detached with minimal displacement (Figs 12.9 III and 12.12). The most common site for this injury is the distal tibia and the prognosis is generally good provided that the fragment can be accurately replaced.

TYPE IV

A fracture extends across the epiphysis, growth plate and metaphysis, fragments of part of both the epiphysis and metaphysis are seen on the films (Figs 12.9 IV and 12.13). Growth arrest and joint deformities are a distinct possibility although the chances are reduced by proper reduction and fixation.

TYPE V

Type V injuries constitute 10 per cent of Salter–Harris fractures and result from a pure crush injury. There is usually no immediate radiographic evidence and they

(a)   *(b)*

Figure 12.13 *(a) AP view of the ankle in a child with a Salter–Harris Type IV fracture through the medial malleolus extending through the epiphysis and metaphysis (short arrows). (b) The same view 18 months later. The fracture has resulted in premature fusion of the growth plate (curved arrow) and attendant growth deformities.*

very commonly lead to shortening and deformity (Fig. 12.9 V).

The majority of injuries are Types I and II and are manifest by displacement of the shaft relative to the ossification centre and widening of the growth plate. Changes may be minimal, necessitating additional or comparative views. In Type II the metaphyseal fragment is easily seen if it is caught in profile on the X-ray, but *en face* may be mistaken for buckling of an incomplete fracture or indeed overlooked. Subtle widening of the growth plate should be looked for and oblique views should be considered. Spontaneous reduction may occur, leaving only the metaphyseal fragment visible.

Apophyseal separations are seen when the apophysis is at a distance from the underlying bone. They may heal by callus bridging the entire gap or a fibrous union may form. Rarely a deformity may result from overgrowth. In fractures that result in deformities, a variable time may elapse between the injury and cessation or relative retardation of growth. Two years must elapse before one can confidently exclude shortening or deformity; therefore, clinical review with repeat X-rays should happen at 3–6 month intervals.

NON-ACCIDENTAL INJURY (NAI)

The clinical condition of non-accidental injury, specifically the association of long bone fractures with subdural haematomas, was first described by Caffey in 1946. Most victims are below the age of 3 years, and 50 per cent of injuries occur in children younger than 1 year of age. Conversely, accidental fractures are rare below the age of 1 year. It is a very important diagnosis to make, because failure to remove the child from the environment of abuse may at least result in long-term physical and psychological damage, and tragically, in some cases, death.

There are both clinical and radiological manifestations of repeated injury. The child may show evidence of burns and bruises, be withdrawn and underweight, and the history given for the injuries is often inconsistent or bizarre. There may be delay or failure to seek medical advice.

The **cardinal radiological sign** is the presence of multiple fractures at different stages of healing. The following sites of fracture are considered to have a high specificity for child abuse: metaphyses, ribs, scapula, outer end of the clavicle, spine, bilateral fractures, complex skull fractures, and finger injuries in non-ambulant children.

The metaphyseal fractures of child abuse are usually very close to the growth plate (unlike accidental metaphyseal fractures which are normally at the diametaphysis) and of the torus type. The fractures occur through the most immature part of the metaphysis and an ossified ring of metaphysis is avulsed with physis giving the characteristic **'corner' fracture** (Fig. 12.14). A less well-known variant of metaphyseal injury is a lucency in the immediate subphyseal region; these have been proven to be true fractures by histological studies. Metaphyseal fractures are most common in the tibia, femur and proximal humerus. The significance of metaphyseal injuries is that they are often caused by the

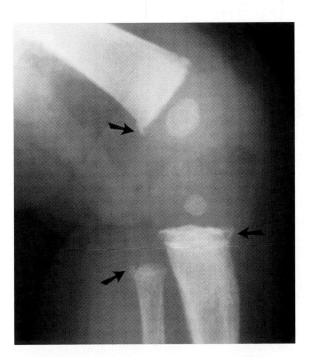

Figure 12.14 *Lateral view of the knee in a toddler. Metaphyseal corner fractures are seen at the distal femur, proximal tibia and proximal fibula (arrowed).*

Figure 12.15 *AP view of the tibia and fibula in an infant. A multilayered periosteal reaction is seen surrounding both the tibia and the fibula in this case of NAI (open arrows).*

infant or child being shaken and are therefore associated with brain damage from subdural haematoma. Even when recent these fractures may be undetectable clinically as they do not commonly cause pain. The only evidence for them is radiological, thus a skeletal survey is indicated. Even in the absence of a skull fracture, shaking may result in haemorrhage leading to raised intracranial pressure and widened sutures. A head CT scan may be indicated to exclude subdural haemorrhage, as may MRI to search for damaged or ischaemic tissue.

Metaphyseal fractures, although said to be specific for child abuse, are in fact much less common than diaphyseal fractures. With the exception of supracondylar fractures, all fractures of the humerus in children under the age of 3 years are strongly suggestive of abuse, and femoral fractures occurring under the age of 1 year are, more often than not, due to abuse. Long bone fractures are often associated with a florid subperiosteal reaction (Fig. 12.15), mimicking metabolic disease or dysplasia. This generally indicates repeated trauma, as do breaches in the outer layer of new bone.

Salter–Harris type epiphyseal injuries may on occasion result from child abuse but are rare. Rib fractures are virtually diagnostic of child abuse, being rarely seen even in severe accidental trauma, such as road traffic accidents. They are more frequent in the posterior and axillary parts of the ribs and are frequently multiple and bilateral. Posterior and neck fractures may be difficult to identify on plain films and may be more readily detected by isotope bone scanning. However, although scintigraphy may be useful to detect some occult injuries, skull fractures may not show increased uptake.

The main differential diagnoses are metabolic bone disease and osteogenesis imperfecta. Rickets and scurvy are readily eliminated by blood tests, and copper deficiency is extremely rare. In osteogenesis imperfecta the severe forms do not cause a diagnostic problem, and the milder manifestations rarely result in fractures until the child is ambulant.

NORMAL FRACTURE HEALING

Fracture healing may be divided into three phases: **inflammatory**, **reparative** and **remodelling**, although there is overlap in the temporal sequence of events. It should be remembered also that in addition to the injured bone there will be an associated soft-tissue injury with haematoma formation. Shortly after the injury the periosteum begins to proliferate and haematoma is transformed into granulation tissue by ingrowth of fibroblasts and capillaries. Metaplasia of the fibrous tissue into cartilage occurs and a layer of woven bone cements itself to the outer layers of the fracture fragments. The cartilage adjacent to bone then becomes ossified and is eventually remodelled into mature bone.

Not all fractures heal at the same rate, or with the same amount of **callus**. More callus is seen in the long bones, in the diaphysis and where distraction is greater. Thus less callus is seen with internal fixation, indeed the formation of significant amounts of callus may suggest either excessive movement or infection. There is also a paucity of callus in bones such as the scaphoid, where the cortex is thin and healing occurs via endosteal or medullary callus formation. The same phenomenon is seen in other intra-articular fractures. Fracture healing may be slow in the elderly, where vascularity is compromised, or where the fragments are widely separated or inadequately immobilized. Corticosteroids will slow healing, but increase the amount of callus seen.

The earliest **plain film** finding of repair is widening and blurring of the fracture line due to resorption of the underlying bone. This is seen by 10–14 days. The next manifestation is the appearance of fluffy and amorphous calcified callus around the fracture site, found initially at the periphery of the haematoma, so it may not be adjacent to the fracture site. As mentioned previously, endosteal or medullary callus is difficult to identify radiologically. Gradually the callus fills in, increasing in both density and quantity, until eventually

(a) *(b)* *(c)* *(d)*

Figure 12.16 *Series of films of the mid shaft of the tibia and fibula (a) A transverse fracture is seen through the tibia. (b) The edges of the fracture line have become slightly blurred and early callus formation is seen together with a periosteal reaction, predominantly on the lateral aspect. (c) More mature callus is seen to surround the fracture, although the fracture line itself remains visible. (d) The callus has largely remodelled and the fracture line can no longer be identified with certainty.*

it becomes mature callus with the texture of bone. It is rare for callus to develop at an equal rate around the circumference of the fracture site, because of variable amounts of periosteal stripping, apposition and so forth. Ultimately the fracture line is entirely obliterated (Fig. 12.16).

Disuse osteopenia is commonly seen following a fracture and is due to immobility and inactivity. There is acute and rapid resorption of both medullary and cortical bone distal to the fracture site in the affected extremity. It can be distinguished from other forms of osteopenia because of the focal nature of the process, the pronounced subcortical linear lucencies from endosteal resorption and the 'spotty' nature of the osteopenia. The changes reverse spontaneously once the patient resumes normal activity. Persistence, or even worsening, of the appearances following removal of a cast may suggest the development of a reflex sympathetic syndrome (**Sudeck's atrophy**). In the elderly, the combination of disuse osteopenia on a background of senile osteoporosis may result in an insufficiency fracture.

Clinical **union** occurs before radiographic union. The latter is evidenced by a continuous external bridge of callus uniting the fracture fragments. The callus should be uniformly ossified with a density approaching that of normal bone. The findings should be present on views taken at right angles to each other, as overlapping fragments may mimic union in one projection. In assessing the healing process it is important to compare the current findings with the previous films. If there is a question about the solidity of a union then stress films may be of value.

Malunion is the healing of a fracture with the fragments in a faulty position, with excessive angulation or rotation. In all except the very young, surgical intervention may be required to correct the deformity. An angular malunion is readily identified on plain films but a rotational abnormality may be harder to define. CT scanning, sometimes with three-dimensional recon-

struction, may help in the anatomical definition of a malunion.

Delayed union is the term used to describe a fracture that fails to unite within a normal time scale for a given site taking the age of the patient into account. There is persistent movement at the fracture site and bridging callus is not complete.

Figure 12.17 *AP view of the tibia and fibula. Following a motorcycle accident, this patient, with extensive compound trauma of the tibia and fibula, has developed a hypertrophic non-union.*

Once the healing process has stopped completely and the fragments are not united, then **non-union** has occurred. Non-union is rare in children. In hypertrophic non-union the margins of the fracture are well defined, smooth and sclerotic (Fig. 12.17). No callus crosses the fracture site and a pseudarthrosis, or false joint, may form. In the much less common atrophic form there is only a fine sclerotic line across the medullary canals of the apposing fragments. An established non-union requires operative intervention with a combination of resection of the fracture line, internal fixation and bone grafting. Small fragments of bone from intra-articular fractures may not unite with the bulk of the fracture, and may cause later complications by remaining free in the joint as loose bodies.

POST-TREATMENT RADIOGRAPHY

The aim of fracture treatment is to produce a united fracture without residual deformity or other complications. In practice, this means reducing the fracture, by open or closed manipulation, and then fixing it by external or internal means. Postreduction films, again in two planes, are therefore important to check for apposition and reasonable alignment, bearing in mind that some remodelling will occur during treatment. It is important to make a careful comparison of the pre- and postreduction films. In cases of dislocation, review films following relocation may reveal fracture fragments that were not evident on the initial films. Separation of the fragments may indicate either interposed soft tissue, or excessive traction, from either fixation devices or muscular spasm.

Following internal or external fixation, the entire length of the appliance must be imaged. Intramedullary nails may fracture through the distal cortex of a long bone and, therefore, the distal joint must also be included. Subsequent films are necessary both to check fracture healing, and also to look for complications of fixation, such as migration of metal work, or infection around pin and screw sites, as evidenced by increasing areas of lucency. Shortening should be checked for, if a butterfly fragment was treated with an intramedullary rod. Rotation may be seen where the rod occupies the entire canal of the fractured segments; this can be prevented by the use of an interlocking nail.

COMPLICATIONS OF FRACTURES

Vascular injuries may be due to either blunt or penetrating injury, the latter often from direct transection or laceration by a bony fragment. The sites of predilection for vascular involvement are where the artery lies close to the bone, or where it is tethered on either side of a joint. A tear of an adjacent artery and vein may lead eventually to pseudoaneurysm formation. If there is clinical suspicion of vascular injury, then arteriography may help to confirm the diagnosis prior to surgery. In trauma associated with catastrophic haemorrhage, such as pelvic fractures, percutaneous embolization may reduce or stop the bleeding.

Soft-tissue infection may occur following a compound fracture. Although plain films are likely to be normal, ultrasound, CT or MRI scanning may show an abscess cavity. With soft-tissue ischaemia or gross contamination of the wound, there is a risk of gas gangrene or other anaerobic infection. This may be seen on plain films if air bubbles are identified in the tissues; often there are linear lucencies tracking along fascial planes. However, small, rounded, pockets of gas may be seen as a normal finding in the early post-traumatic or postsurgical period.

Fat embolism was first described by Bergmann in 1873, and pathological studies suggest that subclinical emboli occur very frequently. Only a small percentage of patients sustaining fractures of the long bones show clinical or radiological manifestations of fat embolism. Symptoms, such as respiratory insufficiency associated with marked desaturation, confusion, pyrexia, petechiae and haemoptysis, normally occur some 48 hours after the injury and are most common in patients with multiple sites of fracture. Radiographic findings are somewhat non-specific and lag a little behind the clinical features. On the chest radiograph, a diffuse mixed alveolar and interstitial pattern with some sparing of the apices, is present bilaterally. Pleural effusions are normally absent. The appearance may be impossible to distinguish from adult respiratory distress syndrome, but in the uncomplicated case spontaneous clearing should occur in 7–10 days.

Osteomyelitis is potentially one of the worst complications of bone trauma, resulting in delayed healing at best, and at worst necessitating amputation or even ending in death. Post-traumatic osteomyelitis is normally due to a focus of infection introduced either at the time of a compound injury, or during open reduction and internal fixation. Very rarely it may be associated with a closed fracture, usually in children with intercurrent sepsis. The dominant symptom of osteomyelitis is an increase in the degree of pain experienced by the patient. From the time the infective process begins, 10–14 days must elapse before the plain film changes are evident. There may be soft-tissue swelling, periosteal new bone formation, and bone destruction with lytic areas, all of which may also be seen with non-infected fractures. Where internal fixation is in place, these lytic areas may occur around the pin or screw sites (Fig. 12.18), a finding which suggests infection. Periosteal reaction is unusual in the presence of non-infected internal fixation devices and, when it does occur, it is almost never layered.

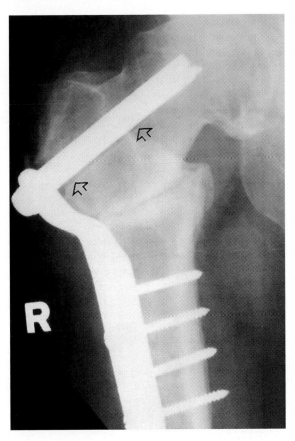

Figure 12.18 *AP view of right hip. Following internal fixation, the patient presented with pain in the hip. A zone of lucency (open arrows) is seen around the pin in the femoral neck, indicating infection around the pin site.*

Figure 12.19 *AP view of the second toe metatarsophalangeal joint in a patient with the classic appearance of Freiberg's disease. Fragmentation, flattening and sclerosis is noted of the second metatarsal head in this young ballet dancer. The spur seen on the lateral aspect of the metatarsal head is almost certainly due to secondary degenerative change.*

Other imaging modalities may assist in the detection of **infection**. Ultrasound may show a subperiosteal abscess; this may be aspirated under ultrasound guidance, confirming the diagnosis and providing microbiological evidence of the cause. MRI may also be useful for showing areas of high signal on the T2-weighted scans, although in the presence of metalwork there may be significant artefact obscuring the site of interest.

Sclerosis, excessive callus formation and the presence of sequestra, or small fragments of dead bone, indicate chronicity. Replacement or complete removal of metalwork may be necessary to effect a cure. Antibiotic beads, particularly gentamicin, are sometimes inserted to deliver a local effect. They are seen on plain radiographs as multiple rounded opacities.

Post-traumatic reflex dystrophy is a poorly understood condition and is difficult to diagnose. It was first described by Sudeck following a penetrating injury, but is most commonly seen following closed, and often trivial, fracture of the extremity. The limb is affected distal to the site of the injury. A variant of the syndrome occurs as a result of repetition injury, often associated with the patient's occupation, and on occasion leads to litigation. Although the precise mechanism is not known, the process is mediated through the sympathetic nervous system, and treatment is aimed at abolishing the sympathetic response. The diagnosis is essentially clinical, based on increasing pain and oedema after the injury. The skin is classically red, hot and shiny. Plain films may show only marked osteopenia, due to the hyperaemia, often starting in aperiarticular distribution, although soft-tissue swelling may be evident. The appearances may progress until there are small erosions and cortical breaks. The only other imaging modality of value is the three-phase radionuclide bone scan, where the affected extremity may show increased uptake on dynamic, blood pool and static images.

Avascular necrosis is the result of compromise of the blood supply to part of the fracture. The affected bone shows a pattern of mixed sclerosis and lysis and may eventually collapse. Where it is the result of repeated minor trauma, a number of eponymous syndromes are described, e.g. **Freiberg's** disease of the second metatarsal head (Fig. 12.19).

Osteochondritis dissecans is common in adolescents and young adults. It is probably due to repeated minor trauma, although the aetiology is uncertain; the patient may present with a history of pain but no definite previous injury. The most frequently affected site is the lateral surface of the medial femoral condyle, and a small, dense fragment of bone is seen lying in a shallow cavity. MRI can be used to demonstrate whether the overlying cartilage is intact and whether the bony fragment is viable. In early stages, arthroscopic pinning may be used to secure the fragment. Occasionally, the fragment may become a loose body. Loose bodies may also result from an osteochondral fragment of bone being separated acutely at the time of injury.

Deep venous thrombosis is relatively common in patients who are immobile following trauma. The imaging of venous thrombosis is discussed on p. 668.

OCCULT FRACTURES

On occasion, there may be a high clinical index of suspicion, whilst plain films do not show any sign of a fracture despite **supplemental plain radiographic views**. Treatment may be decided on the basis of clinical findings alone but it may be necessary to define a fracture more clearly. At some sites, such as the scaphoid, a delayed film after 10–14 days may show sclerosis or a clearly defined lucency, which were not seen at the time of presentation. The patient may be treated symptomatically in a plaster cast until that time.

A useful procedure in selected cases is the **radionuclide bone scan**. This highly sensitive technique detects fractures at a very early stage and is useful for confirming injury in equivocal cases. It can also be used to confirm stress fractures that may be difficult to identify on the plain films at presentation.

Plain films may suggest that a fracture is present; for example, a lipohaemarthrosis in the knee indicates that a fracture must have occurred in order to allow marrow fat into the joint space.

Because of the ability to scan in the axial plane and excellent anatomical resolution for bone, **CT** is extremely useful in confirming and defining fractures, particularly in the spine, pelvis, knee and foot. Reconstructions in multiple planes and three-dimensional reconstructions aid the surgeon in planning his approach.

Ultrasound is of limited value in the diagnosis of bony injuries although it may demonstrate an effusion and therefore lend support to the suspicion of a fracture. Rarely a fracture fragment may be identified.

MRI can be used to detect a fracture line, seen as a dark line across the normal, bright signal of marrow fat with associated oedema being of high signal on T2-weighted scans. MRI has been shown to be more sensitive than radionuclide scanning in the detection of occult fractures of the femoral neck.

FOREIGN BODIES

A careful history from the patient should indicate whether there is a risk of a foreign body, and the presence or absence of a foreign body following penetrating injury can usually be imaged. Even tiny metal density fragments are easily seen as they are extremely dense. Glass fragments are variably dense but fragments over a couple of millimetres in size can usually be found. Wood and thorn splinters are not radiopaque and plain films are not, therefore, of value, but ultrasound is sensitive in locating such foreign bodies. Appropriate imaging should be repeated following removal of fragments to confirm that no significant residual foreign bodies remain.

MUSCLE TEARS

A muscle tear is frequently the result of sports injury and cannot usually be identified on plain films. Ultrasound, performed using a 7.5 MHz linear array probe, gives excellent resolution of muscle fibres. The appearances can be graded, from minor separation of the muscle fibres, to a tear along the fascial attachment, and complete rupture of the muscle substance (Fig. 12.20). The latter is normally associated with a significant **haematoma**, seen as a hypoechoic region within the muscle bulk and disruption of the normal anatomy. A haematoma lying in the subcutaneous soft tissues has a similar appearance. MRI can also be used to demonstrate muscle tears but is more expensive,

Figure 12.20 *Longitudinal ultrasound scan through the hamstring muscle in a middle-aged cricketer. The normal muscle fibres are shown as multiple longitudinal and obliquely positioned striations. A haematoma cavity is identified (curved open arrows) and some torn muscle fibres are identified superficial to this (fine arrows).*

Figure 12.21 *A series of X-rays taken over a 2-month period show an area of maturing ossification in the posterior aspect of the thigh in this patient who had suffered soft-tissue trauma.*

Figure 12.22 *Longitudinal ultrasound scan of the patellar tendon in a 24-year-old professional footballer who complained of pain at the inferior patellar pole. P = patella; T = tendon. There is an area of highly reflective material (arrows) contained within a more diffusely hypoechoic area (open arrow) in the proximal patellar tendon representing calcific, and therefore moderate to severe, tendinitis.*

less readily available and less sensitive to the different types of tear.

A soft-tissue haematoma may heal with calcific and eventually ossific changes, and is then called **myositis ossificans** (Fig. 12.21). After 2–3 weeks, amorphous calcifications are seen within a soft tissue mass. The mass may appear attached to the underlying bone and a periosteal reaction can be seen. This combination of findings may resemble a malignant neoplasm. Often the history of antecedent trauma is forgotten and a tentative diagnosis of tumour is made. The characteristic finding of post-traumatic myositis is that the new bone becomes more mature, a feature that can be demonstrated on subsequent films from 6 to 8 weeks following the injury. In contrast to parosteal osteosarcoma there is also mature bone on the inner aspect of the lesion. Full radiological maturity occurs at 5–6 months when there may be some shrinkage and separation from the underlying bone. It is important to recognize the condition as post-traumatic in nature, as the histology can also appear malignant and early resection may lead to a recurrence. Myositis ossificans can also be seen in association with burns and around the hips in approximately one third of paraplegic patients.

TENDON INJURIES

Tendon injuries are often the result of sporting endeavour, from a repetition injury or occurring as an acute rupture. The Achilles tendon and patellar tendon are most commonly affected. Ultrasound is able to show the integrity of ligaments and the changes of tendonitis: the normal tendon is relatively hyperechoic with internal fibrillary structure well shown provided that a 7.5 MHz probe is used. Features of tendonitis are: a hypoechoic area at the bony insertion of the tendon; fusiform thickening of the tendon; and a peritendinous effusion indicating a tenovaginitis. Calcific deposits may form in severe cases (Fig. 12.22). A full thickness rupture is readily identified. Again the changes are visible on MRI but grading the severity of the lesion may be difficult.

SPECIFIC REGIONAL INJURIES

HAND

Avulsion fractures are common in the hand, are easily missed and are functionally important. The **mallet finger** results from forcible flexion of the extended finger and the common extensor tendon is avulsed. There is, therefore, a fracture of the dorsal aspect of the base of the distal phalanx. A **volar plate** fracture results from a hyperextension injury and displaces a fragment from the palmar aspect of the base of the middle phalanx (Fig. 12.23). Collateral ligaments are found at all the small joints; the most common injury is the avulsion of the ulnar collateral ligament of the metacarpophalangeal joint of the thumb, or **skier's thumb** (**gamekeeper's thumb** being a chronic instability). This fracture may cause an intra-articular fragment at the base of the proximal phalanx on the ulnar side. Otherwise stress views may be required to demonstrate the lesion. A commonly missed fracture in children is a **greenstick fracture of the diametaphysis of the**

(a)   *(b)*

Figure 12.23 *Volar plate fracture. (a) Lateral view of middle finger showing a dorsal dislocation at the proximal interphalangeal joint of the middle finger. (b) On the postreduction film, bone fragments are identified deep to the head of the proximal phalanx, with a small defect at the base of the middle phalanx (arrow).*

Figure 12.24 *AP view of carpometacarpal joint of thumb in Bennett's fracture. The fracture line runs obliquely through the base of the thumb disrupting the proximal intra-articular cortex (arrow).*

proximal phalanx after a hyperextension injury. A sudden angulation in the cortex indicates its presence.

It is important to differentiate between intra- and extra-articular fractures of the thumb as the former require open reduction. **Bennett's fracture** forms 30 per cent of thumb metacarpal fractures; it is a fracture dislocation with an oblique intra-articular fracture at the base of the metacarpal, and dorsal dislocation of the large fragment of metacarpal (Fig. 12.24). Bennett's fractures usually require treatment by open reduction and internal fixation. Less common is the **Rolando fracture**, a markedly comminuted but impacted fracture with a separate dorsal fragment. Fixation is generally not of value in the presence of such marked impaction.

WRIST

A fall on the outstretched hand results in different injuries depending on the age of the patient: greenstick or torus fractures of both bones in a young child; a Salter–Harris II fracture of the distal radius in an older child; scaphoid fracture in a young adult and fractures of the distal radius, commonly **Colles' fracture**, in the elderly. The Colles' fracture is a fracture of the distal

2–3 cm of the radius with dorsal angulation. A **Smith's fracture**, on the other hand, has volar angulation. Distal radial fractures may be radiographically occult, and a clue may be the presence of the pronator quadratus sign, in which the fat pad in front of the pronator muscle is displaced in a palmar direction.

Distal radioulnar dislocation may be suggested by an abnormal position of the head of the ulna in the ulnar notch. This may be seen as part of a **Galeazzi fracture**,

(a)   *(b)*

Figure 12.25 *Barton's fracture. (a) AP and (b) lateral view of the wrist. In addition to the slight posterior displacement of the distal fragments, there is clearly an intra-articular fracture of the distal radius (arrow), thus distinguishing this from an ordinary Colles' fracture.*

Figure 12.26 *AP film of the wrist. Note the normal alignment of the two rows of the carpal bones.*

Figure 12.27 *Lateral view of the wrist showing a perilunate dislocation. The lunate (L) lies in its normal position with respect to the radius. The scaphoid is in two fragments (s) and there is also a fracture of the triquetral (t). This is, therefore, a trans-scaphoperilunate fracture.*

in which the radius is also fractured. A **Barton's fracture** is an intra-articular fracture of the dorsal lip of the radius, with the carpus following the dorsal fragment (Fig. 12.25). As this is an unstable fracture, frequently requiring internal fixation, it is important to differentiate from a Colles' fracture, where there is a fracture of the distal radius with volar angulation producing the classic 'dinner-fork' clinical deformity.

Wrist injuries are ten times more common than carpal injuries; the latter are rare in children under the age of 12. Fractures of the scaphoid form 60–70 per cent of injuries, 10 per cent are dislocations or fracture dislocations, and 10 per cent are dorsal chip fractures, the vast majority being from the triquetral, and these are only identified on the lateral view. On the PA view the width of the intercarpal joints should be about 2 mm; three parallel arcs have been described to assist in evaluating the alignment (Fig. 12.26).

- along the proximal articular margins of the proximal carpal row;
- along the distal articular margins of the proximal carpal row;
- along the proximal articular margins of the distal carpal row.

The lunate is trapezoidal in shape on the PA film; if it appears triangular then it is abnormally rotated. On the lateral view there should be a co-axial arrangement of the articular surfaces of the radius, lunate, capitate and third metacarpal.

Up to 70 per cent of **scaphoid fractures** are at the waist and undisplaced. As the blood supply to the proxi-

mal pole enters at the waist, these fractures are at risk of delayed or non-union and of avascular necrosis. It may take up to 2 years for radiographic union to occur. Lunate fractures are difficult to identify, but again there is a risk of avascular necrosis; findings of mixed sclerosis and lysis, with cortical collapse (**Keinbock's disease**), are thought to be due to previous trauma.

Carpal dislocations can be identified by disruption of the normal anatomical arcs described above, and loss of the co-axial appearance on the lateral. Fracture dislocations are more common than pure dislocations, so the films should be carefully examined for a fracture line. In a **perilunate dislocation** (Fig. 12.27), the capitate articular surface is dorsally dislocated from the lunate, while the lunate maintains its normal articulation with the radius. In a **mid-carpal dislocation** the lunate tilts in a volar direction but is not dislocated from the radius. The capitate is dislocated from the lunate, but is not placed as posteriorly as above. In a **lunate dislocation** (Fig. 12.28), there is loss of the lunate articulation with both the capitate and the radius and it is displaced volarly with a 90° angulation. The capitate remains in alignment with the radius but drops down towards it.

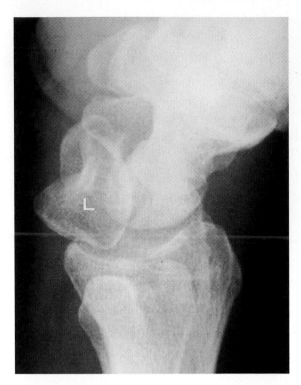

Figure 12.28 *Lateral view of the wrist showing lunate dislocation. Unlike the previous film, the lunate (L) has been displaced anteriorly and has lost its normal articulation with the radius.*

Ligamentous injury can cause instability without a frank dislocation. The PA film should be examined for diastasis that is over 2 mm at the scapholunate joint and lunate tilt: the **Terry-Thomas sign** (Fig. 12.29), which indicates capholunate dissociation and may be associated with rotatory subluxation of the scaphoid. Other forms of instability are complex and may only be identified at fluoroscopy with either ulnar or radial stresses or distraction applied. Wrist arthrography may be necessary to identify a ruptured triangular fibrocartilage complex or interosseous ligaments. Contrast injected in between the scaphoid and radius should normally be contained within the radiocarpal compartment. Contrast entering the distal radioulnar joint indicates a triangular fibrocartilage complex tear; if contrast enters the mid-carpal joint there is a rupture of one of the interosseous ligaments. Degeneration of these ligaments and the triangular fibrocartilage complex is a normal ageing phenomenon and renders evaluation by MRI prone to false positives. If surgery is contemplated then arthrography is the recommended method of evaluation.

ELBOW

In the normal patient the radius articulates with the capitellum and the ulna articulates with the trochlea. On a true lateral film a line, the anterior humeral line, drawn along the anterior humeral cortex, should intersect the capitellum in its middle third. With the elbow in any position a line, the radiocapitellar line bisecting the proximal radial shaft, intersects the capitellum; if not, there is a radial head dislocation. The anterior fat

Figure 12.30 *Lateral view of the elbow showing a radial head fracture. Both anterior (arrow) and posterior (open arrow) fat pad signs are identified around the distal humerus. In addition, the fragments from the radial head can be seen lying in the anterior joint space (fine arrow).*

Figure 12.29 *AP view of wrist showing the 'Terry-Thomas' sign. Note the wide space in between the scaphoid (S) and lunate (L) indicating disruption of the scapholunate ligament.*

pad should normally be identified in the coronoid fossa on the lateral film and the posterior fat pad is not seen. In the presence of an effusion, the anterior fat pad is convex and the posterior fat pad can be identified. Multiple views may be necessary to identify an associated fracture.

In children 60 per cent of elbow fractures are **supracondylar**; almost all have posterior displacement of the condyles and an abnormal anterior humeral line. In adults 50 per cent of elbow fractures are of the **radial head** and this is the commonest cause of a positive fat pad sign in an adult (Fig. 12.30). Of elbow dislocations, 80–90 per cent are posterolateral and are often associated with fractures of the coronoid process or radial head. An isolated dislocated radial head is rare in adults and there may be an associated ulnar fracture (**Monteggia fracture**).

SHOULDER AND STERNOCLAVICULAR JOINT

The normal clavicular articular surface extends above the manubrium so the sternoclavicular articulation has an unusual and confusing appearance, but it should be symmetrical. Anterior **dislocation at the sternoclavicular joint** is more common than posterior, but the latter may compress the great vessels and therefore necessitate surgery; thus accurate diagnosis is mandatory. A limited CT scan of the area is probably the most accurate method of diagnosis.

Acromioclavicular joint separation may involve the acromioclavicular joint itself, with a tear of the acromioclavicular ligament as well as the coracoclavicular ligaments. The acromioclavicular joints are both X-rayed, with and without hand weights. The width of the acromioclavicular joint is normally 3–5 mm but may be up to 8 mm; the disparity between the two sides should be no greater than 3 mm. The length of the coracoclavicular ligament is 11–13 mm, with no greater than 5 mm difference between sides.

Shoulder dislocations are common owing to the shallow joint; 95 per cent are anterior or subcoracoid. The posterolateral portion of the humeral head may impact on the antero-inferior part of the glenoid. Particularly after repeated dislocations, this may produce a wedge-shaped **Hill–Sach's defect** of the humeral head, seen best on the Stryker view (Fig. 12.31). The corresponding chip fracture of the glenoid is called the **Bankart lesion**. If only the labrum is involved, it is best seen on double-contrast CT arthrography, although some may be seen on MRI which also allows accurate evaluation of the anterior glenohumeral ligament. It is important to identify these lesions as they may be associated with instability.

Posterior dislocations are usually secondary to fits or electroconvulsive therapy. The humeral head is usually locked in internal rotation, and this gives the **light bulb**

(a)   *(b)*

Figure 12.31 *Bilateral Stryker's views of the shoulders. (a) The right shoulder shows a large Hill–Sach's defect of the humeral head (arrowed). The glenoid cavity is, however, normal. (b) The left humeral head is normal.*

appearance where the humeral head is seen as symmetrical and round (Fig. 12.32). The congruity of the joint space is lost. These are, however, relatively subtle signs and many posterior dislocations are missed. The abnormality is obvious on an axial view of the shoulder, or if this cannot be obtained, a 'Y' view of the scapula will show the dislocation. A reverse Hill–Sach's, and/or reverse Bankart lesion may be seen. The rare inferior dislocation results in the articular surface being dislocated inferiorly to the glenoid with fixed abduction of the shaft.

The rotator cuff consists of the supraspinatus, infraspinatus and teres minor muscles which insert on the greater tuberosity, and the subscapularis muscle which inserts on the lesser tuberosity. The supraspinatus muscle and subacromial bursa occupy the space between the humeral head and the acromion; thus it is the supraspinatus tendon that is most commonly torn. **Tears of the rotator cuff** can be acute or chronic. In the latter, plain films may show a reduction in the subacromial space, sometimes with erosion of the inferior surface of the acromion from mechanical forces; however, in the acute tear, radiographs are normal. The diagnosis is frequently made on MRI where a disruption of the normal black signal of the supraspinatus tendon is seen in association with an effusion and retraction of the belly of the supraspinatus muscle (Fig. 12.33). Ultrasound is also used to make the diagnosis and both of these techniques have superseded the use of arthrography. Clinical signs suggestive of a rotator cuff tear, painful and limited abduction in acute trauma, may be due to an avulsion of the greater trochanter. Avulsion of the lesser trochanter by the subscapularis tendon is rare and difficult to see on plain films, and diagnosis may be aided by ultrasound.

(a)

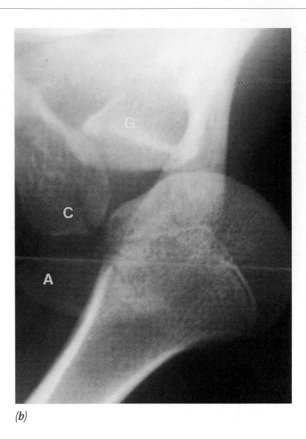

(b)

Figure 12.32 *Posterior dislocation of the shoulder. (a) AP view of the shoulder. The configuration of the humeral head is more rounded than on the normal AP view. (b) However, the abnormal position of the humerus, displaced posteriorly with respect to the acromion (A), clavicle (C) and glenoid (G) is more evident on the axial view.*

Figure 12.33 *T2-weighted paracoronal MRI through the right shoulder. A small area of bright signal under the acromioclavicular joint represents an effusion in the subacromial bursa (curved arrow). The high signal defect in the distal supraspinatus tendon is also readily identified (arrow).*

Proximal **humeral fractures** are common, especially in osteoporotic bone. **Neer's four segment classification** helps in guiding treatment and suggesting prognosis. The four segments are: humeral head, humeral shaft, greater and lesser trochanters. If any of the segments is displaced by over 1 cm or 45° then it is significantly displaced; if none of the fragments is displaced then it is undisplaced, irrespective of the degree of comminution. A lateral film must be obtained since anterior angulation is relatively common and is not identified on the other views. If one segment is displaced it is a two-part fracture; if two are displaced it is three-part, etc. Pseudo-subluxation may occur from haemarthrosis or weakness of the deltoid and rotator cuff muscles.

PELVIS

Pelvic fractures and dislocations may be difficult to diagnose. The films should be evaluated with particular attention to the following structures: the iliopubic and ilio-ischial lines should be intact, as should both anterior and posterior acetabular rims. **Judet**, or 45° oblique, views of the acetabulum are very useful: the posterior oblique view shows the posterior column and anterior acetabular rim, while the anterior view shows

Figure 12.34 *AP view of pelvis in a child showing an unstable pelvic fracture. The pubic symphysis is diastased (curved arrow). In addition, there is disruption of the left sacroiliac joint (arrows). The double break in the pelvic ring indicates that the fracture is unstable.*

Figure 12.35 *AP view of right hip in a young adult showing ischial tuberosity avulsion. A fragment of bone has separated from the ischial tuberosity and is pulled laterally and inferiorly by the attached hamstring muscles (open arrow).*

the anterior column and posterior rim. Femoral head subluxation and dislocation can be checked, as can disruption in the dome of the acetabulum, with medial migration of the femoral head, **protrusio acetabuli**.

Sacral fractures and **sacroiliac joint disruptions** are particularly hard to identify on the plain films. An apparent single break in the pelvic ring, or a fracture of the transverse process of L5 should alert one to the possibility of sacral or sacroiliac joint injury. The symphysis pubis and sacroiliac joints should not be diastased. The former may be up to 10 mm in children but not more than 5 mm in adults, and the sacroiliac joints should be 2–4 mm wide in adults.

Two thirds of **pelvic fractures** are stable and are single breaks along the peripheral margins: avulsion, iliac wing fracture, sacral fracture, or pubic rami fracture. Pelvic disruption in two or more places constitutes an unstable pelvic fracture (Fig. 12.34). The most common is the vertical shear, or **Malgaigne fracture**; this is usually a sacral fracture with ipsilateral inferior and superior pubic rami fractures. Another is the **straddle fracture**, involving both the superior and inferior pubic rami bilaterally. These unstable fractures are associated with a significant risk of haemorrhage and visceral damage, and often require internal fixation.

CT is unnecessary in routine evaluation of stable pelvic fractures but is useful for unstable injuries, sacral and saroiliac joint fractures. CT may show more extensive disruption to the posterior ring than is seen on the plain films. CT is also of value in searching for intra-articular loose bodies which may prevent adequate reduction following hip dislocation.

Isolated traumatic sacral fractures are usually transverse and result from a direct blow; when seen in conjunction with complex pelvic trauma they are usually vertical and disrupt the sacral foramina and neural arches.

Apophyseal avulsion injuries are common in adolescents around the pelvis. The anterior superior iliac spine is the origin of the sartorius muscle, the anterior inferior iliac spine the origin of the rectus femoris, the ischial tuberosity is the origin of the hamstring muscles (Fig. 12.35), and the inferior pubic ramus, at the symphysis, is the site of origin of the adductor muscles. In the early stages, apophyseal avulsion injuries may be difficult to diagnose, and amorphous new bone formation may be confused with an osteogenic tumour. Occurrence at characteristic sites, together with an appropriate history, and gradually maturing bone, should lead to the correct diagnosis.

HIP

The AP film should show the hip in slight internal rotation. The neck of the femur is thus elongated, the greater trochanter is seen in profile and the lesser trochanter is partly hidden. A true lateral view can be difficult to obtain but may be important in order to confirm a subtle fracture line. Comment is sometimes made about the fat planes surrounding the hip, but displacement of these lines is not useful in confirming the presence of an effusion.

Hip fractures are rare in the young and middle-aged, unless there has been severe trauma. Because of senile osteoporosis, however, they are extremely common in the elderly, and subcapital fractures are twice as common as intertrochanteric fractures. The **subcapital fracture** may be obvious as a change in angulation or as disrupted or angulated trabeculae or, if impacted, it may be seen as a line of increased density, or an irregularity at the outer cortex at the junction of the head and neck. A ring of osteophytes on the superior border of the greater trochanter may be mistaken for an impacted fracture. The blood supply to the femoral head enters through the neck in an adult, and therefore the blood supply is easily compromised in the presence of a subcapital fracture, leading to avascular necrosis in up to 30 per cent. Subcapital fractures are thus commonly treated by hemiprosthetic replacement, although on occasion, if there is significant acetabular degenerative change, the surgeon may elect to perform a total hip replacement.

Intertrochanteric fractures occur in a slightly older age group than subcapital fractures; they may be two, three or four part, depending on the involvement of the trochanters. The oblique fracture usually runs from the greater trochanter superiorly to the lesser trochanter inferiorly, with the greatest amount of comminution seen posteriorly. The fractures are normally internally fixed with a dynamic hip screw. This allows some settling and impaction, and shortening of the screw maintains tension across the fracture. In a severely osteoporotic patient there is a risk of the screw cutting out the femoral head and neck, so the tip of the screw should be placed as posteriorly and inferiorly as possible. Avascular necrosis is rare in intertrochanteric injury.

Avulsion fracture of the lesser trochanter is not an uncommon injury in children and adolescents. If the fragment is pulled up over the pelvis it may not be seen, and the lesser trochanter may just seem to have 'disappeared'. If found as an isolated fracture in an adult, then it is usually pathological and metastatic in nature.

Hip dislocation is the occasional result of severe trauma and is most often posterior. The head is located superiorly and there may be an associated acetabular rim fracture. It may be difficult to recognize, although lack of congruity of the joint surfaces and a smaller femoral head on the affected side may be seen. The femoral head can often be palpated in the buttock. Early diagnosis is imperative as the risk of avascular necrosis increases with time: 50 per cent after 24 hours.

Slipped capital femoral epiphysis is seen in 10–16-year-olds. Male, overweight or black patients are more commonly affected; 20 per cent are bilateral, but they are rarely synchronous. Slipped capital femoral epiphysis occurs at the age of rapid growth during which the alignment of the femoral neck changes from valgus to varus, thus producing a factor of shear stress in the growth plate. The slip may, therefore, be precipitated by minor trauma, but it is also more common in the presence of

Figure 12.36 *AP view of pelvis in an adolescent showing slipped capital femoral epiphysis. The left capital femoral epiphysis is displaced medially and posteriorly as compared with the right (arrowed).*

infection, congenital hip dislocation or metabolic bone disease. On the AP film the epiphyseal plate appears wider with indistinct margins, and the epiphysis appears shorter (Fig. 12.36). A line drawn along the lateral aspect of the femoral neck intersects no more than a small portion of the femoral head. The frog-leg lateral will confirm the findings. The treatment is to pin the slip *in situ*. Avascular necrosis develops in 10 per cent, and this complication is more often seen in severe slip and where open reduction has been attempted.

KNEE

Most knee injuries involve only the soft tissues, to which the only clue may be the presence of an effusion. The lateral view is sensitive to the presence of an effusion. In the normal knee, the fat pad posterior to the quadriceps tendon is divided in two by a line of soft-tissue density, the suprapatellar bursa, which should be no more than 5 mm wide. An anterior cruciate ligament avulsion may, however, be associated with an avulsion injury of the anterior tibial spine, an injury more commonly seen in children and adolescents than adults, because at this age the ligaments are stronger than the bony attachments. Avulsion of the posterior cruciate ligament may result in avulsion of a sliver of bone from the posterior tibia.

The most sensitive imaging method for detecting an **internal derangement** is MRI, although on occasion it may still be necessary to perform arthrography on a patient who is unable to undergo MRI. Cruciate ligament tears, collateral ligament tears, extensor mechanism pathology and meniscal tears are all readily identified. The normal tendons, ligaments and menisci give low signal (black) on MRI, and tears may be seen as linear high signal (white) extending through these structures (Fig. 12.37). The popliteal tendon runs obliquely long the

Figure 12.37 *T2-weighted sagittal MRI of the knee showing a meniscal tear. The normal triangular shape of the posterior horn of the medial meniscus is disrupted by a line of high signal running through it (curved arrow).*

posterior part of the lateral meniscus and may be confused with a tear. The normal menisci are 'bow-tie' shaped in sagittal images, and the medial is thicker posteriorly than anteriorly; a discoid meniscus, usually the lateral, is uniformly thick throughout, and is associated with pain, tears and locking. Meniscal cysts often occur peripherally in the meniscus and are readily identified.

Many surgeons proceed directly to arthroscopy if there are strong clinical indications of an internal derangement, but the equivocally abnormal knee, following previous surgery, discoid meniscus, or persistent symptoms following an apparently normal arthroscopy, may all be indications for an MRI to be performed first. Bone bruises and other subchondral pathologies can be seen at MRI but not at arthroscopy, while ultrasound is useful for delineating a **Baker's cyst**, showing a large, fluid-filled posterior lesion, and may show the site of a connection with the joint space.

Epiphyseal injuries around the knee are rare, but complications are frequent; 70 per cent are Salter–Harris Type II, and 15 Type III. The latter usually involve the medial condyle and are due to valgus stress. They are often undisplaced and therefore occult. The knee is the most common site of Salter–Harris Type V fractures; they are usually seen in the proximal tibia and are associated with tibial shaft fractures. As the rate of growth plate disturbances is so high, prognosis should be guarded, and a careful search maintained for early diagnosis of bony bridging across the physis.

Tibial plateau fractures are common in road traffic accidents involving pedestrians, as the tibial plateau is at the level of a car bumper: 80 per cent are confined to the lateral plateau as they are the result of valgus stress. They may be subtle but it is important to establish the extent of tibial plateau depression as a depression over 1 cm or a widely separated (5 mm) vertical split will probably need internal fixation.

Sixty per cent of **patellar fractures** are transverse from indirect force, such as a violent contraction of the quadriceps tendon. The majority of the remainder are stellate due to a direct blow. Beware the bipartite or multipartite patella: the separate fragments are commonly seen on the superolateral aspect of the patella and have well corticated margins. The pattern may be symmetrical. Patellar dislocation is usually lateral, a tendency dictated by the presence of the following anatomical variants: patellar tilt, lateral patellar displacement and patella alta (the ratio of the normal length of the patellar tendon to the length of the patella should be between 0.8 and 1.2).

ANKLE

The lateral margin of the tibia has a fibular notch into which the fibula should fit snugly. If the fibula is shortened after a fracture, the more bulbous distal part of the fibula does not articulate properly with this notch. This in turn leads to lateral shift of the talus, reducing the congruity of the joint, and early degenerative change. Therefore, only 2–3 mm of fibular shortening is acceptable. The joint space should be even across the entire ankle mortise; over 2 mm widening at any point is abnormal. In stress views, valgus and varus force is applied to the calcaneus. There is a wide range of normal ankle laxity, with talar tilt of up to 20° in exceptionally lax ankles, so on occasion comparison views may be necessary. MRI may be helpful to delineate ligamentous injury.

The **Weber classification** is used as it correlates well with treatment and prognosis. It uses the level of the fibular fracture to deduce the injury to the tibiofibular ligaments. The Weber A is a transverse avulsion fracture of the lateral malleolus at, or distal to, the tibiofibular joint and thus does not involve the tibiofibular ligament complex. It may be associated with an oblique fracture of the medial malleolus. The Weber B is a spiral fracture of the lateral malleolus beginning at the level of the ankle joint. This leads to a partial disruption of the tibiofibular ligament complex and so the diastasis of the mortise depends on the severity of the injury. It may be associated with a transverse or slightly oblique fracture of the medial malleolus below the ankle joint or with a deltoid ligament rupture. The Weber C is a fibular fracture proximal to the ankle joint, which invariably tears the tibiofibular ligament complex and leads to lateral talar instability. The medial malleolus is avulsed just below the level of the ankle joint, or the deltoid ligament may be torn (Fig. 12.38). Exact anatomic, stable reconstruction of the mortise is essential to prevent post-traumatic arthritis.

Osteochondral fractures of the lateral or medial dome of the talus can occur during ankle trauma and

Figure 12.38 *AP view of lower leg showing a Weber C ankle fracture. The fibula is fractured in the proximal to mid-shaft (open arrow). There has been an avulsion of the medial malleolus (closed arrow) and therefore there is lateral talar instability.*

Figure 12.39 *(a) Normal lateral view of the calcaneum illustrating Bohler's angle (large asterisk). The normal range is 28–40°. (b) The patient has an intra-articular fracture of the calcaneum and Bohler's angle is markedly reduced (small asterisk).*

may not be evident on the plain films at the time of injury. There is a high incidence of avascular necrosis, and plain film, CT or MRI may aid diagnosis. With any fracture resulting in widening of the mortise, there may be an associated tear of the proximal tibiofibular ligament and fracture of the proximal fibula, the **Maisonneuve fracture**. The entire fibula should therefore be X-rayed under these circumstances.

Fusion of the distal tibial epiphysis starts at 12–13 years of age; it begins centrally and proceeds medially and then laterally. The unfused portion is often confused with a fracture. The **juvenile Tillaux fracture** may be seen during this pattern of fusion. This injury is a Salter–Harris Type III fracture of the lateral portion of the distal tibial epiphysis that occurs after fusion of the medial part. The **triplane fracture** also occurs in children; it involves the lateral half of the distal tibial epiphysis and a posterior triangular metaphyseal fragment.

The base of the fifth metatarsal should be included on the lateral ankle film, as a fracture at this site (**Jones' fracture**) may be mistaken clinically for an ankle injury because they both may follow inversion injury (Fig. 12.6, p. 310).

FOOT

Several normal appearances can be confused with trauma: notably, the calcaneal apophysis and the navicular may appear dense and fragmented in the normal growing skeleton and the proximal epiphysis of the proximal phalanx of the great toe may be bifid.

The articulations of the tarsals and metatarsals may seem confusing, but normal alignment is important to exclude mid-foot dislocations, which may quickly compromise the vascular supply to the forefoot.

On the AP film;

- the lateral border of the first metatarsal should align with the lateral border of the medial cuneiform;
- the medial border of the second metatarsal should align with the medial border of the middle cuneiform.

On the lateral oblique film:

- the lateral border of the third metatarsal should align with the lateral border of the lateral cuneiform;
- the medial border of the fourth metatarsal aligns with the medial border of the cuboid;
- the base of the fifth metatarsal articulates with the cuboid but extends lateral to the lateral border of the cuboid.

The base of the second metatarsal is recessed between the medial and lateral cuneiform in a lock and key configuration.

Fractures of the calcaneus may be seen best on the axial, or Harris view. They are classified as either intra- or extra-articular. The presence of an intra-articular, crush, fracture is denoted by a decrease in **Bohler's angle** (Fig. 12.39): 10 per cent are bilateral and 10 per cent are associated with thoracolumbar fractures, the **Don Juan fracture**, so called because the common mechanism is a fall from a height, such as hurrying through a window! A talar fracture may occur through the neck and may be associated with a talar dislocation.

The **Lisfranc fracture dislocation** is a dorsal dislocation at the tarsometatarsal joints with a fracture of the base of the second metatarsal. It is either homolateral, with lateral dislocation or neutral position of the great toe metatarsal, or divergent, with medial subluxation of the great toe metatarsal. Continued weight-bearing leads to progressive displacement. The injury is frequently a manifestation of a neuropathic foot. Early changes may be subtle and require CT for diagnosis.

The nail bed of the great toe is attached to the periosteum at the level of the proximal metaphysis, and in a child a stubbed toe may result in a Salter–Harris Type I or II fracture and/or osteomyelitis.

FURTHER READING

Apley, A.G., Solomon, L. 1993: *Apley's system of orthopaedics and fractures* (7th edition). Oxford: Butterworth Heinemann.

Harris, J.H., Mirvis, S.E. 1995: *The radiology of acute cervical spine trauma* (3rd edition). Philadelphia, PA: Lippincott, Williams and Wilkins.

Keats, T.E. 1996: *Atlas of normal roentgen variants that may simulate disease* (6th edition). Mosby Year Book. St Louis, MO: Mosby.

Ogden, J.K., 1999: *Skeletal injury in the child* (3rd edition). Edinburgh: Springer Verlag.

Rogers, L.F. 1992: *Radiology of skeletal trauma* (2nd edition). Edinburgh: Churchill Livingstone.

Bones, joints and soft tissues

ASIF SAIFUDDIN, SARAH BURNETT

This chapter covers the major acquired diseases of bone, joints and soft tissues, excluding skeletal trauma; congenital or developmental syndromes are beyond the scope of this book.

BONE

INFECTIONS

ACUTE PYOGENIC OSTEOMYELITIS

Acute osteomyelitis is typically a disease of childhood and most commonly due to haematogenous spread of *Staphylococcus aureus* from a distant focus. Other less common organisms include *Salmonella* spp., particularly in patients with sickle-cell anaemia, and *Pseudomonas* spp. in drug abusers. Less commonly, infection is due to direct spread from soft-tissue infection or follows penetrating injury (traumatic or iatrogenic).

The site of infection within a bone depends on age. Acute haematogenous osteomyelitis in childhood typically involves the metaphysis of a long bone, because here the blood flow is sluggish and the metaphyseal vessels do not cross the growth plate. Therefore, involvement of the epiphysis and joint is rare. The femur and tibia are involved in 65–75 per cent

of cases. Up to 1 year of age, the metaphyseal vessels penetrate the growth plate and therefore epiphyseal and joint involvement may accompany metaphyseal osteomyelitis in the infant. This may result in slipped epiphysis, dislocation and growth deformity. Multifocal osteomyelitis is also relatively common in neonates. In adults, the growth plate is closed and terminal metaphyseal vessels anastomose with epiphyseal vessels. Joint infection is, therefore, relatively common in association with metaphyseal osteomyelitis, although in adults the spine and small bones are the commonest sites of involvement.

Initially there is inflammation and pus formation in the medulla with associated vascular thrombosis. Infection then spreads through the adjacent cortex, resulting in subperiosteal abscess formation and periosteal elevation. Necrosis of cortical bone may result, producing a sequestrum, while subperiosteal bone formation results in development of an involucrum. Extension of the infective process may occur subperiosteally, both along and around the shaft of the bone. If pus escapes through the periosteum (resulting in cloaca formation), soft-tissue abscesses may develop.

Initial **plain film** findings include soft-tissue swelling with loss of fat planes within the first week. Bone changes are not seen until 10–14 days and consist of osteopenia and poorly defined lytic areas in the metaphysis together with, typically, a single layer of periosteal reaction (Fig. 13.1). This usually develops by 2 weeks

Figure 13.1 *Acute pyogenic osteomyelitis. There are poorly defined lytic and sclerotic areas in the proximal tibial metaphysis and a single layer of periosteal reaction (arrow).*

after the initial symptoms. Areas of cortical destruction and multilayered periosteal reaction may also be seen.

Involvement of the epiphysis may result in diminished size or absence of the epiphysis. Sequestrum formation is identified as one or more areas of dense, necrotic cortical bone, while soft-tissue abscesses may be manifest as gas in the soft tissues and soft-tissue swelling.

Subperiosteal pus collections can be identified with ultrasound well before plain film bone changes occur and ultrasound can be used to guide aspiration/biopsy.

Bone scintigraphy with ^{99m}Tc-methylene diphosphonate (MDP) can demonstrate abnormality in bone within hours to days. Within the first 3 days, there may be a 'cold' area from vascular thrombosis in the medulla, but this progresses to increased activity. Scintigraphy is the method of choice for identifying multifocal osteomyelitis. Gallium-citrate scans and labelled WBC scans are more specific for osteomyelitis than ^{99m}Tc-MDP bone scans.

MRI is also abnormal early and is very sensitive, demonstrating bone oedema as areas of reduced signal on T1-weighted images and increased signal on STIR and T2-weighted images. Ultrasound, CT and MRI are all of value in identifying soft-tissue abscess formation.

Acute osteomyelitis secondary to soft-tissue infection may result in focal, poorly defined bone destruction and periosteal reaction. If plain films are normal, three-phase bone scintigraphy can help to differentiate osteomyelitis from cellulitis, since the latter will show

minimal or no uptake in bone on the delayed (static) images. MRI will also be able to differentiate cellulitis from osteomyelitis.

CHRONIC OSTEOMYELITIS

If treatment of acute osteomyelitis is delayed or inadequate, chronic osteomyelitis may develop. This is characterized pathologically by a prominent involucrum, sequestra and cloaca with sinus formation to the skin. It is the presence of infected dead bone which results in recurrent infection.

Typical radiographic findings include thick sclerotic periosteal reaction and the demonstration of a sequestrum which appears as relatively dense bone that may lie within the medullary cavity (Fig. 13.2).

Additional imaging is aimed at demonstrating a sequestrum as a source of recurrent infection, and at identifying active infection. A sequestrum, if not identified on plain films, is best demonstrated with thin-section CT. Demonstrating activity is more difficult. Increased uptake on ^{99m}Tc-MDP bone scanning is non-specific. However, if ^{99m}Tc-MDP scanning is combined with ^{67}Ga-citrate scanning, infection is likely to be

Figure 13.2 *Chronic osteomyelitis of the humerus. There is concentric thickening of the cortex. A sequestrum is identified within the medullary cavity (arrow).*

Figure 13.3 *Brodie's abscess of the tibia appearing as an oval lytic area in the metaphysis with surrounding sclerosis.*

Figure 13.4 *Tuberculous osteomyelitis of the left proximal femur appearing as a well-defined lytic lesion without marginal sclerosis or periosteal reaction. The location adjacent to a tuberosity is characteristic.*

present, if the uptake on the gallium scan exceeds that on the MDP scan. MRI may also be useful in assessing activity by identifying medullary inflammation. Sinography, CT and MRI are all useful for identifying sinus tracts.

Complications of chronic osteomyelitis include amyloidosis and malignant transformation in a chronic draining sinus tract, usually 10–20 years after the initial infection.

Brodie's abscess

The term 'Brodie's abscess' refers to a particular form of chronic osteomyelitis in which the infection is closely contained resulting in a chronic medullary abscess composed of pus or jelly-like granulation tissue. Radiographs demonstrate a well-defined lytic lesion in the medulla with variable surrounding sclerosis and periosteal reaction (Fig. 13.3). The lesion usually occurs in children in the metaphysis of a long bone. Occasionally, a Brodie's abscess rises within the cortex, where it may elicit a marked sclerotic reaction, mimicking osteoid osteoma. MRI is highly specific in the diagnosis, demonstrating a thin enhancing margin on postcontrast T1-weighted images (the 'penumbra' sign).

TUBERCULOUS OSTEOMYELITIS

Bone and joint tuberculosis usually results from haematogenous spread from lung infection. However, in up to 50 per cent of cases no radiological evidence of active or healed pulmonary tuberculosis is found. The incidence of tuberculous osteomyelitis is relatively high in patients of African and Asian origin and in those with AIDS.

Tuberculosis results in a much more indolent infection than pyogenic osteomyelitis so that, even though symptoms are much less severe, there is usually obvious radiological abnormality at the time of presentation.

Infection is most common in the spine, followed by the large joints. Other sites include the metaphyseal regions of long bones and, rarely, diaphyseal lesions or involvement of bones, such as the sternum, calcaneus, rib and skull. Soft-tissue infection may also result in bursitis or tenosynovitis.

The typical radiological features of tuberculous bone infection include irregular, destructive lesions in the metaphysis without marginal sclerosis and little, if any, periosteal reaction (Fig. 13.4). Involvement of the epiphysis is relatively common. Sclerosis occurs as healing takes place.

Rarer forms of tuberculous osteomyelitis include **dactylitis**, resulting in expansion and thinning of the metacarpals or metatarsals (spina ventosa), and **cystic tuberculosis** resulting in multiple well-defined lytic lesions in the shafts of long bones and in flat bones.

MISCELLANEOUS INFECTIONS

Chronic recurrent multifocal osteomyelitis

This is a rare condition of unknown aetiology occurring in children and young adults, with a female predominance. It typically presents with episodes of pain and swelling at affected sites with or without low-grade fever. The clinical course of exacerbations and remissions has been reported to last up to 15 years. There is an association with pustulosis palmaris and plantaris. Bone biopsy demonstrates a non-specific subacute or chronic osteomyelitis and culture of biopsy material is invariably negative. There is a predilection for the metaphyseal ends of long bones, particularly the tibia and femur. Other common sites include the clavicle, particularly the medial end, fibula, radius and humerus, but many other sites of involvement have been reported.

The initial radiographic finding is a lytic area in the metaphysis, adjacent to a growth plate, associated with periosteal reaction, which may become very thick and dense. Lesions may be symmetrical. The multifocal nature of the condition is well demonstrated by bone scintigraphy. CT or MRI will exclude the presence of an associated soft-tissue mass.

Diabetic foot

Osteomyelitis in the diabetic foot is often difficult to diagnose because of the common coexistence of cellulitis, vascular insufficiency and neuropathy.

Bone infection usually occurs secondary to cellulitis. Plain radiographs may now show osteoporosis and periosteal reaction (the classical findings in acute haematogenous osteomyelitis). Also, bone destruction may be a consequence of neuropathy, making the diagnosis even more difficult. ^{99m}Tc bone scanning will show increased activity in both neuropathy and infection, but a negative bone scan virtually excludes the possibility of osteomyelitis. Increased specificity for osteomyelitis may be obtained with labelled-leucocyte scans and, possibly, MRI.

Syphilis and yaws

Syphilis is now so rare that yaws lesions of bone are more common, particularly in patients from Africa, South America and the Far East. Syphilis may be congenital or acquired, but congenital transmission of yaws does not occur.

The bone changes in congenital syphilis consist of a periostitis and an osteitis, which are usually symmetrical. The periosteal reaction is initially laminated, then consolidates to new bone. The commonest site is the tibia, resulting in a 'sabre tibia'.

The osteitis is due to intraosseous granulomata, usually in the metaphysis. This may be associated with widening of the growth plate and metaphyseal lucent bands. The upper tibia and humerus are common sites. Granulomas may also be found in the skull and digits, the latter causng a dactylitis that resembles tuberculosis.

In acquired syphilis, the periostitis may be either laminated or more local and hypertrophic. The osteitis results in a mixed sclerotic/lytic change, usually within the diaphysis of a bone, associated with periosteal reaction.

The bone lesions of yaws are virtually identical to those of acquired syphilis. Once again, common sites include the long bones, skull and digits.

Leprosy

Leprosy is relatively common in Africa, Central and South America, the Indian subcontinent and the Far East. Bone disease may be due either to direct infection or, more commonly, to neuropathy.

Lepromatous osteitis results initially in osteoporosis. Destructive lesions usually affect the small bones of the hands and feet, and are accompanied by periosteal reaction.

Neuropathic changes manifest as bone resorption, usually from the distal ends of the phalanges and metatarsals. The tips of the resorbed ends may be sharply pointed. Superadded infection results in osteoporosis and bone destruction, with periosteal reaction. Calcification of the peripheral nerves is a rare, but pathognomonic finding.

Fungal infections

There are many fungi which may affect bone, either by direct spread from soft-tissue lesions or from disseminated disease, in which case infection arises in the marrow cavity, resulting in areas of permeative bone destruction, periosteal reaction and variable sclerosis. Sequestrum formation tends not to be a feature.

Recognized causes of fungal osteomyelitis include actinomycosis, streptomyces, histoplasmosis, blastomycosis, coccidioidomycosis and cryptococcosis. They all tend to occur in the Tropics and some areas of North America.

Hydatid disease

Hydatid disease is classically associated with sheep farming. Less than 30 per cent of infected individuals develop bone infection, most commonly in the long bones, pelvis and spine. The intraosseous cyst causes pressure atrophy from within the bone as it enlarges.

Radiographs therefore show a well-defined lytic lesion that expands the bone. Lesions may be multiple and, when long-standing, can develop a sclerotic rim and provoke some cortical thickening.

BONE TUMOURS

GENERAL ASPECTS

Bone tumours commonly present with localized pain and swelling or pathological fracture. Following initial clinical evaluation, a plain radiograph will be obtained. Various radiographic features of the lesion need to be considered and, when combined, may produce a specific diagnosis or a good indication of whether the lesion is aggressive or not.

When a specific radiological diagnosis, such as simple bone cyst or non-ossifying fibroma, can be made, no further action may be necessary. Similarly, a specific diagnosis of osteoid osteoma can allow definitive treatment to be instituted. In most cases, however, biopsy is required for an unequivocal diagnosis.

Radiological assessment of bone tumours

Clinical and radiographic features that must be considered in the assessment of a bone lesion include the following:

Age
Age is one of the most important factors in the evaluation of a solitary bone lesion and is considered in detail under individual tumours.

Site
Both the site within the skeleton and the site within the individual bone are important. These, again, are dealt with in detail under individual tumours.

Pattern of bone destruction
This may be described as either geographic, moth-eaten or permeative:

- A **geographic pattern** of bone destruction appears as a lytic area with well-defined, sharp margins. Such an appearance indicates a slow rate of growth and is commonly seen with benign tumours and tumour-like conditions. Some malignant lesions, notably myeloma, may produce this pattern of destruction. Other malignancies rarely appear so well-defined.

- A **'moth-eaten' pattern** of destruction implies a more aggressive process. The term refers to multiple, small, lytic areas of varying sizes with intervening normal cancellous bone. The lesion has a poorly defined margin and the medullary involvement by tumour is always more extensive than that indicated by the radiograph. Most malignant tumours can produce this type of destruction, along with some benign conditions such as osteomyelitis and Langerhan's cell histiocytosis (LCH).

- A **permeative pattern** of bone destruction is the most aggressive pattern. It appears as multiple, tiny, lytic areas throughout the bone and may sometimes be difficult to appreciate. The extent of medullary involvement is poorly determined on the plain film. Most malignant lesions can produce this appearance, as can osteomyelitis and eosinophilic granuloma.

Margin of lesion
The appearance of the margin of the lesion gives an indication of its rate of growth. The presence of a sclerotic rim indicates a relatively slow rate of growth, since the surrounding bone has had time to react. The thicker the margin of sclerosis, the slower the growth rate. Faster growing lesions may have a well-defined border but no sclerosis, whereas lesions with the most rapid rate of growth will have poorly defined, non-sclerotic margins.

Matrix
The matrix of a lesion is the cellular material produced by the tumour cells. It may be either osteoid, chondroid, collagenous or myxomatous and is only radiographically visible when calcified. Osseous matrix appears cloud-like or hazy and is seen in bone-forming tumours (e.g. osteosarcoma). Cartilaginous matrix may show punctate calcification or rings and arcs of calcification.

Periosteal reaction
The presence and type of periosteal reaction can give clues to the nature and aggressiveness of the associated underlying lesion. A **single layer** of periosteal reaction may be seen with osteomyelitis, LCH, Ewing's sarcoma and osteosarcoma. These same conditions can produce multilayered (onion-skin) periosteal reaction.

Solid periosteal reaction indicates a slow process and is almost always associated with benign lesions. However, periosteal reaction may become solid in malignant tumours that have responded to treatment.

A **spiculated** periosteal reaction may be of either the perpendicular ('hair-on-end') type or the 'sunburst' type. The former is commonest with Ewing's sarcoma whereas the latter is usually seen in osteosarcoma. Both may be seen with metastasis.

A **Codman's triangle** refers to the radiographic appearance of elevated periosteum at the junction with

(a)

(b)

(c)

Figure 13.5 *Osteosarcoma of the femur. (a) The plain radiograph gives little indication of the extent of medullary abnormality or extraosseous mass. (b) Sagittal T1-weighted MRI scan showing the intraosseous tumour as a region of low signal intensity compared to the normal high signal of the marrow. (c) Axial T2-weighted MRI scan clearly demonstrates the extent of extraosseous tumour as a high signal intensity region. The normal left side is shown for comparison.*

the cortex. It indicates the extraosseous margin of a lesion and can be seen in any benign or malignant process that elevates the periosteum.

It should be noted that the periosteum is only visible radiographically owing to mineralization of its deep layer, which usually takes 10–21 days from the onset of the initial insult, whether infection, trauma or tumour. Some tumours may be so aggressive that they do not allow time for this mineralization to occur, and therefore periosteal reaction is not identified radiographically.

FURTHER IMAGING OF PRIMARY BONE TUMOURS

As a rule, **plain radiography** is the most specific technique for establishing a prebiopsy diagnosis of a focal bone lesion using the signs described above. Many benign lesions require no further imaging for adequate treatment. However, in the case of a malignant tumour, the plain film does not indicate accurately the extent of intramedullary spread, the size of extraosseous mass or its relationship to surrounding structures, and the presence or absence of bony or pulmonary metastases. The major role of further imaging is therefore in the local and distant staging of a malignant bone lesion.

MRI is the most accurate technique for local staging

of a tumour (Fig. 13.5). T1-weighted scans clearly indicate the intramedullary extent since tumour tissue has low signal intensity, which contrasts well with the high signal of adjacent medullary fat. T2-weighted scans are ideal for assessing the extraosseous component, since tumour tissue is generally hyperintense compared to surrounding muscle. The relationship to adjacent neurovascular bundles can also be assessed. MRI is relatively poor at demonstrating subtle cortical erosion and small calcifications. These are better identified by CT. Following chemotherapy, MRI can be used to assess response and to define the extent of residual tumour.

^99m^Tc-MDP **bone scanning** is used to identify bone metastases at presentation. These are reported to occur in approximately 10 per cent of Ewing's sarcomas and 2 per cent of osteosarcomas. In the latter case, pulmonary metastases may also be identified if large enough. It is important to realize that the bone scan is generally of limited value in the assessment of the primary lesion, since it cannot differentiate accurately between neoplastic and non-neoplastic conditions, or between benign and malignant neoplastic lesions.

The major role of **CT** is in the identification of pulmonary, pleural and mediastinal metastases, since CT is much more sensitive than the plain chest radiograph. CT may also be useful for biopsy guidance in areas such as the pelvis and spine.

The preoperative investigation of a primary malignant bone tumour should therefore include plain radiography and MRI of the primary lesion, whole body bone scintigraphy, chest radiography, and spiral CT of the thorax.

BENIGN BONE TUMOURS AND TUMOUR-LIKE CONDITIONS

Osseous lesions

Osteoma and enostosis (bone island)

Osteomas and bone islands are hamartomatous conditions producing well-defined, purely sclerotic lesions. Both lesions are non-aggressive. Osteomas usually arise from the outer table of the skull or paranasal sinuses. Multiple osteomas are associated with familial polyposis coli (**Gardner's syndrome**). Bone islands occur within the medullary cavity and any bone may be affected. They must be differentiated from sclerotic metastases.

Osteoid osteoma

Osteoid osteoma occurs most commonly in the second to third decade, being three times more common in males than females. It accounts for approximately 12 per cent of primary benign bone tumours. Patients classically present with focal bone pain which may be

Figure 13.7 *Typical CT features of an osteoid osteoma of the femoral diaphysis. The nidus appears as a round lesion of soft-tissue density containing central calcification. It is surrounded by dense periosteal new bone.*

worse at night and relieved by aspirin. The tumour may be cortical, medullary or, rarely, subperiosteal in location. Cortical lesions are commonest and usually occur in long bone diaphyses but have been described in most bones. Intramedullary osteoid osteomas are usually intra-articular, the commonest site being the medial aspect of the femoral neck.

The classic radiological appearance of a long bone osteoid osteoma is of a region of dense, well-defined

Figure 13.6 *Osteoid osteoma of the medial femoral neck appearing as a small lucent nidus (arrow) surrounded by dense cortical thickening.*

Figure 13.8 *Typical scintigraphic appearance of an osteoid osteoma in the posterolateral tibial cortex demonstrating the 'double density' sign.*

cortical thickening containing a small (usually < 1 cm), lucent nidus which may be calcified (Fig. 13.6). The nidus represents the actual tumour tissue. Occasionally, the sclerotic response is so marked that the nidus is obscured. In these cases, thin section CT is the best technique for identifying the nidus (Fig. 13.7).

Scintigraphy also shows a characteristic appearance: a focal area of intense activity (the nidus) surrounded by a more diffuse area of less increased uptake from reactive sclerosis, the 'double-density' sign (Fig. 13.8). A normal radionuclide bone scan virtually excludes the diagnosis.

Tumours in an intra-articular location may produce a periosteal response that is distant from the lesion, and also result in synovitis and joint effusion. Radiographically, such lesions produce diffuse osteopenia and the nidus may not be seen. In these cases, bone scintigraphy will typically show a focal area of intense activity. CT can then be used to demonstrate the nidus.

CT is also now used to guide percutaneous excision biopsy of this tumour. MRI is less sensitive at identifying the nidus but will identify adjacent marrow and soft-tissue reactive changes.

Osteoblastoma

Histologically, osteoblastoma resembles osteoid osteoma but the nidus is larger (usually > 1.5 cm). Most lesions occur in the spine, where they typically result in painful scoliosis (40–50 per cent), flat bones or long bones in young adults (second to third decade).

Radiologically, the lesions are usually lytic and expansile with well-defined sclerotic margins. Variable matrix mineralization occurs. They may occasionally behave in an aggressive manner. The lesions show intense activity on bone scintigraphy because of their osteoblastic nature.

Cartilaginous lesions

Osteochondroma (exostosis)

Osteochondroma is a very common benign neoplasm that results from the displacement of a fragment of growth plate cartilage into the metaphyseal region. The underlying bone is normal and the osteochondroma develops as an outgrowth which is continuous with the cortex and marrow cavity at its site of origin. The surface of the lesion consists of a cartilage cap.

Osteochondromas may extend from the host bone on a stalk (pedunculated) or be much more broad-based (sessile). They are usually discovered in the first or second decades; 90 per cent are solitary and 95 per cent are found in the major long bones, especially around the knee. They arise in the metaphysis and, with growth, point away from the adjacent joint (Fig. 13.9). The stalk has the appearance of normal bone and the cap may show chondroid-type calcifications. The lesion ceases to grow at the time of skeletal maturity.

Figure 13.9 *Pedunculated osteochondroma of the medial distal femoral metaphysis. With time, the lesion grows away from the adjacent joint.*

Occasionally, a bursa may form over the cartilage cap, which can be demonstrated by ultrasound or MRI.

Complications of osteochondromas include growth abnormalities, mechanical problems and malignant degeneration. Malignant change occurs in less than 1 per cent of solitary lesions and is suggested by the development of pain or further growth after skeletal maturity.

Diaphyseal aclasis is an autosomal dominant condition in which there are multiple osteochondromas. This condition is associated with a relatively high incidence of sarcomatous degeneration (up to 10 per cent).

Enchondroma (chondroma)

Enchondromas are usually solitary tumours occurring most commonly in the medulla of tubular bones (40 per cent in hands, 10 per cent in feet, 20 per cent in long bones) or in the flat bones or spine. They are asymptomatic unless complicated by fracture or malignant degeneration.

Multiple lesions occur in multiple enchondromatosis (**Ollier's disease**) or in association with soft-tissue haemangiomas (**Maffucci's syndrome**). The malignant potential is estimated at 1–5 per cent.

Radiologically, they appear as geographic, lytic lesions which may be expansile, especially in the hands and feet. They have thin, sclerotic borders and a calcified matrix (Fig. 13.10). Differentiation from low-grade central chondrosarcoma may be impossible, necessitating biopsy of suspicious lesions. Rarely, chondromas may occur in a juxtacortical location.

Chondroblastoma

Chondroblastomas are uncommon tumours typically occurring in children: 65 per cent present in the second decade. The commonest sites include the proximal humerus and femur and around the knee joint.

Figure 13.10 *Enchondroma of the middle phalanx appearing as a well-defined, expansile lytic lesion with punctate matrix calcification.*

Figure 13.11 *Chondroblastoma of the proximal humeral epiphysis appearing as a well-defined lytic lesion with thin surrounding sclerosis. Multilayered periosteal reaction is present.*

Plain radiographs show a geographic, lytic lesion with thin, marginal sclerosis located in a long bone epiphysis (Fig. 13.11). Matrix calcification and periosteal reaction may be seen. Lesions occurring after closure of the growth plate may extend into the metaphysis. They rarely metastasize. MRI commonly shows reactive bone oedema. An aneurysmal bone cyst may develop in a chondroblastoma, which can be

demonstrated on MRI by the identification of fluid levels.

Chondromyxoid fibroma

Chondromyxoid fibromas are very rare tumours classically presenting as a geographic, lobulated lytic lesion in the proximal tibial metaphysis with surrounding sclerosis. Matrix calcification is rare. Other sites include proximal and distal femur, flat bones and tarsals.

Giant cell tumour

Approximately 80 per cent of giant-cell tumours occur in the third to fifth decades. The tumour may behave either in a totally benign fashion, may be locally aggressive or, rarely, may metastasize. The majority of these tumours affect the subarticular regions of long bones, with 50 per cent occurring around the knee. The distal radius is another frequent site. Tumours that arise in an unfused skeleton occur in the metaphysis, adjacent to a growth plate or an apophysis. The flat bones and spine are less commonly affected.

Plain radiographs typically demonstrate a lytic subarticular lesion with an indistinct zone of transition, usually without surrounding sclerosis (Fig. 13.12). Trabeculation is a feature of larger lesions. The lesion is eccentric and thins the cortex, not uncommonly breaking through to form an extraosseous mass. Periosteal reaction is rare.

Figure 13.12 *Giant cell tumour of the lateral tibial plateau appearing as a purely lytic lesion with a moderately well-defined margin. Extension to the articular surface is characteristic.*

Fibrous lesions

Fibrous cortical defects and non-ossifying fibroma

The appearance, location and histology of these two lesions is identical. They are differentiated only by their

Figure 13.13 *Non-ossifying fibroma of the distal tibia appearing as a lytic cortically based expansile lesion. The appearances are characteristic.*

Figure 13.14 *Fibrous dysplasia of the right femoral neck. The lesion is expansile and trabeculated. The 'ground-glass' appearance to the matrix is indicative of a fibrous lesion.*

size, with larger lesions (> 2 cm) being designated non-ossifying fibroma; 95 per cent occur before the age of 20 and 90 per cent involve the lower limbs, especially the tibia and fibula. Most lesions are found incidentally and are of no significance, but larger lesions may present with pathological fracture.

Non-ossifying fibroma is typically metaphyseal, appearing as a geographic, lobulated, intracortical, lytic lesions that may expand into the medulla (Fig. 13.13). When multiple, some cases are associated with neurofibromatosis. The plain film findings are usually so characteristic that biopsy is unnecessary.

Fibrous dysplasia and osteofibrous dysplasia
Fibrous dysplasia is a relatively common, non-neoplastic condition that may present in a wide age group, but most commonly manifests in the second and third decades; 70 per cent are monostotic, the commonest sites include the metaphyseal regions of the femur and tibia, the ribs (where it represents the commonest benign lesion), the pelvis, skull base and paranasal sinuses. When polyostotic, the condition tends to present in childhood and 90 per cent of lesions are unilateral. Polyostotic fibrous dysplasia may be associated with pigmentation and precocious puberty in young girls (**Albright's syndrome**).

The radiological appearances are very variable. Rib and long bone lesions tend to be expansile with a well-defined, thin, sclerotic rim. The matrix may be predominantly fibrous, giving rise to a 'ground glass' appearance (Fig. 13.14), or show variable mineralization. Deformity is also a feature. Lytic areas within the lesion may represent cystic change, which predisposes to pathological fracture. Pelvic lesions may be very

expansile and bubbly. Lesions in the skull and facial bones are often densely sclerotic. Periosteal reaction may accompany pathological fracture. The lesions tend to remain quiescent throughout life, with only a small proportion continuing to enlarge after skeletal maturity.

Osteofibrous dysplasia is a rare lesion similar to fibrous dysplasia, classically occurring in the anterior tibia of young children.

Other connective tissue tumours

Desmoplastic fibroma
Desmoplastic fibromas are rare intraosseous lesions, histologically identical to soft-tissue aggressive fibromatosis (extra-abdominal desmoid tumour). The condition may involve various sites, appearing as an expansile lytic lesion.

Cortical desmoid
Cortical desmoids are not true neoplasms, but are a post-traumatic fibroblastic response at the insertion of the adductor magnus muscle on the posteromedial cortex of the distal femur. Cortical erosion, soft-tissue mass and periosteal reaction are seen, features that may mimic a surface osteosarcoma.

Figure 13.18 *Classic osteosarcoma of the distal femoral metaphysis. Note the Codman's triangle (arrow) and matrix mineralization.*

Figure 13.19 *Parosteal osteosarcoma of the femur appearing as a juxtacortical mass of dense tumour bone. The posterior distal femoral metaphysis is a classic site.*

in the metadiaphysis, initially without periosteal reaction. It has a better prognosis than conventional osteosarcoma.

Parosteal osteosarcoma is a variant of osteosarcoma generally occurring in the 20–40-year age group and has a better prognosis than conventional central osteosarcoma. The majority of lesions affect the distal femur, the tibia or proximal humerus.

Radiographs typically demonstrate a dense mass of mature tumour bone wrapping round the metaphysis of a long bone (Fig. 13.19) with a thin, lucent line separating the tumour bone from the cortex. The bone at the periphery of the tumour is less well formed. Initially, the medulla is not involved but extension through the cortex can occur later. Such extension is best identified by CT or MRI.

Periosteal osteosarcoma is a rare lesion with a prognosis in between that of conventional central osteosarcoma and parosteal osteosarcoma. The distal femoral or proximal tibial diaphyses are most commonly involved. The condition occurs usually in the second to third decades.

The tumour is hemispherical and closely applied to the cortex of the bone. Perpendicular spicules of new bone lie within the tumour and there may be periosteal

thickening at its base. The extent of the tumour and status of the medullary cavity, which should not be involved, are best assessed by MRI.

High-grade surface osteosarcoma, which has the same prognosis as conventional central osteosarcoma, has a radiological appearance very similar to periosteal osteosarcoma. The diagnosis is made histologically.

Paget's sarcoma

Sarcomatous degeneration occurs in less than 1 per cent of patients with Paget's disease. Of these, 50 per cent are osteosarcomas, 25 per cent fibrosarcomas and 25 per cent anaplastic sarcomas or other cell types.

Paget's sarcomas are usually seen in the femur or pelvis and manifest radiologically as a poorly defined area of bone destruction with a soft-tissue mass. Tumour bone formation may be seen. The prognosis is extremely poor.

Cartilaginous lesions

Chondrosarcoma

Chondrosarcoma is the third most frequent primary bone malignancy. It may arise *de novo* within bone or may be secondary to a pre-existing lesion, usually an

Figure 13.20 *Chondrosarcoma arising from the left inferior pubic ramus. There is a large extraosseous mass containing typical chondroid-type calcification.*

enchondroma or an osteochondroma, rarely within chondromyxoid fibroma or chondroblastoma. The tumours may therefore be either central, i.e. within the medulla, or peripheral. The mean age at presentation is 50 years with a slight male predominance. The commonest sites include the pelvis, proximal femur and proximal humerus.

The typical radiographic features in long bone lesions include a relatively well-defined, lytic lesion causing endosteal scalloping and mild bony expansion. There may be associated matrix calcification and marked cortical thickening, which is characteristic. Periosteal reaction is variable. In more aggressive tumours, cortical destruction occurs. Pelvic lesions are classically associated with large extraosseous components (Fig. 13.20), which are best delineated with CT or MRI.

Difficulties may arise in the diagnosis of secondary chondrosarcoma. This is suggested clinically when a known benign lesion (osteochondroma or enchondroma) becomes painful and enlarges. Radiological features suggesting malignant change include growth or destruction of part of a calcified cartilage cap or bony stem of an osteochondroma, or enlargement of an enchondroma. The thickness of the cartilage cap can be assessed by ultrasound, CT or, ideally by MRI. The thicker the cap, the more likely that malignant change has occurred. Occasionally, chondrosarcoma may dedifferentiate, usually into malignant fibrous histiocytoma. This is associated with a poorer prognosis.

Other rare varieties of chondrosarcoma include juxtacortical, mesenchymal and clear-cell types.

Fibrous lesions

Malignant fibrous histiocytoma and fibrosarcoma

These are uncommon primary bone sarcomas which usually present in the fourth to fifth decades. Most tumours arise around the knee. Malignant fibrous histiocytomas may also arise in soft tissues and invade bone secondarily. These tumours may also complicate Paget's disease, chondrosarcoma, bone infarction and sinus tracts in chronic osteomyelitis.

Radiographs typically demonstrate a poorly defined, lytic lesion in a long bone metaphysis, occasionally with associated matrix calcification and little periosteal reaction.

Vascular lesions

Haemangiopericytoma

Most haemangiopericytomas are primary soft-tissue neoplasms which may erode the bony cortex. Very rarely, they arise within bone producing a moth-eaten or permeative area of bone destruction. The lesions is monostotic and occurs most commonly in the axial skeleton or in a long bone metaphysis.

Haemangioendotheliomas

Haemangioendotheliomas are rare primary bone tumours occurring in the second to third decade. They are usually polyostotic with lesions tending to involve multiple bones of a single extremity, usually hand or foot. Individual lesions are relatively well-defined and purely lytic. Metastases to the lungs are occasionally seen.

Angiosarcomas

These are rare primary tumours of bone which usually occur in the fourth and fifth decades. The commonest sites of origin include the major long bones and pelvis. Radiographs demonstrate a permeative lytic lesion with associated soft-tissue mass. The tumour is multifocal in approximately 40 per cent of cases.

Malignant round cell tumours

The term malignant round cell tumour of bone includes Ewing's sarcoma, primitive neuroectodermal tumour, metastatic neuroblastoma and primary lymphoma.

Ewing's sarcoma

This is a rare, highly malignant tumour which presents most commonly at 5–15 years of age. The common sites include the major long bones, pelvis and ribs. In the long bones, extensive involvement of the diaphysis is typical, although 25 per cent of cases may arise in the metaphysis.

The medullary lesion causes poorly defined, permeative destruction, which may be difficult to identify. Periosteal reaction is a common feature and may have a single layer or multilayered ('onion-peel') appearance. A perpendicular type of periosteal reaction may also occur (Fig. 13.21). Characteristically, a very large extraosseous component is present and this is best defined by MRI, as is the extent of medullary involvement. Mineralization of the extraosseous mass is not a feature. Ewing's sarcoma

Figure 13.21 *Ewing's sarcoma of the distal femoral metaphysis. The permeative medullary bone destruction, perpendicular periosteal reaction and large extraosseous mass are all characteristic. A Codman's triangle is seen at the margin of the lesion (arrow).*

of a flat bone is more commonly densely sclerotic, due to reactive new bone. Once again, a large extraosseous component is characteristic. Bone metastases at presentation occur in up to 10 per cent of patients.

Primitive neuroectodermal tumours

These occur primarily in soft tissues or bone and produce radiographic changes that may be indistinguishable from Ewing's sarcoma. The diagnosis is made by specialized immunohistochemical techniques.

Metastatic neuroblastoma

This typically occurs in children under 5 years of age who are already known to have a primary abdominal mass. Radiographs may show multiple sites of permeative bone destruction in the metaphyses of the long bones similar to leukaemia or multifocal osteomyelitis. Alternatively, diffuse infiltration of a long bone similar to Ewing's sarcoma may occur. Infiltration of the cranial sutures is relatively common.

Lymphoma of bone

Osseous **Hodgkin's lymphoma** is almost always secondary to primary lymph node disease. Radiographic

evidence of bone disease is seen in 20 per cent of patients. The majority of cases (75 per cent) affect the axial skeleton, especially the spine. Two thirds of cases are multifocal. The radiographic appearances can be either purely lytic with a permeative pattern, sclerotic or mixed. An associated soft-tissue mass is common.

Non-Hodgkin's lymphoma can produce either focal lytic permeative lesions or generalized osteopenia.

Primary lymphomas of bone (reticulum cell sarcoma). The diagnosis of primary lymphoma of bone depends upon involvement of a single site in bone without evidence of extraskeletal lymphoma. The mean age at presentation is in the fifth decade, but the age range is wide. The diaphyses of long bones are most commonly affected, but flat bones are also involved.

Radiographs demonstrate an area of permeative bone destruction, commonly with some reactive sclerosis. Rarely, a purely sclerotic tumour is seen. A large associated extraosseous mass is characteristic. Once again, MRI most accurately defines medullary extent.

Leukaemia

Acute leukaemia is the commonest malignancy of childhood and, consequently, radiographic demonstration of bone lesions is not infrequent. In adults, chronic leukaemias predominate and bone lesions are uncommon.

The neoplastic proliferation of white cells initially results in trabecular and endosteal bone destruction which may be followed by extraosseous spread.

The radiographic changes in children are as follows. Metaphyseal lucent bands are a non-specific feature, most commonly seen in the distal femur, proximal tibia and distal radius. The medullary destruction by tumour is of a permeative type similar to Ewing's sarcoma. Endosteal erosion and cortical destruction follow. Focal osteolytic lesions may occur, usually in long bone diaphyses, in over 60 per cent of cases. However, osteosclerotic lesions are rare. These are seen in the metaphysis, either spontaneously or as a consequence of treatment. Periosteal reaction may be due either to subperiosteal tumour or haemorrhage.

As with other malignant marrow tumours, the extent of local involvement is best demonstrated by MRI. The radiographic features described above are not specific to leukaemia, but may also be seen with metastatic neuroblastoma and multifocal osteomyelitis.

Leukaemic bone lesions in adults are rare and have appearances almost identical to a primary malignant tumour or metastasis.

Multiple myeloma and plasmacytoma

Myeloma is a neoplasm of plasma cell origin and is the commonest primary malignancy of bone; 95 per cent of patients are over 40 at presentation, with a peak

Figure 13.22 *Multiple myeloma affecting the humerus, radius and ulna appearing as well-defined, 'punched-out' lytic lesions without marginal sclerosis.*

incidence at 60–70 years. Men are affected twice as often as women. The axial skeleton and proximal ends of long bones, the sites of red marrow in adults, are usually affected.

The classic radiological findings are multiple, well-defined, 'punched-out' lytic lesions throughout the skeleton (Fig. 13.22). Marginal sclerosis may be seen with healing. Other findings include diffuse osteopenia (15 of cases) and pathological fractures, especially in the spine. Rarely, myeloma may result in sclerotic or mixed lytic and sclerotic lesions.

Myeloma is the commonest cause of a false-negative ^{99m}Tc bone scan or 'cold' lesion, presumably owing to the lack of osteoblastic response to the tumour cells. Scans are positive in 25–40 per cent of myeloma lesions.

The main differential diagnosis is metastatic carcinoma. Features favouring myeloma include presence of an associated soft-tissue mass and involvement of the mandible.

Plasmacytoma, the solitary lesion of myeloma accounting for 30 per cent of cases of myeloma, affects the same sites as multiple myeloma. Radiographs usually demonstrate a well-defined, expansile lesion over 5 cm in diameter with cortical thinning and an associated soft-tissue mass. Plasmacytoma may progress to multiple myeloma.

METASTATIC DISEASE

Metastatic deposits from carcinoma are by far the commonest malignant lesions of bone, being 25 times commoner than primary bone tumours. They are solitary in 9 per cent of cases and, therefore, in a middle-aged or elderly patient, a solitary metastasis is more common than a primary bone tumour.

The commonest carcinomas to metastasize to bone are prostate and breast, followed by bronchus (especially small cell tumours). However, primary gastrointestinal and genitourinary carcinomata not uncommonly produce bone metastases.

The most frequent sites involved are those bones containing red marrow. Metastases are, therefore, usually found in the spine, pelvis, ribs, skull and proximal humeri or femora; 50 per cent of peripheral metastases are secondaries from bronchial neoplasms.

Figure 13.23 *Lytic metastasis of the right inferior pubic ramus.*

Bone metastases have a varied **radiographic** appearance. Most arise within the medulla, producing multiple lytic lesions without sclerotic borders. They may not be visualized until they reach 2 cm in size or until the adjacent bony cortex has been destroyed (Fig. 13.23). Periosteal reaction and extraosseous extension are occasionally seen. Some carcinomas,

Figure 13.24 *Widespread osteoblastic metastases in the pelvis, proximal femora and spine from a primary prostatic carcinoma.*

Figure 13.25 *Typical appearances of multiple metastases on ^{99m}Tc-MDP bone scintigraphy. Rib lesions are characteristically linear along the length of the rib, whereas vertebral lesions tend to be focal and related to the pedicles.*

particularly prostate, produce predominantly sclerotic metastases owing to an osteoblastic response to the tumour (Fig. 13.24). Breast carcinoma may show a lytic, sclerotic or mixed appearance. Expansile lytic lesions are occasionally seen with renal and thyroid metastases.

In a patient with a known carcinoma and bone pain but normal plain radiographs, **bone scintigraphy** should be performed, since it is far more sensitive than plain radiography. If positive, **CT** or preferably **MRI** will demonstrate the lesion, if there is doubt about the interpretation of the scintigram. Scintigraphy may also demonstrate multiple skeletal lesions and can show a characteristic appearance of multiple areas of increased activity in the spine, ribs and pelvis (Fig. 13.25). In a small proportion of cases the bone scan is normal or shows a focal region of reduced activity. Diffuse osteoblastic metastatic involvement of the skeleton may result in a 'superscan', a term which refers to widespread increase in skeletal uptake. MRI is the most sensitive technique for demonstrating skeletal metastases, but is non-specific, lesions appearing as relatively well demarcated areas of low signal intensity on T1-weighted images and increased signal intensity on T2-weighted images, although osteoblastic metastases also show low signal intensity on T2-weighted images.

METABOLIC BONE DISEASE

OSTEOPOROSIS

Osteoporosis is a condition of unknown aetiology in which there is an abnormal reduction in the quantity of bone. However, the bone that remains is normally mineralized and appears normal histologically. There is no associated abnormality of bone biochemistry.

The commonest cause is senile generalized osteoporosis, which typically affects postmenopausal women: 30–50 per cent of women over 60 years of age will show evidence of significant bone loss. The commonest sites affected include the spine, femur (subcapital neck and intertrochanteric region), distal radius and proximal humerus.

Radiographic changes are first seen in the spine but require up to 30–50 per cent of bone loss. There is reduction of bone density owing to loss of horizontal trabeculae with accentuation of the vertical trabeculae. There is also thinning of the cortex. In the femoral neck, there may be accentuation of the major stress-bearing trabeculae. Complications include wedge-compression fractures in the spine, and stress fractures as well as complete fractures at other sites, especially the femoral neck and distal radius. Bone mass may be assessed quantitatively either by dual energy X-ray absorptiometry or quantitative computed tomography.

Disorders associated with osteoporosis include excessive endogenous or exogenous corticosteroids, hyperthyroidism, acromegaly, homocystinuria, alcoholism, osteogenesis imperfecta and some drugs. **Idiopathic juvenile osteoporosis** is a rare, specific condition affecting children aged 8–12 years.

Localized forms of osteoporosis include those due to disuse, **reflex sympathetic dystrophy syndrome** (**Sudeck's atrophy**) and transient regional osteoporosis. In disuse and the reflex sympathetic dystrophy syndrome, the radiographic appearances may be very aggressive with a moth-eaten pattern of bone loss, intracortical tunnelling indicating rapid bone remodelling, and metaphyseal lucent bands. Changes are typically periarticular (Fig. 13.26). The reflex sympathetic dystrophy syndrome is characterized by increased activity in all phases of a triple-phase bone scan.

Transient regional osteoporosis is a self-limiting condition that takes two forms. The migratory form typically occurs in middle-aged males and usually affects the knee, ankle and foot. It resolves within a year but may recur in another joint. Transient osteoporosis of the hip affects either women in late pregnancy, in which case the left hip is typically involved, or one or other hip in males. MRI is sensitive, but non-specific, showing the appearances of bone oedema. Scintigraphy will demonstrate increased activity but is also non-specific.

Figure 13.26 *Sudeck's atrophy of the hand. The severe periarticular osteoporosis is a characteristic finding.*

RICKETS AND OSTEOMALACIA

Rickets and osteomalacia are characterized by a normal amount of osteoid; this, however, shows reduced mineralization. The abnormality of mineralization is related to a deficiency of metabolically active vitamin D. This may be due to dietary causes, malabsorption, liver disease, renal disease, drugs, or, rarely, it may be associated with a variety of tumours (oncogenic osteomalacia).

Both conditions are associated with generalized osteopenia from a decrease in the number of trabeculae, and a coarsening of trabeculae from osteoid deposition without adequate mineralization.

Rickets occurs in childhood with changes predominating at sites of rapid growth, notably the proximal humerus, distal radius, distal femur and both ends of the tibia. Radiographs show widening of the zone of provisional calcification and irregularity and cupping of the metaphyses (Fig. 13.27). Slipping of the epiphysis, bowing of the long bones and vertebral compression fractures may also occur.

Conditions that may mimic rickets include hypophosphatasia and metaphyseal chondrodysplasia (Schmid type).

Osteomalacia is characterized by Looser's zones (pseudofractures) which appear as wide transverse lucent bands, perpendicular to the cortex, that may be incomplete. Characteristic sites include the pubic rami (Fig. 13.28), ribs, axillary borders of the scapulae, medial margin of the proximal femora and posterior border of the proximal ulnae. Bone scintigraphy may

Figure 13.27 *Typical features of rickets in the wrist with widening of the zone of provisional calcification (arrow) and splaying and irregularity of the metaphyses.*

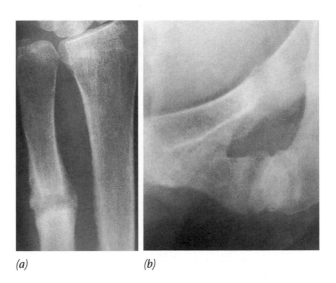

(a)   *(b)*

Figure 13.28 *Radiographs of (a) the wrist and (b) pubic rami in a patient with osteomalacia. Looser's zones appear as lucent bands perpendicular to the cortex. Periosteal reaction occurs as they heal.*

show focal lesions representing Looser's zones and/or a generalized increase in bone uptake with reduced or absent renal activity (superscan).

HYPERPARATHYROIDISM

Hyperparathyroidism may be either primary (90 per cent of primary cases are due to adenomas) or secondary owing to renal dysfunction. Bone pain and tenderness occur in 10–25 per cent of patients.

Radiographically, skeletal abnormalities are seen in 50 per cent of cases. Skeletal manifestations include generalized osteopenia from excessive bone resorption. Subperiosteal resorption is a classic feature, affecting the radial aspects of the phalanges, especially the middle phalanx of the middle and index fingers, terminal tufts (acro-osteolysis) (Fig. 13.29) and medial cortices of the proximal humerus, femur and tibial shafts. Trabecular resorption is best seen in the diploë of the cranium, resulting in a characteristic 'pepperpot' skull. Subchondral resorption may result in subchondral collapse and sclerosis with apparent joint space widening. The sacroiliac, temporomandibular, acromioclavicular joints and the symphysis pubis are most commonly affected. Subligamentous resorption is especially seen in the pelvis and calcaneus.

In some patients, bone formation predominates over bone resorption, resulting in patchy or diffuse osteosclerosis. This is much commoner in secondary hyperparathyroidism.

Brown tumours are now an uncommon finding in primary hyperparathyroidism and represent localized accumulation of osteoclasts. Radiographically, they are lytic and expansile, but may become sclerotic after treatment.

Soft-tissue changes include chondrocalcinosis, periarticular, soft-tissue and vascular calcification most commonly seen in dialysis patients with secondary hyperparathyroidism.

Chronic renal failure results in a combination of bone abnormalities due to rickets/osteomalacia and secondary hyperparathyroidism, known as **renal osteodystrophy**. Also, patients on dialysis may develop bone changes secondary to aluminium poisoning and amyloid.

PAGET'S DISEASE

Paget's disease of bone is a condition of unknown aetiology, typically occurring after 40 years of age with a male predominance. Pathologically, there is simultaneous abnormal osteoclastic and osteoblastic activity, causing abnormal bone remodelling resulting in thickened, disorganized, fragile trabeculae. The condition is often asymptomatic but may cause local bone pain and

Figure 13.29 *Classic appearances of hyperparathyroidism in the hands, manifest as subperiosteal bone resorption predominantly on the radial side of the digit (fine arrows) and acro-osteolysis of the terminal tufts (arrow).*

a variety of other symptoms. Common sites of occurrence include the spine (75 per cent of cases), pelvis (70 per cent), cranium (65 per cent) and tubular bones (35 per cent).

Radiographically, there are three sequential stages, although they may coexist. Initially, there is a predominance of bone destruction. The second stage shows mixed lysis and sclerosis with gradual bony enlargement and deformity. In the third phase, there is further sclerosis with increasing enlargement and deformity.

In the initial phase, radiographs show a geographic area of bone lysis. In the skull, this lytic phase is termed **osteoporosis circumscripta** and usually involves the frontal or occipital areas. In long bones, the lysis typically commences in a subarticular region and extends with a flame-shaped leading margin into the diaphysis (Fig. 13.30). Rarely in the tibia, the disease may commence in the diaphysis.

Following the lytic phase, areas of sclerosis develop which, in the skull, produce a 'cotton-wool' appearance. In the long bones, sclerosis is due to a combination of cortical and trabecular thickening. In the pelvis, the initial manifestation is thickening of the iliopectineal line. This progresses to patchy or diffuse sclerosis, corti-

Figure 13.30 *Paget's disease of the proximal tibia. The disease starts at the articular surface and extends into the diaphysis with a 'flame-shaped' leading edge (arrow). Cortical and trabecular thickening are typical features.*

Figure 13.31 *Paget's disease of the left femur and left hemipelvis. There is marked cortical thickening and coarsening of trabeculae. The femur is bowed and multiple stress fractures are seen on the convex aspect of the shaft (arrows).*

cal thickening with loss of corticomedullary differentiation and enlargement of the bone. Deformities occur, since the bone is abnormally soft. This may result in bowing of long bones (Fig. 13.31), basilar invagination and protrusio acetabulae.

Complications of Paget's disease include stress fracture, osteoporosis (if immobilized), arthropathy and sarcomatous degeneration.

The **scintigraphic** appearances of Paget's disease are also characteristic, with marked increased activity in the involved bone (Fig. 13.32). Scintigraphy is useful in assessing response of the disease to treatment but may be insensitive at identifying stress fractures or sarcomatous change.

SCURVY

Scurvy is due to a deficiency of vitamin C, resulting in abnormal collagen formation. There is a tendency toward haemorrhage and abnormal bone formation. It is rarely seen before 6 months of age.

In the infant, subperiosteal haemorrhage raises the periosteum resulting in extensive subperiosteal bone formation. Abnormal bone formation affects particularly the costochondral junctions and ends of long bones. Radiographs demonstrate increased density and widening of the zone of provisional calcification (white line of Frankel), a dense epiphyseal rim (Wimberger's sign), metaphyseal spurs or corner fractures (Pelkan's sign) and generalized osteopenia.

Radiographic abnormalities in adults are limited to osteopenia and pathological fractures.

MISCELLANEOUS BONE DISORDERS

HAEMOPHILIA

Haemophilic arthropathy is considered in detail in the section on joints. The major non-arthropathic manifestation is the **haemophilic pseudotumour**, which occurs secondary to an intraosseous, subperiosteal or soft-tissue haemorrhage. The commonest sites are the femur, pelvis and tibia.

Radiographs demonstrate an extrinsic and/or intrinsic scalloping and pressure erosion of the affected bone

Figure 13.32 *⁹⁹ᵐTc-MDP bone scintigraphy in two patients showing characteristic features of Paget's disease. In the long bones, the disease starts in a subarticular location and spreads into the disphysis. In the flat bones and spine, the whole of the bone tends to be involved. Enlargement and deformity are also seen.*

Figure 13.33 *Typical features of thalassaemia in the hands with expansion of the tubular bones, generalized osteopenia and thinning of the cortices.*

with sharp, sclerotic margins. Other features include a soft-tissue mass and periosteal reaction. As the name implies, this lesion is readily confused radiographically with an aggressive tumour.

SICKLE CELL ANAEMIA AND THALASSAEMIA

Both conditions can result in similar bony abnormalities. Chronic anaemia results in marrow hyperplasia, which manifests as osteopenia with coarsened trabeculae, widening of the tubular bones (Fig. 13.33), ribs, mandible and diploic spaces of the skull. Such changes are most spectacular in thalassaemia major. Conversely, osteonecrosis, owing to vascular occlusion, is more commonly seen in sickle cell disease (HbSS). Sites of involvement include the small tubular bones of the hands and feet, producing a dactylitis in 10–20 per cent of cases, diaphyses of long bones, vertebral end-plates and femoral and humeral heads. There is also a predilection for osteomyelitis, which may be indistinguishable from osteonecrosis. Staphylococcal infection is commonest, but an increased incidence of salmonella

osteomyelitis is recognized. Patients with sickle cell trait (HbAS) have very few musculoskeletal manifestations, but bone infarcts are occasionally seen.

Sickle cell haemoglobin C disease (HbSC) is associated with marrow hyperplasia of the skull and avascular necrosis.

Chronic anaemia owing to **hereditary spherocytosis** or **iron deficiency** is rarely associated with radiographic bone changes. Occasionally, widening of the diploic spaces is seen, usually in children or infants.

Bone infarction is also an occasional complication of **polycythaemia rubra vera**, resulting from increased blood viscosity from the excessive red cell mass.

The marrow hyperplasia or reconversion that occurs in chronic anaemic states is most sensitively demonstrated by MRI as either diffuse or focal areas of medullary low signal on both T1- and T2-weighted spin-echo sequences.

MYELOFIBROSIS

Myelofibrosis is a primary disease of marrow resulting in fibrosis of areas of the skeleton normally involved in haematopoiesis. This stimulates reconversion of fatty marrow in long tubular bones to red marrow, which subsequently becomes involved in the fibrotic process. The radiographic features include bone marrow sclerosis, seen in 40 per cent of cases, or patchy increased density with cortical thickening in the involved regions (usually spine, pelvis and ribs). The marrow fibrosis will be manifest on MRI as diffuse or patchy areas of reduced signal on all pulse sequences.

MASTOCYTOSIS

Mastocytosis is a rare proliferative disorder of mast cells. Bone abnormalities include generalized or, rarely, focal osteoporosis owing to histamine release, and focal or, rarely, generalized osteosclerosis from the host response to marrow infiltration.

GAUCHER'S DISEASE

Gaucher's disease is a sphingolipid storage disorder resulting in accumulation of Gaucher cells in the reticuloendothelial system and marrow. The commonest form is seen in children and young adults. Bone abnormalities include expansion of the distal femur, the so-called Erlenmeyer flask deformity, and osteonecrosis, especially of the femoral head. Generalized osteoporosis with vertebral end-plate fractures, marrow infarctions and focal lytic areas are also seen. There is an increased susceptibility to osteomyelitis.

SARCOIDOSIS

Sarcoidosis is a systemic granulomatous disorder of unknown aetiology that affects the bones in 1–15 per cent of cases. Bone involvement in most cases occurs only in the presence of lung and skin lesions. The skeletal manifestations are varied and include generalized osteopenia. Focal lytic lesions with lace-like trabeculae are seen, usually in the middle and distal phalanges, whereas the terminal tufts may show sclerosis. A focal or generalized osteosclerosis is also recognized. The associated clinically apparent arthropathy usually shows no radiographic abnormality.

RADIATION-INDUCED DISORDERS

Radiotherapy is reported to cause a variety of skeletal disorders, including radiation osteitis and osteonecrosis, neoplasia and growth disorders.

In cases of **radiation-induced osteitis** and **osteonecrosis**, the initial radiographic changes may be limited to local osteoporosis. In the later stages of frank osteonecrosis, which usually requires a latent period of several years, local increased bone density containing multiple, small, lytic areas is the characteristic finding. Such bone is brittle and is liable to spontaneous pathological fracture, which is the usual mode of presentation. Calcification in the adjacent soft tissues is common. Typical sites of fracture include the upper humerus and upper ribs following treatment for breast cancer, and the pelvis and proximal femora after treatment for pelvic malignancies.

Large focal osteolytic areas may also occur secondary to radiotherapy and may be confused with osteolytic metastases.

Radiation-induced sarcoma is also a well-recognized, although uncommon, complication. The majority of early cases were due to radiotherapy as a treatment for various benign bone lesions, but now most cases are due to the incidental irradiation of bone during treatment of a primary soft-tissue malignancy. There is usually a latent period of at least 4 years. The commonest radiation-induced sarcoma is osteosarcoma and the tumour has no characteristic radiological features to differentiate it from spontaneous osteosarcoma, although evidence of radiation osteitis may be present.

Growing bone at sites of endochondral ossification is particularly radiosensitive. Radiotherapy may therefore produce various growth disorders because of premature epiphyseal fusion, including limb length inequalities and scoliosis.

JOINTS

OSTEOARTHRITIS

Osteoarthritis is the commonest joint disease and is characterized pathologically by non-inflammatory cartilage loss accompanied by new bone formation. It may be either primary (where no previous joint pathology is identified) or secondary to a number of predisposing causes, including trauma, inflammatory arthropathy and osteonecrosis.

The **radiological manifestations** of primary and secondary osteoarthritis, however, are essentially the same. Cartilage loss is always present and tends to be focal, typically in the primary weight-bearing portion of the joint. It is manifest radiographically as reduction in joint space. Erosive changes are not seen, whereas new bone formation, stimulated by abnormal mechanical forces, is common and manifests as osteophyte formation, subchondral sclerosis and cortical buttressing. Osteophytes are small bony protuberances that are in continuity with the underlying medullary cavity and typically occur at the joint margins, though they may be intra-articular. Subchondral sclerosis manifests as focal increased bone density immediately deep to the articular surface. Cortical buttressing is particularly evident along the medial aspect of the neck of femur and appears as thickening of the cortex. Subchondral cyst formation is also common. Cysts usually occur in weight-bearing areas and have thin, sclerotic margins. intra-articular osteocartilaginous loose bodies are also a relatively common finding. The periarticular bone density is typically preserved.

Soft-tissue abnormalities are not a prominent finding, although chondrocalcinosis can occur. Joint deformities owing to osteoarthritis may result in secondary ligamentous abnormalities, such as contractures and laxity, which may produce instability and further degenerative changes.

The common joints involved in primary osteoarthritis are the distal interphalangeal and proximal interphalangeal joints of the hand, the first carpometacarpal and scaphoid–trapezium–trapezoid articulations of the wrist, the hip, knee and first metatarsophalangeal joint. Involvement of the lower cervical spine and lumbar facet joints is also common.

In the **hand**, **Heberden's** and **Bouchard's nodes** refer to osteophytes at the distal and proximal interphalangeal joints, respectively. The metacarpophalangeal joints are less commonly involved. In the **wrist**, involvement of the first carpometacarpal joint may result in radial subluxation of the thumb.

In the **hip**, cartilage loss is usually focal with superior or superolateral migration of the femoral head in 80 per cent of cases. Medial migration with associated protrusio acetabulae is seen in 20 per cent of cases and should suggest the possibility of underlying inflammatory disease, such as rheumatoid arthritis. Typical sites of osteophyte formation are the lateral margin of the acetabulum and in the lateral and medial subcapital region. Subchondral cyst formation is particularly well seen in the weight-bearing portion of the acetabulum. As mentioned previously, cortical buttressing of the medial femoral neck is a classic feature (Fig. 13.34). Superior flattening of the femoral head may occur in advanced disease, simulating osteonecrosis.

In the **knee**, any of the three joint compartments may be involved, in isolation or in various combinations. Medial compartment disease is commonest and may be associated with a varus deformity and lateral subluxation of the tibia. Patellofemoral osteoarthritis usually involves the lateral facet, and may be associated with lateral compartment disease and relative sparing of the medial compartment. Osteophytes may be identified arising from the tibial spines. Osteocartilaginous loose bodies are particularly common in the knee.

Osteoarthritis of the elbow, shoulder and ankle is uncommon and usually secondary to trauma or rheumatoid disease.

Erosive osteoarthritis is an arthropathy seen most commonly in middle-aged women who experience distinct inflammatory episodes, with red, swollen joints similar to rheumatoid arthritis. The distal and proximal

Figure 13.34 *Classic appearances of primary osteoarthritis of the hip with superolateral joint space narrowing, marginal osteophytosis, subarticular sclerosis and cyst formation (short arrow) and cortical buttressing of the medial neck of the femur (long arrow).*

interphalangeal joints are involved. Radiographs show loss of joint space, subchondral sclerosis, erosions which tend to be central in the joint, and marginal osteophytes. The appearance may progress to ankylosis. Typical osteoarthritis of the first carpometacarpal and scaphoid–trapezium–trapezoid articulation in the wrist help to differentiate the condition from psoriatic arthropathy.

INFLAMMATORY ARTHROPATHIES

The inflammatory arthropathies comprise a group of disorders that are characterized by synovial inflammation (of unknown aetiology) which results in cartilage destruction and cortical bony erosion. They may be subdivided into seropositive (rheumatoid arthritis, some juvenile chronic arthritides) and seronegative (psoriatic arthritis, Reiter's disease, ankylosing spondylitis, enteropathic arthritis) arthropathies. Since the underlying pathology is similar, the radiographic manifestations at a particular joint are similar, with the pattern of joint involvement being an important factor in differential diagnosis.

The cardinal radiographic signs of inflammatory arthropathies are periarticular soft-tissue swelling, loss of joint space, periarticular osteopenia, marginal erosions and, later, joint deformity and generalized osteopenia (Fig. 13.35).

The initial radiographic abnormality is periarticular soft-tissue swelling, which is due to a combination of synovial inflammation, oedema and effusion. Loss of joint space, which tends to be relatively uniform, is due to cartilage destruction by hypertrophied, inflamed

Figure 13.35 *Classic features of inflammatory arthropathy. There is periarticular soft-tissue swelling (white arrows), joint space narrowing and marginal erosions (black arrows).*

synovium (termed 'pannus'). Periarticular osteopenia is a manifestation of the acute stage of the disease and is due to hyperaemia. Erosions are initially manifest as loss of the fine white line of the articular cortex. Larger erosions tend to occur later and are located at joint margins where the bone is not covered by articular cartilage, commonly near capsular or ligamentous attachments. Erosions are due to the direct effect of pannus. Later in the disease, joint deformities occur due to laxity of supporting structures and eventually fibrosis. With chronic disuse, generalized osteopenia is seen; this may be accentuated by steroid therapy.

RHEUMATOID ARTHRITIS

Rheumatoid arthritis is the commonest of the inflammatory arthropathies. Onset is usually in young or middle-aged adults with females affected two to three times more commonly than males. Rheumatoid factor is positive in 90–95 per cent of cases. Extra-articular manifestations include subcutaneous or tendon-sheath nodules, tenosynovitis or bursitis, pleural effusions, rheumatoid pulmonary nodules and diffuse interstitial fibrosis.

The **radiographic findings** are as described above. In addition, subchondral cysts may be seen, particularly in the hips and knees. These are continuous with the synovium and tend not to have sclerotic borders. Juxta-articular synovial cysts are also a recognized feature and are well imaged with ultrasound or MRI. Bony ankylosis is a rare feature, limited to the carpus and tarsus.

Any synovial joint may be involved by rheumatoid arthritis, although there is a predilection for certain sites. The disease is characteristically a symmetrical polyarthritis.

In the **hand**, the metacarpophalangeal and proximal interphalangeal joints are involved early with relative sparing of the distal interphalangeal joints. Characteristic deformities are ulnar deviation and volar subluxation at the metacarpophalangeal joints (Fig. 13.36),

Figure 13.36 *Typical features of long-standing rheumatoid arthritis in the hand with ulnar deviation at the metacarpophalangeal joints, 'hitch-hiker's thumb' deformity, ulnar translocation of the carpus and erosion of the ulnar styloid.*

hyperextension at the proximal interphalangeal joints and hyperflexion at the distal interphalangeal joints (**swan-neck deformity**) or, conversely, hyperflexion at the proximal interphalangeal joints and hyperextension at the distal interphalangeal joints (**Boutonnière deformity**). First metacarpophalangeal joint flexion with interphalangeal joint extension (**hitchhiker's thumb**) is also seen. In the **wrist**, early erosions are seen at the distal radioulnar joint, radial and ulnar styloids, scaphoid waist, triquetrum and pisiform. Intercarpal changes occur later. Wrist deformities include ulnar translocations of the carpus, where more than 50 per cent of the lunate articulates with the ulna, radial deviation of the hand, scapholunate dissociation and other patterns of carpal instability.

In the **shoulder** girdle, early changes include erosions of the distal end of the clavicle, the insertion of the coracoclavicular ligament and marginal erosions at the humeral head. Later signs are those of rotator cuff tear, with elevation of the humeral head and concavity of the undersurface of the acromion.

In the **foot**, erosive changes typically affect the metatarsophalangeal joints. Associated abnormalities include lateral deviation and/or hyperextension at the metatarsophalangeal joint, and flexion of the proximal or distal interphalangeal joints (**hammer toes**). Intertarsal erosions are a late finding. Calcaneal spurs and retrocalcaneal bursitis are also recognized findings. Involvement of the ankle is relatively uncommon.

In the **knee**, suprapatellar effusions and **popliteal (Baker's) cysts** are characteristic soft-tissue abnormalities. There tends to be symmetrical involvement of all three joint compartments, unlike osteoarthritis. The commonest deformity is a valgus knee.

In the **hip**, again uniform joint space loss helps to distinguish rheumatoid from osteoarthritis. Protrusio acetabulae is also seen.

JUVENILE CHRONIC ARTHRITIS

Juvenile chronic arthritis comprises a group of disorders that includes the various forms of juvenile rheumatoid arthritis and juvenile ankylosing spondylitis. Psoriatic and inflammatory bowel disease associated arthropathies may also be seen in children.

Juvenile rheumatoid arthritis

This disease complex includes Still's disease (~ 20 per cent), pauciarticular disease (~ 40 per cent), seronegative polyarticular disease (~ 25 per cent) and seropositive polyarticular disease (~ 5 per cent).

Still's disease is an acute systemic illness occurring in children under 5 years of age. The polyarthritis is accompanied by a fever, anaemia, hepatosplenomegaly and lymphadenopathy. In the acute stage, radiographic changes may be minimal, but 25 per cent progress to chronic destructive arthritis. **Pauciarticular juvenile rheumatoid arthritis** usually occurs in young girls. One to three joints are involved, usually knee, ankle or elbow, and chronic iridocyclitis occurs in 25 per cent of cases.

Seronegative polyarticular juvenile rheumatoid arthritis is also commoner in females. Both small and large joints are affected in a symmetrical fashion.

Seropositive polyarticular juvenile rheumatoid arthritis is generally found in teenage girls. Polyarticular changes typical of adult rheumatoid arthritis are seen.

The radiographic features are similar in all forms of juvenile rheumatoid arthritis. Soft-tissue changes include muscle wasting and fusiform periarticular swelling. Hyperaemia and disuse lead to osteoporosis, and metaphyseal lucent lines may be seen during active disease. Periosteal reaction is also an early manifestation. Later findings include loss of joint space owing to cartilage destruction, erosive changes and ankylosis, most commonly in the carpus and interphalangeal joints. Joint deformity from ligamentous rupture is common.

Figure 13.37 *Juvenile rheumatoid arthritis affecting the right knee, manifesting as enlargement of the epiphyses and intercondylar notch (arrow). Similar changes may be seen with haemophilic arthropathy and tuberculous arthritis and are due to chronic hyperaemia and synovitis.*

Chronic hyperaemia results in overgrowth of the epiphyses leading to enlargement of the joints involved (Fig. 13.37), and squaring of the carpal and tarsal bones and of the patella. Advanced skeletal maturation results in premature fusion, limb length deformities and overall shortening of limbs. Chronic synovitis also produces distinctive changes, including enlargement of the trochlear notch of the elbow and intercondylar notch of the knee. In the hip, coxa valga and protrusio acetabulae are seen. Hypoplasia of the iliac wings and small size of the femoral shaft may make prosthetic replacement difficult. Spinal disease is also common, as is involvement of the temporomandibular joint, leading to micrognathia.

Juvenile ankylosing spondylitis

This results in bilateral symmetrical sacroiliac joint and lumbar spine changes in adolescent males. However, other joints, particularly the hips, may be involved prior to sacroiliac joint disease, delaying the diagnosis. Also, diagnostic difficulty arises due to the appearance of normal sacroiliac joints in adolescents, which are wide with indistinct cortices.

ANKYLOSING SPONDYLITIS

Ankylosing spondylitis is the commonest of the seronegative inflammatory spondyloarthropathies, involving primarily the sacroiliac joints, spine and large joints. It is commoner in males (4–10:1/male:female ratio) and usually presents at ages 15–35 years. More than 90 per cent of patients are HLA-B27 positive.

Figure 13.38 *Ankylosing spondylitis involving the left hip. There is concentric loss of joint space, typifying an inflammatory arthropathy, and early osteophyte formation.*

- symmetric polyarthritis resembling rheumatoid arthritis;
- oligoarthritis;
- spondyloarthropathy, occurring in 30–50 per cent of patients with psoriatic arthritis.

The joints commonly involved are the small joints of the hands and feet. In the **hands**, the interphalangeal joints, together with the intercarpal joints, are involved, commonly in an asymmetrical pattern. Terminal tuft resorption is also a feature. In the **foot**, the interphalangeal and metatarsophalangeal joints are predominantly involved. Associated retrocalcaneal bursitis and erosions at the insertions of the Achilles tendon and plantar aponeurosis are seen. In 30–50 per cent of cases the sacroiliac joints are involved and spondylitis is also a feature. Involvement of larger joints is much less common.

Characteristic **radiographic features** include fusiform soft-tissue swelling, leading to a 'sausage' digit if the whole finger is involved. Bone density is generally normal. Early erosions are marginal in location but may progress to the subchondral regions, occasionally producing a 'pencil-in-cup' deformity (Fig. 13.39).

Extra-articular manifestations include iritis, aortic incompetence and upper lobe pulmonary fibrosis.

In addition to spinal and sacroiliac joint changes, (*see* Fig. 3.67, p. 90), involvement of the large joints is relatively common. Up to 50 per cent of patients have hip involvement with concentric loss of joint space owing to chondrolysis, mild erosions, protrusio acetabulae and ring osteophytes (Fig. 13.38). Bilateral but asymmetric involvement may be seen. The glenohumeral joint, symphysis pubis, sternomanubrial joint and costovertebral joints are also relatively commonly involved. Joint ankylosis is a late complication. Other radiographic features include enthesopathy, namely the development of bony spurs at sites of ligamentous and tendinous attachments which is particularly common in the pelvis, calcaneum and patella.

PSORIATIC ARTHRITIS

Psoriatic arthritis occurs in 0.5–25 per cent of patients with psoriasis. It generally occurs in young patients with skin disease, but joints may be affected prior to skin changes in 20 per cent of patients. Five distinct forms are described:

- polyarthritis predominantly of distal interphalangeal joints;
- arthritis mutilans (deforming type);

Figure 13.39 *Psoriatic arthritis affecting the hand. Bone density is generally preserved. There is periarticular soft-tissue swelling and central erosion, resulting in a 'pencil-in-cup' deformity (arrow).*

Figure 13.40 *Reiter's disease affecting the calcaneus, manifesting as erosion at the Achilles tendon insertion (white arrow) and plantar aponeurosis (black arrow).*

Periosteal reaction and, later, joint ankylosis are also features.

REITER'S DISEASE

Reiter's disease is a syndrome consisting of non-specific urethritis (cervicitis in females) in 85 per cent of cases, conjunctivitis in 60 per cent and arthritis. It typically affects young males, with extra-articular manifestations usually occurring initially. The joint involvement is predominantly distal lower limb (Fig. 13.40). Spondylo-arthropathy identical to that of psoriasis is seen in 10–40 per cent of cases. The radiographic abnormalities in the joints are similar to those described for psoriatic arthritis.

ENTEROPATHIC ARTHROPATHY

Sacroiliitis and spondylitis identical to that of ankylosing spondylitis may accompany ulcerative colitis, Crohn's disease and Whipple's disease. Peripheral joint disease is unusual and limited to a mild synovitis with osteopenia, often occurring in conjunction with exacerbation of the bowel disease. Erosive arthritis is rare.

CRYSTAL DEPOSITION DISEASES

GOUT

Gout is a disease caused by the intra-articular and periarticular deposition of monosodium urate crystals secondary to chronic hyperuricaemia. The latter may be idiopathic, secondary to enzyme defects or chronic diseases such as myeloproliferative disorders, renal disease and diuretic therapy.

Acute attacks usually begin in the fourth decade and typically affect the first metatarsophalangeal joint. No radiographic abnormalities may be seen apart from osteopenia and soft-tissue swelling. The classic **radiographic findings** of chronic tophaceous gout occur after several years, namely the development of deposits of sodium urate crystals within soft tissues (**tophi**), commonly within the olecranon bursa and adjacent to joints. The tophi typically appear as non-mineralized soft-tissue masses that occasionally calcify. Tophi may also be intraosseous, appearing as subchondral lucent lesions. Bony erosions may be intra-articular, typically eccentrically located at the joint margin, or extra-articular, related to overlying soft-tissue tophi. The erosions have well-defined sclerotic margins and an overhanging edge is characteristic (Fig. 13.41). The bone density is usually preserved and loss of joint space is only a late feature owing to the development of secondary osteoarthritis. Chondrocalcinosis is rare but is a recognized finding.

The commonest joints involved are the first metatarsophalangeal joint and, to a lesser extent, the other

Figure 13.41 *Chronic tophaceous gout of the hand showing multiple calcified tophi and erosions with sclerotic margins and characteristic overhanging edges (arrow).*

small joints of the foot. Involvement of the hand, wrist, knee, elbow and, occasionally, sacroiliac joints is also seen.

CALCIUM PYROPHOSPHATE DIHYDRATE (CPPD) CRYSTAL DEPOSITION DISEASE

This condition results from the intra-articular deposition of CPPD crystals. It may manifest as chondrocalcinosis (cartilage calcification) or pyrophosphate arthropathy. The condition is seen in the middle-aged and elderly population and is usually idiopathic.

It presents in several ways, the commonest being as pseudogout (acute self-limiting attacks resembling gout or infection) or a chronic progressive arthropathy with exacerbations. In 10–20 per cent of patients there are no symptoms. Rarely, a rapidly destructive arthritis simulating neuropathic arthropathy may occur. Joint aspiration may yield CPPD crystals.

Radiographic findings include chondrocalcinosis, which occurs in both the articular hyaline cartilage and in the fibrocartilaginous structures, such as the menisci of the knee and triangular fibrocartilage in the wrist. Common sites include the knee, wrist, symphysis pubis and acetabular labrum. CPPD crystals may also be deposited in synovium, capsule, tendons and ligaments. The disease resembles osteoarthritis with loss of joint space, osteophytes, subchondral sclerosis and osteochondral fragments. Subchondral cysts are common and may be very large, simulating neoplasm.

The major differentiating feature from classic osteoarthritis is the specific pattern of joint involvement. In the **knee**, the patellofemoral joint is typically involved with relative sparing of the femorotibial compartments (Fig. 13.42). In the **wrist**, the radiocarpal joint is involved and may be associated with scapholunate dissociation and proximal migration of the capitate. In the hand, the second and third meta-

carpophalangeal joints are typically involved. The hip, shoulder and elbow are less common sites of disease. Severe degenerative changes in the spine may also occur.

In patients with **haemochromatosis** 50 per cent develop an arthropathy due to CPPD crystal deposition. The pattern of joint involvement and radiographic features are very similar to those of pyrophosphate arthropathy. Beak-like osteophytes from the second and third metacarpal heads, osteoporosis, extra-articular manifestations and a younger age of onset favour the diagnosis of haemochromatosis.

Other conditions associated with CPPD crystal deposition and chondrocalcinosis include osteoarthritis, trauma, gout, hyperparthyroidism, Wilson's disease and ochronosis.

CALCIUM HYDROXYAPATITE DEPOSITION DISEASE

Calcium hydroxyapatite deposition disease is due to the periarticular deposition of hydroxyapatite crystals. It is usually monoarticular and presents as joint pain in a middle to elderly age group. The commonest joint involved is the shoulder. Other sites include the elbow, wrist and MCP joints.

Radiographs typically demonstrate cloudy or homogeneous periarticular calcification in tendons, ligaments, capsules and bursae, with a normal underlying joint (Fig. 13.43).

Figure 13.43 *Calcium hydroxyapatite deposition in the supraspinatus tendon (arrow) (calcific tendinitis). The underlying joint is normal.*

Figure 13.42 *Calcium pyrophosphate dihydrate deposition disease of the knee. Patellofemoral osteoarthritis predominates. There is calcification of the synovium and menisci.*

Plate 13 *(left) (Chapter 25, page 628) Duplex ultrasound scan showing the bifurcation of a normal common carotid artery into the internal and external carotid arteries.*

(a)

(b)

Plate 14 *(Chapter 25, page 635) Arterial occlusion shown with colour Doppler ultrasound. (a) Start of the occluded segment. No flow is visible in the occlusion (upper arrows). The presence of a large collateral (lower arrow) is useful confirmation of occlusion. (b) Lower end of the occluded segment. Collateral vessels are visible (arrow) supplying blood to the open vessel beyond the block. (c) Spectral Doppler ultrasound from the patent vessel beyond the occlusion, showing marked reduction in peak velocity and damping of the velocity waveform. (Compare with the normal femoral artery flow pattern in Plate 2.)*

(c)

Plate 15 *(Chapter 25, page 635) Duplex ultrasound scan showing a colour change from red to blue in a femoropopliteal vein graft due to turbulent flow at the site of a significant stenosis.*

Plate 16 *(Chapter 25, page 635) Duplex ultrasound scan showing a fistula in a femoropopliteal vein graft.*

Plate 17 *(Chapter 27, page 666) Colour Doppler ultrasound showing the normal confluence of the profunda femoris (PFV) and superficial femoral (SFV) veins. The superficial femoral artery is also shown (SFA).*

Plate 18 *(Chapter 27, page 668) Thrombus in the common femoral vein. Colour Doppler ultrasound in the same patient as in Figure 27.8. The thrombus is outlined by blood flow into the common femoral vein from the long saphenous vein (curved arrows).*

Plate 19 *(right) (Chapter 27, page 669) Colour Doppler ultrasound in calf vein thrombosis. Paired posterior tibial veins (V) are seen on either side of the posterior tibial artery (A). Flow is absent from one vein (arrows) due to thrombosis.*

Plate 20a *(Chapter 27, page 671) Long saphenous vein incompetence. At rest, flow (represented as blue) in the long saphenous vein is towards the heart.*

Plate 20b *(Chapter 27, page 671) When the patient performs a Valsalva manoeuvre, the flow reverses in direction, the representation then changing to orange, confirming venous incompetence.*

Figure 13.49 *Hypertrophic form of neuropathic arthropathy with increased bone density, periarticular bony fragments and a Lisfranc-type tarsometatarsal dislocation.*

disease is usually monoarticular, the joint affected depending upon the underlying cause. Diabetes, syringomyelia, tabes dorsalis and leprosy are common causes. Clinically, the patient presents with a swollen, unstable but pain-free joint.

The radiographic features depend upon whether the arthropathy is predominantly **hypertrophic** (20 per cent), **atrophic** (40 per cent) or **mixed** (40 per cent). The typical features of the hypertrophic variety are increased bone density, swelling, multiple periarticular bony fragments and a disorganized, dislocated joint (Fig. 13.49). The atrophic variety manifests as relatively well-defined bone resorption adjacent to the joint.

The commonest joints involved include the talo-navicular and tarsometatarsal joints in diabetes (usually atrophic or mixed type), the shoulder in syringomyelia (almost always atrophic) and the knee in tabes dorsalis (usually hypertrophic).

An important differential diagnosis of atrophic neuroarthropathy is septic arthritis. The distinction may be particularly difficult in the diabetic foot.

HAEMOPHILIC ARTHROPATHY

Haemophilia is a bleeding disorder caused by deficiency of Factor VIII (haemophilia A) or Factor IX (haemophilia B). The condition is only found in males since it is an X-linked recessive disorder. Joint changes are a consequence of recurrent haemarthroses which result in synovitis and chronic hyperaemia. The synovitis manifests as soft-tissue swelling, which may appear relatively dense due to haemosiderin deposition in the synovium. Hyperaemia in turn results in osteoporosis, epiphyseal overgrowth and early epiphyseal fusion, resulting in short bones.

Cartilage destruction, erosions and subchondral cysts are also seen and secondary osteoarthritis eventually develops. The commonest joints involved are the knee, elbow, ankle, hip and shoulder. The radiographic appearances are similar to those seen in juvenile rheumatoid arthritis.

HYPERTROPHIC OSTEOARTHROPATHY

Hypertrophic osteoarthropathy is a condition of unknown aetiology that presents as an arthropathy but manifests radiologically as symmetrical periosteal reaction along the distal borders of the radius and ulna and tibia and fibula (Fig. 13.50), and occasionally affects the digits. The condition is associated with a variety of

Figure 13.50 *Hypertrophic osteoarthropathy manifesting as fine linear periosteal reaction along the distal tibia and fibula.*

Figure 13.51 *Loosening of both acetabular and femoral components of a left total hip replacement, manifesting as lucency at the cement–bone interface and subsidence of the femoral stem.*

intrathoracic and abdominal diseases, the commonest being carcinoma of the bronchus.

EVALUATION OF JOINT PROSTHESES

Causes of a painful hip prosthesis include infection, mechanical loosening and heterotopic ossification. The latter condition manifests as well-developed bone, bridging the space between the greater trochanter and lateral margin of the acetabulum.

Difficulties arise in the differentiation between **septic** and **mechanical** loosening. Plain **radiographic features** of loosening include increasing radiolucency at the cement–bone interface and change of position of the components with time (Fig. 13.51), cement fracture and cystic resorption of bone around the femoral component. The presence of periosteal reaction or large amounts of heterotopic ossification are suggestive of infection.

⁹⁹ᵐTc-MDP bone scintigraphy has been used extensively to detect loosening and infection. The bone scan remains 'hot' for about 9–12 months postoperatively, then activity gradually subsides. Increased activity at the tip and adjacent to the neck of a femoral prosthesis may

be seen with mechanical loosening, whereas infection tends to result in generalized increase in uptake. However, the lack of specificity or these findings reduces the value of routine bone scanning. Increased sensitivity and specificity for infection may be obtained using gallium or labelled white cell scanning.

CT and MRI have no role to play in the assessment of a painful prosthesis because of the artefact caused by the metal implant.

The most specific preoperative technique for diagnosing infection and loosening is the arthrogram, which can confirm loosening by identifying contrast medium within lucent spaces at the cement–bone interface. Aspiration of the joint prior to contrast injection may identify infected prostheses.

OSTEONECROSIS AND THE OSTEOCHONDROSES

Osteonecrosis and the osteochondroses are considered here because they frequently present with pain or abnormality related to joints.

OSTEONECROSIS

Osteonecrosis is a term that signifies death of bone due to interruption of blood supply in the absence of infection. When a subarticular site is involved, the term 'avascular necrosis' has been used, whereas the term 'bone infarct' has been used for osteonecrosis involving the metaphysis or diaphysis.

The loss of blood supply may be idiopathic or due to trauma, vascular thrombosis or obstruction, or vascular compression. Other causes include corticosteroid therapy, sickle cell disease, Gaucher's disease, pregnancy, causes of fat embolism (including alcohol and pancreatitis) and caisson disease. The commoner sites of involvement include the femoral and humeral heads, the scaphoid, lunate, talus and shafts of long bones. Idiopathic osteonecrosis is a specific condition usually involving the femoral head or medial femoral condyle.

The plain **radiographic** features of osteonecrosis are characteristic. In a subarticular site, the findings include an arc-like subchondral lucent line (the 'crescent' sign), which progresses to patchy sclerosis and lysis, cyst formation and eventually collapse of the articular surface (Fig. 13.52). Initially, there is preservation of the joint space but secondary osteoarthritis may complicate femoral head collapse.

Metaphyseal bone infarcts typically appear as poorly defined lucent areas with peripheral sclerosis that do not expand the bone (Fig. 13.53), whereas osteonecrosis affecting smaller bones, such as the scaphoid or

Figure 13.52 *Osteonecrosis of the femoral head. There is subarticular sclerosis and cyst formation (arrow). The joint space is maintained.*

Figure 13.53 *Typical appearances of medullary bone infarct in the distal tibia identified as a region of peripheral serpiginous calcification. Absence of endosteal cortical erosion is a typical feature.*

lunate, results in mixed sclerosis and lysis with eventual collapse (Fig. 13.54). These changes occur several months after the onset of symptoms and plain radiographs are therefore insensitive for the detection of early disease.

Bone scintigraphy is far more sensitive and will be abnormal in the presence of normal radiographs. Initially, there may be an area of diminished uptake but this is followed within weeks by increased activity. **CT** is also more sensitive than plain radiographs, but it has now been replaced by **MRI**, which is currently the most sensitive technique for imaging osteonecrosis. Within days there is poorly defined reduced signal intensity on T1-weighted scans and increased signal intensity on T2-weighted scans from oedema associated with acute infarction. This is, however, a non-specific pattern and must be correlated with clinical findings. The MRI findings in chronic infarction are much more characteristic.

Early detection of osteonecrosis of the femoral head by MRI or scintigraphy, at a time when radiographs are normal, allows treatment with core decompression, which may prevent progression to collapse and secondary osteoarthritis.

Figure 13.54 *Osteonecrosis of the lunate (Kienböck's disease). There is mixed sclerosis and lysis with early collapse of the distal articular surface.*

THE OSTEOCHONDROSES

The osteochondroses comprise a heterogeneous group of conditions that are characterized by involvement, typically in children, of an epiphysis, apophysis or growth plate. The aetiology may be ischaemic, traumatic, either single or repetitive, or due to chronic stress. It is also recognized that some conditions included in this group are normal variants of ossification, e.g. Sever's disease of the calcaneus.

Each of the conditions discussed below appears to be associated with an abnormality of endochondral ossification. Radiologically, they are characterized by fragmentation, collapse, sclerosis and, frequently, gradual re-ossification.

Legg–Calve–Perthes' disease

This condition affects the femoral capital epiphysis. It is a true infarction, usually occurring in the 4–8-year-old age range when the vascular supply to the femoral head is most at risk. It is commoner in boys and bilateral in 10 per cent of cases, although usually there is asymmetrical involvement. The first radiographic sign may be a joint effusion. The initial bony abnormality is the presence of a subchondral lucent line, best seen on a frog-leg lateral view since it involves the superolateral aspect of the femoral head. Progression leads to fragmentation, sclerosis and collapse of the femoral head. Metaphyseal cyst formation and irregularity of the acetabulum are also features.

With healing, there is resorption of dead bone and gradual reossification of the femoral head. Coxa magna and coxa vara may eventually result.

A poorer prognosis is seen in children presenting at an older age and in girls (who are skeletally more mature). Another poor prognostic sign is lateral extrusion of the femoral head ossification centre, when bone fragments are seen lateral to the acetabular rim. This indicates lack of coverage of the femoral head, leading to incongruity between the head and acetabulum (Fig. 13.55). Surgical treatment is aimed at containing the femoral head within the acetabulum to allow optimal development of the head as the child grows. Prior to surgery, hip arthrography is of value in determining the position of maximum congruity and stability. It will also show that the overlying articular cartilage is intact.

The differential diagnosis of Perthes' disease includes other causes of ischaemic necrosis, such as Gaucher's disease and sickle-cell disease, and other causes of fragmented epiphyses, such as hypothyroidism and multiple epiphyseal dysplasia.

Freiberg's disease

This disease is also a true necrosis, usually involving the second or third metatarsal heads (less commonly, the first and fourth). It is usually seen in teenage females.

Köhler's disease

A dense, fragmented tarsal navicular may be a normal variant of ossification. Therefore, Köhler's disease should only be suggested when there is fragmentation of a previously normal bone in association with pain.

Osgood–Schlatter's disease

Osgood–Schlatter's disease is thought to be due to traumatic avulsion of the tibial tubercle. The diagnosis is made clinically. Radiographs show soft-tissue swelling and fragmentation of the tibial tubercle.

Sinding–Larsen–Johanssen's disease

This entity is due to traumatic avulsion of the inferior pole of the patella.

Blount's disease

Blount's disease is due to involvement of the medial aspect of the proximal tibial epiphysis growth plate with resulting varus deformity of the knee. The commoner infantile type occurs from a worsening of the normal physiological bowing of the lower extremity with weight-bearing. The increased pressure results in fragmentation of the medial aspect of the metaphysis, which causes epiphyseal deformity. More than 50 per cent of cases are bilateral.

Normal variants of ossification that simulate osteochondroses occur at the lateral femoral condyle posteriorly, calcaneal apophysis, trochlea, lateral epicondyle and ischiopubic synchondrosis.

Figure 13.55 *Typical features of Perthes' disease of the left femoral head. The epiphysis is fragmented, flattened and sclerotic. Lateral extrusion is a poor prognostic sign (arrow).*

DEVELOPMENTAL DYSPLASIA OF THE HIP (DDH)

Hip instability in the neonatal period is a relatively common clinical finding. However, in 75–95 per cent of cases, the hip will become stable within a few weeks. The incidence of DDH after the neonatal period is approximately 1:1000.

Radiography in the neonatal period, before ossification of the femoral capital epiphysis, has now been replaced by **ultrasound** which can demonstrate the dysplasia of the acetabular roof and the degree of coverage of the femoral head. Also, because imaging can be performed in real-time, subluxation or dislocation of the femoral head can be viewed directly. Ultrasound becomes difficult after approximately 6–9 months of age, when ossification begins in the femoral head.

Radiographic signs include slanting of the acetabular roof and acetabular anteversion and, in established dislocation, superior and lateral displacement of the femoral head. The capital epiphysis itself is small compared to the normal side (Fig. 13.56).

Following the initial diagnosis of dislocation and subsequent reduction, follow-up radiographs are obtained to check that reduction is maintained, the acetabulum is developing and ossification of the femoral head is progressing. **Osteonecrosis** is a recognized complication of treatment for DDH and manifests as cessation of epiphyseal growth, sclerosis and fragmentation of the epiphysis.

Figure 13.56 *Developmental dislocation of the right hip. There is supero-lateral subluxation of the femoral head. The capital epiphysis is small and the acetabulum dysplastic.*

HAEMATOMA

Haematomas may occur secondary to trauma (including iatrogenic trauma) or spontaneously in patients with coagulation deficiencies. CT may be diagnostic in the early stages since fresh blood has a higher density than muscle. As a haematoma resolves, it becomes cystic centrally and therefore must be included in the differential diagnosis of a cystic mass. The MRI appearances of haematoma can also be characteristic and vary with the age of the lesion (Fig. 13.57).

SOFT TISSUES

SOFT-TISSUE MASSES

The commonest causes of a soft-tissue mass include haematoma, abscess and tumour. It is important to realize that, although plain radiography can demonstrate bone/calcification, air and fat, soft tissue and fluid cannot be distinguished. Ultrasound is the most simple initial technique. Demonstration of a cystic mass by ultrasound can be followed by ultrasound-guided aspiration.

CT and MRI are more sensitive at demonstrating amounts of fat that are too small to see on plain films. However, MRI is relatively poor at identifying gas and calcification compared with CT. MRI is the technique of choice for demonstrating the local relationships of a mass because of its multiplanar imaging capability and also its ability to distinguish solid masses from normal muscle by signal differences on T2-weighted sequences. Generally, a solid mass has the same density as muscle on CT.

Figure 13.57 *Coronal T1-weighted MRI scan of a resolving haematoma of the thigh. The high signal within the mass is due to subacute haemorrhage. The thin hypointense capsule is characteristic.*

Figure 13.58 *Lipoma of the forearm identified due to the relatively low radiographic density of fat (arrows).*

the underlying bone, showing smooth pressure erosion in the case of a slowly growing lesion or frank cortical destruction by an aggressive lesion. Ultrasound is of value in the differentiation of solid from cystic masses. CT is tissue-specific only in tumours with a fatty component (lipoma, liposarcoma). Other soft-tissue tumours tend to be of muscle density. Similarly, MRI has the ability to demonstrate fat as high signal on T1-weighted scans and may indicate lesions with a predominantly fibrous nature, such as aggressive fibromatosis, because these tend to have low signal on both T1- and T2-weighted sequences. The majority of soft-tissue tumours on MRI are of intermediate signal on T1-weighted sequences and of high signal on T2-weighted sequences.

It is also important to realize that, in the absence of local invasion or distant metastases, the differentiation between benign and malignant neoplasms cannot be confidently made. It is evident, therefore, that a large proportion of soft-tissue tumours will need biopsy for a preoperative diagnosis. This is easily accomplished with either ultrasound or CT guidance. Once a diagnosis of a malignant lesion has been made, further staging includes chest radiography and CT to look for pulmonary metastases, and bone scintigraphy to identify skeletal metastases, although these are rare at presentation.

ABSCESS/INFLAMMATORY MASS

The imaging features of an infective inflammatory mass or abscess are also non-specific, although the demonstration of gas in the lesion is suggestive. Initially, the mass may appear solid but, as liquefaction occurs, the central area becomes cystic. This may be identified clearly with ultrasound, CT or MRI. Percutaneous catheter drainage can be performed using ultrasound or CT guidance.

TUMOURS

There are many benign and malignant soft-tissue tumours; only a few have specific features that allow a plain film diagnosis. Examples include **lipoma**, with its characteristic low density (Fig. 13.58), and **vascular tumours**, which may be identified by the presence of phleboliths.

Plain radiographs can, nevertheless, be useful for assessing the effect of a **primary soft-tissue neoplasm** on

FURTHER READING

Lang, T., Augat, P., Majumdar, S., Ouyang, X., Genant, H.K. 1998: Noninvasive assessment of bone density and structure using computed tomography and magnetic resonance. *Bone* **22**(5, Suppl.), 149S–153S.

Ma, L.D. 1999: Magnetic resonance imaging of musculoskeletal tumors: skeletal and soft tissue masses. *Current Problems in Diagnostic Radiology* **28**, 29–62.

Mirra, J.M., Brien, E.W., Tehranzadeh, J. 1995: Paget's disease of bone: review with emphasis on radiologic features, Part II. *Skeletal Radiology* **24**, 173–84.

Ridley, N., Shaikh, M.I., Remedios, D., Mitchell, R. 1998: Radiology of skeletal tuberculosis. *Orthopedics* **21**, 1213–20.

Sammak, B., El Bagi, M.A., Al Shahed, M. *et al.* 1999: Osteomyelitis: a review of currently used imaging techniques. *European Radiology* **9**, 894–900.

Various authors. 1993: Imaging of bone tumours. *Radiologic Clinics of North America* **31**(2), 237–447.

Various authors. 1996: Arthropathies. *Radiologic Clinics of North America* **34**(2) 195–456.

Spine

TIM JASPAN

Imaging the spine and spinal canal contents represents one of the most common indications for a radiological examination, and selection of the most appropriate imaging modality is very important. Spinal imaging has been revolutionized over the past decade following the introduction of magnetic resonance imaging (MRI). The radiological anatomy of complex spinal lesions can now be analysed non-invasively in detail, providing greater insight into the pathophysiology of a variety of spinal disorders without recourse to the use of ionizing radiation. In this chapter a broad perspective of the commoner conditions affecting the spine will be covered, placing emphasis on the most relevant imaging modality and radiological features. Clinical correlation must, however, be made to avoid the risk of 'treating the images rather than the patient'.

IMAGING TECHNIQUES

PLAIN RADIOGRAPHS

Anteroposterior and lateral views of the spine, supplemented by extra projections in certain cases, remain the standard initial assessment of spinal trauma. Plain films retain an important role in the investigation of complex vertebral anomalies, spinal deformities and in monitoring the results of treatment including surgical instrumentation. The place of plain films in the assessment of degenerative and inflammatory spinal disorders has diminished with the advent of the newer imaging modalities. Conventional tomography is helpful in certain situations (e.g. complex craniovertebral anomalies) where bone detail may not be fully appreciated by the newer imaging techniques. Plain films give a significant radiation dosage and provide little information about the intraspinal contents.

RADIONUCLIDE EXAMINATION

The place of radionuclide bone scanning has receded, although it is still used for the detection of metastatic disease, assessment of solitary vertebral osseous lesions and discovertebral infection. MRI is more sensitive and detects these lesions earlier.

MYELOGRAPHY

MRI has largely replaced myelography, which is now reserved for selected cases. MRI may be ambiguous or equivocal in the presence of metallic surgical spinal fixation devices and also for the assessment of cervical spondylosis. Myelography is invasive, carries a high radiation burden, is operator-dependent and may precipitate neurological deterioration in the presence of a complete spinal block.

COMPUTED TOMOGRAPHY

Excellent spatial resolution and detailed bony anatomy is provided by CT, which is particularly useful in studying acute spinal trauma. CT also plays an important role in the investigation of degenerative spinal disease (sometimes in combination with myelography), vertebral tumours and complex vertebral anomalies where multiplanar two- or three-dimensional reconstructions may facilitate interpretation. There is, however, a relatively high radiation burden.

SPINAL ANGIOGRAPHY

Spinal angiography requires selective injections into the arteries supplying the spinal column and contents in order to investigate suspected intraspinal vascular malformations, and certain intraspinal and vertebral body tumours. Therapeutic procedures, such as embolization of spinal vascular malformations and tumours, may be undertaken. Spinal angiography is time-consuming, requires a high level of operator skill and good quality digital subtraction angiographic equipment, and carries a small but not insignificant risk of causing or exacerbating a neurological deficit.

INTRAOPERATIVE SPINAL ULTRASONOGRAPHY

Coupled with colour Doppler imaging, this technique enables real-time intraoperative spinal monitoring. Scanning is performed with a sterilized hand-held transducer, which is immersed in the saline-filled operative site. High-quality images may be obtained with the dura either intact or opened. Intraoperative ultrasound is particularly helpful in the management of trauma, tumour and vascular lesions.

MAGNETIC RESONANCE IMAGING

Since the early 1980s, MRI has become the major imaging technique for the investigation of spinal disorders. The multiplanar capabilities, wide range of pulse sequences, high spatial resolution and sensitivity to pathological processes have revolutionized spinal imaging. Furthermore MRI is non-invasive and avoids ionizing radiation.

TRAUMA

ACUTE SPINAL INJURY

Acute spinal trauma is initially assessed by plain radiographs. In approximately 10 per cent of cases there are multiple levels of injury. Significant injuries, especially when spinal instability or disruption of the spinal canal is suspected, should be investigated by

high-resolution, thin-section CT scanning with supervision by suitably qualified personnel during the transfer of the patient to and from the scanner table. The presence of a neurological deficit is an indication for MRI to demonstrate any surgically remediable lesion (e.g. a disc protrusion or extramedullary haematoma) and to document the presence of spinal cord injury.

The spine is particularly vulnerable to injury at the thoracolumbar and cervicothoracic junctional regions where the relatively rigid thoracic spine, which is splinted by the thoracic cage, interacts with the more mobile cervical and lumbar segments. A significant proportion of cervical spine injuries also occurs at the atlantoaxial level, particularly in patients suffering major craniofacial trauma in whom the spinal component of the patient's injuries may be easily overlooked.

Late neurological deterioration following spinal injury or progressive spinal deformity is best investigated by a combination of plain radiographs and MRI. It is desirable that non-ferromagnetic metallic instrumentation is used at the time of primary stabilization following acute injury so that subsequent assessment by MRI may be possible.

A classification based on the mechanism of injury may be employed based on four major types of injury:

- flexion
- extension
- axial (burst) compression
- rotation–translation

Although each type may occur in isolation, the spine is often subjected to a combination of these forces. Certain types of injury occur more frequently at specific regions of the spine. Of major importance is the assessment of the stability of the spine following acute trauma. The risk of inducing or aggravating neurological injury by inappropriate handling of a potentially unstable spine calls for careful analysis of all images, which should include CT as well as plain radiographs, whenever a significant injury is suspected.

Spinal stability depends upon the integrity of various osteoligamentous components, which can be analysed in terms of three columns (Fig. 14.1). In general,

Figure 14.1 *The three-column spine. 1 = annulus; 2 = nucleus pulposus; 3 = pedicle; 4 = transverse process; 5 = lamina; 6 = spinous process.*

fractures involving a single column (e.g. wedge compression fractures) are stable. Disruption of two or more columns, especially the middle and posterior columns, is associated with a high risk of instability. The most unstable injuries include facet joint fractures and/or dislocation and major translational injuries where there is *en bloc* displacement of the spine in the lateral and/or antero-posterior plane.

Flexion injuries

Flexion injuries occur at sites of maximum spinal mobility, typically the lower cervical spine and the cervicothoracic and thoracolumbar junctional zones. Vertebral body compression or wedging is the predominant feature. More significant forces disrupt the posterior ligamentous column, resulting in facet joint distraction and transient or fixed vertebral displacement (Fig. 14.2). The addition of rotational forces increases the risk of facet joint distraction and ligamentous injury.

Extension injuries

Hyperextension injury occurs most commonly in the cervical region. Fractures involve the spinal canal ring and, particularly, the facet joints. Stability is particularly compromised if the anterior column complex is disrupted.

Figure 14.2 *Hyperflexion injury with fracture dislocation at C5/6. Note widened interspinous gap (circle) and subluxed articular facet joints (arrow).*

Axial (burst) compression injuries

Vertical transmission of forces results in splaying or bursting of the vertebral body and posterior elements, particularly the pedicles or lateral masses. Common sites of involvement include C1 and the lower cervical, thoracolumbar and upper lumbar regions. Retropulsion of bony elements into the spinal canal may compress neural structures, with a high incidence of major irreversible cord damage in cervical injuries. CT not infrequently demonstrates involvement of both the middle and posterior columns indicating potentially unstable injuries.

Rotation–translation injuries

A combination of factors including hyperflexion and hyperextension that, when combined with lateral or rotational forces, result in major spinal disruption or instability. The cervical, upper and lower thoracic regions are the most common sites for this type of injury.

Acute spinal injury may be considered according to the three spinal regions.

Cervical injuries

Upper cervical injuries are often unstable with a high incidence of associated severe neurological compromise or death and are often associated with a major head injury. However, because the spinal canal is relatively capacious (and if further instability is prevented), the late outcome may often be good. Injuries to the atlas include axial compression bursting injuries (**Jefferson fractures**), in which cord damage is rare. CT clearly demonstrates the disruption of the anterior and posterior arches of C1. **Atlanto-occipital dislocation**, usually fatal, is recognized by widening of the gap between the tip of the odontoid peg and the basion (anterior lip of the foramen magnum) to above 12.5 mm. Atlanto-axial dislocation usually occurs in association with fractures of the upper cervical spine and disruption of the transverse ligament.

Fractures of the axis (C2) may either involve the odontoid process or the lateral masses (**hangman's fracture**). Odontoid fractures are common and are classified into type I (tip), type II (base of dens) and type III (C2 body). Type II are the most common, being seen as a horizontal lucency at the base of the dens on the open mouth projection or cortical disruption on a lateral view. Non-union can occur in up to 72 per cent of cases with an increased risk of atlanto-axial instability. A hangman's fracture represents a traumatic spondylolysthesis with fractures through the pars interarticularis produced by a hyperextension injury. The neural arch becomes separated from the body, which subluxes anteriorly. Although this fracture is responsible for death in judicial hanging, in clinical practice

Figure 14.3 *T2-weighted sagittal MRI of an acute hyperflexion injury. Disruption of the C5/6 posterior annulus and posterior ligamentous complex (✲) is present along with some cord contusion (curved arrow), seen as ill-defined high signal in the cord. There is an anterior extradural haematoma (arrows).*

Figure 14.4 *Cervical axial burst fracture at C3 with vertebral body cleavage (small arrows) and left-sided facet joint fracture dislocation (arrow).*

neurological damage is uncommon as the spinal canal becomes effectively widened.

From C3 to C7 hyperextension, hyperflexion and axial compressive injuries predominate. Flexion injuries which leave the middle and posterior columns intact result in simple wedge fractures. More severe flexion forces, as occur in contact sports or diving accidents where the neck becomes flexed whilst the head is relatively fixed, lead to disruption of the posterior longitudinal ligament and posterior column osteoligamentous complex with a significantly increased risk of anterior subluxation or dislocation (Fig. 14.3). The posterior disc space and interspinous distance at the affected level become widened. Uni- or bilateral facet joint fracture–dislocation may also occur with this type of injury. Oblique views are useful but CT is more effective in demonstrating the full extent of the injury. The risk of cord injury is high with cord contusion and/or compression.

Extension injuries range from whiplash soft-tissue injuries without disruption of the spinal column to more significant trauma, in which the anterior ligamentous complex is disrupted and there may be avulsion fractures of the anterior vertebral bodies or compression fractures of the posterior arch. The disc space becomes widened anteriorly and there is often an associated prevertebral soft-tissue swelling. Severe hyperextension 'sprain' injuries may result in transient subluxation with resulting cord impaction and a central cord syndrome, in the absence of overt malalignment. These injuries are, however, unstable in extension. Axial loading compression fractures (e.g. falls onto the vertex in diving accidents) result in major disruption of the vertebral body with bursting and cleavage of the vertebral body (Fig. 14.4). Retropulsion of vertebral body bony elements posteriorly into the cervical spinal canal often results in major cord damage (Fig. 14.5).

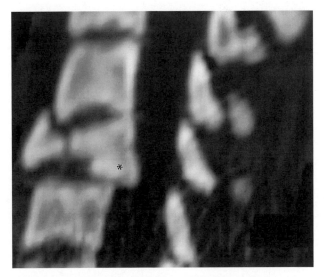

Figure 14.5 *Sagittal CT reconstruction in the midline showing a retropulsed vertebral body fragment (✲) encroaching upon and narrowing the spinal canal. MRI demonstrated cord compression and contusion.*

Thoracic injuries

Fractures in the thoracic spine are less common than in the cervical and thoracolumbar regions. Axial loading compression injuries may result in burst fractures. With major trauma the sternum and/or ribs are often fractured and there is an increased incidence of translational injuries with anterior displacement and acute angulation of the spine. Major cord disruption not infrequently accompanies these injuries.

Thoracolumbar injuries

Injuries in this region account for approximately a third of all spinal trauma, L1 being the most commonly affected. Flexion injuries occur most commonly, often accompanied by compressive forces. Loss of vertebral height anteriorly and increased kyphosis are seen on lateral radiographs. As the middle and posterior columns are usually intact, these are stable injuries. Axial compression forces result in herniation of disc through the end-plate with subsequent bursting of the vertebral body. Lateral splaying of the pedicles, with or without a vertical fracture through the vertebral body, is seen on the frontal views with loss of height of the posterior part of the vertebral body on the lateral views. CT scanning is most valuable in demonstrating comminuted bone fragments, which are most often derived from the posterosuperior part of the vertebral body, spinal canal narrowing and integrity of the posterior neural arch. CT demonstrates the frequent involvement of both the middle and posterior columns and thus the inherently unstable nature of these lesions (Fig. 14.6). Involvement of the conus accounts for the not infrequently associated paraplegia.

Figure 14.6 *L1 burst fracture with splaying of the pedicles (P), right-sided facet joint fracture dislocation (arrow) and 60 per cent narrowing of the spinal canal by a large retropulsed fragment of the vertebral body (*) compressing the conus.*

Figure 14.7 *Plain radiograph of a 'Chance' fracture, a horizontally orientated fracture through the body of L1 extending into the left transverse process (arrows).*

Flexion–distraction forces may result in disruption of the middle and posterior columns with annular tears resulting in vertebral body subluxation and the frequently associated neurological deficits. Hyperflexion forces result in horizontal slicing injury, which may extend through the vertebral body and posterior neural arch and/or ligaments or may pass through the disc space. This type of injury, known as a **Chance or 'seat-belt' fracture dislocation**, is uncommon but is important to recognize because of the high incidence of associated major visceral damage. Neurological deficits are, however, uncommon. Plain radiographs or conventional tomography may define the horizontally orientated fracture through the vertebral body or posterior neural arch (Fig. 14.7). The horizontal orientation of these fractures may lead to difficulty in interpretation with CT, unless multiplanar reconstructions are made.

Flexion–rotation and shearing fracture–dislocation injuries are uncommon, highly unstable injuries which involve all three spinal columns and are usually accompanied by paraplegia. There may be varying degrees of AP or lateral vertebral body displacement and locking. CT best demonstrates the degree of spinal canal involvement and the presence of facet joint dislocation.

SOFT-TISSUE INJURIES

Cord and root injury

Injury to the spinal cord may result from:

- stretching of the cord at the time of hyperextension injury;

Figure 14.8 *Nerve root avulsion. CT myelogram demonstrating a right-sided post-traumatic meningocoele (arrow) with no identifiable nerve root within it; C = spinal cord.*

- focal cord compression or laceration of the cord as it is trapped between the neural arch posteriorly and vertebral body elements anteriorly, particularly in association with a dislocation;
- direct impact by a disc protrusion or bony fragment upon the cord.

Neurological evidence of spinal cord injury when there is incomplete loss of or recovering motor or sensory function, or a neurological deficit in the absence of obvious bony injury, merits further investigation by MRI. Both haemorrhagic and non-haemorrhagic contusional injury may be readily identified as may cord compression by vertebral elements or disc protrusion. Reversible cord injury can arise from cord

concussion and oedema, and carries a more favourable prognosis than a haemorrhagic contusional injury. With non-haemorrhagic contusion the cord appears isointense on T1-weighted images; it may appear swollen and on T2-weighted images demonstrates focal hyperintensity (Fig. 14.3). Haemorrhagic contusion may show high signal on both T1- and T2-weighted images. There is less indication for MRI in completed spinal injuries; however, major cord disruption or transection may be confirmed and identifying any remediable pathology above the site of injury may prevent ascending neurological damage.

Traumatic brachial plexus injuries may be detected with equal accuracy (approximately 60–70 per cent) by myelography and MRI. Root avulsion is most easily identified if there is an accompanying meningocoele or an enlarged empty root sleeve (Fig. 14.8). Brachial plexus injuries frequently involve more than one root.

Traumatic disc protrusion and intraspinal haematoma

Both these injuries may occur in the absence of associated vertebral fractures and are best demonstrated with MRI. The herniated disc may be of high signal intensity owing to the presence of blood products and oedema. With advancing age, spondylosis becomes more prevalent. In the cervical region, this results in narrowing of the spinal canal. The spinal cord is thus particularly vulnerable to hyperflexion injuries in these cases with resultant disc protrusions or spondylotic bars impacting upon and damaging the cord. Acute spinal haemorrhage may demonstrate variable signal characteristics

Figure 14.9 *(a) Sagittal and (b) axial T2-weighted images 5 months following a hyperflexion injury. Note the small left posterolateral disc protrusion (arrow head) and central cord hyperintensity (arrow), indicative of myelomalacia or gliosis probably following an acute disc-related contusional injury to the cord.*

(a)   *(b)*

Figure 14.10 *Sagittal T1-weighted MRI showing a large cervical hydrosyrinx (small arrows) above an old C6/7 fracture dislocation (long arrow).*

depending on the age, size and compartment into which the haemorrhage has occurred. Acute haemorrhage may be difficult to demonstrate on MRI. Subacute haemorrhage (> 48 h) may be of high or mixed high and low signal intensity on both T1- and T2-weighted images because of the presence of blood degradation products at differing stages of evolution. Extrinsic compression of the spinal cord by sub- or extradural haematoma is readily identified.

Extraspinal soft tissue injury

Disruption of the anterior and posterior ligamentous complexes may accompany major spinal injury or occur in isolation, such as occurs with whiplash injuries of the neck. MRI clearly defines the extent of the injuries (Fig. 14.3).

CHRONIC SPINAL INJURY

Assessment of the late sequelae of spinal trauma is required when there is late or evolving neurological deterioration and/or a progressive spinal deformity. MRI can detect early cord damage, such as cystic myelomalacia (Fig. 14.9), which may progress to frank cord cavitation (post-traumatic hydrosyringomyelia), accounting for an ascending pattern of neurological dysfunction (Fig. 14.10).

Progressive spinal deformity may occur either in isolation or associated with cord cavitation. Plain radiographs can be used to monitor the spinal deformity.

TUMOURS

Neoplastic diseases of the spine and spinal cord may be classified by location into:

- extradural
- intradural extramedullary
- intramedullary (Fig. 14.11).

Imaging of these lesions has been transformed by MRI, which can clearly define the relationship of the lesion to the spinal cord and assess the extent of the tumour. Plain radiographs supplemented by conventional tomography, radionuclide studies and plain CT may be useful in certain osseous tumours.

EXTRADURAL TUMOURS

These tumours may be benign or malignant. Metastases to the spine are the most common malignant spinal tumours.

Benign tumours

One of the commonest benign tumours is the vertebral body **haemangioma**, which is often multiple and is increasingly seen as an incidental finding on MRI, with a reported incidence of 11 per cent in autopsy cases. Haemangiomas occur with increasing frequency from middle age. All of part of the vertebra is affected and any part of the spine may be affected, particularly the lower thoracic region. Plain radiographs demonstrate a coarse trabeculated pattern, whilst small punctate densities within a discrete area of reduced attenuation may be seen with CT. On MRI fibroadipose stroma within these vascular hamartomatous lesions leads to heterogeneous high signal intensity on both T1- and T2-weighted images (Fig. 14.12). Less commonly, extraosseous extension into the neuroforaminal or spinal canal may lead to compression of neural tissue.

Tumours in younger patients, usually in their second and third decades, include **osteoid osteomas**, which occur particularly in the posterior neural arch. Although an osteoid osteoma may be difficult to appreciate on plain films, the tumour shows a focal area of intense increased uptake on a radionuclide scan. CT demonstrates a small radiolucency within an area of dense sclerosis and corresponding low signal intensity on MRI.

Osteoblastomas also tend to involve selectively the posterior neural arch, appearing as well-defined expanded lucent lesions.

Osteochondromas occur most commonly in the cervical spine, particularly C2, arising from the spinous or transverse processes. Although rarely producing

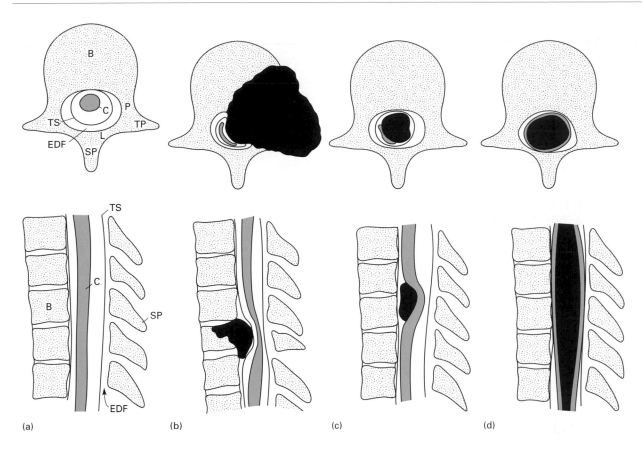

Figure 14.11 *Schematic transverse axial and sagittal sections of the thoracic spine. (a) Normal, where B = vertebral body; C = spinal cord; EDF = extradural fat; TS = thecal sac; L = lamina; P = pedicle; TP = transverse process; SP = spinous process. (b) Extradural metastatic tumour. Extrinsic compression of the thecal sac and spinal cord, which are compressed to an ellipse and displaced away from the tumour. (c) Intradural extramedullary tumour. The tumour is contained within the undisplaced thecal sac but compresses and displaces the spinal cord. (d) Intradural intramedullary spinal cord tumour. The spinal cord is expanded but undisplaced. There is little or no visualization of the cerebrospinal fluid in the thecal sac around the spinal cord.*

Figure 14.12 *T6 vertebral body haemangioma. (a) Coronal T1-weighted and (b) sagittal T2-weighted MRI showing heterogeneous high signal intensity on both sequences, a coarse trabeculated internal structure (circles) and paravertebral soft-tissue involvement (arrows).*

neurological symptoms, they can grow into the spinal canal and compress the cord. Osteochondromas appear as sessile or pedunculated masses. The cartilaginous cap may exhibit punctate calcifications on CT and heterogeneous signal characteristics on both T1- and T2-weighted images (Fig. 14.13).

Aneurysmal bone cysts are non-neoplastic expansile lobulated soft-tissue mass lesions with a highly vascular stroma, occurring most often in the second and third decades. The posterior elements are usually involved but extension into the vertebral body, across adjacent disc spaces or into the spinal canal may occur. MRI demonstrates altered blood products resulting in high signal intensity on both T1- and T2-weighted images, internal septations and fluid levels with a low signal intensity rim.

Malignant tumours

Metastases, particularly from carcinoma of the breast, lung and prostate, are the most common extradural tumours. The posterior part of the vertebral body is most frequently affected. Extension into the adjacent

(a)

(b)

(c)

Figure 14.13 *Osteochondroma of C3. (a) Plain radiograph showing primary involvement of the spinous process. (b) CT more clearly defines the extent of the tumour in the spinous process (S), posterior neural arch (N) and region of the right foramen transversarium (✳). (c) T2-weighted sagittal MRI shows posterior cord compression and early cord signal alteration (arrow).*

paraspinal soft tissues, the neuroforaminal canals and the spinal canal is commonly seen. Plain radiographs may demonstrate lytic foci or collapse of one or more vertebral bodies, pedicular destruction or a paraspinal soft-tissue mass. However, metastases from carcinoma of the prostate or breast, particularly following treatment of breast cancer may appear as sclerotic or mixed lytic and sclerotic lesions.

Whilst 40–50 per cent of the affected bone mass must be destroyed before changes become evident on the radiograph, radionuclide bone scanning is sensitive to a much smaller degree of bone destruction (approximately 10 per cent) and is thus commonly employed as the screening method of choice for the detection of metastases. MRI employing specific pathology-sensitive sequences such as STIR is an even more sensitive alter-native for the detection of metastases (Fig. 14.14). MRI has the additional advantage of being able to assess the spinal canal and location of any intraspinal tumour (Fig. 14.15). Metastases from other primary tumours, such as Hodgkin's and non-Hodgkin's lymphoma may arise within the paraspinal and extradural soft tissues and secondarily involve the vertebral bodies. In children spinal metastases most commonly arise from a neuroblastoma.

The vertebrae are frequently involved in **multiple myeloma**, with peak incidence in the fifth to seventh decades. Focal or diffuse lytic lesions with vertebral collapse may be seen on plain films. The MRI features are multiple lesions which show heterogeneous signal characteristics (Fig. 14.16). Fat-suppressed sequences are helpful in distinguishing between myeloma and

(a)   (b)

Figure 14.14 *(a) Sagittal T1 and (b) STIR images demonstrating metastases in the body of T9 and spinous processes of L1. The STIR sequence demonstrates that the heterogeneity of the signal-related changes on the T1 sequence elsewhere is age-related and is not further deposits.*

Figure 14.16 *Multiple myeloma. T2-weighted MRI showing extensive patchy destructive changes with heterogeneous signal from the vertebral bodies. There is partial collapse of L1 and collapse of T5 (arrow) with spinal cord compression.*

(a)   (b)

Figure 14.15 *Renal cell carcinoma metastasis of the C4–6 vertebral bodies. (a) Sagittal T1-weighted and (b) T2-weighted MRI demonstrating extradural tumour (✳) compressing the spinal cord. There is signal reduction in the vertebral bodies on the T1-weighted images and corresponding high signal on the T2-weighted images.*

patchy fatty marrow replacement, a phenomenon which is increasingly prevalent with advancing age. Myeloma is also accompanied by vertebral body collapse.

The spine may be directly invaded by tumour arising from adjacent structures. The tumour often extends into the spinal canal entering via a neuroforaminal canal (Fig. 14.17).

Other malignant tumours include **chordomas**, which arise from intraosseous notochordal remnants. Over 50 per cent of chordomas occur in the sacrococcygeal region, 35 per cent at the skull base and 15 per cent in vertebral bodies, mainly in the upper cervical region; they appear on CT as expansile lytic masses containing punctate calcifications. Chordomas are typically hypointense on T1-weighted sequences and hyperintense on T2-weighted images, demonstrating internal septations and strong contrast enhancement (Fig. 14.18).

INTRADURAL EXTRAMEDULLARY TUMOURS

The most common intraspinal mass lesions are extramedullary intradural tumours, of which menin-

Figure 14.17 *Axial T1 image in a patient with a Pancoast tumour, which invades the spinal canal and infiltrates the vertebral body and paraspinal musculature.*

(a)

(b)

Figure 14.18 *Chordoma centred upon C2. (a) Sagittal T1, (b) T2, (c) postcontrast T1 images demonstrate an inhomogeneous mass destroying the dens and extending cephalad to involve the clivus. Enhancement is patchy and relatively sparse.*

(c)

giomas and nerve sheath tumours account for 80–90 per cent. Other benign tumours and cystic masses are relatively uncommon and are largely represented by developmental tumours, e.g. dermoid cysts, lipomas, neurenteric cysts, teratomas and arachnoid cysts. Most are associated with spinal dysraphism (see below). Intrathecal malignant tumours occur as a result of metastatic dissemination of tumour cells shed into the CSF, usually from an intracranial malignant mass in direct contact with the ventricular system or subarachnoid spaces.

Benign tumours

Nerve sheath tumours such as **schwannomas** and **neurofibromas** are the most common benign tumours. They present usually in the third to fifth decades and occur anywhere in the spine, most often the thoracic region. Although usually solitary, multiple lesions may occur particularly in association with neurofibromatosis type I. Approximately 75 per cent of the tumours are intradural in location, 15 per cent are both intra- and extradural ('dumbell') and 10 per cent may be entirely extradural. Pedicular erosion, posterior vertebral body scalloping (which may be localized in relation to tumour) or generalized (from dural ectasia), kyphoscoliotic deformities and paraspinal soft-tissue masses may be seen on plain radiographs, particularly in neurofibromatosis. Malignant degeneration occurs in 5–10 per cent of neurofibromas.

MRI is particularly useful in the assessment of neurofibromas, being ideally suited to demonstrate the intra- and extraspinal components, multiple lesions and any secondary cord changes, e.g. hydrosyringomyelia. The tumours appear as isointense well-circumscribed masses on T1-weighted images and corresponding high signal intensity on T2-weighted images (Fig. 14.19). Strong enhancement with contrast is common.

Meningiomas typically arise in the thoracic spine with a 4:1 female to male preponderance, usually after the fifth decade. Over 90 per cent of the tumours are intradural, the remainder being either 'dumbell' or entirely extradural in nature. As plain films are usually unremarkable, MRI is the most useful imaging technique. These lesions usually appear relatively isointense on both T1- and T2-weighted sequences (Fig. 14.20). Modest contrast enhancement is seen with contrast.

Malignant tumours

This group is largely represented by CSF spread of deposits from bronchogenic or breast carcinoma and non-Hodgkin's lymphoma. In children, dissemination occurs from primary neuraxial, especially posterior fossa, tumours such as primitive neurectodermal tumours (PNETs), ependymomas, glioblastoma multi-

Figure 14.19 *Thoracic schwannoma. (a) Axial T2 (b) postgadolinium T1 images show a large 'dumbell' tumour with cystic/necrotic degeneration resulting in heterogeneous hyperintensity and variable enhancement.*

Figure 14.20 *Left-sided C3/4 meningioma (M) showing mild enhancement on (a) parasagittal and (b) axial T1-weighted MRI. The spinal cord (arrow) is tightly compressed by the tumour.*

forme and germ cell tumours. The lesions may appear either as nodular masses on the surface of the cord and/or nerve roots, particularly in the region of the cauda equina, or as sheet-like masses over the surface of the cord. Myelography has been superseded by MRI, which is more sensitive and much safer, particularly in the presence of intracranial disease. Whilst T2-weighted sequences may provide an excellent 'myelographic' effect that may be diagnostic, contrast-enhanced T1-weighted images are more sensitive for the detection of these lesions, particularly the extensive sheet-like lesions

coating the cord and nerve roots (Fig. 14.21) which may not be appreciated on T2-weighted images.

INTRAMEDULLARY TUMOURS

Spinal cord gliomas are by far the commonest intramedullary tumours, representing over 90 per cent of this group. Haemangioblastomas and metastases make up most of the remainder. MRI is the imaging modality of choice, demonstrating these lesions with a high degree of sensitivity.

Figure 14.21 *Leptomeningeal metastases. Pre- and postcontrast T1-weighted sagittal MRI showing flowing enhancement over the cauda equina (arrows).*

Astrocytomas occur most frequently in children; they are low-grade lesions often extending over many vertebral body segments. The cord is often diffusely expanded, showing hypo- or isointensity on T1-weighted images, hyperintensity on T2-weighted sequences and variable heterogenous enhancement with contrast. Tumour-related cysts are common. Extension into the brain stem and cerebellar hemispheres is not uncommon with cervical lesions (Fig. 14.22).

Spinal **ependymomas** are the commonest lesions in adults, accounting for 90 per cent of tumours arising in the region of the conus medullaris and filum terminale. They may also occur in the cervical region, particularly in association with neurofibromatosis type II, appearing as well-circumscribed strongly enhancing masses. There is often extensive oedema and/or cystic change in the adjacent spinal cord. As these lesions are slow-growing, focal expansion of the spinal canal may be seen with posterior vertebral body scalloping on plain films. MRI demonstrates a discrete mass related to the conus, isointense with the cord on a T1-weighted sequence and showing marked enhancement on images after contrast. T2-weighted images often demonstrate strongly hyperintense foci indicating intratumoral cyst formation or haemorrhage (Fig. 14.23).

Metastases to the spinal cord are uncommon and often solitary. The primary source is most commonly carcinoma of the breast or lung (Fig. 14.24). The metastases are usually well defined and enhance strongly. Multicentric or metastatic primary CNS lymphoma may also occur in the spinal cord or over the surface of

(a)

(b)

Figure 14.22 *(a) Sagittal T1-weighted and (b) T2-weighted MRI in a child with a cervical astrocytoma (A) extending into the brain stem, expanding the spinal cord and canal.*

(a)

(b)

Figure 14.23 *Conus ependymoma. (a) T1-weighted MRI shows the tumour (T). (b) After gadolinium the tumour enhances strongly (arrows) and reveals a cystic component (C) within the tumour.*

the cord and may involve the whole of the cord. **Haemangioblastomas** are highly vascular tumours, which are usually solitary. Von Hippel–Lindau disease is associated with 30 per cent of cases. The lesions are often accompanied by marked cord expansion, which may be due to oedema or highly proteinaceous tumour cysts. MRI demonstrates a strongly enhancing tumour nodule or nodules, which are often surprisingly small (Fig. 14.25).

Figure 14.24 *Metastasis to the thoracic cord from a primary breast carcinoma. Sagittal T1-weighted image following gadolinium shows a strongly enhancing well-circumscribed lesion. Note the extensive oedema seen as diffuse hypointensity in the adjacent cord.*

(a)   (b)

Figure 14.25 *Haemangioblastoma (a) Sagittal T2- (b) postgadolinium T1-weighted images demonstrating an expanded cord with a multiloculated cyst extending from C1 to C6 and adjacent cord oedema. Note the small irregular strongly enhancing mural nodule.*

DEGENERATIVE DISORDERS

Degenerative spinal disorders are the commonest cause of chronic pain and loss of working days in most developed countries. Approximately 60–80 per cent of the adult population will develop low back pain at some point in their lives, although in over 90 per cent of cases it is a self-limiting process, resolving without medical intervention. The effective diagnosis and management of these patients presents a major undertaking with far reaching socioeconomic implications.

Degenerative changes can be recognized on plain films as disc-space narrowing, end-plate sclerosis and osteophyte formation. Although frequently requested, plain films add very little to diagnosis and management, as disc protrusion cannot be detected and there is little correlation between the plain film findings and the patient's symptoms. Prior to the era of CT scanning, myelography was the diagnostic mainstay. CT extended diagnostic accuracy, particularly when used in combination with myelography, and also offered a non-invasive alternative for the assessment of suspected disc herniation and spondylosis in the lumbar region. MRI provides increased sensitivity in the study of degenerative disc disease, in associated thoracic and cervical cord compromise and in the postoperative 'failed back' syndrome.

Figure 14.26 *L4/5 and L5/S1 disc degeneration with a posterior annular tear seen as a focal hyperintensity on a sagittal T2-weighted MRI at L4/5 (straight arrow) and a small subligamentous posterior protrusion at L5/S1 (curved arrows).*

DISC DEGENERATION AND PROTRUSION

There is a well-recognized age-related pattern of normal disc dehydration and degeneration that commences over the age of 20 years. This is associated with a reduced water-binding capacity of the disc, a reduction of large molecular proteoglycans and progressive disc fibrosis. These changes are best seen with MRI as signal reduction in the disc on T2-weighted images. There may be an accompanying loss of disc height. Lengthening of annular fibres results in diffuse disc bulging. Focal radially orientated tears in the annulus, recognized as small hyperintensities on T2-weighted images (Fig. 14.26) or foci of enhancement on T1-weighted scans, may result in disc herniation. Discal herniations may be contained by the posterior longitudinal ligament (subligamentous) or rupture through the ligament to enter the spinal cord.

Disc protrusions vary from minimal focal disruptions of the posterior annulus to larger posterior, posterolateral or far lateral herniation of disc material (Fig. 14.27). The protruded disc can migrate a considerable distance and become detached (sequestrated) from the parent disc. Most disc protrusions in the lumbar spine occur at the L4/5 and L5/S1 levels (Fig. 14.28). The region of the conus and lower thoracic spine should, however, be inspected carefully as compressive lesions in this region may present initially as low back pain. Intraspinal fat encases the thecal sac

and exiting nerve root sheaths. Loss of visualization of the fat is a helpful sign in the recognition of subtle or far lateral disc protrusions in the neuroforaminal canal. These lesions cannot be assessed by myelography and are far more sensitively detected by CT or MRI. Over 60 per cent of lumbar disc herniations involve the posterolateral margin of the disc and tend to compress the exiting nerve root. However, it should be noted that disc protrusions are often asymptomatic, particularly when the patient is over 50 years.

Disc protrusions in the thoracic spine are now often identified incidentally during MRI of the spine, particularly in the lower thoracic spine. Whilst most disc protrusions in the thoracolumbar region are degenerative in nature, there is also a significant relationship to trauma.

In the cervical region the intervertebral discs are smaller and assessment of disc status is more difficult. CT-assisted myelography has been regarded as the 'gold standard'; however, improved MR pulse sequences, surface coil design and the ability to obtain thinner slices has increased the sensitivity of MRI. In many centres MRI alone is now considered sufficient for preoperative assessment. Plain films retain a role in correlating osteophytes projecting into the spinal and neuroforaminal canals with the abnormalities demonstrated on MRI, since small bony abnormalities can be difficult to assess with MRI. Plain films are also of value for confirming the vertebral level prior to surgery and

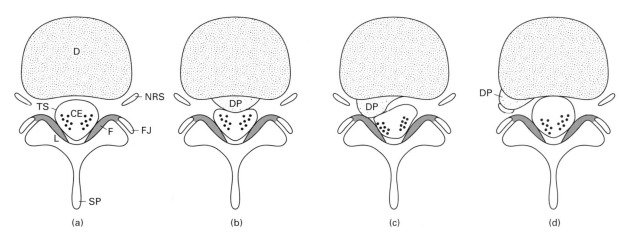

Figure 14.27 *Schematic transverse axial sections taken at the disc space level. (a) Normal where CE = cauda equina; D = intervertebral disc; F = flaval ligament; FJ = facet joint; L = lamina; NRS = nerve root sleeve; SP = spinous process; TS = thecal sac. (b) Central posterior disc protrusion (DP). Disc material indents the thecal sac; however, there is no root compression. (c) Paracentral disc protrusion (DP) compressing the thecal sac and the exiting nerve root just before it enters the nerve root sleeve. (d) Lateral disc protrusion (DP) compressing the nerve root sleeve within the neuroforaminal canal.*

Figure 14.28 *Sagittal T2-weighted MRI showing a large central posterior disc protrusion at L4/5 rupturing through the posterior longitudinal ligament, compressing the thecal sac (arrow). The L5/S1 disc is degenerate and narrowed.*

(a)   *(b)*

Figure 14.29 *Type 2 end-plate and marrow changes at L4/5 with (a) high signal on T1-weighted images and (b) mild hyperintensity on T2-weighted MRI. Note the associated disc degeneration, also present in the adjacent discs.*

assessing the position of metallic fixation devices or bone grafts following surgery. If the MR study is equivocal, the patient should be referred for CT or CT-assisted myelography.

Over 90 per cent of protrusions occur at the lower three cervical disc space levels. Central posterior protrusions are readily identified on MRI, indenting the anterior thecal sac and cord. Laterally situated disc protrusions can be more difficult to detect. Associated findings are asymmetrical appearances of the epidural fat and CSF in the lateral part of the spinal canal and in the neuroforaminal canal.

END-PLATE CHANGES

Striking end-plate changes may be seen on MRI in association with disc degeneration, probably resulting from fissuring of the end-plate regions with subsequent

Table 14.1 *Modic classification of end-plate changes in degenerative disease*

Type	Pathology	T1 signal	T2 signal	Disc signal	Enhancement
Type 1	Granulation tissue deposited in end-plates	Low	High	Low	Mild/moderate
Type 2	Granulation tissue replaced by fat	High	Mildly increased	Low	Mild
Type 3	End-plate/marrow sclerosis	Low	Low	Low	None

ingrowth of granulation tissue (Fig. 14.29). A classification (Modic) has been proposed based upon the MR appearances of the end-plates (Table 14.1).

SPONDYLOSIS AND FACET JOINT ARTHROPATHY

These two conditions are also associated with low back pain. The facet joints are richly innervated and may give rise to pain when associated with inflammation. There may also be direct compression of the exiting nerve root sheath in the exit canal as a result of facet joint hypertrophy or osteophyte formation. Juxta-articular synovial cysts may occasionally project into the spinal or neuroforaminal exit canal compromising the thecal sac or exiting nerve root. Increased facet joint laxity may lead to degenerative spondylolithesis, resulting in spinal or exit canal narrowing.

Cervical spondylosis occurs as a consequence of disc degeneration. Posteriorly directed vertebral body osteo-phytes, often associated with reversal of the normal spinal curvature, impinge upon and compress the spinal cord, resulting in focal hyperintensities on T2-weighted MRI, probably as a consequence of chronic repetitive microtrauma and ischaemic damage (Fig. 14.30). Osteophytes arising from the uncal processes encroach upon the neuroforaminal canal and may compress the exiting nerve root. The degree of compromise of the nerve root may be difficult to assess by MRI. Axial gradient-echo sequences are usually employed but may overestimate the extent of narrowing of the exit canal. Oblique thin slice images may help to assess the exit canals more effectively.

SPINAL CANAL STENOSIS

Acquired or degenerative spinal stenosis is usually caused by a combination of spondylosis, disc bulge/herniation, facet joint and flaval ligament hypertrophy. There is often an underlying predisposition owing to constitutional narrowing of the central spinal

(a)   *(b)*

Figure 14.30 *Cervical spondylosis with localized reversed curvature. (a) Osteophytic cord impingement at C5/6 is demonstrated on the T1-weighted image. (b) Focal cord hyperintensity (arrow) indicative of gliosis is best seen on T2-weighted imaging.*

Figure 14.31 *Axial CT following myelography. Focal canal stenosis with large degenerate facet joints (arrows), thickened ligamenta flava (F) and posterior annular disc bulge (arrowheads) compressing the opacified thecal sac.*

Figure 14.32 *Lower lumbar canal stenosis associated with a degenerative spondylolithesis at L4/5 (arrow). Sagittal T2-weighted MRI showing anterior and posterior compression of the thecal sac and poor visualization of the CSF.*

Figure 14.33 *Pre- and postcontrast T1-weighted axial MRI at L4/5 demonstrating enhancing postoperative scar tissue surrounding the proximal left L5 root sheath (arrow). Note some compression of the thecal sac (TS) has occurred.*

canal and the lateral recesses. The AP and lateral dimensions of the spinal canal are reduced and the thecal sac is concentrically compressed. CT scanning is particularly well suited to defining the canal dimensions and precise contribution of any associated spondylosis (Fig. 14.31), whereas MRI best defines the degree of cord or thecal sac compression and the number of disc space levels involved (Fig. 14.32). In the cervical spine, ossification of the posterior longitudinal ligament may contribute towards the overall degree of spinal canal narrowing.

Spinal canal stenosis in the thoracic region is relatively uncommon; however, when present, it is not infrequently associated with calcification or ossification of the ligamenta flava and/or hypertrophy of the articular facet joints. These changes are particularly well demonstrated by CT-assisted myelography. MRI now offers a more acceptable non-invasive alternative.

FAILED BACK SYNDROME

Recurrent signs or symptoms following spinal surgery constitute a difficult diagnostic and therapeutic dilemma. Common causes are recurrent disc protrusion at the operative level or another disc space, extradural fibrosis and scarring that may involve a nerve root sheath, nerve root inflammation, arachnoiditis, spinal canal stenosis, facet joint arthropathy, discitis or extradural abscess. In the first few weeks following surgery, soft-tissue swelling, extradural haematoma and residual disc fragments or protrusions are commonly encountered. In the subacute and chronic phase the principal differential diagnosis to be made is between residual/recurrent disc protrusion and postsurgical scarring. MRI can be of great help particularly when T1-weighted images are employed before and after intravenous contrast administration. Protruded disc material tends to show some mass effect and variable degrees of rim enhancement. Scar tissue may or may not produce mass effect but enhancement following contrast administration is often intense (Fig. 14.33).

End-plate changes are not usually seen following uncomplicated disc surgery. High signal intensity on T2-weighted or STIR sequences with corresponding signal loss on T1-weighted images should alert the physician to the possibility of infection, particularly if enhancement is seen following contrast administration.

INFLAMMATION AND INFECTION

INFLAMMATION

Inflammatory processes affecting the spinal cord are mostly due to multiple sclerosis, transverse myelitis and neurosarcoidosis. In **multiple sclerosis** approximately

(a)   *(b)*

Figure 14.34 *Demyelinating plaque in the upper cervical cord shown on (a) sagittal and (b) axial T2-weighted MRI. The high signal intensity plaque (arrow) is situated centrally in the dorsal aspect of the cord. Cranial imaging revealed multiple cerebral and cerebellar plaques.*

(a)   *(b)*

Figure 14.35 *Transverse myelitis. Acute presentation with paraparesis and a high thoracic sensory level. (a) Sagittal T2-weighted image demonstrating a long segment of cord expansion and hyperintensity. (b) Postgadolinium sagittal T1-weighted image demonstrates strong focal enhancement within the lesion.*

one third of patients manifest signs or symptoms of spinal involvement. Post-mortem studies frequently demonstrate cord lesions in all MS patients. Detecting small cord plaques employing current MR pulse sequences remains problematic; proton density weighted or FLAIR imaging may increase the sensitivity to some degree. Standard T2-weighted images may demonstrate focal or more diffuse lesions of high signal intensity (Fig. 14.34). Solitary lesions presenting acutely may simulate a cord tumour; however, lesion multiplicity is more common. Enhancement with gadolinium may help to identify acutely demyelinating lesions. Demonstration of further lesions in the brain helps to confirm the diagnosis of multiple sclerosis.

Transverse myelitis is an inflammatory process, which may be either idiopathic or associated with infections, immune system disorders (such as SLE), vaccination, or as an acute manifestation of MS. The lesion in transverse myelitis develops rapidly and may demonstrate an ascending pattern of involvement. The cord may be normal in size or mildly expanded, but myelitis is often identified by diffuse cord expansion extending over several vertebral body segments. The lesion appears hypointense on T1-weighted images and hyperintense on T2 imaging. Enhancement is moderate to marked following contrast administration making differentiation from tumour difficult (Fig. 14.35). MRI later in the course of the disease may show the cord returning to a normal appearance, but more often it will appear atrophic.

There is a wide range of potential causative agents for **arachnoiditis** that result in an inflammatory process involving the spinal arachnoid. Foremost amongst these is surgery, often in association with previous myodil myelography. Other causes include past infection or subarachnoid haemorrhage and spinal anaesthetic agents. MRI is now the modality of choice for investigating this condition, which may show clumping together of adherent roots either centrally or peripherally in the thecal sac. Peripheral aggregation of the roots may leave an appearance of an 'empty' thecal sac (Fig. 14.36). Occasionally a mass-like soft-tissue lesion may fill and obstruct the thecal sac, and may be associated with dense calcification (**arachnoiditis ossificans**), best identified on axial CT.

Leptomeningeal thickening and enhancement is seen with sarcoidosis (Fig. 14.37) or malignant pachymeningitis. Cord involvement with peripheral enhancing cord lesions may also be seen with sarcoidosis.

INFECTION

Infection may involve the vertebral bodies, disco-vertebral complexes, epidural space, leptomeninges or spinal cord.

Infection of the vertebral bodies (**spondylitis** or **vertebral osteomyelitis**) often coexists with discal

(a)

(b)

Figure 14.36 *Arachnoiditis. (a) Sagittal and (b) axial T2-weighted images in the lumbar region demonstrating an 'empty' thecal sac, the roots of the cauda equina being adherent to the theca. Note the L4 laminectomy and hypointensity in the thecal sac at L5/S1 from past Myodil myelography (arrows).*

Figure 14.37 *Neurosarcoidosis. Sagittal T1-weighted image following gadolinium administration. There is plaque-like intramedullary and pial enhancing tissue at the cervicothoracic junction (large arrow) with further delicate small enhancing nodules and plaques on the dorsal surface of the cord in the cervical and thoracic regions (small arrows).*

(a)

(b)

(c)

Figure 14.38 *Culture-negative discitis in 2-year-old child. (a) Sagittal T1 and (b) T2-weighted images in the acute phase shows hypointensity in the vertebral bodies adjacent to the L5/S1 disc space on the T1 image, and corresponding hyperintensity both within the vertebral bodies and the disc on the T2 image. (c) Sagittal T2 image 3 months later demonstrates almost complete resolution of the signal abnormalities and residual endplate irregularity.*

infection. In children infection usually commences in the richly vascular disc and then spreads to the vertebral body (Fig. 14.38). The subchondral portion of the vertebral body is more typically affected in the adult with subsequent infection of the rest of the vertebral body and the adjacent disc. The course of discitis is more benign in children than in adults. A wide variety of pathogens may be involved, with *Staphylococcus aureus*, Enterobacteriaceae and *Escherichia coli* being most common. Needle biopsy, however, may fail to demonstrate a pathogen in 50–70 per cent of patients. Plain radiographs are frequently normal in the acute phase; disc-space narrowing and end-plate irregularities occurring after 1–2 weeks. Radionuclide scanning previously had an important role in the diagnosis of these lesions. However, MRI is considerably more sensitive and demonstrates the disease at a very early stage. The narrowed disc appears hyperintense on T2-weighted images as does the adjacent vertebral body. Contrast administration may demonstrate subligamentous or epidural spread (Fig. 14.39).

Figure 14.39 *Vertebral osteomyelitis and discitis. Postcontrast T1-weighted MRI showing infected tissue, which is enhancing (arrows), extending into the anterior epidural compartment and compressing the spinal cord (C).*

(a)

(b)

(c)

Figure 14.40 *Tuberculosis osteomyelitis. (a) Sagittal T2, (b) pre- and (c) postgadolinium T1 images demonstrate destruction of the posterior vertebral bodies and a large extradural craggy enhancing abscess compressing the thecal sac.*

Tuberculosis is the most common cause of vertebral body infection worldwide. Spread of the mycobacterium to the vertebra is haematogenous from a pulmonary source. Infection often occurs anteriorly in the vertebral body but is not infrequently seen posteriorly, and in 50 per cent of cases extends to the adjacent vertebral body via the disc space (Fig. 14.40). Subligamentous spread may lead to distant vertebral involvement. Secondary involvement of the meninges or cord may occur, typically in patients under 30 years of age. In contrast with other bacterial spondylitides, tuberculous disease is characterized by greater bony destruction, less frequent involvement of the posterior vertebral body elements, large paraspinal soft tissue masses (which frequently calcify late in the disease) and severe end-stage kyphoscoliotic deformities. The onset and subsequent progress of the disease is more insidious than that of pyogenic spondylitis.

Epidural abscesses are uncommon, occurring by haematogenous spread or following spinal puncture or penetrating injuries. *Staphylococcus aureus* is the most common pathogen. The abscess may involve several vertebral body segments (Fig. 14.41). MRI shows a mass compressing the thecal sac and cord. T2-weighted images show variable hyperintensity depending on the degree of liquefaction and pus formation.

Leptomeningeal infection most frequently occurs as a consequence of pyogenic cerebral meningitis or secondary to infected spinal dysraphic lesions such as dermal sinuses. Postcontrast T1-weighted MRI may show enhancement over the surface of the cord and nerve roots, particularly in the cauda equina or enhancing nodular filling defects. There may be thick rind-like enhancement of the thecal sac (Fig. 14.42).

Figure 14.41 *Extradural abscess. Postgadolinium sagittal T1-weighted images showing an extensive lesion anterior to and compressing the cord with peripheral enhancement and non-enhancing pus centrally (arrows). Staphylococcus aureus was cultured from the pus.*

Figure 14.42 *Leptomeningeal infection in a patient with an infected anterior sacral meningocele. Sagittal T1-weighted image demonstrating enhancement of the walls of the meningocele and thecal sac (arrows) and nerve roots (arrowhead).*

Figure 14.43 *Thoracic dural arteriovenous fistula in a middle-aged male. Sagittal T2-weighted image demonstrating tubular flow voids in the CSF dorsal to the cord (arrows). The cord is mildly expanded and hyperintense indicative of secondary congestive venous myelopathy.*

VASCULAR LESIONS

Vascular lesions affecting the spine are relatively uncommon. The two main pathologies are vascular malformations and spinal cord ischaemia/infarction.

VASCULAR MALFORMATIONS

Most spinal vascular malformations are intradural arteriovenous malformations, of which 40 per cent occur within the cord, or arteriovenous fistulae, which are predominantly dural in location. They occur most frequently in the thoracic region. Myelography has been the basis for the detection of these lesions; however, MRI is now considered to be superior, not only for their diagnosis but also for the assessment of any associated cord damage. MRI identifies serpiginous filling defects representing the tortuous arterialized draining veins as flow voids or as enhancing structures following contrast administration. MRI demonstrates the secondary effects of vascular steal or chronic venous hypertension, which may appear as cord swelling or atrophy (Fig. 14.43). Spinal angiography is definitive and mandatory for operative or endovascular treatment (Fig. 14.44). An extensive search for all the feeding arteries is required as well as identification of the normal spinal arterial anatomy, specifically the artery of Adamkiewicz in the thoracic region.

The increased use of MRI has resulted in the detection of cavernous haemangiomas, which cannot be demonstrated by angiography. Vertebral body cavernous haemangiomas account for approximately 30 per cent of all spinal vascular malformations and may be asymptomatic incidental findings. Spinal cord cavernous haemangiomas are, however, rare. They may present with a progressive painful cord syndrome, particularly if there has been haemorrhage into the lesion.

(a)

(b)

(c)

Figure 14.44 *Cervical perimedullary arteriovenous malformation in a child. (a) Sagittal T2-weighted image demonstrating tubular flow voids in the thecal sac with a large sac-like venous aneurysm (arrow). (b) Selective thyrocervical trunk angiogram demonstrating the dilated perimedullary venous drainage and venous aneurysm (arrow). (c) Following embolization (30 per cent N-histyl cyanoacrylate/lipiodol) the malformation is obliterated.*

CORD ISCHAEMIA AND INFARCTION

Severe atherosclerotic disease, aortic dissection and aortic or spinal surgery are usually responsible for cord ischaemia or infarction. Clinical presentation is often acute with para- or tetraparesis, with or without accompanying pain. Vascular watershed areas between the major arterial territories are most frequently affected, specifically the cervicothoracic junction and lower thoracic cord. MRI may demonstrate focal cord expansion and hyperintensity on T2-weighted images with subsequent progression to late cord atrophy. Chronic venous ischaemia occurs not infrequently with vascular malformations; however, acute venous infarction may follow partial or complete spontaneous thrombosis of an underlying vascular malformation with vascular flow voids accompanying a swollen cord.

Intraspinal haemorrhage

Trauma accounts for the majority of causes of intraspinal haematoma. Extradural haematoma are usually focal and of heterogeneous signal characteristics on MRI. Extradural and subdural haemorrhage (SDH) may also be idiopathic in nature and may present with sudden onset pain and rapid onset of neurological dysfunction. SDH may be iatrogenic (Fig. 14.45) and tends to be extensive with imaging characteristics similar to intracranial SDHs. Subarachnoid haemorrhage may occur following rupture of an intraspinal vascular malformation or following distant (usually intracranial) surgery.

CONGENITAL DISORDERS

Developmental abnormalities of the spine are generically known as spinal dysraphism. The basic defect is abnormal formation or fusion of neural (**myeloschisis**) and mesenchymal (**spina bifida**) elements in early gestation. The majority of these abnormalities occur in the lumbosacral region. MRI has now become the imaging modality of choice for this group of lesions, but spinal ultrasound in the first few months of life may be a useful screening tool, and CT-assisted myelography

(a)

(b)

Figure 14.45 *Spinal subdural haematoma 3 days following intracranial surgery. (a) Sagittal (b) T1-weighted images demonstrating extensive hyperintense haematoma. Note the trefoil-like compression of the subarachnoid fluid space on the axial section.*

may be of use in certain cases. There are three major types of lesions: spina bifida aperta, cystica and occulta.

OPEN SPINAL DYSRAPHISM (SPINA BIFIDA APERTA)

This group is represented by the incomplete closure of the neural tube with exposure of neural tissue which may lie flush to the skin (**myelocele**) or is elevated by an underlying herniating CSF sac (**myelomeningocele**). Both are associated with wide defects in the posterior neural arches of contiguous vertebrae. Varying degrees of kyphoscoliosis are often seen. Presentation at birth is with an exposed lesion, which usually requires primary repair. Secondary dysraphic lesions are not uncommon, particularly diastematomyelia (see below). There is an almost invariable presence of a Chiari II malformation and various congenital intracranial abnormalities. Hydrocephalus frequently develops following closure of the defect.

Syringohydromyelia occurs in 30–50 per cent of patients and may affect the whole spinal cord (Fig. 14.46). When the dysraphism is severe secondary neurological dysfunction may develop and may also lead to progressive kyphoscoliotic deformities.

CLOSED SKIN COVERED CYSTIC MASS (SPINA BIFIDA CYSTICA)

The commonest lesion in this group is the **lipomyelomeningocele** in which there is a large lipomatous mass continuous with the subcutaneous fat. This is associated with herniation of a CSF sac, containing spinal cord, into which the lipomatous mass enters

(a)

(b)

Figure 14.47 *Dual arachnoid-dural sac diastematomyelia demonstrated on (a) sagittal and (b) axial T2-weighted MRI. The spinal cord extends down to the lower border of L3 (arrows) with a complex posterior neural arch defect at L2. Note the bony spur interposed between the two sacs and hemicords (curved arrow).*

Figure 14.46 *Chiari II malformation. Sagittal T2 image demonstrating cervicomedullary descent through the foramen magnum, basilar impingement from the dens, an enlarged and elongated fourth ventricle (IV) and multiseptated hydrosyringomyelia.*

Figure 14.48 *Sagittal T2-weighted MRI showing a low spinal cord tethered by a thickened filum terminale (curved arrows). An intraspinal dermoid cyst (arrow) is also present and there is a slender high signal syrinx (S) in the cord.*

Figure 14.49 *Intraspinal lipoma. Sagittal T1-weighted image showing a large hyperintense lipoma (L) filling the sacral cul-de-sac, tethering the spinal cord (arrow).*

Figure 14.50 *Malignant sacrococcygeal teratoma in an 11-month-old child. Sagittal T2-weighted image demonstrating a very large heterogeneously hyperintense lesion filling and expanding the lumbosacral spinal canal, scalloping the posterior vertebral bodies.*

and merges. Multiple posterior neural arch defects are present and in 30–50 per cent of cases a distal cord hydrosyrinx develops.

OCCULT SPINAL DYSRAPHISM (SPINA BIFIDA OCCULTA)

This group contains a wide spectrum of abnormalities and represents the most commonly encountered lesions. The skin is intact but there may be cutaneous stigmata such as a hairy patch, haemangioma or deep skin pit. In many cases there is little or no neurological deficit or associated spinal deformity, and these patients often escape detection during life. Symptomatic patients tend to present in late childhood or early adulthood with a wide range of problems including pes cavus, leg length inequality, lower limb and sphincter dysfunction or progressive spinal deformity. **Diastematomyelia** is the partial or complete splitting of the spinal cord and associated clefting abnormalities of the vertebral bodies and posterior neural arches. The pial lined split 'hemicords' may be contained within a single arachnoidural tube or each hemicord may lie within its own arachnoid-dural envelope (Fig. 14.47). The latter type has a fibrous or bony spur interposed between the two hemicords and is more frequently symptomatic. The cord is tethered and secondary hydrosyringomyelia develops over 50 per cent of the cases. A thickened filum terminal is often present, further tethering the cord distally.

Other lesions include a simple thickened filum terminale (which may contain a lipoma) often tethering a low lying spinal cord (Fig. 14.48); dorsal dermal sinus (an epithelial lined tract that extends from the skin surface to the spinal column, thecal sac or into the sac to merge with a low spinal cord) and intraspinal lipoma (a fatty mass intimately related to the dorsal aspect of the cord and tethering the cord to the thecal sac – Fig. 11.49).

In all these conditions imaging attempts to demonstrate the defect prior to possible surgery and to define any features, such as tethering of the spinal cord, cord cavitation or intraspinal sepsis owing to communication with the skin or bowel.

Sacrococcygeal teratoma is a congenital tumour probably arising from the distal coccyx. It is the most common tumour of the newborn infant. Most are of mixed solid and cystic elements with variable degrees of malignancy. They may be small or huge (Fig. 14.50).

FURTHER READING

Bundschuh, C.V. 1993: Imaging of the postoperative lumbosacral spine. *Neuroimaging Clinics of North America* **3**, 499–516.

Colombo, N., Berry, I., Norman, D. 1992: Infections of the spine. In Manelfe, C. (ed.), *Imaging of the spine and spinal cord*. New York: Raven Press, pp. 489–512.

Dennis, F. 1983: The three column spine and its significance in the classification of acute thoracolumbar spinal injuries. *Spine* **8**, 817–31.

Enzmann, D.R. 1990: Infection and inflammation. In Enzmann, D.R., DeLaPaz, R.L., Rubin, J.M. (eds), *Magnetic resonance imaging of the spine*. St. Louis: C.V. Mosby, pp. 260–300.

McCormick, P.C., Stein, B.M. 1990: Intramedullary tumours in adults. *Neurosurgical Clinics of North America* **1**, 609–30.

Milette, P.C. 1997: The proper terminology for reporting lumbar intervertebral disc disorders. *American Journal of Neuroradiology* **18**, 1860–6.

Modic, M.T. 1989: Degenerative disorders of the spine. In Modic, M., Masaryk, T., Ross, J. (eds), *Magnetic resonance imaging of the spine*. Chicago: Year Book Publishers.

Naidich, T.P., Zimmerman, R.A., McClone, D.G. *et al.* 1996: Congenital anomalies of the spine and spinal cord: embryology and malformations. In Atlas, S.W. (ed.), *Magnetic resonance imaging of the brain and spine*. Philadelphia: Lippincott-Raven, pp. 1265–339.

Pardatscher, K., Fiore, D.L., Lavano, A. 1992: MR imaging of transverse myelitis using Gd-DTPA. *Journal of Neuroradiology* **19**, 63–7.

Pathria, M.N., Petersilge, C.A. 1991: Spinal trauma. *Radiologic Clinics of North America* **29**, 847–65.

Rodesch, G., Berenstein, A., Lasjaunias, P. 1992: Vasculature and vascular lesions of the spine and spinal cord. In Manelfe, C. (ed.), *Imaging of the spine and spinal cord*. New York: Raven Press, pp. 565–98.

Ross, J.S. 1999: Newer sequences for spinal MR imaging: Smorgasbord or succotash of acronyms? *American Journal of Neuroradiology* **20**, 361–73.

Twohig, M., Sze, G. 1990: Spinal tumours. In Cohen, M.D., Edwards, M.K. (eds), *Pediatric magnetic resonance imaging*. Philadelphia: Decker, pp. 463–98.

Skull and brain

DONALD M. HADLEY

In no other area of the body are so many of the available imaging modalities used to provide complementary information. The information may be structural, functional or a mixture of both. Unfortunately the increasing sensitivity of the more recently introduced examinations has not been matched by improved specificity. Fundamental radiological criteria based on a thorough knowledge of the common sites of the possible lesions, their structure and growth patterns are still essential to narrow the differential diagnosis. In many patients a final diagnosis will only be obtained when the radiological findings are matched with the microscopic examination of tissues obtained by image-directed biopsy or surgical resection.

Technical developments in therapeutic radiological intervention have already revolutionized the treatment of many intracranial and intraspinal vascular lesions and promise to change the role of the clinical neuroradiologist in the care of patients presenting with CNS symptoms.

IMAGING TECHNIQUES

Since the development of computed tomography (CT) and magnetic resonance imaging (MRI), plain skull radiographs now seldom give additional information in the evaluation of CNS disease and have lost their pivotal role as the initial examination of the brain and skull. Plain radiography may be justified:

- to assess conditions that affect the density of the skull (Fig. 15.1);
- to assess conditions that cause remodelling of the skull secondary to either local destruction or increased intracranial pressure;
- to assess cases of gross facial and skull fractures;
- to exclude radiopaque foreign bodies, e.g. before MRI.

Intravenous contrast agents are used with CT and MRI to assess the vascularity of lesions and their effect on the **blood–brain barrier**, a functional barrier formed by the tight junctions in the capillary endothelial cells of the brain and spine. This barrier, which prevents hydrophilic molecules from entering the interstitial compartment by passive diffusion from the vascular space (as happens in the rest of the body), is disrupted by most neoplasms, infections, inflammation, infarction and certain stages of maturation of haemorrhage. With CT, iodinated agents show patterns of increased attenuation in areas of blood–brain barrier breakdown, whilst with MRI, paramagnetic agents, such as those based on gadolinium, result in an increased signal on T1-weighted images. These enhancement characteristics help to narrow the differential diagnosis, provide information about the 'activity' of a lesion and can show abnormalities invisible on unenhanced images.

Tissue contrast in the brain on CT is inferior in comparison to MRI and iodinated intravenous contrast is frequently required. However, CT has advantages:

Figure 15.1 *Langerhan's cell histiocytosis. Plain lateral skull radiograph showing a well-defined punched-out lytic lesion with a bevelled appearance of the inner margins (arrows). The extent of the skull lesion is more apparent on a plain film than on CT but even with a typical pattern there are still several differential diagnoses.*

- It is widely available and well understood.
- It can be performed quickly and is relatively inexpensive.
- It is excellent in the examination of patients with:
  - suspected acute subarachnoid haemorrhage;
  - acute trauma;
  - acute stroke to exclude haemorrhage;
  - subtle bony abnormalities, such as those in the temporal and facial regions;
  - calcified intracranial lesions;
  - contraindications to MRI, e.g. patients with a cardiac pacemaker.

MRI is now an alternative to CT for the investigation of nearly all cranial disorders and competes with angiography and ultrasound for the non-invasive assessment of the larger extra- and intracerebral arteries and veins. The increased tissue contrast and spatial resolution produced by MRI together with the multiplanar imaging capability allows earlier detection of many intracranial lesions. This is especially so in regions enclosed by dense bone, such as the middle and posterior fossae which degrades the CT image. However, MRI has disadvantages:

- It is relatively insensitive to calcification.
- It is more expensive and tends to be less readily available than CT.
- It requires more patient preparation.
- It is contraindicated in those patients with electronic implants, such as cardiac pacemakers, most aneurysm clips and any metallic foreign bodies in the orbits.

SCALP AND SKULL

Imaging can play a role in defining the origin and extent of lesions presenting in the scalp. The skin, subcutaneous tissue, galea (epicranial aponeurosis) and subaponeurotic areolar layer overlying the skull are all shown on CT when soft-tissue windows are used, but are better seen on MRI (Fig. 15.2). Haematomas and infection usually result from trauma and can involve any of these layers or the underlying bone. Imaging is not usually required to define the commonly found sebaceous cyst or lipoma but, if there is any clinical doubt or the lesion is unusually large, its morphology can be shown on CT or MRI. Differentiation from dermoids, which usually occur at the outer upper angle of the orbit and may have an intracranial component, is important. A full imaging evaluation is mandatory for midline abnormalities as they may represent the superficial portion of an intracranial lesion such as a cephalocele or meningomyelocele.

Focal involvement of the inner and outer tables of skull may be shown on plain radiography. If the lesion lies posteriorly, a Towne's view will best show the occipital bone. Tangential views of the lesion may be required to assess bone erosion or calcification but these features are better shown on CT, which will also show any additional involvement of the intracranial contents. Plain films often give a better geographical overview of the site and extent of the lesion, but plain films are now being superseded by the use of the digital 'scout' view obtained routinely with CT.

Normal variants producing focal areas of **decreased bone density** include venous lakes, parietal foramina,

(a)

(b)

Figure 15.2 *Subcutaneous occipital scalp lump on (a) proton density and (b) T2-weighted axial sections. The lump is a cyst which contains fatty components. Note intact outer skull table (arrows) under the lesion.*

pacchionian granulations and parietal thinning. These normal findings have to be differentiated from epidermoids, haemangiomas, eosinophilic granulomas and multiple myeloma. Slowly growing lesions, or those producing a long-standing pressure erosion, tend to be well demarcated with some reactive sclerosis in their margins. The lesions of untreated multiple myeloma appear 'punched out' and sharply delineated without sclerosis. Metastatic lesions in the skull are nearly all lytic, although the same primary may produce sclerotic lesions elsewhere. Metastases are poorly marginated, irregular in size and shape, may be single or multiple and produce varying destruction of the inner or outer table of the skull with infiltration of the diploë. Common primary tumours that metastasize to the skull are carcinomas of the breast, thyroid and prostate.

Hyperostosis frontalis interna is a common normal variant seen most frequently in middle-aged women which results in sclerosis and thickening of the inner table and diploë of the frontal bone with relative sparing of the midline. This density change must be differentiated from fibrous dysplasia which produces sclerotic, lytic or mixed lesions involving mainly the outer table. Fibrous dysplasia usually shows 'ground-glass' appearance on plain film; it causes expansion of the bone which may encroach on the paranasal sinuses or skull base foramina. Meningiomas may induce secondary effects which result in hyperostosis and increased density with eventual obliteration of the diploë of the adjacent involved bone. Enlarged vascular grooves on the inner table of the skull may be noted running to the lesion. These are formed by hypertrophied external carotid artery branches supplying this dural-based tumour. Occasionally, destructive changes are found, and a meningioma may be indistinguishable from a solitary metastasis (Fig. 15.3). Osteomas and exostoses show typical densities on imaging and can arise from the inner or outer tables of the skull.

Lesions producing **mixed density** include the various stages of Paget's disease. Its lytic phase involves the frontal or occipital bones and spreads to the vertex affecting the outer table of the skull. The sclerotic phase shows recalcification and dense skull thickening that often produces compression of the skull base foramina. The new bone is soft, and basilar invagination causes compression at the cervical medullary junction. Infection of the skull may be the result of direct extension from surrounding soft tissues, from the paranasal sinuses or mastoids, or from blood-borne infection. Infection causes resorption of bone and a lytic lesion may be shown associated with periosteal reaction and a soft-tissue mass. The main

(a)

(b)

(c)

Figure 15.3 *Meningioma presenting as skull lump in a 60-year-old. (a) Digital lateral CT 'scanogram' shows a calcified mass expanding through the skull. (b) Soft-tissue tangential plain radiograph shows 'eggshell' thinning and expansion of the outer skull table. (c) Axial CT through the lesion shows craggy calcification associated with the dural-based mass expanding through the skull provoking only minimal oedema in the adjacent brain.*

reason for cross-sectional imaging in bony osteomyelitis is to define any intracranial spread so that adequate decompression and appropriate antibiotic therapy is instituted. Occasionally a 'button' sequestrum will form with an island of bone in the lytic area. This is unusual as the skull has such a good blood supply; sequestrum formation occurs most often with tuberculous osteitis and staphylococcal infections. Sclerotic lesions occur when the infection is chronic, as may happen with an inadequately treated acute osteomyelitis or with infections from organisms that have a low virulence, such as fungi, spirochaetes and tuberculosis.

Trauma is now the commonest cause of a skull lesion. Fractures and their effects will be discussed in the section on craniocerebral injuries.

Calcification in the pineal, choroid plexus and habenula, if sufficiently dense, is seen on plain films and must not be mistaken for a lesion. Occasionally, displacement of these normal calcifications reveals the presence of an intracranial mass lesion, although this is more readily demonstrated by CT or MRI.

In young children **increased intracranial pressure** may cause widening of sutures. After suture fusion the effects of chronic increased intracranial pressure may be shown on plain lateral and anterior skull views as thinning of the cortex of the dorsum sellae extending to the floor of the sella turcica. Eventually enlargement of the whole sella may be seen. Although thinning of the calvarium may occur and prominent convolutional markings may develop, these findings may also be seen in normal people. These signs of raised intracranial pressure are only found after a considerable period of raised pressure, but are often seen at first presentation. CT or MRI is required to assess the cause of the increased pressure and the size of the ventricles. If fontanelles are not closed, they can be used as a window for ultrasound to assess ventricular size.

Cranial synostosis, the premature fusion of one or more of the sutures, results in deformity of the skull. An overview of the skull shape and assessment of the sutures is usually made on plain films. CT, or ideally MRI, is used to document the effect on the brain and

(a)

(b)

(c)

Figure 15.4 *Bilateral coronal synostosis producing turricephaly in a 9-month-old infant. (a) Plain lateral radiograph shows the typical skull shape, whilst CT with (b) bone and (c) soft-tissue windows shows that the coronal sutures are fused while the lambdoid and sagittal sutures are normal (arrows); the brain has formed normally and there is no hydrocephalus.*

ventricles. The bone adjacent to the fused suture becomes thickened with a band of increased density parallel to the suture. Involvement of the sagittal suture, the commonest fusion, results in compensatory overgrowth of the sutures perpendicular to it, namely the lambdoid and coronal, producing an elongated narrow skull (dolichocephaly or scaphocephaly). Unilateral coronal synostosis, which is the most common fusion to be treated, results in elongation of the orbit and greater wing of sphenoid producing an oblique-shaped or plagiocephalic skull. With bilateral coronal synostosis there is general shortening of the skull, with compensatory upward growth, resulting in turricephaly (Fig. 15.4). Lambdoid synostosis similarly can be bilateral or unilateral and result in turricephaly or plagiocephaly. Follow-up examinations, plain films, CT or MRI may be required after surgical treatment. Changes in ventricular size are noted particularly.

CONGENITAL STRUCTURAL ABNORMALITIES OF THE BRAIN

Normal mature brain structure depends on incredibly complicated repeated cycles of development and remodelling. Disturbance at a particular stage occurs in up to 1 per cent of live births, although only in less than half can an identifiable genetic, vascular or infectious cause be found. A wide range of congenital malformations may be recognized by using ultrasound in the fetus and infant.

MRI is the optimal imaging modality once the fontanelles close because of the propensity for lesions to lie in the sagittal plane and because of the excellent soft-tissue definition and multiplanar sections possible with MRI.

The abnormalities may be classified according to the timing of the insult with disturbances of dorsal induction (3rd and 4th week of gestation), ventral induction (5th to 10th week), neuronal proliferation, differentiation and histogenesis (8th to 16th week) and neuronal migration disorders (2nd to 5th month) producing distinct groups of lesions. Over 2000 malformations have been described but only the commonest ones with a radiological interest will be discussed here.

DORSAL INDUCTION

Failure of dorsal induction causes the neural tube defects, which include cephaloceles, the Chiari malformations and spinal dysraphic abnormalities (p. 388). These abnormalities are best shown on midline sagittal T1-weighted MRI but suspicious features on a routine axial CT such as an abnormal fourth ventricle, a 'full' foramen magnum and absent cisterna magna must be recognized and followed up with MRI.

Chiari I malformation

Chiari I is the mildest of the hindbrain malformations and is characterized by displacement over 5 mm downwards of deformed cerebellar tonsils through the foramen magnum. The brain stem and fourth ventricle retain their normal position although the ventricle may be small and slightly distorted. A Chiari I malformation is not usually associated with other cerebral abnormalities, but a syrinx may be found in the spinal cord in up to 25 per cent of cases.

Chiari II malformation

A Chiari II malformation is a more extensive and complex abnormality than the Chiari I malformation with infratentorial and supratentorial abnormalities. The cerebellar tonsils, inferior vermis, fourth ventricle and brain stem are herniated from a shallow posterior fossa through a wide foramen magnum (Fig. 15.5). There is nearly always a meningocele or meningomyelocele with some associated hydrocephalus. Partial or complete agenesis of the corpus callosum is found in many patients. A degree of spinal dysraphism is usually present together with a tethered cord and filum lipoma.

Chiari III malformation

A Chiari III malformation is very rare. There is herniation of the posterior fossa contents into an associated occipital or high cervical cephalocele, together with the other features of a Chiari II malformation.

Cephalocele

The term cephalocele refers to an abnormal protrusion of an intracranial structure through a skull defect. It can include brain, ventricles, cerebrospinal fluid (CSF) and

Figure 15.5 *Midline sagittal T1-weighted section showing a Chiari II malformation associated with hydrocephalus.*

meninges either alone or in combination. A cephalocele is commonest in the occipital region in the Caucasian population, but may also occur through the frontal, basal and parietal bones. Although large occipital, parietal and frontal cephaloceles are usually diagnosed on clinical examination, small cephaloceles may be misdiagnosed as a skull lump and should therefore be imaged before biopsy or excision. They usually lie in the midline and T1-weighted MRI is the best way to identify their contents and any connection with intracranial structures. Cephaloceles involving the nasofrontal or sphenoethmoidal bones may present to the otorhinolaryngologist as masses with a wide clinical differential diagnosis. Imaging is essential to prevent possible biopsy of the frontal lobe protruding through a defect. Axial or reformatted sagittal CT sections show the bony defect, but T1-weighted coronal and sagittal MRI scans show the whole lesion more clearly.

VENTRAL INDUCTION

Ventral induction results in the formation of the brain and face. Disorders of ventral induction result in holoprosencephaly, septo-optic dysplasia and the Dandy–Walker syndrome. The Dandy–Walker syndrome is the commonest and the most important.

Dandy–Walker syndrome and variant

The Dandy–Walker syndrome comprises partial or complete cerebellar vermis aplasia, so that the cerebellum is displaced and the fourth ventricle replaced by a cyst which does not communicate with the subarachnoid CSF. The condition is thought to be due to obstruction of CSF flow at the foramina of Luschka and Magendie. More than 50 per cent of patients have other congenital anomalies including agenesis of the corpus callosum, holoprosencephaly, schizencephaly, polymicrogyria, cephaloceles and grey matter heterotopia. The clinical signs and symptoms usually relate more to these associated conditions than to the main defect.

The Dandy–Walker variant is a less severe form of the complex in which the vermis and fourth ventricle are better developed. Communication between the fourth ventricle and the posterior fossa cyst is variable. Hydrocephalus, heterotopias and callosal dysgenesis occur much less commonly in the variant. CT axial sections show the CSF space and the cerebellar dysplasia, but these are all best shown with MRI using sagittal and axial sections of the posterior fossa and foramen magnum. The many associated anomalies are readily shown on MRI.

The Dandy–Walker syndrome and variant must be differentiated from a giant cisterna magna, which is a normal variant, and a posterior fossa arachnoid cyst not communicating with the fourth ventricle, and is not associated with other anomalies.

NEURONAL PROLIFERATION, DIFFERENTIATION AND HISTIOGENESIS

Disorders of these stages of development result in neoplastic and vascular malformations often with cutaneous manifestations, hence they are also called neurocutaneous disorders or phakomatoses.

Neurofibromatosis I

Neurofibromatosis I is the commonest type of neurofibromatosis accounting for 90 per cent of cases. The defect is known to lie on the long arm of chromosome 17 and in half the patients the disorder is transmitted as an autosomal dominant; it is sporadic in the remainder. In this type of neurofibromatosis there are prominent skin manifestations associated with tumours of neurones and astrocytes often with distinctive osseous and dural lesions, such as sphenoid dysplasia or vertebral scalloping and lateral meningoceles. Spinal neurofibromas, which are often small and single, may develop.

Neurofibromatosis II

Neurofibromatosis II is much less common than neurofibromatosis I and the cutaneous manifestations are less marked. Neurofibromatosis II is also an autosomal dominant disorder but the defect is on chromosome 22. There are associated tumours of the meninges and Schwann cells, the hallmark of the condition being bilateral acoustic schwannomas. Ependymomas and astrocytomas of the spinal cord may develop.

Von Hippel–Lindau disease

Von Hippel–Lindau disease is an autosomal dominant multisystem disorder in which the short arm of chromosome 3 has been implicated. Screening has been implemented for at-risk families. Patients usually develop posterior fossa or spinal haemangioblastomas associated with retinal angiomas, renal cell carcinomas, phaeochromocytomas, and cysts of the kidney, pancreas and liver. Multiple haemangioblastomas, which develop in the third or fourth decades, are pathognomonic.

The cerebellar tumours are seen with CT and MRI either as a strongly enhancing mass (20 per cent) or a cystic lesion with an enhancing mural nodule (80 per cent). They are usually located in the vermis, the brain stem being a less common site; cerebral hemisphere lesions are rare. The cystic component usually gives a higher signal than CSF on T1-weighted MRI because of its raised protein content. Vertebral angiography may define a vascular blush in the nodule. Angiography can assist in differentiating a haemangioblastoma from a cystic astrocytoma or metastasis.

Spinal cord lesions are seen with MRI in 8–35 per cent of patients. These are similar to the intracranial haemangioblastomas but may be associated with larger, more syrinx-like cysts. Angiography may be required to define the vascular supply.

Sturge–Weber syndrome

The Sturge–Weber syndrome is characterized by a vascular naevus of the face, the so-called 'port-wine stain', which occurs in one or more divisions of the fifth cranial nerve. The accompanying intracranial lesion is an ipsilateral angioma of the meninges, which results in hemiparesis, seizures and mental retardation. Typically, unilateral curvilinear calcification in the gyri in the occipitoparietal regions may be seen on plain films and CT, which also demonstrates cerebral atrophy.

Tuberous sclerosis

Tuberous sclerosis is characterized by multisystem hamartomatous tumours. Cranial involvement results in mental retardation, seizures and adenoma sebaceum of the face with calcified retinal hamartomas. Intracranial hamartomas are seen most typically as subependymal lesions, which usually undergo calcification, best detected by CT. In 10–15 per cent of patients malignant transformation into a subependymal giant cell astrocytoma occurs within a hamartoma located at the foramen of Monro. Cortical tubers are best appreciated on MRI, appearing as iso- or hypointense areas on T1-weighted images and hyperintense foci on a T2-weighted sequence (Fig. 15.6). Lesions may also be seen in the kidneys, heart, lung, liver, spleen and bones.

MIGRATION DISORDER

Migration disorder occurs between 2 and 5 months of intrauterine life when there is a disorder of the systematic migration of the proliferating neurones from the periventricular region to the cortex and deep nuclei, resulting in schizencephaly, agyria, pachygyria, heterotopia and dysgenesis of the corpus callosum. Although MRI can now clearly define the abnormal brain structure, functional imaging with positron emission tomography or single photon emission computed tomography (SPECT) may be required for assessment of associated abnormal function such as epilepsy. Corpus callosum abnormality is associated with many of the other lesions already mentioned and is discussed in more detail below.

Dysgenesis of the corpus callosum

During months 3 and 4 of fetal life the corpus callosum develops from the front to the back beginning with the genu. An interruption of growth affects the body, splenium or rostrum. Agenesis results from an insult before 12 weeks of gestation and is associated with many anomalies including Dandy–Walker, Chiari malformations and midline lipoma (Fig. 15.7). CT and MRI show absence or underdevelopment of the corpus callosum with separation of the lateral ventricles and elevation of the third ventricle between them.

INTRACRANIAL NEOPLASMS

Primary tumours can arise from any intracranial cell line other than mature neurones, which do not divide, except for aesthesioneuroblastoma which is derived from still

Figure 15.6 *Tuberous sclerosis. T2-weighted axial section in a 2-year-old showing hypointense subependymal calcified tubers (arrows) and hyperintense cortical hamartomas (arrowheads).*

Figure 15.7 *T1-weighted midline sagittal section showing hyperintense lipoma of the corpus callosum.*

Figure 15.8 *Intense* [201]*Tl uptake in a deep left temporoparietal glioma; baseline assessment before resection.*

dividing neural tissue in the olfactory mucosa. Metastatic disease is commonest from lung, breast, kidney, melanoma and colon tumours while prostatic secondaries and myeloma are found in the dura and calvarium.

CT is still the first modality for the investigation of most patients presenting with signs or symptoms of a tumour, but the advantages of MRI in terms of increased contrast sensitivity, direct multiplanar capability and lack of bone artefact are now being realized. MRI is especially useful for detecting and managing tumours in the brain stem, middle and posterior cranial fossae. Angiography is still used to assess the vascularity of selected tumours, such as meningiomas, and may be combined with presurgical embolization. SPECT with ^{201}Tl shows selective uptake in malignant tumours (Fig. 15.8), as well as meningiomas, and thallium scanning is useful both for measuring the functional volume of the tumour before and after treatment, and in the differential diagnosis between radiation necrosis and recurrent tumour, both of which may be present as enhancing masses on CT or MRI.

Tumours are characterized on CT and MRI by showing a central mass causing variable displacement (or mass effect) on adjacent normal structures which can lead to obstructive hydrocephalus. Tumours are frequently surrounded by oedema, the most severe oedema being seen with fast-growing and aggressive tumours. In general, the density of the mass on CT is reduced compared to normal brain, and after intravenous contrast, if there is blood–brain barrier breakdown due to 'leaky' immature neovascularity, various patterns (homogeneous, ring, patchy) of enhancement are identified. On MRI the T1- and T2-relaxation times of tumour are increased, so it appears hypointense on T1-weighted and hyperintense on T2-weighted images.

(a)

(b)

Figure 15.9 *Intermediate grade glioma in a 29-year-old with personality change, headaches and papilloedema. (a) T2-weighted axial and (b) T1-weighted coronal post-gadolinium enhancement sections show a left frontal cystic mass surrounded by oedema with an enhancing irregular solid nodule and cyst wall, together with marked ventricular compression and displacement.*

Any surrounding oedema follows a similar but more pronounced set of signal patterns, which can sometimes make it difficult to separate tumour mass from oedema. Blood–brain barrier breakdown can be highlighted in a similar way to that with CT, with intravenous gadolinium-based contrast agents; these cause a shortening of T1-relaxation time resulting in increased signal on T1-weighted images (Fig. 15.9). It is important to avoid equating the extent of a tumour shown radiologically with the limits of its growth, because CT and MRI stereotactic biopsy studies have shown that malignant cells often extend into the peritumoral oedema beyond the enhancing margins of the mass.

Neoplasms are generally classified according to their site and original cell type:

- **Intra-axial: glial tumours**
  - astrocytoma
    - ▸ low-grade astrocytoma
    - ▸ anaplastic astrocytoma
    - ▸ glioblastoma
  - oligodendroglioma
  - ependymoma
  - choroid plexus tumour
- **Intra-axial: non-glial tumours**
  - haemangioblastomas
  - primitive neuroectodermal tumour (PNET)
  - lymphoma
  - metastasis
  - hamartoma
- **Intraventricular**
  - colloid cyst
  - choroid plexus tumour
  - ependymoma
  - astrocytoma
  - meningioma
  - subependymal giant cell astrocytoma
- **Extra-axial**
  - meningioma
  - nerve sheath tumours
    - ▸ schwannoma
    - ▸ plexiform neurofibroma
  - glomus tumour
  - chordoma
  - chondroma, chondrosarcoma
  - epidermoid
  - dermoid
  - teratoma
  - arachnoid cyst
  - pituitary tumours
  - metastatic tumours.

Unfortunately the cell type is only known with certainty after histological examination and often requires specialist immunological stains directed at individual cellular components. It is sometimes possible to identify a particular tumour type with a high degree of confidence on both CT and MRI but, since many tumours contain calcification, haemorrhage, cysts or necrotic areas, it is not surprising that there is a huge overlap in the appearance of the different types of tumour.

Once a tumour is imaged the first critical decision, which will narrow the differential diagnosis, is whether it is an intra-axial lesion arising from brain substance or an extra-axial lesion arising in the dura, meninges, or extradural or intraventricular space. On CT or MRI extra-axial lesions buckle the cortex and white matter, displace the subarachnoid veins inwards, expand the ipsilateral subarachnoid space and sometimes cause reactive bone changes. Axial lesions lie within the brain and expand the cortex with no separation by the underlying leptomeninges. They spread across parenchymal boundaries and the dura is seen to lie peripherally. If a lesion is aggressively invasive the distinction between an intra- or extra-axial lesion may be blurred and, rarely, a dural meningioma invades the brain while a parenchymal metastasis may invade the meninges.

INTRA-AXIAL TUMOURS

Intra-axial tumours include metastases, glial and non-glial neoplasms. Glial tumours, which cause up to 45 per cent of primary brain tumours, arise from astrocytes, oligodendrocytes, ependymal cells and the choroid plexus. The non-glial tumours include those arising from primitive bipotential precursors (primitive neuroectodermal tumour or PNET), mesenchymal cells (haemangioblastoma), the lymphoreticular system (lymphoma) and those associated with the phakomatoses.

Developmental tumours (dermoid/epidermoid tumours) although strictly extra-axial are frequently seen within the brain substance and are considered in this section.

Metastases

Metastases are usually multiple, well-defined, enhancing masses that characteristically grow from the grey–white matter junction (Fig. 15.10). They are typically low density on non-contrast CT unless haemorrhagic or hypercellular. On T1-weighted MRI they are either hypointense or isointense, while on T2-weighted sections they have variable intensity depending on cellularity, haemorrhage, necrosis and cyst formation. Nearly all metastases enhance to some degree on CT and MRI in either a homogeneous ring, or patchy manner, MRI being more sensitive to tiny lesions. The surrounding oedema is often out of proportion to the size of the metastases.

Glial tumours

Astrocytomas
Astrocytomas are graded from I to IV depending on their malignant potential with the grade IV type being considered as **glioblastomas**. The lowest grade tumours have variable CT appearances with mixed attenuation and poorly defined margins in which tumour and oedema merge. Calcification may be present. MRI shows these low-grade tumours as areas of hyperintensity on T2-weighted and hypointensity on T1-weighted scans with mild enhancement following intravenous contrast.

Figure 15.10 *Metastases in a 67-year-old with a previous resection of a colonic carcinoma presenting with ataxia, left-sided sensory symptoms and headache. CT with contrast shows multiple small ring-enhancing masses surrounded by extensive disproportionate oedema.*

Figure 15.11 *T1-weighted contrast-enhanced sagittal section showing an ependymoma (arrows) involving the exits of the fourth ventricle causing an obstructive hydrocephalus.*

Calcification, if dense, will produce signal voids. MRI is usually no better at showing tumour margins than CT. Cystic astrocytomas are low grade and are most often seen in children, frequently in the cerebellum. Occasionally cyst wall or nodular enhancement will be seen on CT or MRI. **Oligodendrogliomas** are slow growing, tend to be large and are mainly found in adults. Calcification is an important diagnostic feature being seen in 80 per cent on CT. They may undergo malignant astrocytic behaviour.

With the most malignant grades such as anaplastic astrocytomas (III) and glioblastomas (IV), CT shows areas of mixed attenuation with central low attenuation often representing necrosis. After intravenous contrast there is marked irregular enhancement. These aggressive tumours invade grey and white matter producing extensive surrounding oedema. MRI demonstrates heterogeneous intensity, which is increased on T2-weighted and decreased on T1-weighted images. Contrast enhancement is even more marked than on CT. Haemorrhage in various states of maturation is often seen on MRI.

Ependymomas
Ependymomas most often arise in the posterior fossa in children, although there is a second smaller incidence in the third decade. An ependymoma presents on CT as a midline mass which shows variable enhancement (Fig. 15.11); 50 per cent show calcification. The tumour is often cystic and may extend into the cerebellopontine angles and the foramina of the fourth ventricle and spread in the subarachnoid space.

Choroid plexus tumours
Choroid plexus tumours are intraventricular and should really be considered as extra-axial. They are unusual in adults and are most commonly found in the atria of the lateral ventricles in children under 5 years old. On CT they appear as well-marginated, lobulated, isodense intraventricular masses that show strong uniform contrast enhancement. There is calcification in up to 80 per cent of the tumours. On MRI both T1- and T2-weighted images may show intermediate intensities, with foci of dense calcification showing as signal voids. The mass enhances strongly. Old haemorrhage seen on T2-weighted images as hypointensity is common. Malignant change should be suspected if the tumour extends into brain parenchyma. Hydrocephalus can be caused by haemorrhage obstructing the flow of CSF or possibly by overproduction of CSF by the tumour. Both the benign and malignant forms can seed through the CSF pathways.

Non-glial tumours

Primitive neuroectodermal tumours
Primitive neuroectodermal tumours now include tumours that pathologists previously classified as medulloblastomas and pineoblastomas in addition to other undifferentiated small cell tumours. Most medulloblastomas are seen on CT as well-defined, hyperdense, midline, posterior fossa masses which nearly all show uniform strong enhancement. A few tumours calcify but haemorrhage is rare. Most patients present because of the accompanying obstructive hydrocephalus. On MRI the features are variable with the mass iso- to hypointense on T1-weighted and iso- to hyperintense on T2-weighted images. Strong contrast enhancement is common. The extent of the mass and its relation to the fourth ventricle is shown best on sagittal sections. Metastases that have seeded via the CSF can be shown

on enhanced T1-weighted images in over 25 per cent of patients. These metastases can involve the cerebral subarachnoid space in addition to the spinal cord, cauda equina and thecal sac.

Pineal region tumours
Pineal region tumours are a heterogeneous group of neoplasms, which includes the primitive neuroectodermal tumours described above in addition to germinomas, teratomas, pineocytomas and tumours arising from other cell types such as gliomas, meningiomas, melanomas and metastases. All are best imaged with MRI using a combination of axial and sagittal plane T1- and T2-weighted sections. MRI also demonstrates the site of the obstruction responsible for hydrocephalus, which is frequently the presenting complaint.

Haemangioblastomas
Haemangioblastomas have already been described earlier as part of von Hippel–Lindau disease (p. 397). Most occur sporadically in young or middle-aged adults and, although a benign tumour, some 25 per cent recur after surgery.

Lymphomas
Lymphomas are uncommon but the incidence is rising with the increasing population of immunocompromised patients with AIDS and from transplant programmes. Lymphoma usually forms a solitary mass but multiple lesions clustered around the ventricles may be seen. On CT there is slightly increased attenuation with marked homogeneous contrast enhancement and surrounding oedema. MRI demonstrates the expected hyperintensity on T2- and hypointensity on T1-weighted images. The mass frequently abuts a CSF surface such as the pia or ependyma of the ventricles. After steroid treatment the mass may temporarily disappear. In patients with possible concurrent infections, such as AIDS-associated toxoplasmosis, a thallium radionuclide scan will show uptake in tumour but not abscess.

Epidermoids
Epidermoids arise from the inclusion of epidermal tissue. They most commonly involve the cerebellopontine angles but are also found in the sylvian fissures or basal cisterns. CT shows a lobulated mass of low attenuation without enhancement, unless there have been reactive changes in the surrounding brain. Occasionally flecks of marginal calcification may be seen. It can be difficult to differentiate these tumours from arachnoid cysts, but an epidermoid mass is extra-axial and invaginates into the brain substance.

Dermoids
Dermoids arise from the inclusion of ectoderm, mesoderm and endoderm and are generally midline tumours frequently involving the posterior fossa.

Dermoids contain varying amounts of fat and calcification. The fat is seen as low attenuation on CT associated with high attenuation due to calcification. Occasionally the fat leaks into the surrounding CSF space to cause a ventriculitis or meningitis. On MRI the fat is seen as a high signal on T1-weighted images. As with epidermoids, dermoids are really extra-axial but are generally seen within brain parenchyma and so are considered here.

Tumours associated with the **phakomatoses** have been discussed under the neurocutaneous syndromes (p. 397).

EXTRA-AXIAL TUMOURS

Extra-axial tumours include neoplasms of mesenchymal cell origin (meningiomas), nerve sheath tumours, schwannomas, tumours related to maldevelopment with inclusions and metastatic neoplasms. Pituitary tumours are also discussed in this section.

Meningiomas
Meningioma is the most common extra-axial tumour. In order of frequency it is found in the parasagittal regions, convexities of the skull vault, sphenoid wing, cerebellopontine angle, olfactory groove and planum sphenoidale. On unenhanced CT more than 50 per cent of these tumours have a higher attenuation than brain with calcification in 20 per cent. The lesions commonly invaginate into and buckle the brain parenchyma but, because they grow slowly, they have less mass effect than would be expected for their size (Fig. 15.12). Some tumours grow *en plaque* along the dura, especially in the posterior fossa and the parasellar regions. Hyperostosis of adjacent bone, which may be appreciated on plain films of the skull, is common. After intravenous contrast there is marked enhancement of the tumour seen on CT, although areas of necrosis or fatty degeneration remain unenhanced. Surrounding oedema is variable with most large tumours invoking oedema, but small tumours may have no oedema, although occasionally they show considerable oedema, especially if adjacent to the skull base. On MRI the signal from the tumour is usually similar to grey matter on both T1- and T2-weighted images, making it difficult to identify small tumours without contrast. Avid enhancement after contrast is seen in meningiomas of all sizes. An adjacent tail of dural enhancement may be seen, which is due to either dural reactive changes or frank invasion, but this appearance is also occasionally seen with other tumours such as metastases and gliomas. Signal voids from flow in enlarged vessel and dense calcification are often seen. As meningiomas grow extra-axially they often have a large external carotid arterial supply with a typical vascular pattern, which can be shown with angiography. Preoperative embolization by the neuro-

(a)

(b)

(c)

(d)

Figure 15.12 *Frontal meningioma in a 54-year-old. CT (a) before and (b) after enhancement shows a dense dural-based mass lesion that enhances strongly after contrast. Selective digital subtraction angiography of the external carotid artery (c) before and (d) after flow-directed particulate embolization shows obliteration of the arteriolar blush (arrows) of the tumour prior to resection.*

radiologist can be used to make subsequent resection easier (Fig. 15.12).

Schwannomas

Schwannomas are the usual cranial nerve sheath tumours, whereas most cutaneous and peripheral nerve sheath tumours are neurofibromas. Schwannomas are associated with neurofibromatosis II. Schwannomas affect the cranial nerves III–XII, most commonly the vestibular division of the eighth nerve known as an **acoustic neuroma**. These tumours are well-defined iso- or hypodense masses which enhance strongly on CT and occasionally calcification is present. On MRI the tumours are hypo- or isointense on T1-weighted and hyperintense on T2-weighted images and show marked enhancement

after contrast (Fig. 15.13). An enlarged internal auditory meatus and canal may accompany the eighth nerve lesion. When screening for tumours, very high definition T2-weighted axial sections are made. Small tumours may be obscured by the high signal from the CSF but the presence of a tumour may be suspected by blurring of the normal outline of the individual nerves; a tumour can be confirmed by contrast-enhanced T1-weighted sections, which will show marked enhancement in tumours as small as 1–2 mm (Fig. 15.14).

Colloid cysts

Colloid cysts, though not neoplastic, are important intraventricular mass lesions that arise in the anterior portion of the third ventricle close to the foramen of

Figure 15.13 *Large acoustic schwannoma in a 49-year-old with left-sided sensorineural deafness. T1-weighted contrast enhanced axial section shows a 28 mm diameter extra-axial cerebellopontine angle enhancing mass compressing the brain stem and fourth ventricle extending from the internal auditory canal.*

Figure 15.15 *Unenhanced axial CT showing a high attenuation colloid cyst in a typical position at the foramen of Monro.*

Monro. Even small colloid cysts can cause an acute obstructive hydrocephalus of the lateral ventricles, which may initially be intermittent. Colloid cysts are well-defined, often pedunculated, round lesions, with increased attenuation on CT owing to their high protein content (Fig. 15.15). On MRI they are usually hyperintense on both T1- and T2-weighted sections. Sagittal and coronal sections are best for defining the lesions which do not usually enhance after contrast.

Metastases

Metastases involving the dura occur most commonly with tumours of the lung, breast, prostate and melanoma. Dural metastases tend to spread as plaque lesions and there may be associated parenchymal lesions. On CT, metastases appear as isodense thickening of the meninges, which enhances after contrast. Increased signal is seen on T2-weighted and decreased signal on T1-weighted MRI

(a)

(b)

Figure 15.14 *Small acoustic schwannoma in a 41-year-old complaining of tinnitus. (a) T2-weighted high-definition axial section shows a 3 × 3 × 2 mm diameter filling defect in the right internal auditory meatus (arrow) displacing the seventh and eighth cranial nerves. (b) T1-weighted contrast-enhanced coronal section confirms the tiny enhancing hyperintense tumour (arrow).*

(a)

(b)

Figure 15.16 *Subarachnoid and pial metastases shown as focal and coalescing hyperintensities over the superior cerebellum and vermis on (a) axial and (b) coronal-enhanced T1-weighted MRI.*

and, again, marked enhancement is a feature. With subarachnoid seeding small plaques or minute foci of tumour may be found with enhanced T1-weighted MRI. CT is considerably less sensitive for the detection of metastases than MRI. Subarachnoid metastases are found typically in the cerebellopontine angles and the basal cisterns but there is a broad differential diagnosis including infection and granulomas (Fig. 15.16).

Chordomas

Chordomas arise from notochord remnants and are most frequently seen in the clivus and sacrum. Chordo-

mas produce focal bone destruction eroding into the adjacent structures, compressing cranial nerves and eventually vessels. CT shows the extent of bone erosion and a mass of inhomogeneous density with focal calcification and patchy enhancement with intravenous contrast. Chordomas are best demonstrated with T1-weighted MRI, where they appear as a mass replacing the normal high intensity marrow signal (Fig. 15.17a). On MRI, chordomas have an inhomogeneous intensity, which is generally hypointense on T1-weighted and hyperintense on T2-weighted images, and show patchy contrast enhancement. Metastatic lesions and bone

(a)

(b)

Figure 15.17 *Differentiation of sellar and parasellar tumours is made easier by identifying the structures involved on sagittal and coronal MRI. (a) Chordoma. T1-weighted sagittal section showing a hypointense mass (circle) replacing the normally hyperintense marrow of the clivus, while the pituitary (arrow) remains intact. (b) Pituitary macroadenoma. T1-weighted contrast-enhanced sagittal section showing an enhancing mass (asterisk) expanding out of the sella to impinge on the optic chiasm (arrow) and floor of the third ventricle.*

tumours such as sarcomas and chondrosarcomas may initially appear very similar to a chordoma.

Pituitary tumours

Pituitary tumours are arbitrarily divided into macroadenomas (> 1 cm) and microadenomas (< 1 cm).

Macroadenomas usually enlarge and expand out of the pituitary fossa to produce symptoms eventually by impinging on the optic nerves and optic chiasm. Endocrine abnormalities are a less prominent feature. Macroadenomas should be recognized on routine axial CT but are better outlined by direct coronal dynamic enhanced CT. Sagittal and coronal MRI T1-weighted sections will define the limits of the mass and its relation to adjacent structures, such as the chiasm, floor of third ventricle, pituitary stalk, cavernous sinuses, intracranial carotid arteries and sphenoid sinus. The tumours are usually homogeneous appearing iso-hypointense on T1-weighted images with hyperintensity on T2-weighted images and show moderate enhancement with intravenous contrast (Fig. 15.17b). The occasional presence of haemorrhage, cysts or necrosis influences the MRI appearances.

Microadenomas are more common than macroadenomas and present with hormone imbalance rather than mass effects. Prolactin-secreting tumours are the most common tumours but adrenocortico-trophic- and growth hormone-secreting lesions are also found. Again high definition, dynamic enhanced direct coronal CT will identify lesions over 5 mm in diameter, which are silhouetted as a low density against the normally enhancing pituitary gland. The pituitary stalk may be displaced away from the lesion and there may be localized erosion of the floor of the pituitary fossa. MRI is more sensitive than CT for the detection of microadenomas. With dynamic enhanced coronal and sagittal T1-weighted thin sections, a microadenoma appears as a non-enhanced focus against a background of enhancing normal pituitary gland (Fig. 15.18). The displaced stalk can be assessed while the relationship of the adenoma to the cavernous sinus and adjacent carotid arteries is clearly displayed. These are important features to note prior to trans-sphenoidal surgery.

HEAD INJURY

Head injuries now represent a major cause of death and disability especially in young otherwise healthy people. The main cause of head injury is still road traffic accidents in spite of seat belt, alcohol and crash helmet legislation reducing hospital admissions by 25 per cent. Falls, assaults and sports injuries form an increasing proportion of the workload in neurosurgical units.

CLASSIFICATION OF INJURIES

With a combination of clinical and imaging information, injuries may be classified into primary lesions, secondary consequences and late sequelae (Table 15.1). Primary lesions are due to damage at the moment of impact and immediate complications. Primary lesions include skull fractures, diffuse axonal injury, contusions, lacerations and intracranial haemorrhage which may be found both intra- and extracerebrally. Secondary consequences occur later and include brain swelling, raised intracranial pressure, ischaemic damage and infarction due to brain herniation or vascular injury. Late sequelae include cerebromalacia, cerebral atrophy, hydrocephalus, CSF fistula, infection and vascular lesions.

CT is still the examination of choice in the immediate assessment of a patient with a head injury. Whilst

Figure 15.18 *Non-enhancing hypointense microadenoma (arrow) shown against the background of the hyperintense enhancing normal pituitary on a dynamic T1-weighted contrast-enhanced thin-section MRI in a patient with Cushing's disease.*

Table 15.1 *Clinical and imaging classification of head injury*

Primary lesions	Secondary consequences	Late sequelae
Skull fracture	Raised intracranial pressure	Cerebromalacia
Diffuse axonal injury		Cerebral atrophy
Contusions	Ischaemic damage	Hydrocephalus
Lacerations	Brain herniation	CSF fistula
Haemorrhage:	Vascular injury	Infection
intracerebral	Infarction	Vascular lesions
intraventricular		
subarachnoid		
subdural		
extradural		

CT is adequate for making acute surgical management decisions, it has become increasingly clear that MRI is more sensitive to minute alterations in cerebral water content and blood products, and MRI can show injuries invisible to CT. MRI is particularly useful in the subacute and chronic phases. Radionuclide scanning can show the functionally disrupted metabolism and ischaemia prevalent in most types of brain injury. The cerebral protection therapies currently under development are directed at potentially reversible damage and confirm the increasing complementary role for functional and structural imaging.

PLAIN SKULL FILMS FOLLOWING HEAD INJURY

Although skull radiographs can sometimes be important in the triage of minor injuries, if CT is indicated on clinical grounds or if neurosurgical referral is already deemed necessary, performing a skull radiograph will just delay the definitive CT examination or hinder the patient's transfer, and give no additional management information. A skull radiograph should now be performed in those patients with a minor head injury to identify a skull fracture so that they may be scanned electively within the following 4 hours.

If a skull radiograph is required, at least two views at right angles should be taken. The lateral view should be taken with the patient supine and a horizontal X-ray beam to ensure that a fluid level may be seen in the paranasal sinuses and that any intracranial air can be detected. Moreover the cervical spine is not moved and the upper cervical region is included on the radiograph. A fluid level caused by blood within the sphenoid sinus is a common indirect sign of a skull base fracture but CT is usually required to show the fracture line. Fractures are shown on plain films as sharply demarcated black lines without corticated margins. Fractures do not branch, tend to run in straight lines and stop at sutures which may themselves be diastased. A depressed fracture may be suspected if there is an area of reduced density, with an associated area of increased density corresponding to displaced bone superimposed upon adjacent normal skull. A tangential view will confirm the degree of displacement.

Plain films and direct coronal CT are used to assess complex facial fractures, but can be delayed until the patient has been stabilized, is fit enough to cooperate or reparative surgery is imminent. Three-dimensional surface reconstruction of a stack of CT sections can give the surgeon a dynamic interpretation of the image, highlighting bony displacements or distortions. However, the algorithms used in the formation of the 3D image can obscure or falsify fracture lines, and the value of 3D reconstruction in patient management is therefore limited.

CERVICAL SPINE INJURY

It may be impossible to exclude a cervical spine injury without radiology in the head-injured patient with a severely impaired conscious level. Lateral and frontal films, which include the craniocervical junction and the first thoracic vertebra, are first obtained. As the cervicothoracic region is frequently not satisfactorily imaged on the plain films, axial thin-section CT from C6 to T2 should be carried out, and midline and oblique sagittal reconstructions obtained to show any fractures or subluxation. MRI may be required to demonstrate or exclude soft-tissue injury involving the cord, ligaments, discs or paraspinal tissues.

CT IN HEAD INJURY

When blood clots, its large protein molecules become compacted, water is excluded and a high electron density develops. This attenuates X-rays more than in normal brain and the clot is displayed as a bright area. Conversely, oedema or ischaemia produce an increase in water content and hence a reduction in electron density. This reduced attenuation is displayed as a dark area. Normal grey and white matter lie between these two extremes.

Patients are usually scanned supine but, if they are restless, a decubitus position may settle them long enough to enable a diagnostic scan to be carried out without sedation or anaesthetic. The scan should extend from the foramen magnum to the vertex. Both soft-tissue and bone-window images can be obtained from the same data set.

MRI IN HEAD INJURY

Now that MRI-compatible cardiorespiratory monitoring and support equipment are available, critically ill patients can be imaged safely at any stage after a head injury. However, if the patient is not unconscious or paralysed and ventilated, a higher degree of patient cooperation is required than for CT. These patients may have sustained multiple injuries and screening is required to exclude ferrometallic foreign bodies or electronic implants, which would preclude MRI.

With appropriate choice of sequence the contrast between normal and pathological tissues can be many times that shown by CT. Certain sequences are very sensitive to acute and chronic haemorrhage. Rapid sequences have been developed recently and the increased speed of acquisition can be used to carry out a quicker study in children or severely injured patients. Alternatively, more acquisitions can be acquired in the same time as a conventional scan to improve anatomical detail markedly.

(a)

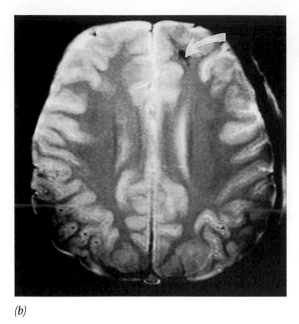

(b)

Figure 15.19 *Diffuse axonal injury in a patient unconscious 8 h after an acute head injury from a road traffic accident. (a) CT normal. (b) T2-weighted MRI section shows the hypointensity of deoxyhaemoglobin in acute haemorrhage in the parasagittal frontal white matter (arrow), one of the hallmarks of diffuse axonal injury.*

RADIONUCLIDE SCANNING IN HEAD INJURY

Radionuclide scanning with agents such as ^{99m}Tc-hexamethyl propylene amine oxime (^{99m}Tc-HMPAO) is used to map regional cerebral blood flow. Because HMPAO is lipophilic, it crosses the blood–brain barrier, where it is rapidly converted into a hydrophilic compound and is trapped for several hours while the distribution is recorded.

PRIMARY INJURY OF THE BRAIN

Diffuse axonal injury

Axonal injury is due to the stresses in the brain caused by severe acceleration and/or deceleration of the head at the moment of injury. Varying degrees of white matter tract disruption may occur often with involvement of adjacent capillaries. It has recently been shown that the lesion may progress, and so treatment to limit its progression is being sought. Sometimes the damage from diffuse axonal injury may be apparent only when diffuse atrophy is found on follow-up examination.

Axonal damage occurs in a 'top-down' pattern. With a mild concussive injury, small lesions with increased water content are seen paramedially at the junction of the cortical grey/white matter on MRI, while on CT these lesions are usually invisible (Fig. 15.19). These lesions are thought to represent the 'gliding contusions' described neuropathologically, although direct correlation is unavailable. With increasing severity other lesions become apparent in the corpus callosum and extend downward into the brain stem. MRI is very sensitive to these lesions even in the absence of macroscopic haemorrhage, a feature that has to be present before the diagnosis can be made on CT. The full classic triad of haemorrhage in the brain stem, the corpus callosum and the cortical grey/white matter junction on CT or MRI is rarely found. Small haemorrhages in the

Figure 15.20 *Thalamic, basal ganglia and grey/white matter interface haemorrhages with intraventricular haemorrhage on acute CT following a 20 m fall. These features are associated with diffuse axonal injury.*

basal ganglia region and intraventricular haemorrhage may also be seen (Fig. 15.20). As the injury ages the blood becomes isodense on CT and, if the CT scan is delayed beyond a few days from the injury, the scan may be falsely interpreted as normal. If the scan is delayed still further, low-attenuation mass lesions may be seen at the site of the resolving haemorrhage. MRI is the best method of detecting haemorrhage and diagnosing the extent of injury.

Contusions and lacerations

Contusions are bruises of the brain formed by coalescing petechial haemorrhages caused by direct contact of the brain with the inner table of the skull. Contusions are seen most frequently on the under surfaces of the frontal and temporal lobes and are the most common complication of head injury. Lacerations are due to direct tearing of the brain by penetrating sharp objects such as bone spicules, bullets or stabbing. A variable amount of ischaemic brain, which further enlarges the area of swelling, surrounds the contusion or laceration. Although blood–brain barrier breakdown occurs in the surrounding ischaemic area, contrast enhancement on CT or MRI adds nothing to the diagnosis and may be toxic to the damaged brain.

Contusions are recognized on CT as areas of low attenuation. Haemorrhage is always present pathologically but may be microscopic and undetectable on CT. However, the amount of blood present varies from a small quantity on the brain surface to substantial collections extending deeply into the subcortical white matter (Fig. 15.21).

INTRACEREBRAL HAEMATOMA FOLLOWING HEAD INJURY

Most intracerebral haematomas develop as a complication of a contusion. On CT, acute haemorrhage is seen as a hyperdense area with a rim of surrounding oedema, which is darker than normal brain. As the haematoma ages it becomes isodense with the brain over the course of the next 1–4 weeks. Occasionally angiography is required to exclude aneurysmal rupture as the cause of an unexplained haematoma.

A penetrating injury should be suspected if a laceration is demonstrated and haemorrhage is seen in a peripheral-to-deep linear orientation or if a foreign body is present (Fig. 15.22).

Delayed haematomas are now being seen more frequently. Patients tend to be scanned soon after their head injury, before the haematoma has time to develop, and then subsequently have a repeat scan. Delayed haematomas usually occur at the site of a contusion but may develop in the extradural or more rarely the

(a)

(b)

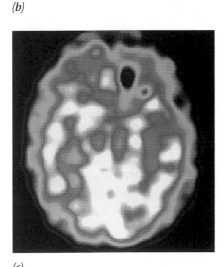

(c)

Figure 15.21 *Bilateral frontal contusions following a fall down steps shown on (a) axial and (b) coronal CT (note the bilateral orbital rim fractures). (c) ^{99m}Tc-HMPAO SPECT section showing bilateral frontal hypoperfusion, worse on the left than the right.*

Figure 15.29 *T1-weighted coronal MRI with a left subdural haematoma causing uncal herniation (arrows) through the tentorial notch.*

Figure 15.30 *Brain swelling and right temporal contusion following severe trauma. Although the basal cisterns contain CSF, the third ventricle is not visible, confirming raised intracranial pressure between 25 and 30 mmHg.*

lesion is small. The fourth ventricle should always be visible, lying centrally in a reasonably well-positioned axial scan. If the fourth ventricle is displaced or compressed, a local cause should be sought and a thin extracerebral collection excluded by viewing the CT scan at different window levels or carrying out MRI.

Large supratentorial masses produce lateral and downward herniation of the brain. There is compression of the ipsilateral ventricle, shift of the midline structures below the falx and dilatation of the contralateral trigone and temporal horn of the lateral ventricle once the foramen of Monro is occluded. This ventricular dilatation is often associated with periventricular oedema and the third ventricle is occluded. At this stage there is usually transtentorial herniation. Transtentorial herniation is well shown on coronal MRI on which subcallosal and uncal herniation can be appreciated (Fig. 15.29). Such downward shift of the brain is associated with raised intracranial pressure and is a life-threatening condition. On the other hand even severe lateral shift can be tolerated if the third ventricle and the basal cisterns remain patent.

Tonsillar herniation cannot be shown directly by CT although it is clearly demonstrated by sagittal sections on MRI. Isolated masses within the posterior fossa can cause an acute obstructive hydrocephalus of the third and lateral ventricles by compressing the fourth ventricle. The earliest sign of hydrocephalus is dilatation of the temporal horns which, in normal young people, are seen only as narrow curved slits. Upward tentorial herniation is unusual because isolated infratentorial traumatic lesions are uncommon.

The midline may remain undisplaced when there are bilateral masses of similar size or if there is general swelling of the hemispheres, but significant downward herniation and raised intracranial pressure can still be present. Normally it should always be possible to identify the third ventricle and basal cisterns as low-attenuation CSF-containing spaces. If either the third ventricle or the basal cisterns are obliterated with less than 5 mm of midline shift, the intracranial pressure lies between 25 and 30 mmHg (Fig. 15.30). If both the third ventricle and basal cisterns are obliterated, the intracranial pressure is over 35 mmHg.

It is not clear whether the generalized hemisphere swelling occurring after head injury is due to hyperaemia or ischaemia. This hemisphere swelling is most commonly seen in children and young adults.

ISCHAEMIC DAMAGE, VASCULAR INJURY AND INFARCTION FOLLOWING HEAD INJURY

On CT, **ischaemia**, which may be reversible, and infarction are both shown as areas of reduced attenuation. Cerebral ischaemia is universal in fatal head injuries, but it is rarely demonstrated by CT in life, as it is almost impossible to separate necrotic brain from the coexistent cytotoxic oedema of ischaemia. The diffuse multifocal ischaemia seen commonly by the pathologist cannot be shown by CT, although it has been demonstrated with radionuclide studies.

Arterial vascular territory ischaemia is the most commonly recognized ischaemic complication. It frequently involves the posterior cerebral artery ipsilateral to a mass lesion causing severe midline shift. Pericallosal artery ischaemia can be produced in a similar way.

Visible middle cerebral territory ischaemia suggests damage to the carotid artery in the neck or skull base, local dissection or embolic thrombosis from more proximal **dissection**. Early angiography will identify lesions that can be treated surgically although treatment for traumatic small vessel dissection or thrombosis remains controversial. Ischaemia in the basilar territory causes diffuse low attenuation on CT in the brain stem and mid brain which is contrasted against the preserved normal density pattern of the cerebellum. Vertebral dissection may show only as infarction in the territory of the ipsilateral posterior inferior cerebellar artery.

All ischaemia is much better visualized with MRI than with CT, especially ischaemia in the posterior fossa and medial aspects of the temporal lobes. Ischaemia appears on MRI as well-defined focal regions of hyperintensity on T2-weighted sequences with corresponding less prominent areas of hypointensity on T1-weighted sections.

Cortical venous infarction can be caused by a fracture involving a major venous sinus or secondary infection, which results in dural venous sinus thrombosis. This can occasionally mimic gliding contusions. Venous occlusion is further discussed on p. 437.

Ischaemia in watershed territories can develop after a period of global hypotension. On CT, areas of reduced attenuation will be seen, whilst MRI shows hyperintensity on T2-weighted images with hypointensity on T1-weighted images. These changes are seen in the watershed area between the anterior and middle cerebral artery territories, in the frontal and parafalcine regions, and in the area between the middle and the posterior cerebral artery territories in the parietal region.

Profound persistent hypotension, ischaemia or generally elevated intracranial pressure usually results in loss of the normal grey/white matter differentiation in both hemispheres and is associated with an apparent increase in the attenuation of the normal cerebellum and tentorium on CT. These appearances are limited to children and young adults and are pathognomonic of a non-perfused cerebrum.

Radionuclide scanning is more sensitive to perfusion changes than CT or MRI, and often shows regions of both abnormally high and abnormally low cortical blood flow. All focal traumatic mass lesions such as contusions and intracerebral haemorrhage show zones of severely reduced cerebral blood flow, which can persist for days to months particularly in the surrounding oedematous areas. Occasionally the abnormal perfusion pattern persists over several months even though the structural appearance on CT or MRI returns to normal. This abnormal perfusion may correlate with some of the late neuropsychological sequelae found after head injury.

CEREBROMALACIA FOLLOWING HEAD INJURY

As contusions heal by progressive degradation and maturation of haemorrhage with eventual gliosis they

Figure 15.31 *CSF fistula shown by leakage of intrathecal contrast (arrow) into the posterior ethmoid air cells on coronal CT.*

shrink to leave a low-attenuation area on CT with loss of cortex and adjacent white matter. This lesion, known as cerebromalacia, is commonly found in a subfrontal and/or temporal location. After the acute space-occupying effects of haemorrhagic contusion have resolved, an *ex vacuo* effect supervenes resulting in enlargement of adjacent sulci and ventricles.

CEREBROSPINAL FLUID FISTULA FOLLOWING HEAD INJURY

An overt CSF leak is present in about 25 per cent of patients with pneumocephalus demonstrated on CT, but in the majority the leak ceases spontaneously within 7–10 days. If it persists or if there is evidence of meningitis, then the fracture site should be sought. Direct coronal high-resolution CT of the anterior fossa is used to investigate **CSF rhinorrhoea**, and axial and coronal high-resolution sections of the petrous bones are used in patients with CSF otorrhoea. If CT fails to demonstrate an opaque sinus adjacent to a bone defect, the examination should be repeated following contrast opacification of the cisternal CSF by instilling 5 ml of non-ionic contrast medium via a lumbar puncture. The contrast is then run up to the basal cisterns and positioned over the appropriate portion of the skull base and the CT repeated to detect any leak (Fig. 15.31).

VASCULAR LESIONS FOLLOWING HEAD INJURY

Penetrating injuries must be recognized in the acute stage and any associated vascular lesion demonstrated by urgent angiography. **Arteriovenous fistula** or a **pseudoaneurysm** can form secondary to a skull fracture and tear of the meningeal vessels. Delayed or recurrent intracranial haematomas can follow penetrating injuries. When the intracavernous segment of the carotid artery is damaged, with or without a skull-base fracture, a **caroticocavernous fistula** may form with unilateral or bilateral pulsing exophthalmos or, much less commonly, a pseudoaneurysm may form. Although either condition can be present at the time of injury, both are more frequent after several weeks have elapsed. Angiography is required for the full definition of the vascular components, but the abnormal vessels will be shown on enhanced CT and MRI. Either an endovascular approach with embolization or a combined neuroradiological–neurosurgical treatment plan is now used to occlude the fistula, aneurysm or parent vessel, preserving as much of the normal vasculature as possible.

HYDROCEPHALUS FOLLOWING HEAD INJURY

Localized dilatation of the ventricles may be seen adjacent to a large area of cerebromalacia following head injury, but generalized hydrocephalus is unusual and most often follows intraventricular or subarachnoid haemorrhage. In hydrocephalus there is disproportionate ventricular enlargement compared to the cortical sulci and cisterns. Although the temporal horns should be involved, care has to be taken as their enlargement can also be a local complication of cerebromalacia. With severe hydrocephalus, CT or MRI may show periventricular white matter oedema. Progressive ventricular dilatation associated with enlarged cortical sulci and cisterns owing to cerebral atrophy, which may be seen 4–6 months after an injury, may be the only sign of diffuse axonal injury.

INFECTION FOLLOWING HEAD INJURY

Infection is still a serious problem but nowadays is usually pre-empted by prophylactic treatment.

Meningitis is a common complication of compound skull fractures. It is diagnosed clinically and a CT or plain film usually simply confirms the fracture site. CT and MRI with intravenous contrast enhancement show generalized meningeal enhancement, although in the acute phase the examination may be normal.

Cerebral abscess may present as an intracranial mass, most often associated with a penetrating injury or a foreign body, even though the primary breach in the dura may not have been suspected.

Bone infection is unusual and is seen most frequently in association with a craniotomy bone flap or an infected scalp wound. Plain films or CT shows the abnormalities once the infection is established.

CEREBRAL ATROPHY, EPILEPSY AND POSTCONCUSSION SYNDROME FOLLOWING HEAD INJURY

Cerebral atrophy usually starts to show around 4 months after a head injury. It may be progressive with ventricular dilatation and enlarged sulci and cisterns. The presence of the enlarged sulci and cisterns differentiates atrophy from the obstructive forms of hydrocephalus.

Epilepsy is commonest in patients who had seizures in the acute phase of a head injury, and in patients who had a depressed fracture or who underwent a craniotomy. Other than defining that an injury has occurred, imaging does not have a role to play in these patients with epilepsy.

Postconcussion syndrome is being increasingly recognized and comprises symptoms such as headache, dizziness, lack of concentration and poor memory. Although the syndrome may relate to minor diffuse cerebral injury, CT and MRI show similar abnormalities in patients with postconcussive syndrome as in patients with no complaints following head injury.

INFECTIONS

Intracranial infections include abscess, encephalitis and meningitis. Imaging plays a central role in the management of abscesses and encephalitis but has a lesser role in meningitis. The brain reacts to an insult such as an infection in a limited way by becoming hyperaemic, swollen and oedematous; consequently many infections have a similar appearance. The blood–brain barrier is breached and shows leakage of contrast following intravenous contrast injection. If there is focal brain damage the tissue shrinks leaving an area of gliosis and malacia in the healing phase.

ABSCESS

Abscesses can be caused by pyogenic, tuberculous, fungal or parasitic organisms. They may lie within brain parenchyma, the subdural or epidural (extradural) spaces or may involve each compartment. Radiological localization is essential prior to biopsy, drainage or definitive resection. Localization can be carried out with a few MRI or CT sections through the lesion with a suitable skull marker in position. Formal stereotactic localization can be performed with CT or MRI now that special frames are available.

An established abscess is a focal parenchymal infection with a central zone of liquefaction and necrosis surrounded by a fibrocollagenous capsule, which localizes the infection. An abscess may be surrounded by

(a)   (b)

Figure 15.32 *T1-weighted postcontrast on (a) axial and (b) sagittal sections of left frontal brain abscess associated with frontal sinus infection and adjacent epidural abscess in a 19-year-old with headache, lethargy and progressive reduction in conscious level.*

oedema. The imaging appearances depend on the maturity of the abscess at the time of scanning. Initially there is a cerebritis with minimal or no CT change. At this stage MRI is more sensitive than CT and shows hyperintensity on T2-weighted sections with irregular enhancement on T1-weighted images. Later the abscess increases in size, becomes rounded and a central necrotic zone develops with a thick wall, which shows irregular enhancement on both CT and MRI. With more maturity the abscess wall becomes thinner and less irregular, while the centre undergoes liquefaction (Fig. 15.32).

Abscesses within the brain substance often occur by spread from the epidural and subdural spaces. Epidural infection is most often the result of spread of infection from the mastoids, paranasal sinuses or cranium. CT shows a focal low-attenuation epidural mass but MRI is more sensitive with hypointensity on T1- and hyperintensity on T2-weighted images. Dural thickening or a ring configuration is seen after contrast enhancement. Epidural infection may cross the midline so differentiating it from a subdural empyema.

Subdural abscesses occur as acute or chronic lesions appearing as extracerebral collections over the convexities and within the interhemispheric fissure. On CT, a subdural abscess shows as a low or isodense extra-axial mass. MRI demonstrates an isointense signal on T1-weighted and hyperintense signal on T2-weighted sections. Depending on the amount of granulation tissue the mass shows contrast enhancement on CT and MRI. The underlying brain may be affected and there may be enhancement of the cortical gyri.

Many **parasitic infections** can invade the brain. **Cysticercosis** from the pork tapeworm is one of the commonest worldwide demonstrated by multiple,

Figure 15.33 *Toxoplasmosis. Multiple small ring-enhancing abscesses shown on a T1-weighted section in a 43-year-old HIV-positive patient.*

small, rounded, ring-enhancing lesions on CT and MRI. **Toxoplasmosis** is a ubiquitous protozoan infection and in immunocompromised hosts, such as in AIDS (p. 422), may reactivate. In toxoplasmosis, abscesses form most commonly in the basal ganglia, corticomedullary junction, white matter or periventricular regions. Ring or nodular enhancement is seen on CT and MRI (Fig. 15.33). **Paragonimiasis** from the lung fluke produces clusters of abscess-like ring-enhancing masses with surrounding oedema. **Hydatid cysts** from the dog tapeworm can produce large cysts of CSF density on CT and MRI without enhancement in cysts that are not secondarily infected.

ENCEPHALITIS

Encephalitis can be caused by a wide variety of organisms (most commonly viruses) or immune-mediated reactions to actual infections (acute disseminated encephalomyelitis). CT shows asymmetrical unilateral or bilateral focal areas of reduced attenuation causing a mass effect especially with herpes encephalitis. The typical distribution involves the temporal lobe, orbitofrontal region and insula. The changes are much better defined with MRI, which shows hyperintensity on T2-weighted and hypointensity on T1-weighted sections. The infection mainly affects the cortical grey matter and later spreads to the subcortical white matter. The basal ganglia are spared. Haemorrhage is not uncommon. Enhancement with intravenous contrast on CT and MRI varies with the stage and severity of disease. SPECT with ^{99m}Tc-HMPAO shows hyperperfusion often before changes are seen on CT or MRI. If imaging is delayed or if the patient does not respond to antiviral therapy, blood–brain barrier breakdown occurs and linear, subarachnoid or gyriform enhancement is seen.

Acute disseminated encephalomyelitis produces a reactive multifocal acute inflammatory demyelination in the white matter of the brain or spinal cord, which may be indistinguishable from an acute episode of multiple sclerosis. MRI is the most sensitive method for assessment. Contrast enhancement distinguishes acute enhancing plaques of demyelination from established non-enhancing more chronic lesions.

MENINGITIS AND VENTRICULITIS

Meningitis and ventriculitis present with inflammation of the meninges or ependyma following haematogenous dissemination of organisms or following direct inoculation after a compound fracture, or, more rarely, following surgery particularly mastoid/paranasal sinus surgery or shunt insertion. The diagnosis of meningitis or ventriculitis is made clinically with bacteriological examination of the CSF and imaging is used only to evaluate complications.

In **acute meningitis**, CT and MRI are usually normal. In severe cases there may be some brain swelling with obliteration of the basal cisterns and sulcal CSF spaces. Leptomeningeal inflammation, showing enhancement extending to the depths of the sulci, develops, and is most clearly seen on T2-weighted coronal postcontrast MRI. The inflammation may cause ischaemia producing further generalized brain swelling, focal infarction or communicating hydrocephalus.

Granulomatous meningitis, such as tuberculosis, produces more prominent meningeal reaction with obliteration of the cisterns and involvement of the branches of the circle of Willis with ischaemia, which often results in haemorrhagic infarction of the basal ganglia.

Ventriculitis is seen on CT or MRI as enhancement of the ependyma. Ventriculitis is often associated with retrograde spread of infection from the meninges, the presence of foreign bodies such as shunts, or rupture of an abscess into the ventricle. Occasionally with severe ventriculitis a pus–CSF level may be seen in the occipital horns of the lateral ventricles, which are the most dependent parts of the ventricular system, when the patient is scanned in the supine position. Ventriculitis can result in an obstructive hydrocephalus.

AIDS AFFECTING THE CNS

The spectrum of disorders includes:

- primary human immunodeficiency virus type 1 infection;
- secondary (opportunistic) processes;
- cerebrovascular disease;
- nutritional and metabolic disorders;
- drug toxicity that affects patients with the AIDS complex.

Differential diagnosis of CNS lesions

When a patient who is infected with HIV-1 presents with neurological signs or symptoms, imaging plays a crucial role in the differential diagnosis, although it can seldom identify the specific cause. Generally patients have opportunistic infections, tumours or cerebrovascular disease in order of frequency. Initial brain imaging can be carried out by CT or MRI with MRI being more sensitive and anatomically easier to interpret. Intravenous contrast enhancement is essential with both examinations for the assessment of the blood–brain barrier. The position of a lesion in relation to the CSF spaces, the brain parenchyma and the ventricles is important and the recognition of mass effect is crucial. The first scan will define whether the brain is normal, shows disproportionate atrophy for the patient's age, has hydrocephalus or has a mass lesion. The patients with normal or atrophic brains should have a screening CSF evaluation, whilst those with hydrocephalus may first require shunting before the CSF is examined. The result of the CSF examination usually defines the cause of their symptoms and appropriate treatment can be instituted. If the cause cannot be determined, the patient is usually observed and rescanned after an interval, if there is no improvement. When the patient presents with a mass, the key decision is whether this is a stable situation or whether the patient is deteriorating and at risk of imminent herniation, when neurosurgical decompression must be considered with resection following open biopsy, unless there is time to carry out a stereotaxic biopsy. The results of the biopsy should allow definitive targeted treatment. If single or multiple mass lesions are found in a stable patient, there is time to carry out a SPECT scan with thallium-201. A positive uptake suggests lymphoma or other high-grade neoplasm and the patient can go on to a confirmatory stereotactic brain biopsy. A negative SPECT will tend to exclude lymphoma and other opportunistic infections must be considered. Toxoplasma serology may be undertaken, but often by this time patients have already been started on antitoxoplasm therapy. If the serology for toxoplasma is negative and there is only a single lesion on imaging, a stereotactic biopsy may be indicated, whilst multiple lesions suggest a trial of antitoxoplasma therapy.

Primary human immunodeficiency virus (HIV) type 1 infection

Infection with the HIV type 1, a lymphotrophic and neurotrophic RNA retrovirus, itself can result in:

- meningitis (acute and chronic)
- subacute encephalitis
- myelopathy
- peripheral neuropathy.

The infection also starts the process that leads to the destruction of CD4+ T lymphocytes – the body's main defence against certain opportunistic infections and some neoplasms. Eventually there are so few CD4+ cells left that the immune system can no longer work effectively. At this point the person becomes prone to a wide variety of illnesses of growing severity and the diagnosis of acquired immune deficiency syndrome (AIDS) can be applied. The virus is both neurotrophic and lymphotrophic infecting neurological tissue early. The interval between the onset of HIV infection and the collapse of cellular immunity varies from 2 to 15 years, but ultimately more than 50 per cent of people infected with HIV develop symptomatic neurological disease with this figure reaching over 90 per cent at autopsy.

Acute and chronic meningitis are frequent but clinically non-specific and may only result in CSF pleocytosis. HIV is the most common cause but cryptococcosis, tuberculosis, syphilis and lymphoma are not uncommon.

Subacute encephalopathy. HIV-associated dementia (AIDS dementia) can produce a progressive dementing illness with minor or major cognitive disorders associated with progressive motor abnormalities. At the time of diagnosis up to a third of ptients will show features of this complex, whilst half with advanced AIDS will develop cognitive impairment.

Imaging is non-specific and just reflects the gross pathology of perivascular demyelination with astrocytic

Figure 15.34 *HIV subacute encephalopathy. A 30-year-old man recently found to be HIV-positive presenting with a dementing illness. T2-weighted axial section shows diffuse deep white matter hyperintensity largely sparing the grey matter, associated with generalized atrophy.*

gliosis and astrocytosis in the cerebral cortex. CT and MRI show brain atrophy, sulcal widening and concomitant ventricular dilatation with diffuse symmetrical widespread white matter abnormality. This produces low attenuation on CT, hyperintensity on T2-weighted and to a lesser extent hypointensity on T1-weighted sections (Fig. 15.34). Contrast enhancement is not present. The key value of imaging is to exclude other cerebral abnormalities.

HIV-associated myelopathy is insidious and causes progressive leg weakness, gait impairment, paraesthesias, bladder, bowel and sexual dysfunction, and is the result of a specific vacuolating myelopathy, which shows loss of myelin and spongy degeneration especially in the dorsal and lateral columns.

The cord remains normal on CT myelography but with MRI the demyelination and microcystic changes produce focal hyperintensity on T2-weighted and proton density-weighted sections. The appearance is usually symmetrical and extends over several segments following the white matter tracts. There is no cord expansion or enhancement with contrast.

Although **peripheral neuropathy** is well documented with electrophysiological studies, imaging does not feature in the diagnosis, except to exclude other mass lesions.

Secondary (opportunistic) processes

Viral infections
These will occur in approximately 30 per cent of patients with AIDS.

(a)

(b)

(c)

Figure 15.37 *A 38-year-old HIV-positive man developed a progressive right hemiparesis. (a) Contrast-enhanced CT on admission shows a non-enhancing non-space-occupying low-attenuation lesion in the left basal ganglial region. (b) Pre- and (c) postcontrast-enhanced CT 6 days later shows that the lesion is now larger, space occupying and surrounded by vasogenic oedema, giving a 'target'-like appearance with an enhancing rim and central nodule. The lesion was slow to respond to antitoxoplasma therapy, and lymphoma and cryptococcosis were considered. A biopsy confirmed toxoplasmosis.*

there is invasion of the parenchyma with enhancement. On MRI these cryptococcomas are easier to define, being hypointense on T1-weighted, and hyperintense on T2-weighted and proton density-weighted sections; they are surrounded by a variable amount of oedema. Gadolinium enhancement is variable but not a feature early in the course of the infection. Double and triple doses of intravenous gadolinium have been advocated to define the lesions better. The lesions may also involve the choroid plexus and cell masses in the ventricles may eventually produce an obstructive hydrocephalus.

Other fungal meningitides can also occur. AIDS patients are susceptible to infection with *Aspergillus*, *Mucor* and *Candida* spp., but these infections are commoner in patients with other causes of immuno-suppression, such as neutropenia, diabetes, leukaemia and lymphoma. *Histoplasma*, *Blastomyces* and *Coccidioides* spp., which occur mainly in North America, cause CNS infection, but only with blastomycosis is HIV infection thought to be a cofactor.

Protozoal infections

Toxoplasmosis is caused by *Toxoplasma gondii*, an obligate intracellular parasite; it is the most common opportunistic infection producing neurological complications of HIV infection. It also causes the most common intracranial mass lesion in an HIV-positive patient. There is a clear distinction between infection with *T. gondii* and toxoplasmosis. Dogs and cats are the key reservoirs of infection, although many other mammals can be incidental hosts. Humans are infected from contaminated food or other material, when the organism in its pseudocyst form is ingested or inocu-lated. In the older child or adult, symptoms of a primary infection may include a rash, fever and lymph node enlargement, with eye signs of chorioretinitis and uveitis. Usually the infection is benign and self-limit-ing, controlled with an effective humoral and cellular immune response, but the organism is not eradicated. With the exception of the retina, these cysts in the majority of patients can remain dormant, typically in

(a)

(b)

(c)

Figure 15.38 *Young HIV-positive child showing multiple cortical and subcortical lesions: (a) T2-weighted, (b) T1-weighted and (c) T1-weighted postcontrast MRI showing vasogenic oedema surrounding enhancing nodules lying immediately subcortically. Biopsy showed a tuberculous caseating abscess.*

the brain and muscle, for the lifetime of the host, but antibodies can be detected in the blood against the toxoplasma antigen.

When the host's immunity is reduced, as in HIV infection, active proliferation of the organism can occur. This develops in up to 30 per cent of AIDS patients who have toxoplasma antibodies. It produces a focal or diffuse necrotizing encephalitis of any part of the brain, but the basal ganglia and the cortico-medullary junction are most frequently affected. Multiple lesions are typical, but solitary lesions are present in up to a third of patients. Pathologically these lesions have three distinct zones and no capsule: a solid coagulated aseptic central zone, surrounded by a hypervascular inflammatory intermediate zone containing many encysted organisms, and an oedematous peripheral zone with few vascular changes and encysted organisms. Although direct meningeal infection can occur, diffuse spread through the leptomeninges is not a feature.

MRI with contrast enhancement is more sensitive than CT with enhancement, but most lesions are seen on either examination. Precontrast there is usually an irregularly marginated lobulated mass lesion showing variable inhomogeneous enhancement centrally with a ring or nodular appearance. An eccentric nodule of more solid enhancement is sometimes present, which can help with the differential diagnosis. On CT the lesion produces an isodense focus surrounded by low-attenuation vasogenic oedema with high-attenuation enhancement (Fig. 15.37). On MRI the central part is often isointense on T1-weighted and T2-weighted sections, with the surrounding oedema showing as hypointense on T1-weighted and hyperintense on T2-weighted and proton density-weighted sections. Rarely some haemorrhage may produce hyperintensity, depending on the timing of the imaging, confusing the hyperintensity shown after enhancement on T1-weighted sections of the central lesion. Treatment is

(a)

(b)

(c)

Figure 15.39 *A severely immunosuppressed 50-year-old man. (a) T2-weighted, (b) T1-weighted and (c) T1-weighted postcontrast MRI shows a multiloculated ring-enhancing lesion extending to the cortical surface and associated with some dural enhancement. Biopsy showed a nocardia abscess.*

usually empirical with antitoxoplasmosis drugs. Imaging is used to monitor the response. If the lesions were caused by toxoplasmosis, there should be a reduction in their size and number and resolution of the enhancement. Occasionally cerebromalacia or calcification may be found. If the lesions do not respond with 2–4 weeks of adequate therapy, an alternative or concurrent diagnosis must be sought such as lymphoma or cryptococcal infection.

Bacterial infections

Mycobacterial infections (*Mycobacterium tuberculosis, Mycobacterium avium-intracellulare*) causing tuberculosis is now the commonest opportunistic infection worldwide.

Reactivation is still the most frequent source of infection in adults although there is an increasing rate of primary infection in these HIV-positive patients. It is often the first AIDS-defining infection in an HIV-positive patient. Disseminated systemic disease is common, but the incidence of CNS infection varies geographically. It is higher in injecting drug abusers and in Africa and Asia. CNS disease includes meningitis, cerebritis, abscess formation and tuberculoma.

CT and MRI can be used to show the lesions but MRI is more sensitive particularly to the enhancement found associated with meningitis. Tuberculosis mainly affects the basal cisterns and the cranial nerves that traverse them. CSF replacement can be seen on non-contrast CT and MRI with the exudate enhancing after intravenous contrast. Abscesses are a rare form of tuberculous CNS disease, which resemble a pyogenic abscess, but are more frequently found in immunosuppressed patients (Fig. 15.38). Ring-enhancing mass lesions surrounded by oedema can be shown on CT and MRI. These changes can result in an obstructive hydrocephalus, which may require shunting. The level of obstruction can best be assessed by MRI where sagittal sections are particularly valuable. In the chronic stages CT may identify calcification.

Syphilis (*Treponema pallidum*) or neurosyphilis can present as a more acute disease in the immunosuppressed patient producing an acute meningitis during the course of the secondary stage. The latent period is reduced, and relapse after adequate treatment has been noted. Imaging may demonstrate the inflamed meninges, but CSF examination is the primary investigation.

(a)   (b)

Figure 15.40 *A 31-year-old HIV-positive man presenting with reduced consciousness and ocular symptoms. (a) Subtle hypo- and iso-intense mass lesions mainly in a periventricular distribution on T1-weighted section. (b) After contrast many but not all of the lesions enhance and are easier to define. There was no improvement on antitoxoplasma therapy but the* ^{201}*Tl SPECT showed some uptake. Biospy confirmed lymphoma.*

Listeriosis (*Listeria monocytogenes*) has a surprisingly low incidence compared with other patients with cell-mediated immunity. *Listeria* produces a meningitis or brain abscess with a predilection for the brain stem. On imaging these cannot be distinguished from other infections.

Nocardia infection (*Nocardia asteroides*) affecting the CNS is the second commonest site of this infection, which is usually due to haematogenous spread from the primary lesion in the respiratory system, producing brain abscesses that are often multiple.

CT and MRI show these ring-enhancing mass lesions with surrounding oedema, and when associated with subependymal nodules and local meningitis this appearance may be suggestive of the diagnosis (Fig. 15.39). Although initial treatment may appear successful, relapse is common and these patients have a high mortality rate of about 80 per cent.

Neoplasms

Primary CNS lymphoma is the most common CNS malignancy to affect HIV-positive patients and it also affects other patients who have reduced cellular immunity, such as transplant recipients and patients with congenital immunodeficiencies. The lymphoma is a non-Hodgkin's B-cell lymphoma thought to be produced by reactivation of latent infection by the Epstein–Barr virus following a self-limiting infection in childhood (infectious mononucleosis) and is found in a younger age group in both men and women, unlike the non-AIDS patients who are older, typically elderly,

men. The tumour is usually situated in the deep grey or white matter or adjacent to the ventricles. Subependymal spread is common.

Precontrast CT often highlights the tumour's hypercellularity, displaying it as a focal or multicentric mass lesion often with increased attenuation. When necrosis supervenes there is inhomogeneous reduced attenuation. Calcification is not a feature. Following intravenous contrast, single or multicentric ring or nodular inhomogeneous enhancement is seen surrounded by low-attenuation vasogenic oedema. Again MRI (Fig. 15.40) is more sensitive than CT and, on T2-weighted sections, it appears as an isointense lesion with surrounding hyperintense vasogenic oedema. If the lesion is necrotic, the signals become inhomogeneous with mixed hyperintensity on T2- and hypointensity on T1-weighted sections. Following intravenous gadolinium contrast, T1-weighted sections show an enhancing mass lesion. SPECT studies with thallium-201 show avid uptake of this potassium analogue from the high cell turnover in lymphoma, helping to differentiate it from other non-neoplastic masses.

Metastatic CNS lymphoma results from spread from aggressive systemic non-Hodgkin's lymphoma. In HIV-positive patients these systemic neoplasms often have a high rate of extranodal disease at presentation, and symptoms are commonly due to CNS disease. A lymphomatous leptomeningitis is frequently found, producing a malignant meningitis or involvement of the cranial nerves (Fig. 15.41a,b). It is thought that this is due

(a)

(b)

(c)

Figure 15.41 *HIV-positive woman with cerebral and spinal signs and symptoms: (a) T2-weighted MRI shows extensive vasogenic oedema surrounding a mixed axial and extra-axial meningeal lesion in the base of the brain and left temporal lobe (arrows). (b) After contrast on T1-weighted sections the full extent of the lesion becomes clear with meningeal and cerebral enhancement, particularly on the left. (c) Postcontrast T1-weighted sagittal section of the cervical and thoracic spine shows extensive nodular-enhancing masses in the subarachnoid space and dura. Biopsy confirmed metastatic non-Hodgkin's lymphoma.*

to direct spread through the dura to the subarachnoid space from adjacent infiltrated bone marrow.

Imaging may show non-specific meningeal enhancement after contrast. MRI (Fig. 15.41c) is more sensitive than CT. In the spine, marrow infiltration can be seen as hypointensity from replacement of the fatty marrow, which would normally produce hyperintensity on T1-weighted sections. Matting of the nerve roots with enhancement may be seen in the lumbar theca. Rarely the whole CSF space is replaced by enhancing neoplasm.

Cerebrovascular disease

Although the incidence of stroke is little different from that found in an age- and sex-matched population, the types of disease are very different in HIV-positive patients with a much larger number of causes. Vasculitides, embolic phenomena and coagulation disorders predominate. HIV infection itself can produce a vasculitis, which can result in focal infarction, whilst the opportunistic infections occasionally produce mycotic aneurysms, which can result in haemorrhage or infarction. Concomitant heart disease with endocarditis is common and can result in emboli, whilst thrombocytopenia has been implicated in haemorrhage.

CT and MRI can show the infarct or haemorrhage whilst high-quality MR angiography can occasionally demonstrate beaded or narrowed vessels in vasculitis or aneurysms associated with a haemorrhage, but contrast angiography will frequently be required if a management option depends on visualization of a vasculitis or aneurysm.

Nutritional and metabolic disorders

Imaging may occasionally be helpful in specific deficiency syndromes, such as Wernicke's and vitamin

B_{12} deficiency, with mamillary body changes and white matter demyelination respectively.

Drug toxicity

Symptoms owing to drug toxicity are common and imaging is used to exclude other causes for the symptoms and signs. Presentations with peripheral neuropathy secondary to the antiretrovirals, mitochondrial myopathy secondary to zidovudine and the neuroleptic malignant syndrome are some of the commonest.

VASCULAR ABNORMALITIES

STROKE

Stroke is a lay term defined as a sudden focal neurological deterioration, which becomes maximal within minutes to several hours. It is one of the commonest causes of hospital admission in the developed world, has a high morbidity and consumes more healthcare resources than nearly any other single disease. Although in widespread use, the term stroke requires the individual event to be investigated and the cause of the deficit precisely defined.

There are five major causes of stroke:

- cerebral ischaemia and infarction
- primary intracerebral haemorrhage (ICH)
- intracranial aneurysms
- subarachnoid haemorrhage (SAH)
- veno-occlusive disorders.

Cerebral ischaemia and infarction

When an area of the brain is deprived of its blood supply, it undergoes infarction, which may be ischaemic or haemorrhagic. Approximately 90 per cent of infarcts are ischaemic and 10 per cent haemorrhagic. Infarcts are often caused by thrombosis occurring in a vessel with a pre-existing abnormality, such as atherosclerosis, dissection or vasculitis, or when there is a hypercoagulability state. A smaller number of infarcts are due to emboli from the heart or proximal vessels. Despite treatment advances, the mortality rate remains at around 50 per cent. It is thought that only preventive public health measures and earlier thrombolytic therapy for these 'brain attacks' can improve this situation. It requires the early accurate identification of patients with acute infarcts and those with transient ischaemia at risk of completing their infarcts. Treatment with tissue plasminogen activator has been shown to be effective only within 3 hours of ischaemic stroke. This short treatment window requires rapid emergency evaluation, diagnosis and treatment. Radiology has a

key role in showing any haemorrhage present and excluding the other differential diagnoses which may mimic ischaemic stroke.

Despite its poor delineation of **acute infarction**, CT is usually the initial emergency imaging undertaken because of its widespread availability, its relative tolerance to patient restlessness and the easy exclusion of haemorrhage. Subtle pointers to the infarction are occasionally present even at this time. Increased attenuation within a major cerebral artery representing vessel occlusion from thrombus to embolus is one of the earliest signs. There is a small but visible increase in attenuation (75 HU to 90 HU) of the stationary clotting blood as it retracts and loses its serum, increasing the net concentration of haemoglobin. This sign is seen most often in the middle cerebral artery (Fig. 15.42a) or basilar artery. Lysis and recanalization of the clot are usually noted within a week. Parenchymal changes on CT depend on the severity of the ischaemia, its duration and site and the eventual size of the infarct. The cytotoxic oedema produced by an infarct can reduce the attenuation of the brain within 2–4 hours and should be visible as reduced attenuation on CT. More commonly with marginal ischaemic perfusion it takes longer to develop and the infarct is not usually seen on early CT scans before 12 hours. These subtle differences in attenuation are seen as a series of boundary losses:

- obscuration of the lentiform nucleus with basal ganglia oedema related to middle cerebral artery territory infarction;
- loss of the insular ribbon (from cytotoxic oedema in the grey matter in the insula) and subsequent loss of the grey matter (white matter boundaries at the lateral margins of the insula);
- reduced parenchymal attenuation, swelling and sulcal effacement, which is often not seen before 24 hours and evolves to a clear-cut territorial wedge-shaped low-attenuation area over 3 days, with maximum swelling between 3 and 4 days.

High-attenuation **haemorrhagic transformation** may be seen particularly in the basal ganglia and cortex at this time, associated with severe ischaemia or if the patient was on anticoagulant therapy prior to the ischaemia.

Routine unenhanced MRI can detect abnormalities within 8 hours of the onset of symptoms of ischaemia without paramagnetic contrast, whereas CT is often normal for at least 12 hours and, if perfusion is not re-established, remains 'bland' for several days. MRI initially shows subtle swelling and hyperintensity particularly on T2-weighted sections (Fig. 15.42b) and usually hypointensity on T1-weighted sections owing to failure of the 'sodium–potassium' pump and increasing intracellular water–cytotoxic oedema. At this stage function

(a)   *(b)*

Figure 15.42 *A 34-year-old man with right Horner's syndrome and left hemiparesis. (a) CT on admission 6 hours after the event shows a dense right middle cerebral artery containing clot (arrow) but no attenuation changes in the arterial territory. (b) T2-weighted MRI just after the CT shows hyperintensity in the middle cerebral artery territory representing the infarct. Final diagnosis was internal carotid artery dissection and thrombosis at the level of the skull base.*

is lost but structure is maintained. It is only with continuing ischaemia that blood–brain barrier breakdown occurs, structural integrity is lost and vasogenic oedema supervenes.

With gadolinium-enhanced T1-weighted sequences, abnormal curvilinear areas of enhancement, thought to represent cortical arterial vessels with markedly slowed circulation, are seen adjacent to infarcted brain. These flow-related abnormalities, the absence of normal flow voids and the presence of arterial enhancement can be detected within minutes of the onset of symptoms. Brain swelling on T1-weighted images without signal changes on T2-weighted images are also detected within the first few hours. There is an evolving pattern of enhancement, reflecting the underlying pathophysiology:

- vascular enhancement – days 1–3, seen in 77 per cent of patients;

(a)   *(b)*

Figure 15.43 *A 58-year-old woman developed a right hemiplegia, dysphasia and increasing drowsiness. (a) T2-weighted and (b) T1-weighted MRI 3 days after the event show a left middle cerebral distal branch territory and posterior watershed territory cortical infarct with swelling and hyperintensity on T2-weighted sections. Fine haemorrhage is seen on the T2-weighted section as a hypointense linear signal following the cortex (arrows) while on the T1-weighted section it is hyperintense.*

(a)

(b)

(c)

Figure 15.44 *A 43-year-old woman with multiple haemorrhagic infarcts. (a) T2-weighted MRI shows multiple hyperintense focal infarcts with acute hypointense haemorrhage within them. (b) The haemorrhage is confirmed on CT but at this stage the infarcts are not well seen. (c) Selective right internal carotid angiogram shows the cause: multiple distal stenotic vessels typical of vasculitis (arrows).*

- leptomeningeal enhancement – days 4–7, seen only in larger infarcts;
- brain parenchymal enhancement – days 7–14, seen in 100 per cent of infarcts.

Enhancement is not noted after 2–3 months.

The concept of a therapeutic window implies that there is a brief period (< 6 h) during which it may be possible to salvage some ischaemic but still viable tissue surrounding the core of the infarct. This has driven the quest for imaging sequences that will produce visualization of the infarct surrounded by its ischaemic penumbra in the very early stages, in addition to being able to show overt haemorrhage, which would preclude treatment with human tissue plasminogen activator. These techniques have only been possible with the development of fast scanning methods such as echoplanar and strong, fast gradients. Diffusion- and most recently perfusion-weighted images are now possible on routine clinical machines and, when combined, are thought to be able to define the ischaemic penumbra.

Once the parenchymal long T1- and T2-weighted signal changes are established (Fig. 15.43), the differen-tial diagnosis must be made in a similar way to conventional CT following consideration of:

- site: vascular territory, watershed region, deep grey or white matter tracts;
- shape: wedge, involving grey and white matter;
- margins: sulcal effacement, blurring of the grey and white matter interfaces;
- resolution of mass effect over 3–4 weeks.

Hypointensity on heavily T1-weighted sequences and the use of gradient echoes or susceptibility mapping can often show petechial haemorrhage in the second week, which is not seen on CT. While frank haemorrhage correlates with a worsening clinical state (Fig. 15.44), small foci of haemorrhage within the infarct do not relate to anticoagulation or indicate a poorer outcome.

The patency of the extracranial and major intracerebral arteries can be assessed on routine MRI sequences as a 'flow void'. Projectional images produced by time-of-flight (Fig. 15.45), phase contrast and contrast-enhanced angiographic sequences are being evaluated as to whether they can replace conventional angiography (Fig. 15.46).

(a)

(b)

Figure 15.45 *A 31-year-old with a transient left hemiparesis lasting 2 hours. (a) Time-of-flight MR angiogram shows an occluded right middle cerebral artery (arrow) and a right carotid siphon intracavernous aneurysm – the presumed source of the occluding embolus. (b) T2-weighted MRI was normal in this young patient with good collateral vessels; the proton density-weighted MRI was also normal.*

Figure 15.46 *A 45-year-old with a small right parietal infarct. Bolus contrast-enhanced subtraction MR angiogram of the aortic arch and great vessels to the level of the skull base showing normal vessels.*

Arterial occlusive disease

Atherosclerosis affects the extracranial carotid or vertebral arteries and is the commonest cause of intracranial artery stenosis. However, the intra- and extracranial vessels may be affected by a variety of conditions including arteritis, sickle cell disease, neurofibromatosis and many rare congenital diseases. Stenosis can lead to territorial or watershed infarction from emboli or ischaemia. The origin of the internal carotid artery is the commonest site for cranial vessel arterial stenosis.

Transient ischaemic attacks

Patients with carotid artery stenosis present clinically with either a transient ischaemic attack or a stroke, which may produce loss of vision, loss of speech, sensory disturbances and/or loss of motor power in an arm or a leg. Recovery occurs within 24 hours in the transient ischaemic attack, but not after a stroke.

The initial investigation of patients with a bruit in the neck from suspected carotid artery stenosis includes duplex ultrasound, magnetic resonance (MR) angiography and intravenous digital subtraction angiography.

Duplex ultrasound is a non-invasive method of imaging the crotid and vertebral arteries in the neck with a high sensitivity and specificity for carotid artery stenosis, but it can still misinterpret a high-grade stenosis as an occlusion. However, ultrasound is now well established as the primary method for detection and quantification of carotid artery disease. The initial stage of the examination is to view the common, internal and external carotid vessels with conventional grey-scale imaging for the presence of plaque, using a 5 or 7 MHz transducer. Plaque is characterized as hypoechoic, echoic or calcified. If the surface of the plaque can be seen clearly, it is classified as smooth or irregular, calcified or non-calcified (Fig.

(a)   (b)

Figure 15.47 *Stenosis of the internal carotid artery (ICA). (a) Grey-scale image of the ICA shows a large, heavily calcified plaque at the vessel origin. (b) Spectral Doppler signal taken from a point within the stenosis, showing elevation of peak systolic (2.21 m/s) and diastolic velocity (0.73 m/s).*

15.47a). Focal pits in the surface of the plaque or hypoechoic areas within it may represent areas of ulceration or intraplaque haemorrhage, which are both associated with transient ischaemic attacks and stroke.

Colour Doppler is used to visualize flow within the vessels. Focal narrowing reduces the lumen width but also produces a local increase in flow velocity, which is visible as a colour change. Turbulence results in a colour mosaic beyond the stenosis, which is the colour Doppler representation of spectral broadening. The severity of narrowing is quantified using velocity measurements made from the spectral display. Peak and end-diastolic velocities are recorded in the common, internal and external carotid arteries and also at the site of maximal velocity within the stenosis (Fig. 15.47b) and these values are compared with reference values to arrive at an estimate of the degree of stenosis, usually quoted as the percentage reduction in vessel diameter.

Magnetic resonance angiography is also a non-invasive method of imaging which has the advantage of being able to demonstrate both the intrathoracic and intracranial vessels, although it also tends to overestimate the degree of stenosis. **Intravenous digital subtraction angiography** is an invasive method of imaging with a lower sensitivity and specificity for carotid artery stenosis than duplex ultrasound and has the disadvantage of demonstrating all the intracranial arteries simultaneously, which overlap on the images.

Patients with a low-grade stenosis of less than 30 per cent are treated conservatively with antiplatelet therapy, such as aspirin, but patients with a high-grade stenosis of over 70 per cent should be considered for surgery or possibly angioplasty (Fig. 15.48). The management of patients with a stenosis between 30 and 70 per cent varies between centres.

Arteriography is performed only in patients being assessed for carotid endarterectomy, because it carries a

Figure 15.48 *Internal carotid artery stenosis in a 57-year-old with transient ischaemic attacks. Carotid angiography shows over 70 per cent stenosis of the internal carotid artery with an atheromatous ulcer (arrow) distal to the stenosis, the source of emboli.*

risk of permanent neurological damage of about 1 per cent in this age group. Selective carotid arteriography may show an atheromatous stenosis or an ulcerating plaque at the origin of the internal carotid artery or, less commonly, a stenosis at the origin of the external carotid artery, in the common carotid artery and occasionally even in the intracerebral arteries. Arch aortography may show an atheromatous stenosis at the origin of one of the great vessels arising from the arch of the aorta; an arteritis with multiple stenoses; occlusions in the carotid and subclavian arteries; or even the subclavian steal syndrome when there is occlusion of the left subclavian artery and reverse flow down the left vertebral artery.

Patients with a pulsatile lump in the neck also require investigation with either duplex ultrasound or carotid arteriography. CT or MRI may help to show the vessel and any associated mass. The lump is commonly due to a tortuous carotid artery in an elderly hypertensive patient, but may be due to a chemodectoma, carotid body tumour or an aneurysm of the internal carotid artery.

Arterial dissection

Arterial dissection is being demonstrated more commonly as a cause of stroke in young people. Dissection usually involves the extracranial internal carotid and vertebral arteries. Angiography or MRI will show the typical tapering of the lumen of the affected vessel.

Primary intracerebral haemorrhage

Intracerebral haemorrhage usually presents acutely and is the primary event in 10 per cent of strokes. The average age is younger than in purely ischaemic stroke. Intracerebral haemorrhage may be associated with some subarachnoid haemorrhage or intraventricular haemorrhage but these are not dominant features. A diverse range of potential causes must be considered when planning the patient's investigation. Several are discussed here with the others being covered in the appropriate sections (Table 15.3).

Hypertension is presumed to be the most common cause of spontaneous intracerebral haemorrhage and, although traditional teaching implicated the rupture of microscopic (so-called Charcot–Bouchard) aneurysms, this has not been sustained by recent histological studies, and the most likely cause is now thought to be degenerative arterial wall changes (lipohyalinosis and fibrinoid necrosis) in small perforating vessels. The commonest sites for hypertensive haemorrhage are in

Table 15.3 *Causes of intracerebral haemorrhage*

Very common	Common	Uncommon
Hypertension	Infarct with	Eclampsia
Aneurysm	reperfusion	Encephalopathies
Trauma	Amyloid angiopathy	(HSV)
Arteriovenous	Coagulopathies	Vasculitides
malformation	Neoplasm	(fungal more
	Venous infarct	often than
	Drug abuse	non-fungal)

Figure 15.49 *Acute hypertensive haemorrhage in a 38-year-old woman. High-attenuation lesion with very little surrounding oedema involves the right putamen and causes mass effect with compression of the frontal horn of the right lateral ventricle.*

the deep regions of the brain: the basal ganglia, particularly the putamen (Fig. 15.49), the thalamus, the brain stem and the dentate nucleus region of the cerebellum. Haemorrhage is very variable in size, is usually solitary and can break into the ventricular system. Occasionally recurrent haemorrhage is found at the same site, but this is more common with amyloid angiopathy.

Rupture of a **berry aneurysm** can frequently produce intracerebral clot, which may dominate the subarachnoid haemorrhage, especially if imaging is carried out a few days after the episode allowing the subarachnoid haemorrhage time to mature and resolve. These associated haematomas occur in typical sites related to the positions of common aneurysms on the circle of Willis (Fig. 15.50).

Arteriovenous abnormalities are the commonest cause of intracerebral haemorrhage in the young adult, but only underlie a third of cases overall. They are further discussed on p. 437.

Traumatic intracerebral haematomas can range in size from extremely large to microscopic and may or may not be associated with contusions (see Fig. 15.21). They are further discussed on p. 409.

Infarction from thrombosis of a major supply artery may produce severe ischaemia and infarction, resulting in brain and microscopic vessel necrosis. When these vessels in the infarct are re-exposed to flowing blood at systolic pressure on reperfusion either spontaneously or following treatment with tissue plasminogen activators, they burst, resulting in intracerebral haemorrhage.

Amyloid angiopathy is associated with deep lobar haematomas particularly in the elderly population (Fig.

Figure 15.50 *A 54-year-old woman with acute headache, who collapsed and became comatose. CT shows a high-attenuation intracerebral haemorrhage extending into the right frontal lobe associated with extensive subarachnoid haemorrhage in the basal cisterns and the sylvian fissures with intraventricular haemorrhage. The intracerebral haematoma has mass effect producing subfalcine herniation, whilst the subarachnoid haemorrhage has produced early hydrocephalus seen as dilatation of the temporal horns. Cerebral angiogram defined a right anterior communicating artery aneurysm.*

Figure 15.51 *A 52-year-old man with hypertension. CT shows high-attenuation haemorrhage in the left centrum semiovale. The slight increased attenuation posteriorly suggests previous haemorrhage, which was confirmed clinically. Final diagnosis was amyloid angiopathy-related intracerebral haemorrhage.*

15.51). Although patchy deposits of amyloid are found in the muscle layers of medium and small cerebral arteries of many elderly people, it is greater in extent, leading to secondary fibrinoid necrosis seen in those patients who have intracerebral haemorrhages. These cerebral amyloid deposits are not related to generalized amyloidosis. If multiple or recurrent haemorrhage is found or if there is a family history of such haemorrhage, amyloid angiopathy should be suspected.

Haemorrhage associated with **anticoagulant therapy** has a similar distribution to hypertensive haemorrhage with the risk increasing as the INR rises above 5.0, but most patients with anticoagulant-related haemorrhage have appropriate therapeutic levels of the drug. The haematoma formed often has a fluid–fluid level with unclotted sedimented red cells lying in the dependent portion of the haematoma below the serum. Similar appearances can occur with haemorrhage in alcoholics who have liver damage with clotting deficiencies, including low platelet counts. The absolute risk of haemorrhage with antiplatelet treatment, usually aspirin, is minimally increased. **Thrombolytic therapy** for non-cerebral thrombosis, such as myocardial infarction, does increase the risk of cerebral haemorrhage, but it is now thought that this occurs most frequently in an area of pre-existing amyloid angiopathy. Myeloid leukaemia may cause haemorrhage but it is rare in other leukaemias. Haemorrhage is possibly related to aggregates of tumour cells producing microinfarcts and leakage in the cortex and subcortical white matter. Disseminated intravascular coagulation is also associated with intracerebral haemorrhage.

Haemorrhage into a **neoplasm** accounts for only 5 per cent of all intracerebral haemorrhage. If the tumour is known about, there is no difficulty with the diagnosis but, if unsuspected, the haemorrhage may be the first indication of a tumour. Haemorrhage is caused either by necrosis, usually in the centre of a tumour, or by rupture of the friable neovascularity around its growing margin.

Haemorrhage associated with a **venous infarct** is now more commonly recognized. It is discussed on p. 437.

Drug abuse with cocaine, amphetamine and phenylpropanolamine or their derivatives is causing an increasing number of intracerebral haemorrhages. Vessel damage with fibrinoid necrosis, hypertension and emboli all contribute to vessel rupture, although underlying vascular anomalies have been found with high frequency in cocaine abusers presenting with intracerebral haemorrhage.

Vasculitis is an uncommon cause of haemorrhage but mycotic aneurysms distant from the circle of Willis, particularly if related to fungal infection, can cause vessel rupture and result in intracerebral haemorrhage.

When acute intracerebral haemorrhage is suspected, CT is generally the most important examination. The

(a)

(b)

(c)

Figure 15.52 *A 26-year-old presenting with 4 weeks of facial numbness and diplopia and with a previous history of a sixth and seventh nerve palsy a year apart. (a) T2-weighted axial MRI shows the typical slightly lobulated hyperintense nidus surrounded by hypointense haemosiderin rim, whilst (b) T1-weighted sagittal section shows the hyperintense nidus and hypointense rim of a cavernous angioma in the posterior aspect of the left side of the pons (arrow). (c) Another patient, a 42-year-old man with multiple small haemorrhages from a left sylvian fissure AVM. T2-weighted MRI showing hyperintensity in the sylvian fissure from residual blood clot and hypointense 'pencil lining' of localized superficial siderosis from the final resolution of haemorrhage when macrophages engulf the methaemoglobin, which is metabolized to haemosiderin.*

haemorrhage will be shown as a high-attenuation lesion with minimal or no surrounding oedema. As the lesion matures over the next 72 hours, the surrounding low attenuation increases. Unless the haemorrhage is associated with a neoplasm, vasogenic oedema is not seen. Fluid levels suggest a coagulation disorder, while the site of the haematoma can hint at the underlying cause. If multiple or recurrent haemorrhage is noted in an elderly patient, amyloid angiopathy must be considered. Contrast enhancement is not required in the acute situation but may be necessary when tumours, arterio-venous malformations (AVMs) or veno-occlusive disease is suspected. Over time the haematoma will mature to isoattenuation and then to reduced attenuation leaving only a tiny slit-like area of malacia filled with low-attenuation fluid. If the haemorrhage resulted from transformation of an infarct, a typical segmental area of malacia will result. The maturation of intrac-

erebral haemorrhage has been discussed in the trauma section (p. 410).

All these features of haemorrhage can be shown with MRI, but it is more difficult to conduct the examination in an acutely ill patient unless full monitoring equipment compatible with the magnetic field is available. In the subacute and chronic stages it is the ideal examination, as it will show haemorrhage at all stages and is often able to define the underlying cause of the haematoma if it is due to a vascular abnormality. Chronic haemorrhage can also be shown when it is not visible on CT (Fig. 15.52). The association of ischaemia and infarction with a haematoma can be shown with greater sensitivity on MRI, especially if FLAIR and diffusion-weighted sequences are used. The maturation of haemorrhage proceeds in an orderly fashion on T1- and T2-weighted scans as described in the trauma section (see Table 15.2).

(a)   *(b)*

Figure 15.53 *Anterior communicating artery aneurysm in a 60-year-old with sudden severe headache, meningism and photophobia. (a) CT shows extensive basal cistern and interhemispheric subarachnoid haemorrhage. (b) Oblique view from a selective internal carotid artery angiogram shows the aneurysm (arrow); its rupture had caused the haemorrhage.*

SPECT has a limited role but ^{99m}Tc-HMPAO may confirm the presence of an infarct or show widespread ischaemia related to the haematoma or AVM. Thallium-201 will show high-grade neoplasms related to haematomas.

If the patient is to have the haemorrhage removed in the acute stage because of severe space occupation and incipient coning, an angiogram is sometimes required to define any underlying vascular abnormality such as an AVM or aneurysm. In the subacute or chronic stage this will still be required in those patients in whom neurosurgery or intravascular intervention is considered appropriate, if a vascular lesion is found. This tends to occur in a patient who is less than 65 years old and not hypertensive and the haemorrhage is not in the deep regions of the brain. As the sensitivity of MR angiography increases this non-invasive examination will gradually replace catheter angiography.

Intracranial aneurysms and subarachnoid haemorrhage

Berry aneurysms occur at the arterial bifurcations in or near the circle of Willis and are due to acquired conditions, such as atherosclerosis superimposed on a congenital propensity to a deficient internal elastic lamina and collagen disorder. These aneurysms show a familial tendency and are associated with inherited conditions such as Ehlers–Danlos syndrome, Marfan's syndrome, neurofibromatosis and polycystic kidney disease. Approximately 33 per cent of intracranial

aneurysms occur on the anterior communicating arteries, 33 per cent at the origin of the posterior communicating arteries, 20 per cent in the middle of the cerebral artery, 5 per cent each at the basilar bifurcation and rest of the posterior fossa, with 1–3 per cent in sites distal to the circle of Willis; 15–20 per cent of patients have multiple aneurysms.

Aneurysms can rupture to cause subarachnoid haemorrhage but may cause symptoms because of mass effect even when only 6 mm in diameter. Posterior communicating aneurysms can present with a third nerve palsy due to direct pressure on the nerve. The aneurysm in this case is usually of sufficient size to be demonstrated by dynamic bolus contrast high-definition CT. Giant middle cerebral and basilar tip aneurysms impinge on adjacent structures and can cause pressure effects.

CT is the best way to demonstrate acute subarachnoid haemorrhage but, if CT is delayed, it is progressive less sensitive as the blood is washed away in the CSF. If subarachnoid haemorrhage is diagnosed on CT (Fig. 15.53), a lumbar puncture and CSF examination are not required. Lumbar puncture could be hazardous if there were an intracerebral mass and raised intracranial pressure. Unfortunately in a patient with clinically suspected subarachnoid haemorrhage, a normal CT examination does not exclude the diagnosis.

CT also shows associated intracerebral haemorrhage and any direct or retrograde spread of haemorrhage into the ventricles that is best appreciated in the dependent trigones and occipital horns. The site of maximal haemorrhage often gives a clue to the site of the

(a)

(b)

Figure 15.54 *Terminal internal carotid artery aneurysm (arrow) demonstrated on (a) MR angiography with (b) conventional common carotid angiogram for comparison.*

aneurysm. MRI can show subarachnoid haemorrhage, but special sequences are required that depend on the increased protein content of bloody CSF. MRI is sometimes useful to identify small associated intra-cranial haemorrhages, which indicate which aneurysm has ruptured when multiple aneurysms have been found at angiography.

Once the patient is stable, angiography is required to identify the cause of the haemorrhage, which is most commonly due to an aneurysm and less commonly to an arteriovenous malformation or other anomaly.

Preshaped catheters are used to catheterize the carotid and vertebral arteries selectively via the transfemoral route. The entire intracranial vascular tree can be visualized in arterial, capillary and venous phases. Aneurysms as small as 1–2 mm may be defined, whilst most are around 5–10 mm. Aneurysms over 10 mm may well contain clot and only the lumen will fill with contrast on the angiogram, thus underestimating its size. A contrast-enhanced CT may well show the organized clot and the enhancing lumen if the aneurysm is sufficiently large.

(a)

(b)

Figure 15.55 *Treatment of a terminal basilar artery aneurysm with microcoils. (a) Lateral view of aneurysm before endovascular introduction of coils and (b) exclusion of the aneurysm from the circulation by the tight coil nest preserving the parent and distal vessels.*

(a)

(b)

Figure 15.56 *CT venography following a bolus of intravenous contrast shows (a) the filling defect in the proximal superior sagittal sinus representing thrombus (arrow) (the delta sign). (b) The filling defect caused by thrombus in the left sigmoid sinus (arrow) can be compared to the normally enhancing right sigmoid sinus.*

MR angiography can also be used to demonstrate aneurysms and the vascular tree non-invasively, using the magnetic properties of flowing blood (Fig. 15.54). Currently, aneurysms as small as 5 mm can be shown reliably but, at the present stage of development of MR angiography, the gold standard remains conventional angiography.

Most aneurysms are treated by isolating them from the circulation with an aneurysm clip at open craniotomy with the use of an operating microscope. Percutaneous transarterial interventional radiological catheter techniques are now being increasingly used to treat increasing numbers of selected aneurysms: platinum microcoils are threaded through the catheter and released in the aneurysm to form a small 'nest' (Fig. 15.55). This invokes thrombosis in the aneurysm and over time the thrombus becomes endothelialized and the aneurysm is excluded from the circulation preventing further haemorrhage.

Subarachnoid haemorrhage is often accompanied by arterial spasm induced by vasoactive substances released in response to the haemorrhage. Spasm can be severe enough to cause ischaemia, infarction and even death. The angiogram will show irregular narrowing of the intracranial vessel usually close to the ruptured aneurysm, but spasm can be extensive involving many vessels. Transcranial Doppler ultrasound can be used to monitor the blood flow in the circle of Willis and can indicate the presence of spasm.

Other causes of subarachnoid haemorrhage include arteriovenous malformation, intracerebral haemorrhage, trauma, dural fistula and, rarely, haemorrhagic infarcts and tumours. CT shows the abnormality, and angiography is required in many of these patients to show the vascular aspects of the lesion.

Veno-occlusive disorders

Although facial and mastoid infection used to be the commonest cause, thrombosis is now most frequently associated with dehydration, often after gastrointestinal infections, on long aeroplane flights, hormone treatment, trauma or tumours directly affecting the sinus. Occlusion of the dural venous sinuses and intracerebral veins with subsequent venous infarction or brain swelling and increased intracranial pressure is much less common than arterial infarction. The imaging appearances are less predictable and a high index of suspicion is required to make an early diagnosis. Dynamic contrast CT will usually show non-enhancement of a whole segment of sinus or may show filling defects in the sinus (Fig. 15.56). On MRI the absence of normal flow phenomenon in the sinus will be seen. MR venography is excellent in the superior sagittal sinus, straight sinus and parts of the transverse sinuses but, around the torcula and the sigmoid sinuses, the normal turbulent flow patterns can easily be confused with partial occlusions. Late views in the venous phase of conventional angiography remain the definitive diagnostic method.

ARTERIOVENOUS ANOMALIES

Arteriovenous anomalies are divided into:

- arteriovenous malformations;
- venous angiomas which are composed entirely of veins;
- cavernous angiomas which show large sinusoidal vascular spaces;
- telangiectases which are tiny capillary angiomas.

(a)   (b)

Figure 15.57 *Arteriovenous malformation in a 14-year-old. (a) CT shows a right frontal intracerebral haematoma. (b) Internal carotid arteriogram shows the malformation is supplied by abnormal branches of the anterior and middle cerebral arteries.*

Arteriovenous malformations, the commonest vascular anomaly, are congenital lesions consisting of a coiled mass of arteries and veins. Arteriovenous malformations generally involve the cerebral hemispheres but may occur anywhere in the brain and can have single or more usually multiple arterial supply. Aneurysms are sometimes found on the feeding arteries. Venous drainage can be by single or multiple veins running to the deep or superficial venous systems. CT shows serpiginous densities that enhance markedly after contrast, representing the draining veins. There may be associated calcification in the lesion but little or no mass effect if the lesion has not bled. Intracerebral and intraventricular haemorrhage and, less often, subarachnoid haemorrhage result if the arteriovenous malformation bleeds (Fig. 15.57). MRI is particularly useful in defining the relationship of the arteriovenous malformation to other midline and posterior fossa structures by observing the flow voids produced by the arteries and veins. MRI is better than CT in defining any subacute and chronic parenchymal haemorrhage that may have occurred. Treatment is by endovascular occlusion, surgical excision, 'gamma knife' stereotactic radiotherapy or a mixture of each, with the aim of obliterating the maximum amount of the arteriovenous malformation while doing least damage to the normal surrounding brain. Angiography enables the normal and abnormal vascular tree to be outlined and the feeding and draining vessels to be identified. In selected patients microcatheters can be guided into the malformation and cyanoacrylate glues or coils introduced to occlude the lesion.

Cavernous angiomas are usually high attenuation-enhancing lesions on CT and usually produce no mass effect. They are often occult and do not show on angiography. Calcification may occasionally be seen within the lesion. On MRI, cavernous angiomas show a typical pattern consisting of a hypointense ring owing to haemosiderin around an inhomogeneous hyperintense lesion on T2-weighted scans. Cavernous angiomas rarely bleed and are usually only removed if they cause symptoms such as focal epilepsy.

HYDROCEPHALUS

CSF is formed from a mixture of plasma ultrafiltrate produced by the choroid plexus and of cerebral extracellular fluid permeating through the ependyma into the ventricles. It functions as a homeostatic medium and provides a protective hydrostatic cushion for the brain. CSF is dynamic, pulsing with the arterial pressure wave, but also circulates from its production site in the ventricles, into the subarachnoid spaces, around the brain and spinal cord with reabsorption back into the vascular system, through the arachnoid villi that project into lacunae along the superior sagittal sinus.

Strictly defined, hydrocephalus just means an increased amount of CSF in the cranial cavity. It is usually associated with enlarged ventricles but not all patients with enlarged ventricles have clinical hydrocephalus as the enlargement may be an *ex vacuo* effect due to loss of brain substance, as in the physiological atrophy of ageing or following head injury, infection or dementia. Hydrocephalus is now usually defined as an imbalance between CSF production, circulation and reabsorption, and radiology plays a key role in defining its presence and cause.

Excessive production of CSF associated with hydrocephalus has been attributed to intraventricular choroid plexus papillomas, but there is increasing evidence that there is obstruction of the foramina of Luschka and Magendie by tumoral haemorrhage, high protein levels or intraventricular debris rather than just overproduction of CSF.

Headaches, nausea and vomiting are the cardinal symptoms of hydrocephalus once it causes increased intracranial pressure in the older child or adult. In the infant, accelerated head growth with widening of the sutures is often the first sign. Gradual increases in intracranial pressure may be accommodated for a short time and the onset of symptoms may be delayed.

Radiology is used to confirm the presence of abnormal CSF circulation and make an estimate of ventricular size. Comparison with previous imaging is essential for progression to be assessed. CT is most frequently used because of its wide availability, but MRI with axial and sagittal sections will give a more complete impression of the disruption to CSF flow. Multiple measurements of ventricular size and shape have been defined, but in routine clinical practice they are seldom used.

With increasing CSF pressure the lateral ventricles first show subtle enlargement of the normally slit-like temporal horns. Their size provides a sensitive indication of increased pressure. There is then symmetrical rounding of the anterior horns leading to an increase in the angle between the frontal horn and the median sagittal plane and finally, if there is no obstruction at the foramen of Monro, the ventricles dilate. The third ventricle is surrounded by relatively compact brain and so dilates later in the presence of increasing intracranial pressure, and tends to be the first region to resume normal size after the pressure is relieved. Sagittal MRI now makes the assessment of the aqueduct easier and dilatation or focal stenosis can be seen directly. The fourth ventricle may also dilate later with increased CSF pressure. It assumes a more rounded shape on axial section, whilst on sagittal sections an enlarged triangular shape is maintained (Fig. 15.58). The caudal foramina must be assessed and those that are seen to be wide and dilated differentiated from those appearing stenotic or closed by a membrane.

Periventricular oedema, seen on CT as a rim of decreased attenuation on T1- and T2-weighted MRI imaging as hypo- and hyperintense signal respectively, may occur with increased intraventricular pressure, especially if there has been an acute pressure rise. Periventricular oedema initially represents the 'damming back' of the transependymal flow of extracellular fluid towards the ventricles, and then with increasing pressure flow reverses with leakage from the ventricles through the damaged, stretched ependyma into the periventricular white matter (Fig. 15.59). When chronic, a degree of demyelination can occur. Hydrocephalus rarely becomes compensated, but a new equilibrium may be established at a higher intracranial pressure owing to the opening of other pathways of

Figure 15.58 *Hydrocephalus in a 55-year-old following meningitis. The lateral, third and fourth ventricles are all dilated owing to obstruction around the basal cisterns.*

absorption through the arachnoid membrane, the stroma of the choroid plexus and, with reversed transependymal flow, through the cortical mantle.

The ventricular dilatation compresses the brain against the skull vault and displaces CSF from the sulci and cisterns. This differentiates hydrocephalus from atrophy where the increase in ventricular size is proportionate to the increase in sulcal and cisternal CSF volumes. Another feature of cortical atrophy is that atrophy causes less dilatation of the third ventricle compared to the lateral ventricles.

The flow pattern and absorption of CSF can be followed directly with radionuclide studies by injecting ^{111}In-DTPA (indium-111 diethylenetriaminepentaacetic

Figure 15.59 *Acute hydrocephalus of the lateral and third ventricles with periventricular oedema (arrows) on T2-weighted axial sections. Arrow heads mark lateral border of the ventricle.*

acid) into the lumbar or cisternal theca and following the activity period over 48 hours. This technique has been largely superseded by the indirect visualization of CSF flow by MRI.

CONGENITAL HYDROCEPHALUS

Congenital hydrocephalus is usually caused by insults during the 3rd and 4th week after conception. It most frequently results from aqueduct stenosis (43 per cent) followed in frequency by forms of communicating hydrocephalus (38 per cent), Dandy–Walker syndrome (13 per cent) and other anatomical lesions (6 per cent). Hydrocephalus is usually recognized on ultrasound but MRI is required for a full anatomical assessment of the site of CSF flow blockage and for detecting any of the frequently associated congenital abnormalities, such as cephaloceles, absent corpus callosum, Chiari malformation and neural tube closure defects.

INTRAVENTRICULAR OBSTRUCTIVE (NON-COMMUNICATING) HYDROCEPHALUS

When the ventricular CSF is unable to communicate with the subarachnoid space, the ventricles proximal to the obstruction dilate. The cause of the obstruction may arise within the ventricular system, such as an ependymoma, glioma or a colloid cyst of the third ventricle, and cause an obstruction of the foramen of Monro; more commonly the abnormality arises outside the ventricular system such as a craniopharyngioma, pituitary macroadenoma or primitive neuroectodermal tumour. A third possibility is a congenital lesion such as an aqueduct stenosis.

EXTRAVENTRICULAR OBSTRUCTIVE (COMMUNICATING) HYDROCEPHALUS

This term is used when the obstruction is distal to the outlets of the fourth ventricle and is due either to impeded flow around the convexities or to impeded reabsorption by the arachnoid villi. The condition most commonly follows subarachnoid haemorrhage when absorption through the arachnoid villi is blocked. Similar blockage may also occur with widespread subarachnoid neoplasm (primitive neuroectodermal tumour, lymphoma, adenocarcinoma) and infections such as purulent or tuberculous meningitis. In some cases the obstruction to free flow will be at the level of the tentorial hiatus or basal cisterns.

For normal absorption to occur there must be a pressure difference across the arachnoid villi of about 3–6 cm of water. If there is venous hypertension or venous sinus thrombosis, absorption is impaired and hydrocephalus supervenes. This can be shown on dynamic contrast-enhanced CT or MR venography.

CONCLUSION

Imaging in hydrocephalus has a key role:

- in deciding whether hydrocephalus is present;
- in categorizing the type;
- in assisting in the choice of treatment;
- in assessing the effect of treatment with shunting or internal diversions;
- in monitoring the side effects of treatment.

CT is usually adequate but MRI will give a more complete understanding of the CSF pathways.

NORMAL AGEING, ISCHAEMIC LESIONS AND NEURODEGENERATIVE DISORDERS

NORMAL AGEING

Atrophy reflects the loss of brain tissue – an inevitable consequence of ageing. This may involve the cortical grey matter, subcortical white matter or the deep grey matter separately or together in the supra- or infratentorial compartments. In people with normal cognition there is a gradual loss of brain substance with age and a concomitant increase in CSF in the ventricles and sulci. This produces a wide spectrum of normal age-related atrophy. Many toxins, drugs and neurodegenerative states, such as alcohol, phenytoin and vascular disease (Fig. 15.60) can accelerate this process. Although there are several indices that describe the

Figure 15.60 *A 48-year-old woman with severe congenital vascular disease leading to dementia: T2-weighted MRI showing atrophy, numerous small subcortical infarcts and a diffuse leucoencephalopathy.*

degree of atrophy and define the extent of ventricular dilatation, they tend to be used only in research studies, with routine clinical reporting dependent on the radiologist's experience and knowledge of the local population. Both CT and MRI can be used to define the degree and extent of any of atrophy present. With atrophy there is sulcal widening and mildly enlarged lateral ventricles appropriate to the size of the sulci, the third ventricle usually has concave lateral walls and the angle of the frontal horns is obtuse.

The differential diagnosis between ventricular dilatation from atrophy and that from impaired CSF absorption (communicating hydrocephalus, normal pressure hydrocephalus) can sometimes be difficult. It may be important because CSF diversion with a shunt may relieve the symptoms when the dilatation is due to poor absorption. CT or MRI will show dilatation of the frontal and temporal horns of the lateral ventricles and the third ventricle, but a normal-appearing fourth ventricle in communicating hydrocephalus with an acute angle to the frontal horns. The hemispheric sulci are small or effaced. Recent MRI techniques may help to select patients for surgical treatment.

ISCHAEMIC LESIONS

Areas of **periventricular low attenuation** on CT, with corresponding focal and confluent hyperintensities on FLAIR, proton density- and T2-weighted MRI sections, and often hypointensities on T1-weighted sequences, do not necessarily represent actual necrosis and infarction but can be due to a spectrum of chronic cerebrovascular insufficiency particularly involving small end-arterioles. This merges with the non-specific white matter changes found in as many as 30 per cent of the normal ageing population over 60 years of age who show no clinical cognitive deficit. These appearances are also seen more commonly in patients with hypertension, diabetes mellitus and coronary artery disease.

Lacunar infarcts may be seen that represent focal areas of infarction less than 1 cm in diameter, which characteristically occur in the territory of perforating arteries arising from the major vessels. Dilated perivascular spaces give a signal owing to CSF and are usually smaller than lacunar infarcts. They typically occur in the basal regions, deep white matter and cortex of the brain. Gliosis may become more confluent around these vessels as the vascular insufficiency progresses, and produces an increased signal on FLAIR or proton density-weighted images and hyperintensity on T2-weighted sections.

These white matter changes seen on CT and MRI (Fig. 15.61) are therefore non-specific and, although seen with increased frequency in ischaemic brains, there is often little or no direct correlation with the clinical state in the individual elderly patient.

Figure 15.61 *A 63-year-old man with hypertension but no cognitive deficit. T2-weighted MRI shows non-specific periventricular focal and coalescent hyperintensity associated with early atrophy and concomitant ventricular enlargement.*

NEURODEGENERATIVE DISORDERS

The neurodegenerative disorders form a heterogeneous group of disorders that tend to occur in the middle-aged and elderly, and are often associated with focal or diffuse atrophy resulting in various degrees of cognitive dysfunction. Dementia affects between 6 and 10 per cent of the population aged over 65 years, and in up to 50 per cent of the population over 80 years. As the elderly proportion of the population is expected to grow considerably in the next 10 years, there is a desperate need in terms of both human suffering and economics to improve the understanding of these diseases. CT, MRI and SPECT studies all have a role in their investigation.

Alzheimer's disease (dementia of the Alzheimer type – DAT) is the commonest of the dementias making up about half the cases examined *post mortem*, and presents with a gradual onset and progression of forgetfulness, resulting in interference with the activities of daily living. It is a primary disorder of nerve cells histologically characterized by neuronal loss, senile plaques and neurofibrillary tangles, and it is thought that the underlying symptoms are caused by a selective loss of cholinergic neurones. This finding underlies the only currently available treatment strategy with acetylcholinesterase inhibitors for mild and moderate dementia, slowing the rate of cognitive decline in 40 per cent of patients. It has no effect on other dementias and it is therefore essential to target the treatment correctly.

On CT and MRI there is diffuse cerebral atrophy with enlarged sulci and ventricles especially in the later stages of the disease. More specific to DAT, the medial temporal lobes show focal, often symmetrical atrophy

Figure 15.62 *CT section through the long axis of the temporal lobes in a 72-year-old woman with dementia of the Alzheimer type, showing the hippocampus measuring less than 11 mm (arrows) and marked temporal atrophy.*

involving the hippocampus (Fig. 15.62), which tends to occur earlier in the course of the disease and often before severe global atrophy is seen. There is a concomitant enlargement of the temporal horns of the lateral ventricles. It is important that this assessment is carried out on sections taken along the long axis of the temporal lobe or, if MRI is used, coronally at right angles to the long axis as well. SPECT with ^{99m} Tc-HMPAO will show the functional effects of the lack of neurotransmitter, and these investigations are essential in supporting the diagnosis of DAT, especially if drug treatment is being considered. A pattern of bilateral hypoperfusion in the posterior temporal and parietal lobes is most commonly seen in association with atrophy (Plate 5b, opposite p. 358).

Lewy body dementia can only be differentiated from DAT *post mortem*. Structural imaging will show atrophy, but in group studies there is less temporal lobe involvement at a similar stage in the cognitive decline than with DAT. SPECT with ^{99m}Tc-HMPAO shows either similar defects to those produced by atrophy or a similar appearance to DAT. The absence of hippocampal atrophy correlates better with Lewy body dementia.

Multi-infarct dementia is caused by multiple small or large infarcts that produce a dementia dependent on the number, size and position of the infarcts. There is a spectrum of disease from the borders of normal in the ischaemic brain to the severely affected. The features are all associated with hypertension and ischaemia and can be superimposed on a background of the other demen-

tias. Treatment that prevents further ischaemia may be available, and it is therefore important to differentiate multi-infarct from other dementias. Extensive periventricular white matter lesions on CT or on T2-weighted MRI do not, however, distinguish between them, but the presence of cortical and basal ganglial lacunar infarcts favours a diagnosis of multi-infarct dementia. SPECT with ^{99m}Tc-HMPAO is more sensitive to cortical ischaemia and may show multiple patchy areas of hypoperfusion or no perfusion representing grey matter infarcts throughout the brain, without the patterns associated with the other dementias, adding weight to the diagnosis.

Pick's disease is an uncommon primary dementing disease with focal lobar atrophy affecting one or more lobes of the brain, leaving the rest relatively unaffected. CT, MRI and SPECT with ^{99m}Tc-HMPAO all show patterns of atrophy affecting most commonly the frontal lobes, while the remainder of the brain is normal.

Primary parkinsonian syndromes include Parkinson's disease, progressive supranuclear palsy and striatonigral degeneration (often associated with olivopontocerebellar degeneration and Shy–Drager syndrome in multisystem atrophy).

Parkinson's disease is relatively common affecting up to 3 per cent of the population at some time in their lives with the commonest age of onset between 50 years and 60 years. There is loss of the neuromelanin-containing neurones, gliosis and Lewy body formation in the substantia nigra, especially in the pars compacta. CT is generally used to exclude other disease as it does not show any specific changes, whilst MRI is more sensitive in excluding other causes of the symptoms; it may also demonstrate decreased width of the pars compacta and an increase in the normal hypointensity found on T2-weighted sections owing to deposition of iron or other paramagnetic substances. As the projection neurones from the substantia nigra go to the basal ganglia, they are also affected and eventually destroyed. Specialized nuclear medicine investigations can show a specific depletion of D2 transporters and these tests can also be used to assess whether there are sufficient D2 receptors left intact for treatment with levodopa to be effective.

DEMYELINATING DISEASES

There are a bewildering number of causes and pathological mechanisms of disease of the white matter. MRI is much more sensitive than CT for diagnosing these disorders and has gained widespread acceptance as the key imaging modality. However, neither MRI nor CT offers much specificity and it is rarely possible for the radiologist to make a specific diagnosis based on imaging findings alone.

The MRI appearances vary with the specific diagnosis. But in general terms, the demyelinated white matter shows hyperintensity on T2-weighted images, with corresponding hypointensity on T1-weighted images.

There are two main groups of disorders:

- A dysmyelinating group known as leucodystrophies, all of which are rare, in which there is a biochemical defect of the production or maintenance of normal myelin. Most cases present in infancy or childhood with delay in milestones, intellectual failure and progressive spastic paresis. In many of the dysmyelinating conditions the diagnosis is made primarily on biochemical findings. A detailed description of the MRI appearances is beyond the scope of this book. The general features are MRI evidence of demyelination (see above) which may be accompanied by atrophy of specific parts of the brain.
- A demyelinating group in which myelin is formed normally but is later destroyed. This group forms the vast majority of adult white matter disease encountered in clinical practice. The most common example is multiple sclerosis.

MULTIPLE SCLEROSIS

Multiple sclerosis (MS) is an idiopathic inflammatory and demyelinating disorder of the central nervous system (CNS). It is now one of the commonest reasons given for requesting MRI in the northern latitudes of the western world and this diagnosis has huge social and economic consequences.

Clinically the disease usually follows a fluctuating course with symptoms varying from paroxysmal and brief to slowly progressive and chronic. The lesions affect single or multiple sites simultaneously, usually involving white-matter tracts, leading to visual loss, numbness, tingling in the limbs, spastic weakness and ataxia. However, clinicopathological correlation is often poor. Diagnosis is made when a combination of signs and symptoms localizes lesions in separate and distinct areas of the CNS, disseminated in time and space. Supportive laboratory and imaging data are now defined for research studies, dividing the disease into clinically definite and probable MS, with or without laboratory support. Although some CT studies using double dose-enhanced delayed imaging have reported sensitivities as high as 70 per cent when patients are in an acute relapse, MRI has considerably greater sensitivity, nearing 100 per cent, especially if the spinal cord is examined at the same time. With the use of intravenous gadolinium-based contrast agents, acute plaques showing blood–brain barrier breakdown can be separated from subacute and chronic lesions. Plaques can occur anywhere in the white matter. They have a predilection for periventricular white matter and callosal fibres.

Although no single MRI sequence will detect all lesions, multifocal supratentorial white-matter abnormalities are ideally shown on moderately T2-weighted or FLAIR images producing hyperintensity, and may be correspondingly hypointense on T1-weighted sequences (Fig. 15.63). MRI is also ideal for the exclusion of other causes of the patients' signs and symptoms, such as Chiari malformations and spinocerebellar degeneration.

(a)

(b)

Figure 15.63 *A 28-year-old woman with multiple sclerosis presenting with optic neuritis, patchy sensory loss and ataxia. (a) T2-weighted and (b) T1-weighted postcontrast MRI show multiple focal and confluent plaques mainly in a periventricular white-matter distribution, with enhancement indicating blood–brain barrier breakdown around the borders of the left frontal plaque, which is in the acute inflammatory stage.*

Table 15.4 *The differential diagnosis of multifocal white-matter lesions on T2-weighted MRI*

Commonest	Common	Uncommon
Virchow–Robin perivascular spaces	Embolic disease	Vasculitis
Normal ageing	Metastases	Postviral demyelination
Atherosclerosis	Trauma, e.g. diffuse axonal injury	Multifocal primary neoplasm, e.g. lymphoma, glioblastoma
Multiple sclerosis		Congenital and acquired leucoencephalopathy
Granulomatous diseases, e.g. sarcoid		Neurocutaneous syndromes

Serial studies may also fulfil the criterion of dissemination in time by showing new, often asymptomatic lesions. The T1- and T2-relaxation time of apparently normal white matter in patients with MS may be increased. Post-mortem studies have confirmed that the lesions with increased T2-relaxation correspond to MS plaques. This sensitivity makes MRI the most appropriate modality for examining a patient with suspected MS.

Unfortunately these multifocal white-matter lesions may be indistinguishable from other conditions that produce demyelination, gliosis or periventricular effusions (Table 15.4) and between 5 and 30 per cent of apparently normal controls older than 50 years have been shown to have white-matter lesions, probably owing to asymptomatic cerebrovascular disease. The patient's age and pattern of lesions can help to improve the specificity of MRI.

The areas of perivenular inflammation and oedema associated with acute MS plaques cause a transient disruption of the blood–brain barrier and allow leakage of intravenous gadolinium contrast agents (Fig. 15.64). This is shown as enhancement on T1-weighted images with hyperintensity within or around the edges of the plaque. Correlation with the lesions seen on T2-weighted sections is good. A small number of cortical or subcortical plaques are seen solely on enhanced T1-weighted images. This enhancement can be made more obvious by using magnetization transfer sequences, where the hyperintensity of the contrast is shown against a 'flatter' generally darker background, thus increasing the contrast to noise ratio. Enhancement is now considered a consistent feature of recogizably new lesions or new parts of existing plaques. The inflammatory demyelination has been shown pathologically to begin in a perivenular distribution and spread centrifugally corresponding with ring enhancement. Gadolinium enhancement is particularly useful in the clear delineation of lesions in the spinal cord and optic nerves, especially if T1-weighted fat saturation chemical shift sequences are used to reduce the high signal from surrounding periorbital fat. STIR sequences are excellent at showing the hyperintensity associated with optic neuritis (Fig. 15.65).

Differences in the enhancement pattern in the two major clinical patient groups – primary and secondary progressive MS – have been identified. The secondary progressive group has more new lesions, of which a larger proportion enhance. This compares with few new lesions (less than four lesions per patient per year), where very few enhance in the primary progressive group when there were no differences over 6 months in the rates of clinical deterioration between the two groups.

Now that new and biologically active lesions can be identified routinely by gadolinium-enhanced T1-weighted scans, the association of blood–brain barrier leakage in some, but not all, multiple plaques shown on T2-weighted images indicates the presence of dissemination in time, and refines the diagnosis of MS. The method using gadolinium enhancement can be used to subdivide clinical groups and is useful in monitoring and possibly shortening the time required for therapeutic trials in MS.

ACUTE DISSEMINATED ENCEPHALOMYELITIS (ADEM)

ADEM is a demyelinating disease which is thought to be an immune-mediated disorder secondary to a recent viral infection (or more rarely to vaccination). It has an acute onset and a monophasic course, which separates it from MS. Most patients recover with few neurological sequelae. This makes it one of the most important differential diagnoses of MS in the acute clinical situation.

Pathologically there is a diffuse perivenous inflammatory process resulting in confluent areas of demyelination mainly in the white matter. These frequently occur at the corticomedullary junction. Large areas of hyperintensity on T2-weighted and hypointensity on T1-weighted sequences are found in both hemispheres but the changes are usually asymmetrical. Although in the acute stage the demyelinating lesions may enhance, the blood–brain barrier quickly returns to normal. Occasionally similar lesions affect the spinal cord. As with MS, MRI is much more sensitive than CT at demonstrating these lesions.

Figure 15.64 *A 34-year-old man with multiple sclerosis followed over 6 months with T2- and postcontrast T1-weighted MRI, (a) and (b) at presentation, (c) and (d) 1 month later, (e) and (f) 5 months later. Plaques wax and wane over this period of time with the acute inflammatory changes shown by oedema on T2-weighted sections and enhancement on T1-weighted sections.*

(a)

(b)

(c)

(d)

(e)

(f)

(a)   (b)

Figure 15.65 *A 27-year-old woman with blurring of vision in her left eye and a patch of sensory loss on her left leg. Oblique parasagittal STIR (short tau inversion recovery) MRI of (a) the right orbit showing a normal optic nerve signal, whilst (b) the left orbit shows hyperintensity of the optic nerve.*

SCHILDER'S DISEASE (MYELINOCLASTIC DIFFUSE SCLEROSIS)

This is a rare but distinctive acute demyelinating condition which can be defined by biochemical, pathological and electrophysiological criteria. There is a severe selective inflammatory demyelination with sparing of the subcortical U fibres, and extensive attempts at remyelination.

White-matter changes on MRI have been described with bilateral involvement of the anterior hemispheres, extensive fluctuating increased relaxation times, mass effect and varying partial ring enhancement indicating changes in blood–brain barrier breakdown. Other leucodystrophies with a similar appearance, such as adrenoleukodystrophy and Pelizaeus–Merzbacher disease, must be excluded by biochemical testing.

POSTINFLAMMATORY RESPONSES (VIRAL, ALLERGIC AND IMMUNE-MEDIATED RESPONSES TO PREVIOUS INFECTION)

Subacute sclerosing panencephalitis is a rare progressive demyelination resulting from reactivation of the measles virus from a defect in immunity, which allowed the virus to remain latent. There is a variable rate of progression with death between 2 months and several years after reactivation. There is perivascular infiltration by inflammatory cells, cortical and subcortical gliosis, and white-matter demyelination progressing from occipital to the frontal lobes and from the cerebellum to the brain stem and spinal cord. This is seen as multifocal patchy white-matter lesions with hyperintensity on T2-weighted and hypointensity on T1-weighted MRI.

Progressive multifocal leucoencephalopathy is a demyelinating disease probably caused by the papovaviruses (e.g. JC). These are dealt with in the section on AIDS, page 421.

POST-THERAPY RESPONSES

Disseminated necrotizing leucoencephalopathy

When patients are treated with intrathecal antineoplastic agents, such as methotrexate, for disseminated lymphoma, leukaemia or carcinomatosis, a necrotizing leucoencephalopathy can occur, despite the fact that the agent does not usually cross the blood–brain barrier. Radiation therapy potentiates this neurotoxicity. This causes a relative tissue ischaemia, demyelination and necrosis. On MRI there is a diffuse increase in T1- and T2-relaxation times with no mass effect and little or no gadolinium enhancement, reflecting only the oedema and demyelination present.

Radiation encephalopathy

The patterns of injury to the white matter from radiation therapy on its own are divided into three stages: acute, early and delayed. In the first days or weeks after therapy, vasogenic oedema may be produced because of transient disruption of the blood–brain barrier, and some enhancement will occur. In the weeks or months following radiation demyelination may occur in a patchy often periventricular distribution that may be asymmetrical, affecting the white matter but generally sparing the corpus callosum, internal capsules and basal ganglia. The grey matter is usually not involved. Delayed effects are less common and can occur months to years after therapeutic irradiation. There is endothelial hyperplasia, fibrinoid necrosis of perforating arterioles and thrombosis. Cerebral necrosis supervenes with blood–brain barrier disruption, oedema and mass effect. MRI at this stage shows a mass having increased T1- and T2-relaxation times and enhancement after intravenous gadolinium and cannot therefore be differentiated from recurrent tumour. Measurement of the lesion's metabolism with ^{18}F-deoxyglucose PET, ^{201}Tl or ^{123}I-methyltyrosine SPECT scan will help to differentiate hypometabolic radiation necrosis from a hypermetabolic malignant tumour.

TOXIC AND DEGENERATIVE

Central pontine myelinolysis produces loss of myelin and oligodendroglia in the central pons, which may extend to the lateral thalamus and mesencephalon sparing the ventrolateral longitudinal fibres. It is usually associated with alcoholics with hyponatraemia too rapidly corrected. The demyelination is shown as hyperintense on T2-weighted and hypointense on T1-weighted sections, with no mass effect and usually no blood–brain barrier breakdown.

Marchiaflava–Bignami disease is characterized by a toxic demyelination of the corpus callosum in alcoholics. In the acute form extensive lesions have been reported in the centrum semiovale and corpus callosum, whilst at the chronic stage only corpus callosum lesions are seen; occasionally there is a favourable outcome. MRI shows these as small areas of increased T1- and T2-relaxation time with no contrast enhancement or mass effect.

Carbon monoxide encephalopathy is due to the displacement of oxygen from the haemoglobin molecule by the binding of carbon monoxide, inducing hypoxia and destroying vulnerable cells. Although the grey matter structures are damaged first, the white matter is also involved, especially when there is episodic or chronic exposure. MRI shows areas of increased T1- and T2-relaxation time in the thalamus, basal ganglia, hippocampus and centrum semiovale. These areas may show enhancement with gadolinium in the acute stage. The lesions are usually bilateral and symmetrical but can be patchy. Laminar necrosis has been reported as hyperintense cortical foci on T2-weighted images.

Substance abuse by inhalation (e.g. heroin vapours: pyrolysate, cocaine) produces a wide variety of acute and chronic neurological signs and symptoms. The effects on the white matter will depend largely on the chemical constituent involved. Toluene (one of the constituents of paint sprays) abuse produces generalized cerebral,

cerebellar and corpus callosum atrophy, with a loss of grey–white matter contrast, associated with diffuse multifocal hyperintensity of the cerebral white matter and hypointensity of the thalami on T2-weighted sequences. With cocaine abuse there is generally neurovascular damage with vasculitis, vasospasm and thrombosis. Eventually cerebral atrophy can be seen.

CONCLUSION

MRI is now the main diagnostic tool in the investigation of white-matter disease. In some conditions its sensitivity is the key to selecting patients for further attention, while in others it identifies more specific features which lead to a final diagnosis. MRI can be used to select patients for treatment and to monitor the effects of this treatment.

FURTHER READING

GENERAL

Atlas, S.W. (ed.) 1996: *Magnetic resonance of the brain and spine*. Philadelphia: Lippencott-Raven.
Bradley, W.G., Bydder, G.M. 1997: *Advanced MR imaging techniques*. London: Martin Dunitz.
Grossman, R.I., Yousem, D.M. 1994: *Neuroradiology, the requisites*. St Louis: Mosby Year Book.
Osborn, A.G. 1994: *Diagnostic neuroradiology*. London: Mosby.
Osborn, A.G., Tong, K.A. 1996: *Handbook of neuroradiology: brain and skull* (2nd edition). St Louis: Mosby Year Book.

HEAD INJURY

Gean, A.D. 1994: *Imaging of head trauma*. New York: Raven Press.
Reilly, P., Bullock, R. 1997: *Head injury: pathophysiology and management of severe closed injury*. London: Chapman & Hall.

NUCLEAR MEDICINE – SPECT

Duncan, R. 1997: *SPECT imaging of the brain*. London: Kluwer Academic Publishers.

STROKE

Nesbit, G.M. (ed.) 1999: Acute ischemic stroke. *Neuroimaging Clinics of North America* **9**(3) August.
Warlow, C.P., Dennis, M.S., Gijn, J. van *et al*. 1996: *Stroke: a*

practical guide to management. London: Blackwell Science.

Wilms, G., Demaerel, P., Bosmans, H., Marchal, G. 1999: MRI of non-ischemic vascular disease: aneurysms and vascular malformations. *European Radiology* **9**(6), 1055–60.

WHITE-MATTER DISEASES

Edwards, M.K. (ed.) 1993: White matter diseases. *Neuroimaging Clinics of North America* **3**(2) May.

Forsting, M. 1999: MR imaging of the brain: metabolic and toxic white matter diseases. *European Radiology* **9**(6), 1061–5.

Miller, D.H., Kesselring, J ., McDonald, W.I., Paty, D.W., Thompson, A.J. (eds) 1977: *Magnetic resonance in multiple sclerosis*. Cambridge: Cambridge University Press.

CONGENITAL LESIONS

American Journal of Neuroradiology 1992. [Whole volume devoted to the developing brain] **13**, 419–832.

Barkovich, J.A. 1996: *Pediatric neuroimaging* (2nd edition). Philadelphia: Lippincott-Raven.

Knaap, M.S. van der, Valk, J. 1995: *Magnetic resonance of myelin, myelination, and myelin disorders* (2nd edition). Berlin: Springer.

TUMOURS

Kleihues, P., Burger, P.C., Scheithauer, B.W. 1993: The new WHO classification of brain tumours. *Brain Pathology* **3**, 255–68.

Lizak, P.F., Woodruff, W.W. 1992: Posterior fossa neoplasms: multiplanar imaging. *Seminars in Ultrasound, CT and MRI* **13**, 182–206.

Ricci, P.E. (ed.) 1999: Brain tumours. *Neuroimaging Clinics of North America* **9**(4) November.

Sartor, K. 1999: MR imaging of the brain: tumours. *European Radiology* **9**(6), 1047–54.

INFECTION

Brugieres, P., Combes, C., Ricolfi, F. *et al*. 1995: Imagery of human immunodeficiency virus (HIV) encephalitis. *Journal of Neuroradiology* **22**(3), 163–8.

Hassine, D., Gray, F., Chekroun, R., De-Truchis, P., Schouman-Claeys, E., Vallee, C. 1995: CMV and VZV encephalitis in AIDS. *Journal of Neuroradiology* **22**(3), 184–92.

Miller, R.F., Lucas, S.B., Hall-Craggs, M.A. *et al*. 1997: Comparison of magnetic resonance imaging with neuropathological findings in the diagnosis of HIV and CMV associated CNS disease in AIDS. *Journal of Neurology, Neurosurgery, and Psychiatry* **62**(4), 346–51.

NEURODEGENERATIVE DISEASES

Barber, R., Gholkar, A., Scheltens, P., Ballard, C., McKeith, I.G., O'Brien, J.T. 1999: Medial temporal lobe atrophy on MRI in dementia with Lewy bodies. *Neurology* **52**(6), 1153–8.

Barber, R., Scheltens, P., Gholkar, A. *et al*. 1999: White matter lesions on magnetic resonance imaging in dementia with Lewy bodies, Alzheimer's disease, vascular dementia, and normal aging. *Journal of Neurology, Neurosurgery, and Psychiatry* **67**(1), 66–72.

Eye and orbit

IVAN MOSELEY

With the development of modern imaging techniques, the orbit can be visualized by:

- plain radiographs
- ultrasonography
- arteriography
- dacryocystography
- computed tomography
- magnetic resonance imaging.

IMAGING TECHNIQUES

Since so many techniques are available, an informed choice is essential.

PLAIN FILMS

Plain films now have very limited applications. They are mainly used in the management of suspected foreign bodies within the orbit, fractures and a few cases where bone disease such as fibrous dysplasia is suspected. There are virtually no indications for 'optic foramen' views. Plain films, however, do offer a simple means of confirming the presence of paranasal sinusitis.

ULTRASONOGRAPHY

The role of sonography is essentially in the investigation of ocular disease. Although it is quick and simple, its use as a 'screening' test in patients with suspected orbital masses does not obviate more definitive studies.

INTRAVASCULAR PROCEDURES

Intravascular procedures have become much less common in recent years. There is now no place for **orbital phlebography** except as part of an interventional procedure. With the very rapid and striking improvements in magnetic resonance angiography, diagnostic **carotid arteriography** is performed less frequently, but it is the examination of choice for interventional procedures, including embolization of vascular malformations and tumours in and around the orbits and cavernous sinus region. Both diagnostic and therapeutic angiograms should be performed and interpreted only by experts.

DACROCYSTOGRAPHY

Dacryocystography has specific indications which are discussed below.

COMPUTED TOMOGRAPHY (CT)

CT is especially suited to examination of the orbit, because the orbital walls and soft-tissue structures have high natural radiographic contrast. It does, however, have the disadvantage that the lens is particularly sensitive to ionizing radiation, so the examination should not be undertaken lightly, especially in children or when repeated studies seem probable. The ophthalmologist should insist on high-quality, high-resolution studies with sections no more than 2 mm thick. Resolution can be increased by 'coning down' on the orbits, but for many orbital problems, particularly unilateral visual loss, it is highly desirable that the pituitary fossa be included in the field of view. The adjacent paranasal sinuses should also be covered, as an apparently intraorbital mass may arise from one of the sinuses. In many institutions it is a general rule that CT is carried out first without intravenous contrast medium and repeated after injection, should that prove necessary. Because of constraints on radiation dose, orbital CT is best performed with contrast medium from the start; the injection rarely assists in diagnosis of orbital lesions, but extension of pathological processes beyond the orbits may be much more accurately assessed. When the orbits are being imaged, it is often helpful to have both bone and soft-tissue 'windows'.

MAGNETIC RESONANCE IMAGING (MRI)

MRI does not use ionizing radiations and is therefore theoretically preferable to CT for examination of the orbit, but the long data acquisition times sometimes necessary for MRI mean that movement of the eyes can occur. Special considerations arise because of the presence of the orbital fat. The high signal from the orbital fat and the major differences in MRI characteristics of the orbital tissues may give rise to chemical shift artefact, so that structures such as the optic nerve have a dense white line along one side and a black one along the other. Special sequences can be employed to reduce these effects. Furthermore, pathological enhancement with intravenous gadolinium is manifest on T1-weighted images as high signal, which paradoxically has the effect of making a mass outlined by high-signal orbital fat less conspicuous. Contrast-enhanced images of the orbit should therefore be obtained using fat-suppression sequences. Mascara contains iron and degrades the images of the anterior orbit; it should be removed before the examination.

TRAUMA TO THE ORBIT

A blow to the orbit can involve the eye, the other soft tissues (including the lids and extraocular muscles) and the surrounding bones. The eye may be subject to blunt trauma or a penetrating injury.

FOREIGN BODIES

One of the commonest indications for imaging is the suspicion of an intraocular foreign body. If it lies within the globe, it should be removed because of the risks of premature cataract and sympathetic ophthalmitis, but small extraocular foreign bodies are usually left *in situ*. Imaging of any kind should follow expert clinical examination, as the detection rate for intraocular foreign bodies is very low when an ophthalmologist believes that none is present.

The basic technique is **plain film radiography**. With advances in vitreoretinal surgery, very precise localization of intraocular particles is less critical than previously, and a simple technique usually suffices. A single lateral film, which shows the corneal surface clearly, is all that is usually required for screening. This must be obtained with the eye open, in the primary position, the side being investigated next to the film. All metallic foreign bodies of sufficient size should be visible, as will the large majority of glass fragments and some other foreign bodies composed of, for example, stone. If no foreign body is visible, the plain film examination is over. When a radiopaque foreign body is identified as a white blob or streak on the film, a postero-anterior film (with the face against the film) is required for localization. A second lateral exposure, with the patient looking up or down, may be helpful if the preceding films do not make it clear that the foreign body is intra- or extraocular (Fig. 16.1). If the fragment moves with the eye, it is within it, although, rarely, a foreign body in one of the extraocular muscles can cause confusion. Simple measurements on the postero-anterior and lateral views, suitably corrected for magnification, can be transferred to a chart for presurgical localization.

When the plain film shows no foreign body in the face of strong clinical suspicion, **ultrasonography** may reveal a fragment that is not radiopaque. If the long axis of a shard of foreign material lies in the plane of the ultrasound beam, however, it can be overlooked.

If the foregoing studies are inconclusive as to the presence and/or intraocular location of a foreign body, or if multiple fragments preclude localization from two films in two planes, **CT** can be employed. Fine (1.5–2.0 mm) axial or coronal sections, with reformats in appropriate planes, are required. Wooden foreign bodies may appear of less than soft-tissue density.

Not only is **MRI** not indicated in a suspected intraocular foreign body, but also any patient who might have a metallic foreign body in the orbit (metal workers, for example) must not undergo MRI of any part of the body, as the movement of the fragment in the magnetic field can cause serious damage. Plain films of the orbits should be obtained before carrying out MRI for other indications in patients at risk. Most, but importantly not all, metal-containing surgical materials placed within the orbits, such as intraocular lenses, wire sutures, retinal tacks, do not contraindicate MRI, as the material is not ferromagnetic. However, ocular implants containing magnets are an absolute contraindication to MRI.

(a)   (b)

Figure 16.1 *Plain film localization of a metallic foreign body. (a) Postero-anterior and (b) double-exposed 'eye-mover' lateral plain films. A metallic fragment is seen laterally in the right orbit; although it might be thought too laterally placed to be intraocular, it does move with eye movement.*

OTHER OCULAR INJURIES

Ultrasonography is the method of choice for the detection of other traumatic injuries such as dislocation or rupture of the lens (Fig. 16.2), intraocular haemorrhage or retinal detachment. CT or MRI may sometimes be necessary for demonstration of rupture of the globe, particularly if the media are opaque. The long-term result of severe ocular trauma is a shrunken globe, with calcification in the coats. On CT or MRI the characteristics of the media are different from those of the opposite eye.

Injuries to other soft-tissue structures in the orbit

Imaging usually plays little part in the assessment of orbital soft-tissue injuries, but CT or MRI can be used to demonstrate division of the extraocular muscles.

Orbital fractures

Other than in major, widespread facial injuries, fractures usually involve the thin floor and medial wall of the orbit. The mechanism of injury is most commonly a direct blow to the eye by a fist or an object of similar size. The major indications for imaging are enophthalmos and/or diplopia, particularly if these features are persistent.

Radiographic examination is not an emergency and may be delayed until some of the overlying soft-tissue swelling has subsided. In the acute phase, plain

Figure 16.2 *Traumatic rupture of the lens: ultrasonography. The probe is positioned at the top of the image. The aqueous and vitreous are very hypoechoic, whereas the retrobulbar fat appears very bright. The nucleus of the lens (arrow) has been extruded through a defect in the posterior capsule.*

radiographs may show direct evidence of downward displacement of the floor of the orbit (a '**blow-out' fracture**), frequently centred on the infraorbital canal. Medial displacement of the lamina papyracea, which separates the orbit from the ethmoid air cells, is more difficult to recognize because of normal bone anterior and/or posterior to the displaced fragment. Indirect signs of fractures include:

- non-specific soft-tissue swelling, evident as increased density of the affected side;
- air within the orbital cavity 'orbital emphysema' (Fig. 16.3) which, in the absence of a penetrating injury, indicates a fracture involving one of the paranasal sinuses;

- protrusion of orbital soft tissues (the 'hanging drop') through the fracture in the orbital floor;
- a fluid level in the maxillary antrum.

In many cases diplopia resolves quite rapidly after injury, but when double vision or enophthalmos persists, CT is the investigation of choice. Thin sections in the direct coronal plane are most useful in order to show not only the details of fractures (particularly those fractures involving the floor of the orbit) but also the position of the extraocular muscles and retrobulbar fat, either of which may become trapped in the fracture (Fig. 16.4).

Investigation and treatment of acute traumatic optic neuropathy are the subject of intense debate. The case for active decompressive treatment is as yet unproven, and there is thus no indication to search for orbital fractures and/or haematomas. It may, however, be wise to examine the orbital apices, where compression or trapping of the optic nerve is most likely to occur, in a patient with normal vision who is to undergo surgical fixation of extensive facial fractures; CT is the technique of choice.

Figure 16.3 *Blow-out fracture; anteroposterior plain film. Orbital emphysema is evident as low-density bubbles within the superior (white arrow) and medial parts of the right orbit. There is a blow-out fracture of its floor, centred on the infraorbital canal, with downward angulation of the fragments medial (two black arrows) and lateral (single black arrow) to it.*

OCULAR LESIONS

The position of a mass relative to the cone formed by the extraocular muscles and eye may give a clue to its nature. Thus, ocular and optic nerve tumours are, by definition, **intraconal**. Some tumours, such as cavernous haemangiomas, most commonly arise within the muscle cone, while others, including those arising from the lacrimal gland, are primarily **extraconal**. Yet others, such as lymphoma and metastases, can arise in either site.

TUMOURS

Primary diagnosis of ocular tumours is by fundoscopy, but imaging may be required if the media are opaque, when a retinal detachment is thought to be secondary to an underlying neoplasm (Fig. 16.5), or when a retrobulbar extension of a tumour is suspected.

In children, **retinoblastoma** is the principal ocular tumour; it may be bilateral. Sonography, CT or MRI can be used to confirm the presence of a fundal mass and to assess any retrobulbar extension, although CT and MRI may necessitate sedation or even general anaesthesia in a young child. Small tumours can be rendered more conspicuous with intravenous contrast medium enhancement on both CT and MRI. Calcification of the tumour, visible on CT and occasionally dense enough to be seen on plain films, is highly suggestive of the diagnosis. Distinction from Coats' disease,

Figure 16.4 *Blow-out fracture of the floor of the left orbit in a patient with persistent restriction of elevation: direct coronal CT. The fracture has occurred in the centre of the floor, with downward displacement of medial and lateral fragments. Orbital fat has herniated into the fracture site, and there is abnormal soft tissue, probably representing scar tissue (arrow), between the inferior rectus muscle and the lateral fragment. There could well be disruption of the medial wall of the orbit, adjacent to the medial rectus muscle. High-density blood is seen in the upper part of the left maxillary antrum, above presumably pre-existing mucosal thickening.*

Figure 16.5 *Ocular tumour causing retinal detachment: ultrasonography. Image configuration as in Fig. 16.2. The leaves of the detached retina (arrows) are clearly seen, and were shown to change position with eye movement. A solid mass underlying the detachment (indicated by asterisks) arises from the posterior surface of the eye.*

Figure 16.6 *Ocular malignant melanoma with subretinal haemorrhage: axial T1-weighted MRI after intravenous gadolinium. The remaining vitreous overlies subretinal fluid, which has divided into high-signal anterior and intermediate-signal posterior (arrow) layers; the high signal of the former is due to methaemoglobin. The retina is still attached in the region of the optic disc (white arrowheads). A contrast-enhancing mass (black arrowheads) is seen in the macular area and behind the posterior pole, indicating trans-scleral extension.*

which is an exudative retinopathy, may be problematic; retinoblastoma, however, tends to give lower signal than subretinal fluid on T2-weighting.

In adults the common ocular tumour is **malignant melanoma of the choroid**. In the early stages this is best imaged by ultrasonography or MRI; these show a localized area of thickening of the choroid. Ultrasonography is much simpler and although MRI may be specific, showing high signal on T1-weighted images due to the T1 shortening effect of melanin, it is less reliable in cases where the clinical diagnosis is in doubt. Similar high signal has been described not only in uveal naevus, for example, but also in choroidal haemangioma, metastases, osteoma and retinal gliosis. Fat-suppressed, contrast-enhanced T1-weighted images may show trans-scleral spread of the tumour, which is a bad prognostic sign (Fig. 16.6). If treatment is to consist of topical radiotherapy, a chest radiograph is essential to exclude dissemination. When the patient with advanced disease presents with a shrunken phthisical eye, the observation on CT or MRI of a retrobulbar mass that also involves the eye itself is highly suggestive of melanoma; invasion of the globe by orbital tumours is very uncommon.

OTHER OCULAR DISEASES

Imaging may be required in **malformations of the globe**. When there is apparent anophthalmos, sonography, CT or MRI may reveal a buried globe, for which surgery may potentially be beneficial. Some malformations, such as colobomas, can be associated with more complex anomalies, such as basal encephaloceles; CT or MRI can be of great importance in showing that an external soft-tissue mass in such cases is not an associated soft-tissue tumour that might be thought suitable for excision, but consists of brain herniating through a bone defect. Some children have a developmentally large (buphthalmic) eye, probably because of congenital glaucoma; differentiation from proptosis may require imaging.

Retinal and choroidal detachments can be documented rapidly and simply by sonography. The classic retinal detachment shows as a fine, V-shaped line whose base is at the optic disc. If the patient is instructed to move the eye during the examination, the mobility of the detached retina, of significance as regards surgical repair, can be assessed. The ultrasonographer can also examine the fundus of the eye to detect a tumour as the cause of the detachment. MRI may be useful for distinguishing a simple detachment from a subretinal haemorrhage. After intraocular tamponade, some investigations, such as ultrasonography or MRI, may be hindered by artefact.

Uveitis can be clinically isolated or found as part of a large spectrum of systemic diseases. Imaging is directed at the latter and can include a plain film of the chest (for sarcoidosis or tuberculosis); sacroiliac joints (for ankylosing spondylitis) and heels (for calcaneal spurs in Behçet's disease). Brain imaging may be required if systemic lymphoma or multiple sclerosis is suspected.

When **scleritis** involves the anterior portion of the globe, the diagnosis can often be made clinically, but imaging techniques can aid in the assessment of posterior scleritis, showing soft-tissue thickening, often centred around the most anterior portion of the optic nerve.

LACRIMAL SYSTEM

In patients who present with epiphora or masses at the medial canthus, **dacryocystography** can be informative. It should be performed only after probing and syringing of the canaliculi by an ophthalmologist. Two major methods are employed, involving either plain radiographs with introduction of positive contrast medium into the lacrimal system, or a gamma camera following instillation of a radioactive material into the conjunctival sac. The former method gives much more precise anatomical detail, but the latter is perhaps more physiological.

With the patient prone and after topical anaesthesia of the conjunctival sac, a soft plastic cannula is introduced into the inferior canaliculus, and an oil-based or water-soluble iodinated contrast medium is injected. A general anaesthetic may be required in children. Films are exposed just before and during injection; digital subtraction equipment can be used. It is customary to inject both sides, for comparison and because asymptomatic contralateral disease is not rare. If obstruction is shown, a further film may be obtained in the erect position. If the inferior punctum cannot be cannulated, the superior one may be employed. The system may be obstructed at any point; the proximal common canaliculus, the lower border of the lacrimal sac (with the formation of a mucocele) (Fig. 16.7) and the inferior ostium of the nasolacrimal duct are common sites. For planning surgery, precise localization of proximal obstructions is required, as the exact site determines the surgical procedure. Filling defects within the system may represent dacryoliths, and are relatively common with fungal infections; however, air bubbles must be considered. Dacryocystography may be particularly informative as regards the patency of the surgical tract when an operation for lacrimal pathway obstruction has been unsuccessful, in order to show re-stenosis, occlusion or formation of a 'sump' in which the tears collect.

CT may be employed to show involvement of the bony portion of the nasolacrimal duct by disease in adjacent structures.

Transnasal balloon dilatation of the lacrimal pathways can be employed as an alternative to surgery.

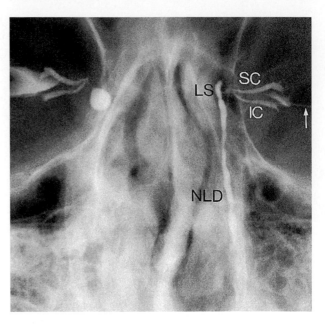

Figure 16.7 *Mucocele of the right lacrimal sac on dacryocystogram: anteroposterior projection during injection. Both inferior canaliculi have been cannulated; note the fine polyethylene catheter (arrow). On the left, the lacrimal system is patent but, on the right, no contrast medium passes further distally than the dilated lacrimal sac. There is considerable reflux of contrast medium, mainly via the superior canaliculus, into the conjunctival sac. IC, SC = inferior and superior canaliculi; LS = lacrimal sac; NLD = nasolacrimal duct.*

MASSES IN THE LACRIMAL GLAND REGION

The superolateral angle of the orbit is a relatively common site for a number of masses, only some of which are associated with the lacrimal gland. The masses include developmental lesions (dermoid cyst), primary tumours (carcinoma, pleomorphic adenoma, lymphoma), inflammatory swellings (acute and chronic dacryoadenitis, orbital pseudotumour, sarcoidosis – often bilateral, primary amyloidosis) and post-traumatic lesions (cholesterol granuloma).

Dermoid cysts may arise anywhere around the orbital margin, or within the orbit, but the lateral canthus is the most common site. If a clinically typical dermoid cyst is freely mobile in all directions on clinical examination surgery can be carried out without imaging, especially in children, but relatively immobile lesions, or those that appear to extend posteriorly, require radiological investigation. Plain radiographs are inadequate; CT is probably the optimal technique, although high-quality MRI may be satisfactory. A dermoid cyst is seen on CT as a mass of water or lower density (depending on the fatty content), with a fine soft-tissue density rim, but larger lesions are frequently more complex. The orbital walls should be carefully

Figure 16.8 *Lateral canthus dermoid cyst on axial CT. A large cyst, whose contents are similar in density to the orbital fat, has displaced the right globe anteriorly and inferiorly. It is clearly seen to communicate with a loculus in the temporal fossa via a cleft in the lateral wall of the orbit.*

Figure 16.9 *Pleomorphic adenoma of the lacrimal gland on direct coronal CT. A rather dense soft-tissue mass occupies the position of the left lacrimal gland. It displaces the globe downwards, flattening its superolateral aspect, and has caused smooth erosion of the adjacent bone (arrows).*

examined for evidence of the cyst extending into a canal in the bone; 'collar-stud' cysts extending from the orbit to the temporal fossa, or vice versa, are not rare (Fig. 16.8).

Carcinomas of the lacrimal gland are most commonly of the adenoid–cystic type, but adenocarcinomas occur. On CT or MRI they are manifest as a soft-tissue lesion, often moulded to the eye. Curiously, calcification within the tumour is more common than with benign lacrimal gland lesions. Infiltrative bone destruction is highly suggestive of the diagnosis of carcinoma. Evidence of deep, often perineural extension towards the orbit, cranial cavity or infratemporal fossa may be present. Follow-up frequently shows spread of this type.

Pleomorphic adenomas ('benign mixed tumours') of the lacrimal gland are characteristically hard. They therefore tend to indent the adjacent globe (Fig. 16.9) and, as they enlarge slowly, have often also caused smooth pressure erosion of the lacrimal fossa by the time of presentation. *En bloc* removal, without biopsy, is the treatment of choice for these tumours, so preoperative diagnosis is important.

Primary orbital lymphoma not uncommonly involves the lacrimal gland region, although it can arise anywhere within the orbit. On CT the tumour appears of soft-tissue density; it may appear infiltrative, but is often rather well defined (Fig. 16.10). Signal characteristics on MRI are variable, but non-specific. The only factor that reliably differentiates lymphoma from benign idiopathic inflammatory disease is that lymphoma may cause bone destruction, but it does so only in a small minority of cases. Either condition may be bilateral, and biopsy is necessary to make the diagnosis.

In **acute inflammatory dacryoadenitis** the diagnosis is usually obvious, but pain is relatively mild in some patients. A chronically inflamed gland may simply be swollen, but if the inflammatory process spreads to the

(a)

(b)

Figure 16.10 *Primary orbital lymphoma. (a) Axial and (b) direct coronal contrast-enhanced CT showing an amorphous, but well-defined, soft-tissue density mass extending across the roof of the anterior half of the left orbit, moulded to the globe, which it has displaced anteriorly and downwards. There are no bone changes. Biopsy would be necessary to distinguish this lymphoma from other infiltrative lesions such as a metastasis or even a benign inflammatory orbital pseudotumour.*

(a)

(b)

Figure 16.11 *Retrobulbar cavernous haemangioma on parasagittal MRI (a) before and (b) after intravenous gadolinium. A strikingly smooth, elliptical mass lies beneath the inferior rectus muscle, with the optic nerve draped over it. The mass shows inhomogeneous contrast enhancement, spreading out from its centre, because of the very slow blood flow within it; for the same reason, these lesions do not 'blush' on angiography. Note the normal contrast enhancement of the extraocular muscles (arrows).*

surrounding tissues, the margins of the gland may become blurred on CT or MRI. In such cases, differentiation from carcinoma or lymphoma will require a biopsy.

When **sarcoidosis** involves the lacrimal glands, the swelling is frequently bilateral and imaging simply shows expansion of the glands. However, this appearance can also be seen in lymphoma. The chest radiograph, showing the classic bilateral hilar adenopathy, may clinch the diagnosis, but the chest radiograph is sometimes normal.

Cholesterol granuloma is thought to be the result of haemorrhage into bone, with formation of a granulomatous reaction around blood products, and progressive bone erosion. The superolateral angle of the orbit is, for unknown reasons, a prime site. Plain films show ragged bone destruction, more suggestive of a malignant tumour. CT reveals that the soft-tissue mass associated with the granuloma projects inferomedially into the orbit and is characteristically of lower density than brain; this is a valuable observation which allows distinction from a carcinoma. MRI shows high signal on both T1- and T2-weighted images. After curettage, imaging procedures may show remarkable resolution of the bone destruction.

PRIMARY ORBITAL NEOPLASMS

Benign orbital neoplasms are relatively uncommon in young children; the most frequent tumour is **rhabdomyosarcoma**. Often presenting with an inflammatory clinical picture, a rhabdomyosarcoma is manifest on imaging as a non-specific and often moderately well-defined orbital mass. Since the tumour arises from primitive rests within the orbit, it characteristically

does not simulate an expanded extraocular muscle. Contrast enhancement on CT or MRI is typically marked. Bone destruction is not characteristic.

The commonest benign retrobulbar tumour is the **cavernous haemangioma** which presents, usually in adult life, with proptosis and occasionally also with visual impairment, particularly if the tumour arises at the apex of the orbit. CT or MRI shows a discrete, rounded retrobulbar tumour, typically lying within the cone formed by the extraocular muscles lateral to the optic nerve. Contrast enhancement is characteristically intense and homogeneous, although rapid imaging may show enhancement spreading through the tumour from a 'hilum' (Fig. 16.11).

Neurofibromas or **neurilemmomas** can arise from the intraorbital branches of the cranial nerves. Imaging procedures show them as solid masses, commonly in the upper half of the orbit. The tumours tend to be more elongated in the anteroposterior plane than haemangiomas and may extend posteriorly through the superior orbital fissure towards the cavernous sinus. Fibrous histiocytoma and haemangiopericytoma also form rounded masses, but are more common in the anterior half of the orbit. Angiography may be indicated, if a mass looks hypervascular or appears pulsatile, to confirm the vascular nature of the tumour and show the origin of feeding vessels; in some cases, preoperative embolization may be possible. Several of these solid tumours also have malignant forms, and primary sarcomas also arise within the orbit. Liposarcoma may be particularly difficult to recognize if its imaging characteristics are similar to those of the adjacent orbital fat.

The orbit is a common site for **metastases**. Their imaging features are very varied, but a poorly defined soft-tissue mass, which fails to respect normal tissue planes, is most common. Some fibrotic tumours, such

Figure 16.12 *Fibrous dysplasia of the orbital walls: axial 'bone-window' algorithm CT. Gross thickening of its lateral wall is encroaching on the right orbit, displacing the globe anteriorly. Note the very characteristic, featureless, 'ground-glass' texture of the abnormal bone. Although the bone surrounding it is involved, the optic canal (arrowheads) is not significantly narrowed. The granular texture of the soft tissues is an imaging artefact typical of high-resolution 'bone-window' imaging.*

as scirrhous carcinoma of the breast, cause volume loss, resulting in enophthalmos.

Meningiomas arising within the orbit, other than from the sheath of the optic nerve, are extremely rare, although it is a common error to include meningioma in the differential diagnosis of discrete intraorbital masses. However, the orbit is not uncommonly invaded by meningiomas of the sphenoid bone, and proptosis and/or visual disturbance may cause the patient to consult the ophthalmologist rather than the neurologist. The cardinal abnormality on imaging is thickening (hyperostosis) and increased density (sclerosis) of the greater wing of the sphenoid; the soft-tissue component may be relatively small, and may be visible on CT only following intravenous contrast medium. The lateral rectus muscle often appears swollen. Differential diagnosis is from other causes of focal bone thickening, such as fibrous dysplasia (in which there is no soft-tissue lesion) (Fig. 16.12) or osteoblastic metastasis.

Mucoceles or tumours of the paranasal sinuses can present as orbit masses, so that adequate imaging for an orbital mass should always include the adjacent sinuses.

OPTIC NERVE AND MENINGEAL COVERINGS

TUMOURS

Glioma

The optic nerve itself effectively gives rise to only one tumour: the optic nerve glioma, which occurs almost invariably in children, and is usually a relatively benign lesion. This uncommon tumour is manifest on CT as a swelling of the optic nerve, often rather bulky by the time of presentation, with a waist between the mass of the tumour and the posterior pole of the globe. Contrast enhancement is variable. Coronal sections sometimes reveal a 'target' appearance, the central portion of the nerve appearing denser than the periphery. Posterior extension to the intracranial optic pathways is an important prognostic observation. It may not be obvious whether a mass, particularly one that is rather elongated in the anteroposterior plane, arises from the optic nerve or lies alongside it; MRI may be particularly helpful in such cases.

Meningioma

The meninges surrounding the optic nerve can give rise to meningiomas. Unlike optic nerve gliomas, meningiomas occur almost exclusively in adults. On CT the optic nerve appears thickened, in a more fusiform manner than in cases of glioma (Fig. 16.13) and plaques of calcification are diagnostic. Abnormally intense contrast enhancement may be seen. MRI is insensitive to calcification of the meningeal sheath of the nerve, but shows intracranial extension of the tumour to better advantage than CT. Since in most patients vision is at least moderately impaired by the time of presentation, surgery on the nerve itself is unlikely to be beneficial, but imaging is particularly important for detection of intracranial tumour, which may compromise not only the chiasm, but also the contralateral optic nerve. Bilateral optic nerve sheath meningiomas are frequently associated with intracranial meningiomas.

Swelling of the optic nerve/sheath complex can also be seen in raised intracranial pressure since the subarachnoid space surrounding the nerve is in continuity with the intracranial cerebrospinal fluid spaces and inflammatory conditions (retrobulbar neuritis, sarcoidosis).

OTHER INTRINSIC DISEASES OF THE OPTIC NERVE

A number of inflammatory and idiopathic diseases can affect the optic nerve without causing morphological changes. These conditions are not generally of surgical significance, but may be revealed by imaging. In **retrobulbar neuritis**, typified by multiple sclerosis, inflammation in the acute stage, gliosis in the chronic stage and plaques of demyelination can be demonstrated on MRI as areas of altered signal, without mass effect. Contrast enhancement is shown in the acute phase. Similar signal changes can be seen in some cases of acute disseminated encephalomyelitis or sarcoidosis, with optic nerve involvement, or conditions such as Leber's hereditary optic neuropathy.

(a)

(b)

Figure 16.13 *Meningioma of the sheath of the optic nerve. (a) Axial CT section in the plane of the optic nerves shows the right nerve/sheath complex to be wider, denser and more irregular in outline than its fellow. Other images showed no evidence of intracranial extension. (b) Coronal contrast-enhanced T1-weighted MRI section through the cranial end of the optic canals in the same patient shows a thin layer of pathologically enhancing tissue (arrowheads) surrounding the optic nerve as it enters the head; it almost reaches the midline, and threatens eventually to involve the contralateral optic nerve (arrow). S = sphenoid sinus.*

INFLAMMATORY DISEASE

PYOGENIC INFECTION OF THE ORBITS

Orbital cellulitis is a condition requiring urgent treatment. Imaging with CT or MRI can be employed to determine whether the disease extends posterior to the orbital septum and, more rarely, whether there is an orbital abscess, although differentiation of confluent cellulitis and abscess may be difficult. Plain films are a simple way of diagnosing associated paranasal sinusitis and may also show an unsuspected orbital foreign body.

Chronic fungal infections may produce large soft-tissue masses in the orbit, which have non-specific appearances on CT, but characteristically give low signal on MRI.

THYROID OPHTHALMOPATHY

Graves' disease characteristically causes swelling of the rectus muscles; the superior oblique may also be involved. Although this is a systemic disease, imaging often shows the muscle involvement to be asymmetrical, or even unilateral (Fig. 16.14); the medial rectus and inferior rectus muscles are most commonly affected. In a relatively small proportion of patients the muscles appear normal, but the retrobulbar fat appears increased in volume. In some patients the expanded muscles show fatty replacement. There is typically marked proptosis with forward herniation of orbital fat. The orbits may be enlarged with medial bowing of the

lamina papyracea on one or both sides. The optic nerve often appears stretched in advanced cases, but optic neuropathy is probably due to compression of the nerve by the expanded muscle bellies near the orbital apex. The superior ophthalmic vein may also be engorged. CT may be useful for determining the anatomical efficacy of surgical decompression.

OTHER IDIOPATHIC INFLAMMATORY CONDITIONS

Idiopathic inflammation of the orbit ('**orbital granuloma**' or '**pseudotumour**') is one of the commonest causes of pain and/or proptosis in adults. By definition, no infective organism is found, although some cases are associated with systemic illness or paranasal sinus disease. Imaging procedures show proptosis, usually unilateral, with a soft-tissue mass that can involve the orbital fat, extraocular muscles, lacrimal gland and optic nerve. The tissue planes around these structures are frequently obliterated and vessels may be prominent in the fat. In some patients, enlargement of a single muscle ('orbital myositis') may be seen. The 'pseudotumour' may show marked contrast enhancement. Extension intracranially via the superior orbital fissure is infrequent but well documented; the cavernous sinus can appear expanded. The process may also extend out of the orbit onto the facial soft tissues and, via the inferior orbital fissure, down to the infratemporal fossa and pterygoid region. Bone erosion is uncommon but in chronic disease the adjacent orbital walls may become

(a)   (b)

Figure 16.14 *Unilateral thyroid ophthalmopathy. (a) Axial and (b) reformatted coronal CT show marked swelling of all the rectus muscles on the right, with exophthalmos and expansion of the orbit. The optic nerve appears stretched and the coronal image shows the potential for compression of the nerve at the apex. Note that on the healthy side only about three quarters of the globe is anterior to an imaginary line joining the anterolateral bony margins of the two orbits.*

thickened. There is considerable overlap between the imaging features of orbital pseudotumour, lymphoma and metastases. Moreover, differentiation on clinical and histological grounds may be problematic. As management of each condition is different, biopsy is essential; localization of the lesion for biopsy is a major contribution of imaging.

Other inflammatory processes can involve the orbit. Quasimalignant diseases, such as **Wegener's granulomatosis** and **lethal midline granuloma**, frequently involve the paranasal sinuses, and can cause widespread bone destruction affecting the orbits.

VASCULAR LESIONS OF THE ORBIT

In young children, **capillary haemangioma** is the commonest developmental vascular lesion. Although congenital, the bluish periorbital mass develops after birth and may enlarge until about the age of 18 months. The nature of the lesion is usually evident clinically; ultrasonography, CT or MRI (Fig. 16.15) usually demonstrates a rather homogeneous soft-tissue mass that shows marked contrast enhancement. Closure of the palpebral fissure in early life threatens

(a)   (b)

Figure 16.15 *Capillary haemangioma in a 15-month-old child. (a) Axial T2-weighted MRI shows a heterogeneous high-signal mass anterior to the left eye, which is displaced laterally. (b) Magnetic resonance angiography shows high-flow intracranial arteries, but no abnormal vasculature related to the slow-flow haemangioma.*

Figure 16.16 *Orbital varices on axial CT. The left globe is displaced forwards and laterally by a mass composed of multiple serpiginous structures, containing a phlebolith (arrow). The left orbit is enlarged.*

to produce amblyopia. Angiography may be helpful prior to surgery and intravascular therapy may be possible.

Venous malformations ('orbital varices') are also relatively common. Plain films may show enlargement of the orbit. CT shows serpiginous or multinodular masses within the orbit, which on MRI characteristically show mixed signal intensity, owing to both fast and slowly flowing blood or thrombus. Phleboliths, evident as small, punctate areas of increased density seen on CT within the mass, are more readily seen on CT than on plain films and are diagnostic (Fig. 16.16).

Paradoxically, arteriography and phlebography are unrewarding investigations. The nosology of 'orbital lymphangioma' is contested; some workers suggest that these lesions are simply chronic venous malformations with lymphocytic infiltration.

The imaging manifestations of **arteriovenous malformations** within the orbit depend on their size and flow characteristics. High-quality superselective arteriography is required for planning treatment (Fig. 16.17). With the development of fine catheters that may be introduced into the branches of not only the external carotid, but also the ophthalmic artery, occlusion by embolization is a serious therapeutic option.

The orbit may also be secondarily involved in patients with arteriovenous fistulae or malformations in the region of the cavernous sinus, in which abnormal drainage occurs via the veins of the orbit. Imaging may show the superior ophthalmic veins to be dilated; there is commonly proptosis and swelling of the orbital soft tissues, notably the extraocular muscles, because of the increased venous pressure within the orbit.

Orbital haemorrhage usually has typical clinical features, particularly a very acute onset. Although bleeding may be secondary to an underlying lesion, such as varices or an arteriovenous malformation, in many cases no source is found. Management is conservative so extensive investigation is not required. In children particularly, the clot tends not to spread through the orbit; the septa within the fat limit the haemorrhage, giving rise to a rounded 'haematic cyst', which can be documented on CT or MRI. The density on CT or signal characteristics on MRI may make its nature unmistakable, especially if a fluid level between solid and liquid components is shown. A follow-up examination usually demonstrates resolution. In the elderly, the laxer soft tissues do not confine the bleeding, which is often manifest clinically as subconjunctival extension.

(a)

(b)

Figure 16.17 *Orbital arteriovenous malformation on digital subtraction angiography, with arterial phase (a) internal and (b) external carotid artery injections. Extensive pathological vessels within the orbit fill from both the ophthalmic artery (open arrow) and several branches of the external carotid artery, mainly the internal maxillary artery (arrow).*

FURTHER READING

Cabanis, E.A., Bourgeois, H., Iba-Zizen, M.T. 1996: *L'imagerie en ophtalmologie*. Paris: Masson.

Gonazález, C.F., Becker, M.H., Flanagan, J.C. 1986: *Diagnostic imaging in ophthalmology*. New York: Springer-Verlag.

Jackson, A. 1996: Magnetic resonance imaging of orbital disease. *Optician* **212**, 18–23.

Kupersmith, M.J. 1993: *Neurovascular neuro-ophthalmology*. Berlin: Springer-Verlag.

Moseley, I.F. 1992: Diagnostic imaging in visual loss: a problem-orientated approach. *Imaging* **4**, 151–5.

Moseley, I., Hadley, D. 1995: Magnetic resonance imaging and the eye. In: Jay, B., Kirkness, C.M. (eds), *Recent advances in ophthalmology*. Edinburgh: Churchill Livingstone, pp. 215–24.

Moseley, I., Gass, A. 1997: Magnetic resonance imaging in optic neuropathy. *Clinical Neuroscience* **4**, 302–19.

Newton, T.H., Bilaniuk, L.T. 1990: *Radiology of the eye and orbit*. New York: Raven Press.

Pérez Moreiras, J.V. 1986: *Patología orbitaria*. Barcelona: Pujades.

Wolff, E. 1957: *Anatomy of the eye and orbit*. London: Lewis.

Maxillofacial region, jaws and salivary glands

JAMES McIVOR

Plain films still have an important role in the initial imaging of the maxillofacial region and jaws and are still the best technique for demonstrating pathological conditions limited to the teeth and adjacent bone. Intra-oral dental films provide very detailed images of a small area, and panoramic radiographic techniques such as orthopantomography will show the whole dentition on a single film. However, CT and MRI are playing an increasingly important role in this region and are of particular value in diagnosing complex fractures and defining the extent and nature of soft-tissue lesions.

FRACTURES OF THE MAXILLA

LE FORT FRACTURES

Maxillary fractures are still classified according to the system of Le Fort (Fig. 17.1) who defined three principal patterns of fracture after applying blunt trauma to the faces of cadavers at the beginning of the twentieth century.

In a **Le Fort I** fracture the tooth-bearing part of the maxilla becomes separated from the rest of the maxilla by fractures through the medial and lateral walls of the maxillary sinuses, and by a fracture through the lower part of the nasal septum.

The **Le Fort II** fracture (Figs 17.2, 17.3) is more extensive and the separated fragment is pyramidal. The apex of the pyramid is the lower part of the nasal bones and the fracture lines run inferiorly and laterally through the medial and inferior walls of the orbits.

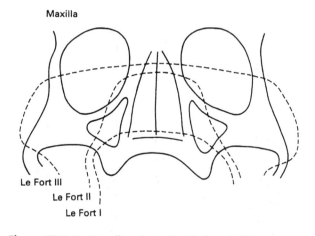

Figure 17.1 *Fracture lines in Le Fort I, II and III fractures.*

In the **Le Fort III** fracture (Fig. 17.4a) there is complete craniofacial disjunction. The fracture line runs through the nasal bones as in the Le Fort II fracture, and then posteriorly and laterally through the medial and lateral walls of the orbits, and through the zygomatic arches.

In practice, many fractures do not fit these descriptions exactly. Fractures caused by sharp-edged objects can produce comminuted fractures. Some fractures are unilateral (Fig. 17.3), and a Le Fort I or II fracture may coexist with a Le Fort III. However, the Le Fort classification is still in general use, as it allows these complicated fractures to be described in a few words, and has the additional advantage of grouping the fractures according to the pattern of subsequent surgical

Figure 17.2 *Le Fort II fracture. The fractures of the inferior margins of the orbits and of the lateral walls of the maxillary sinuses can be seen (arrows) but the fracture of the nasal bones is not visible on this projection.*

(a)

Figure 17.3 *Axial CT of a Le Fort II fracture of the right maxilla. There are fractures of the anterior and posterolateral walls of the right maxillary sinus.*

(b)

Figure 17.4 *Combined Le Fort II and Le Fort III fractures. (a) There are fractures of the nasal bones, lateral orbital margins, inferior orbital margins and zygomatic arches (arrows). There is a fluid level in the right maxillary sinus and opacification of the left maxillary sinus. (b) The fracture is reduced by metallic dental splints and interosseous pins in the skull base.*

management. In Le Fort I and II fractures the detached maxillary fragment is usually wired or plated to the zygomatic arches, but if the arches are fractured, as in a Le Fort III fracture, it may be necessary to resort to a more complicated type of pin and rod fixation to the skull vault (Fig. 17.4b).

FRACTURES OF THE ZYGOMA (FIG. 17.5)

The zygomatic bone contributes to the lateral and inferior margins of the orbit, the lateral wall of the maxillary sinus and the anterior end of the zygomatic arch. A fracture of zygomatic bone results in fractures of these regions (Fig. 17.6). It is usually impossible to see all four fractures on a single film but the presence of even one fracture should raise the suspicion that

Figure 17.5 *Usual sites of fracture of the zygoma and of the zygomatic arch. O = orbit; MS = maxillary sinus.*

Figure 17.6 *Displaced fracture of the zygoma (arrows).*

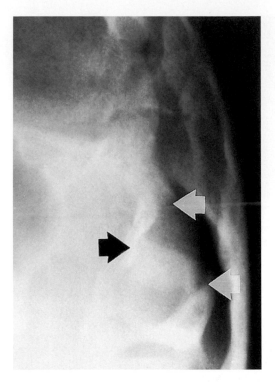

Figure 17.7 *Fracture of the zygomatic arch (arrows).*

other fractures are present and is an indication for further imaging.

The zygomatic arch may be fractured in association with a fracture of the zygoma as described above, or it may be fractured as a result of direct trauma, when it fractures in three places (Fig. 17.7).

Fractures of the zygoma also occur in Le Fort II and III fractures.

BLOW-OUT FRACTURES OF THE ORBITAL FLOOR

A 'blow-out' fracture of the orbital floor is an uncommon sequel to blunt trauma applied to the front of the orbit. The orbital rim remains intact, but the temporary increase in pressure within the orbit causes the thin floor to fracture and the soft tissues of the orbit to herniate through the defect into the maxillary sinus.

The herniated orbital contents may show as a soft-tissue shadow in the upper part of the maxillary sinus on a plain radiograph, but the fractured bony floor rarely shows. If a blow-out fracture is suspected, coronal CT of the orbital floor is indicated as it will demonstrate soft-tissue herniation and the fractured orbital floor (Fig. 17.8).

The clinical importance of a blow-out fracture is that the inferior rectus and oblique muscles become attached to the orbital floor by fibrous tissue, resulting in permanent limitation of upward rotation of the eyeball and permanent diplopia on looking upwards. The changes are best shown by coronal MRI imaging.

Figure 17.8 *Coronal CT scan showing a blow-out fracture of the floor of the left orbit with posterior displacement of the globe of the eye.*

Fractures of the orbital floor can occur in association with Le Fort II and III fractures and with zygomatic fractures (Fig. 17.9).

RADIOLOGICAL INVESTIGATION OF MAXILLARY FRACTURES

The initial radiographic investigation of a patient with a suspected fracture of the maxilla should be limited to three films: a standard occipitomental, a 30° occipitomental and a lateral film centred on the maxilla. These films may provide the diagnosis but further imaging is often necessary.

Figure 17.9 *Coronal CT of a comminuted fracture of the left zygoma showing a fracture of the orbital floor and herniation of the orbital contents into the maxillary sinus.*

Figure 17.10 *Fracture of the nasal bones on a lateral radiograph.*

Recent undisplaced or 'crack' fractures may be difficult or impossible to demonstrate even on plain films of the highest quality and one should be very cautious about 'excluding' a recent, undisplaced fracture on the basis of a normal plain film examination.

Fractures of the nasal bones which occur in Le Fort II and III fractures are best shown on standard lateral films of the nasal bones (Fig. 17.10).

Fractures of the teeth and alveolar bone show most clearly on non-screen intraoral dental films.

CT is indicated if the fractures cannot be satisfactorily demonstrated on plain radiographs or if there is a discrepancy between the clinical findings and the fractures shown on the plain films.

Axial slices parallel to the occlusal plane of the teeth are convenient for detecting maxillary fractures as slices in this plane can be repeated at a later date and artefacts

produced by metallic dental restorations will be limited to a few slices. Thin slices of 2 mm at 5 mm intervals are adequate in most cases.

Direct coronal slices at right angles to the occlusal plain demonstrate fractures of the orbital floor more clearly than axial slices but coronal views suffer from the disadvantage that the neck has to be fully extended and this may not be possible in elderly, uncooperative or recently injured patients.

Three-dimensional CT reconstruction is a very elegant technique demonstrating fractures of the facial skeleton and can provide an excellent overview of a complex fracture (Fig. 17.11). The main disadvantages are that a high-quality reconstruction requires the patient to remain completely immobile for 10–20 slices and the radiation dose is about twice as high as a standard CT examination of the same region.

INDIRECT SIGNS OF MAXILLARY FRACTURES ON PLAIN RADIOGRAPHS

Soft-tissue swelling and opacification of the maxillary sinus are two radiological abnormalities that are often

(a)

(b)

Figure 17.11 *(a) Comminuted fracture of the left zygoma on axial CT. There are multiple fractures of the anterior, posterolateral and medial walls of the maxillary sinus. (b) Three-dimensional CT reconstruction of the left zygoma.*

Figure 17.12 *Fracture of the condylar neck of the mandible on an anteroposterior radiograph showing displacement of the condyle (C) of the mandible out of the glenoid fossa.*

Figure 17.13 *Fracture of the ramus of the mandible on coronal CT (arrow).*

due to maxillary fractures, but which may occur in other conditions. Thus, their presence in patients with a history of facial trauma should increase the suspicion that a fracture is present, and should be an indication for further films.

Soft-tissue swelling is a common and non-specific sign which is almost invariably present if there is a recent fracture.

Opacification of the maxillary sinus is usual in fractures that involve its wall (Le Fort I, II and III fractures, zygomatic fractures) and a fluid level is occasionally seen (see Fig. 17.4a). Both these abnormalities should suggest haemorrhage into the sinus.

FRACTURES OF THE MANDIBLE

CLASSIFICATION

Fractures of the mandible are classified according to the site of fracture. The most common sites are the condylar neck (Fig. 17.12), the ramus (Fig. 17.13), the angle (Fig. 17.14) and the body (Fig. 17.15), but fractures can occur elsewhere. Pathological fractures secondary to tumours (Fig. 17.15), osteomyelitis (see Fig. 17.31, p. 473) and large cysts are uncommon but do occur.

Undisplaced fractures of the body and angle are classified as being 'vertically favourable' if the fracture line runs inferiorly and anteriorly, as the muscles attached to the fragments tend to pull them together. Conversely, a fracture running inferiorly and posteriorly is described as vertically 'unfavourable', as the fragments tend to be pulled apart by the muscles inserted into them (Fig. 17.16).

Figure 17.14 *Vertically unfavourable fracture through the angle of the mandible. The two radiolucent lines represent fractures through the inner and outer plates.*

Figure 17.15 *Pathological fracture of the right side of the mandible secondary to carcinoma of the oral mucosa that has extended into the mandible.*

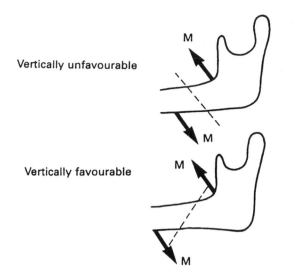

Figure 17.16 *Fracture lines in vertically favourable and unfavourable fractures of the body of the mandible (M). Arrows indicate the direction of muscle pull on the anterior and posterior fragments.*

Fractures through the tooth-bearing part of the mandible are almost invariably compound into the mouth but, despite this, osteomyelitis is very rare unless the patient is immunologically compromised (Fig. 17.17).

The mandible is commonly fractured at two sites, as the bone is U-shaped and held firmly at both ends by the capsules of the temporomandibular joints. A fracture of the body on one side is often accompanied by a fracture of the condylar neck on the other.

RADIOLOGICAL INVESTIGATION OF MANDIBULAR FRACTURES

Recent, undisplaced fractures of the mandible can be difficult to demonstrate and may not show on plain films until some days after the injury, when there will be some resorption at the fracture site. The initial films should consist of a posteroanterior view of the facial bones, plus oblique views of the injured side of the mandible. If the patient is able to cooperate, a panoramic radiograph of the mandible should also be taken.

Coronal CT should be used to demonstrate undisplaced fractures of the mandibular ramus and condyle that may be impossible to demonstrate on plain films (*see* Fig. 17.13).

BENIGN CYSTS

Benign cysts of the jaws differ pathologically from benign cysts in other bones as they are usually of dental origin. Cysts are common lesions, which usually present when they rupture into the oral cavity and become infected.

In general, benign cysts and tumours displace the roots of adjacent teeth without resorbing them, but malignant tumours often resorb the roots of teeth. Benign cysts can become very large before they present clinically.

The surgical treatment of benign cysts is usually curettage, followed by primary closure, but large cysts are occasionally marsupialized into the oral cavity. As in other bone lesions, the final diagnosis depends on a combination of the clinical, radiological and histological features.

Figure 17.17 *Osteomyelitis following a vertically unfavourable fracture of the angle of the mandible. There is bone rarefaction around the fracture lines and subperiosteal new bone formation (arrowed). The patient was HIV positive.*

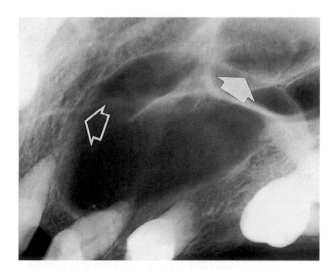

Figure 17.18 *Apical dental cyst arising from an upper canine tooth. The cortical margin of the cyst has been partially destroyed anteriorly (open arrow) by infection but is intact posteriorly (solid arrow).*

Figure 17.19 *Large residual dental cyst which has expanded into the right maxillary sinus. The radiopaque line at the upper margin of the soft-tissue shadow (arrows) indicates that the lesion has originated outside the maxillary sinus and expanded into it.*

Figure 17.20 *Dentigerous cyst around the crown of an unerupted lower third molar tooth (T).*

A **dental cyst** (periodontal cyst) is the most common cyst of the jaws, and accounts for almost half of all radiolucent jaw lesions. It develops at the root apex of a non-vital permanent tooth, and can present at almost any age above 18 years (Fig. 17.18). Large cysts expand the cortical outline of the maxilla or mandible, and maxillary cysts may expand into the maxillary sinus (Fig. 17.19). Some cysts appear multilocular radiologically, but they are always unilocular at operation.

A **residual dental cyst** (residual periodontal cyst) is an apical or lateral dental cyst that was left behind when the tooth from which it developed was extracted. It is, therefore, more common in the older age groups (Fig. 17.19).

A **dentigerous cyst** develops from the enamel-forming tissue (enamel organ) of a developing permanent tooth. These cysts usually present during the second decade and commonly develop around the crowns of lower third molars (Fig. 17.20). The cortical outline is continuous in the absence of infection. Adjacent teeth are often displaced, but their roots are rarely resorbed. Dentigerous cysts can become very large and may develop a multilocular appearance on plain radiographs. However, they are always unilocular at operation.

An **incisive canal cyst** (nasopalatine cyst) arises within the incisive canal of the maxilla. The diagnosis can be made with some confidence if the diameter of the incisive canal measures over 20 mm and should be suggested if the diameter if over 15 mm. These cysts usually present as painless, palatal swellings.

A **globulomaxillary cyst** is an uncommon fissural cyst which develops at the junction between the premaxilla and maxilla, where it appears as a radiolucent area between the roots of the lateral incisor and the canine teeth.

Odontogenic keratocysts (primordial cysts) occur most commonly in the ramus of the mandible, and are often associated with a missing lower third molar.

However, keratocysts can arise from any tooth-bearing part of the jaws. The diagnosis depends entirely upon the histological appearance of the lining, which consists of a thin layer of keratinized, stratified, squamous epithelium. Microscopic daughter cysts are occasionally seen beyond the bony margin of the main cyst, and this may account for the high rate of recurrence of about 10–20 per cent after simple curettage. Multiple odontogenic keratocysts are a feature of Gorlin's syndrome.

The **non-epithelial bone cyst** (solitary bone cyst, haemorrhagic bone cyst, traumatic bone cyst, unicameral bone cyst) is always located in the body of the mandible below the premolar and molar teeth. They are rare lesions which are usually discovered incidentally in young adults. These lesions should not really be classified as cysts, as they have no epithelial lining. The pathology is uncertain and it has been suggested that they are bone infarcts. There are a few reports of untreated 'cysts' resolving completely on follow-up radiographs.

BENIGN TUMOURS

Benign tumours of the jaws are rarer than benign cysts. The radiological abnormalities produced by benign tumours are similar to cysts, but tumours are more likely to be multilocular and are more likely to resorb teeth.

The **giant cell tumour** (**osteoclastoma**) is an uncommon tumour of the jaws and, like giant cell tumours elsewhere, usually occurs in adults aged between 20 and 40 years. Radiologically it appears as an expanding multilocular lesion with a scalloped margin. Recurrence after excision is common.

The **giant cell reparative granuloma** is peculiar to the jaws and has the same radiological features as a

Figure 17.21 *Giant cell reparative granuloma of the right maxilla on axial CT showing the typical multilocular appearance.*

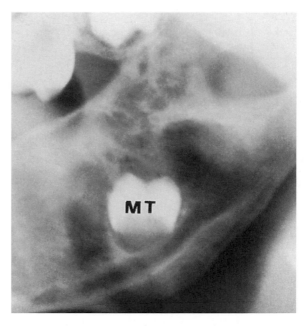

Figure 17.23 *Haemangioma of the body and ramus of the mandible in a child aged 6 years. The developing second molar tooth (MT) has been displaced posteriorly.*

giant cell tumour (Fig. 17.21). However, it occurs in a younger age group (10–25 years) and, although it grows more rapidly than a giant cell tumour, it rarely recurs after removal.

Ivory osteomas and **osteochondromas** occasionally arise from the maxilla and mandible, and have the same features as in other bones (Fig. 17.22). Multiple ivory osteomas are a feature of Gardner's syndrome.

The **chondroma** is a rare tumour of the maxilla, which usually develops after the age of 40 years. It appears as an area of bone destruction and often erodes the roots of teeth without displacing them. Complete excision is difficult, and recurrence is common.

The **fibromyxoma** is a rare tumour of children and young adults, and appears radiologically as a multilocular expanding lesion.

Haemangioma of the mandible is an extremely rare tumour that appears radiologically as a multilocular radiolucency (Fig. 17.23), with occasional ring opacities in the soft tissues owing to calcified phleboliths. It is important to diagnose haemangiomas as they can result in torrential haemorrhage if teeth are extracted from the affected bone, and the diagnosis should always be considered for any multilocular radiolucent lesion in the mandible.

A **neurilemmoma** or **neurofibroma** occasionally arises from the inferior dental nerve, and may cause widening of the inferior dental canal.

Fibromas, **lipomas** and **ganglioneuromas** may rarely develop in the maxillofacial region.

AMELOBLASTOMA

Ameloblastoma (**adamantinoma**) is a remarkably well-known tumour despite the fact that it accounts for only 1–2 per cent of tumours in the maxillofacial region. Radiologically it appears as an expanding multilocular radiolucent lesion, which may erode the roots of adjacent teeth.

Recurrence is common after simple curettage, so the tumour should be removed along with a margin of apparently normal bone. These tumours are slow growing and can reach an enormous size. Ameloblastoma is a locally invasive tumour and its behaviour has been compared to basal cell carcinoma. Pulmonary metastases have been reported in a few cases. Large tumours are best shown by CT (Fig. 17.24).

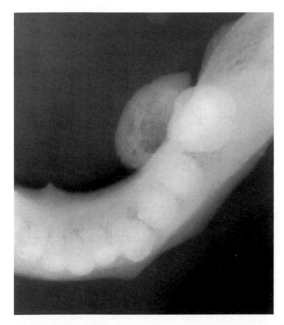

Figure 17.22 *Benign 'ivory' osteoma arising from the lingual plate of the mandible.*

(a)

(b)

Figure 17.24 *Ameloblastoma of the right maxilla. (a) Axial CT shows the tumour has extended through the posterolateral wall of the sinus into the infratemporal fossa and through the medial wall of the sinus into the nasal cavity. (b) Coronal CT shows tumour extension into the maxillary sinus and the ethmoid sinuses on both sides, and destruction of the bony floor of the right orbit. (Courtesy of Dr Otto Chan, The Royal London Hospital, London.)*

Ameloblastomas usually present in early adult life, but can occur at any time after the age of 12 years.

NON-NEOPLASTIC BONE LESIONS

An **odontome** is an abnormal growth of calcified dental tissue, which behaves like a hamartoma rather than a neoplasm and stops growing when the individual stops growing.

A **complex composite odontome** is a mass of enamel, dentine and cementum that shows as a dense radiopacity with an irregular but clearly defined margin (Fig. 17.25). Sometimes there are small radiolucencies within this radiopaque mass due to small cysts.

A compound composite odontome is a mass of small 'denticles', most of which contain enamel, dentine and cementum (Fig. 17.26). It is more commonly situated anteriorly than posteriorly. Multiple compound composite odontomes have been described in association with Gardner's syndrome.

Dilated composite odontomes and germinated composite odontomes are abnormally formed teeth.

Fibrous dysplasia in the maxillofacial region is usually monostotic but can be a feature of polyostotic fibrous dysplasia or of Albright's syndrome. Fibrous dysplasia is more common in the maxilla than the mandible, and presents as painless bony swelling, usually in adolescence.

Fibrous dysplasia begins as an expanding radiolucent lesion. Sclerotic areas soon develop within the

Figure 17.25 *Complex composite odontome in the upper premolar and molar regions which appears as a very dense radiopacity with a well-defined lobulated margin.*

Figure 17.26 *Compound composite odontome in the incisor region. It appears as a mass of 'denticles' or small deformed teeth and has delayed the eruption of an upper first incisor tooth.*

Figure 17.27 *Carcinoma of the left mandibular ramus on axial CT showing irregular destruction of the medial cortex (arrow), destruction of trabecular bone and marked soft-tissue swelling laterally.*

radiolucency and gradually enlarge and coalesce until there is dense, homogeneous opacification of the expanded bone, sometimes described as a 'ground-glass' appearance.

CT shows generalized expansion of the affected bone with thickened irregular trabeculae plus sclerotic and radiolucent areas.

The teeth in the affected bone are often displaced. The eruption of developing teeth is usually delayed or prevented.

Paget's disease can affect the maxilla and the mandible, and is usually bilateral. In most cases it is preceded by Paget's disease of the skull vault. As in other bones, the radiological features are bone expansion with a coarse trabecular pattern. Areas of dense bone sclerosis may develop, and masses of radiopaque cementum may develop adjacent to the roots of teeth (**hypercementosis**).

MALIGNANT TUMOURS

Carcinoma is the most common malignancy of the maxillofacial region and usually presents in the middle-aged and elderly, with pain, anaesthesia and loosening of teeth. Most tumours are squamous cell carcinomas

(a)

(c)

(b)

Figure 17.28 *Osteogenic sarcoma of the right mandible. (a) Axial CT shows bone destruction in the molar region and new bone formation ('sun-ray' spiculation) in the soft tissues laterally (open arrow). (b) On T2-weighted axial MRI, the high signal areas medially and laterally indicate soft-tissue extension (open and closed arrows) but a high signal is also produced by fat. (c) On fat-suppressing STIR sequence axial MRI the high signal areas medially and laterally (open arrows) indicate soft-tissue tumour extension. (Courtesy of Dr Otto Chan, The Royal London Hospital.)*

or adenocarcinomas. The carcinoma usually arises from the oral mucosa, but occasionally develops within the mandible or maxilla.

Radiologically, carcinomas are purely destructive and there is little evidence of bone expansion or of subperiosteal new bone formation. The margin of the lesion is irregular (Fig. 17.27) and erosion of the roots of teeth is common.

Osteogenic sarcoma is the most common malignant tumour of the jaws in young adults, and usually presents between the ages of 15 and 30 years, with pain, local anaesthesia and loosening of the teeth. Radiologically it appears as an ill-defined area of bone destruction, often associated with resorption of the roots of adjacent teeth and with thickening of their periodontal membranes. In a few cases, sclerosis is more marked than bone destruction, and these tumours are said to have a slightly better prognosis. However, the most striking bone abnormality is the presence of subperiosteal new bone, which may have a lamellar (onion-skin) or spiculated (sun-ray) appearance (Fig. 17.28a). Histologically the tumour is always much more widespread than the bone abnormalities suggest, and MRI is currently the best technique for demonstrating extension into the soft tissues (Fig. 17.28b,c).

Metastatic carcinoma rarely affects the maxillofacial region, but when it does the primary tumour is usually situated in the breast, bronchus, colon or kidney. Radiologically there may be a single ill-defined area of bone destruction, or multiple coalescing radiolucent areas scattered throughout the maxillofacial bones. Occasionally a single metastasis lodges in the inferior dental canal and widens it.

Multiple myeloma may produce multiple radiolucencies in the mandible in the absence of similar radiolucent areas of the skull vault.

Burkitt's lymphoma of the maxilla and mandible is very common in some parts of Africa, where it affects children of all ages. Radiologically it is a highly destructive lesion, usually accompanied by massive soft-tissue swelling, with patchy radiolucencies, destruction of the cortex, resorption of the lamina dura and destruction of the developing teeth.

INFECTION

A **dental alveolar abscess** results from bacterial infection spreading from the pulp of a tooth through the root apex into the periapical bone. The earliest radiological change is widening of the radiolucent periodontal membrane around the tooth root and this is followed in a few days by localized rarefaction of the periapical bone and bone destruction (Fig. 17.29).

Pyogenic osteomyelitis of the mandible is usually precipitated by local conditions, such as a dental abscess or a fracture. Considering the frequency of dental

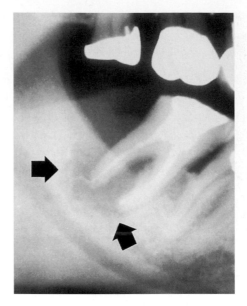

Figure 17.29 *Dental alveolar abscess (arrows) around the root apices of a root-treated lower molar tooth.*

alveolar abscess, osteomyelitis is surprisingly rare. The infecting organism is usually a staphylococcus.

Acute osteomyelitis in children may complicate severe infections such as measles and typhoid, and is presumably a blood-borne infection. Acute osteomyelitis may also be a complication of local pyogenic infections such as tonsillitis. The incidence of infection is higher after radiotherapy (osteoradionecrosis, see below) and in HIV-positive patients (see Fig. 17.17).

As in other bones, the radiological features do not appear until the clinical symptoms of pain, tenderness and soft-tissue swelling have been present for some days. The earliest change is an ill-defined area of bone rarefaction,

Figure 17.30 *Acute osteomyelitis of the ramus of the mandible with a periosteal reaction laterally (arrow).*

Figure 17.31 *Chronic osteomyelitis around an infected unerupted tooth with a pathological fracture through the angle of the mandible.*

which rapidly progresses to more extensive bone destruction. Subperiosteal new bone formation develops in most cases (Fig. 17.30). Sequestra are inevitable, unless the appropriate antibiotic is given early, and appear as opacities lying in cavities. A pathological fracture may occur if the mandible is seriously weakened (Fig. 17.31).

Chronic osteomyelitis may follow acute osteomyelitis and has similar radiological features, with patchy osteoporosis, patchy sclerosis and sequestra lying in cavities. Subperiosteal new bone is a relatively uncommon feature.

Garré's osteomyelitis (subperiosteal sclerosing osteomyelitis) presents as a tender bony swelling and often responds to antibiotics and conservative surgery.

The dominant radiological feature is the formation of dense subperiosteal new bone. There is sometimes patchy sclerosis in the underlying bone and, rarely, patchy rarefaction and sequestrum formation.

Osteoradionecrosis is the name given to a particularly intractable form of chronic osteomyelitis, which can occur following radiotherapy. Radiotherapy itself rarely produces any radiological change in the bone pattern of the maxilla or mandible, but very high doses occasionally result in rarefaction or sclerosis. The radiological abnormalities produced by this infection are widespread patchy sclerosis, with areas of rarefaction and multiple sequestra.

TEMPOROMANDIBULAR JOINT

The temporomandibular joint is a synovial joint, divided into upper and lower compartments by a fibrocartilaginous disc. These compartments may communicate through acquired disc perforations.

INTERNAL DERANGEMENT

The fibrocartilaginous disc may become displaced and is then often associated with pain, tenderness, limited opening and 'clicking'.

Magnetic resonance imaging is the best technique for demonstrating the disc and its relationship to the glenoid fossa. T1-weighted images are taken in an oblique parasagittal plane with the mouth closed and open. Techniques have been described for obtaining images of the joint in intermediate positions to give a dynamic picture of movements of the disc and mandibular condyle. Coronal images can also be obtained. T2-weighted images will demonstrate soft-tissue inflammation around the joint as a high-signal area.

Figure 17.32 *Disc displacement without reduction. Parasagittal T1-weighted image with the mouth open showing anterior displacement of the disc (arrow), against the anterior wall of the glenoid fossa. There is limited forward movement of the condyle (C) on mouth opening. (Courtesy of Dr Richard Nakielny, Royal Hallamshire Hospital, Sheffield.)*

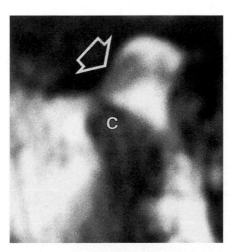

Figure 17.33 *Disc displacement with reduction. T1-weighted parasagittal MRI taken with the mouth open. There is anterior displacement of the disc against the anterior wall of the glenoid fossa (arrow) and the condyle (C) has moved anterior to the displaced disc, on opening. (Courtesy of Dr Richard Nakielny, Royal Hallamshire Hospital, Sheffield.)*

In **disc displacement without reduction**, the disc is fixed against the anterior wall of the glenoid fossa with the posterior margin of the disc anterior to the superior convexity of the articular surface of the mandibular condyle. Anterior movement of the condyle on opening is considerably reduced (Fig. 17.32).

In **disc displacement with reduction**, the disc is also fixed against the anterior wall of the glenoid fossa anterior to the superior convexity of the articular surface of the condyle when the mouth is closed, but the condyle moves anterior to the displaced disc when it opens (Fig. 17.33).

The **pain-dysfunction syndrome** is the clinical diagnosis most frequently applied to patients with temporomandibular joint pain. The aetiology is uncertain, but most cases are probably due to internal derangement of the joint. The joint is usually normal on plain radiographs.

ARTHRITIS

Inflammatory arthritis due to systemic disease is uncommon, but can be a feature of connective tissue diseases such as rheumatoid arthritis and psoriasis. Erosions develop in the articular surface of the condyle and they can be very extensive. The glenoid fossa remains radiologically normal.

Degenerative arthritis (osteoarthritis) (Fig. 17.34) can occur in the elderly and eventually results in the same abnormalities as osteoarthritis in other synovial joints, namely joint-space narrowing, sclerosis and osteophyte formation. The sclerosis is confined to the mandibular condyle and osteophytes arise only from the anterior margin of the condyle. The articular surface of the glenoid fossa remains normal.

Ankylosis of the temporomandibular joint may follow infective arthritis or traumatic haemarthrosis. As these disorders usually occur in childhood, most cases are complicated by hypoplasia of the mandibular condyle owing to the epiphyseal cartilage of the condylar neck having been damaged at the same time. CT is usually required to demonstrate bony ankylosis between the temporal bone and the mandibular condyle.

DISLOCATION

The diagnosis of dislocation is made clinically rather than radiologically as the mandibular condyle may move anterior to the maximum convexity of the articular eminence in normal individuals. The role of imaging in dislocation is to exclude a fracture or some other pathology such as a bone tumour. Recurrent dislocation may be a feature of Marfan's syndrome and the Ehlers–Danlos syndrome.

SALIVARY GLANDS

IMAGING THE SALIVARY GLANDS

Lesions of the gland parenchyma such as tumours and abscesses are best shown by CT, MRI or ultrasound, which can usually distinguish between lesions situated in the salivary glands and those situated in adjacent structures.

Imaging is particularly useful in lesions of the parotid glands as the retromandibular vein (posterior facial vein) can often be identified on **axial CT images** (Fig. 17.35) and **T1-weighted MR** images. This vein is a useful anatomical landmark for the facial nerve (seventh cranial nerve), which supplies the facial muscles and runs immediately lateral to the vein. The facial nerve divides the parotid gland into a large

Figure 17.34 *Degenerative arthritis (osteoarthritis). There is flattening and sclerosis of the mandibular condyle (C).*

Figure 17.35 *Normal parotid glands on axial CT. The glands (G) have a lower attenuation than the surrounding muscles owing to the presence of fat. The retromandibular vein on the right has been arrowed.*

Figure 17.36 *Normal submandibular glands (G) on a coronal T1-weighted MRI.*

Figure 17.37 *Benign pleomorphic adneoma of the superficial lobe of the left parotid gland on axial CT. The lesion is homogeneous and has a higher attenuation than normal gland parenchyma. The border is well defined.*

superficial lobe and a much smaller deep lobe. The clinical importance of this distinction is that tumours in the superficial lobe can be surgically removed with little risk of damaging the nerve, but tumours in the deep lobe have to be dissected from the nerve and its branches and there is always a risk of temporary or even permanent nerve damage.

Coronal MRI is particularly useful for showing the submandibular glands and adjacent structures (Fig. 17.36).

Disorders of the duct systems, such as calculus, stricture and sialectasis of the parotid and submandibular glands, are best demonstrated by **sialography**. The examination should be preceded by plain radiographs to show any radiopaque calculi. Cannulation of the parotid ducts is usually straightforward, but the orifices of the submandibular ducts can be extremely difficult to identify and cannulate. Water-soluble low-osmolar media should always be used as any extravasation into the soft tissues is relatively painless and has no complications.

Delayed radiographs should be taken 10 minutes after the cannula has been removed, as the presence of contrast medium remaining within the duct system indicates duct obstruction or reduced function.

Disorders of function and some inflammatory conditions are best shown by **radionuclide scanning**. 99mTc-pertechnetate will outline normally functioning parotid, submandibular and sublingual glands, as the isotope is excreted in the saliva. Most tumours produce a localized area of reduced uptake.

Gallium scanning with 67Ga citrate is an effective technique for diagnosing infectious and inflammatory processes such as sialadenitis, sarcoid and benign lymphoepithelial infiltration.

(a)

(b)

Figure 17.38 *Benign cystic pleomorphic adenoma (arrow). (a) Axial T1-weighted MRI shows the adenoma as a low-signal area. (b) Coronal T2-weighted MRI shows the adenoma as a high-signal area (arrowed) owing to fluid in the cyst. (Courtesy of Dr R. Phillips, St Bartholomew's Hospital, London.)*

TUMOURS

Salivary gland tumours can develop at any age, and usually present as a painless swelling. They are more

Figure 17.39 *Huge mucoepidermoid carcinoma (arrows) of the right parotid gland on enhanced axial CT. The lesion contains an area of low attenuation and has a poorly defined margin which merges with adjacent structures.*

per cent of all tumours. CT usually shows a well-defined homogeneous lesion with a higher attenuation than in normal parotid gland parenchyma (Fig. 17.37). Malignant change occurs rarely and usually results in an area of low attenuation within the tumour and blurring of the tumour margin. Sialography of benign lesions shows displacement of the intraglandular ducts but malignant lesions may occlude ducts. Myxoid tissue or fluid in the stroma of benign and malignant pleomorphic adenomas will produce a characteristically high signal on T2-weighted MR images (Fig. 17.38a,b).

Adenocarcinomas are rarely true adenocarcinomas and usually have a distinctive histological appearance. The commonest histological types are **adenoid cystic carcinoma** and **mucoepidermoid carcinoma**. These tumours grow slowly but are difficult to eradicate, and the 10-year survival rate is less than 50 per cent. The larger tumours often contain areas of low attenuation on CT and have an irregular border which merges with adjacent structures (Fig. 17.39). Sialography usually shows obstruction of the intraglandular ducts and there may be complete absence of a normal duct system in the affected part of the gland (Fig. 17.40a). Ultrasound usually shows an ill-defined area of reduced and mixed echogenicity (Fig. 17.40b).

Rare tumours include the **benign adenolymphoma (Warthin's tumour)**, which has a high uptake on radionuclide scanning, and **malignant lymphoma**, which is characteristically hypoechoic on ultrasound.

common in the parotid than in the submandibular glands. The overall incidence of malignancy is 10–20 per cent, being higher in the submandibular gland than in the parotid. The pathological classification is complex.

Benign pleomorphic adenoma is the commonest tumour of the salivary glands and accounts for over 50

(a)

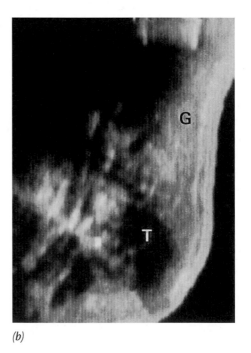

(b)

Figure 17.40 *(a) Parotid sialogram of an adenoid cystic carcinoma of the lower pole of the left parotid gland which has destroyed the duct system. G = upper pole; T = tumour. (b) The ultrasound examination (slice in the coronal plane) shows an area of reduced and mixed echogenicity (T) in the lower part of the gland. The lesion has poorly defined margins, which is typical of a malignant tumour.*

Figure 17.41 *Submandibular sialogram showing two calculi in the main duct (Wharton's duct). The calculi appeared radiopaque on the preliminary films taken before contrast medium was injected.*

Figure 17.42 *Multiple strictures of the main parotid duct (Stensen's duct) on sialography (arrows).*

CALCULI AND DUCT STRICTURES

Calculi are more common in the submandibular region than in the parotid region, and are usually a sequel to infection or stasis. Most calculi are radiopaque on plain films but show as relatively radiolucent lesions on sialography (Fig. 17.41).

Strictures of the main ducts and of the intraglandular ducts are usually due to infection or calculi, and predispose to sialectasis and calculus formation. Strictures at the orifices of the parotid ducts may be caused by cheek biting, and strictures at the anterior ends of the submandibular ducts may be caused by trauma from an ill-fitting denture.

Sialography will demonstrate strictures quite clearly (Fig. 17.42) and may show dilatation of the duct system behind the stricture.

SIALECTASIS

Sialectasis is usually associated with recurrent infection and describes a radiological appearance. The terms 'punctate' or 'globular' are sometimes used to describe small regular cavities measuring less than 2 mm in diameter (Fig. 17.43), and the term 'cavitary' to describe larger cavities with irregular walls (Fig. 17.44). A cavity which is over 5 mm in diameter is likely to be an abscess. Infective sialectasis can produce any of these abnormalities, and may be accompanied by calculus formation in the main duct or in the sialectatic cavities within the gland.

Sjögren's syndrome and other connective tissue diseases are also associated with sialectasis. Most patients with Sjögren's syndrome have sialectasis and there is often dilatation of the main duct.

Figure 17.43 *Parotid sialogram showing punctate sialectasis localized to the inferior pole of the gland. The area of clinical swelling has been outlined with a radiopaque wire.*

Figure 17.44 *Parotid sialogram showing 'cavitary' sialectasis throughout the gland.*

Figure 17.45 *Benign lymphoepithelial infiltration of the parotids on axial CT. The glands are grossly enlarged and contain multiple round areas of low attenuation.*

Figure 17.46 *Extravasation of contrast medium from the left parotid duct into the soft tissues. The duct had been damaged at surgery 2 weeks earlier.*

MISCELLANEOUS CONDITIONS

Infective sialadenitis of viral or bacterial origin causes generalized glandular enlargement and there is usually increased attenuation on CT. Abscess formation will produce an area of low attenuation on CT and an area of low echogenicity on ultrasound. Sialography in cases of recurrent infection may show calculus, duct stricture or sialectasis.

Benign lymphoepithelial infiltration can occur as an isolated abnormality (Mikulicz's disease) but is more commonly a feature of Sjögren's syndrome or HIV disease. The CT appearance in advanced disease is quite characteristic. The glands are grossly enlarged and contain multiple well-defined areas of low attenuation (Fig. 17.45). The condition is not as benign as the name implies; it is complicated by malignant lymphoma in 5 per cent and anaplastic carcinoma in about 1 per cent of patients.

Trauma to the main parotid duct, or to one of its larger intraglandular branches, occasionally results from penetrating facial injury and is a very rare complication of surgery. Sialography will show extravasation of contrast medium from the duct system into the soft tissues (Fig. 17.46).

FURTHER READING

Gibilisco, 1992: *Stafne's oral radiographic diagnosis*. Philadelphia, PA: W.B. Saunders.

Langlais, R.P., Kasle, M.J. 2000: *Exercises in oral radiographic interpretation* (2nd edition). Vol. 1. Philadelphia, PA: W.B. Saunders.

Mancuso, A.A., Hanafee, W.N. 1985: *Computed tomography in magnetic resonance imaging of the head and neck* (2nd edition). Baltimore, MD: Williams & Wilkins.

Whaites, E. 1996: *Essentials of dental radiography and radiology* (2nd edition). Edinburgh: Churchill Livingstone.

White, S.C., Pharoah, M.J. 2000: *Oral radiology* (4th edition). St Louis, MO: Mosley.

Sinuses

IAIN R. COLQUHOUN

Conventional radiographic examinations have a limited role for investigation of sinus pathology. A single occipitomental (OM) view is recommended for assessment of inflammatory disease. This film is taken with the patient erect with a horizontal X-ray beam to demonstrate fluid levels. More detailed assessment of the sinuses requires computed tomography (CT) or magnetic resonance (MRI) imaging.

ANATOMY

The sinuses develop as pouches from the nasal cavity, lined by ciliated columnar epithelium. The maxillary and ethmoid sinuses are present at birth, but fluid-filled. The ethmoid sinuses reach near adult size by 12 years of age. The maxillary sinuses have two major growth periods at 0–3 and 7–12 years. The frontal sinuses, usually derived from the anterior ethmoid sinuses, are visible by the age of 2 and well pneumatized by the age of 12. The sphenoid sinuses pneumatize from the age of 3.

The maxillary sinuses drain via a single ostium into the middle meatus, lateral to the middle turbinate. Accessory ostia within the medial maxillary wall occur in 15–40 per cent of patients. In general the frontal, anterior and middle ethmoid sinuses also drain via the middle meatus. Each sphenoid sinus drains via a single ostium, which is located 10–15 mm above the floor of the sinus, into the sphenoethmoidal recess in the superior meatus, where the posterior ethmoid sinuses also drain.

Sinus anatomy is ideally demonstrated with coronal CT, developed as a 'road map' to facilitate functional

Figure 18.1 *Normal coronal sinus CT through the osteomeatal complex. N = infraorbital nerve; M and I = middle and inferior turbinates; O = maxillary ostium; U = uncinate process; S = middle meatus; B = ethmoidal bulla. O, U and S together form the 'osteomeatal complex'.*

endoscopic sinus surgery. One key structure for endoscopic sinus surgery is the 'osteomeatal complex' within the middle meatus, where the frontal, ethmoid (anterior and middle) and maxillary sinuses drain (Fig. 18.1). Obstruction to the osteomeatal complex typically results in opacification of this group of sinuses (Fig. 18.2).

INFLAMMATORY DISEASE

Sinusitis can be related to acute or chronic infection, allergy, altered immunity or a combination of these

Figure 18.2 *Coronal CT in acute sinusitis demonstrating unilateral osteomeatal complex disease (curved arrow) and consequent opacification of the maxillary and middle ethmoid sinuses. Anterior ethmoid and frontal sinus opacification is also present.*

Figure 18.3 *Coronal CT in gross polyposis with opacification of all the sinuses, resulting in marked loss of definition of the bony septa.*

factors. In the absence of trauma, fluid levels usually denote acute infection. The degree and extent of mucosal thickening are very variable. Involvement of a single sinus usually denotes **infection**, whereas multiple sinus and nasal mucosal involvement, often with polypoidal mucosal thickening, suggests an allergic aetiology. Chronic sinusitis usually produces thickening and sclerosis of the bones surrounding the involved sinus. Infective, as opposed to **allergic**, mucosal thickening will exhibit enhancement with intravenous contrast on both CT and MRI. This enhancement is typically peripheral as opposed to the solid or uniform enhancement of tumours. Inflammatory mucosal thickening is markedly hyperintense on T2-weighted MRI sequences, whereas tumours are of more intermediate intensity. However, in chronic sinus disease, resorption of water will result in variable signal intensities, making exclusion of a tumour difficult on MRI. The major complication of sinus infection is spread of infection to the orbit, brain or cavernous sinus.

Because of the excellent contrast between bone, soft tissue and air, CT is the most suitable technique for assessment of inflammatory sinus disease. The major disadvantage of MRI is that neither cortical bone nor air produces a signal, thereby reducing anatomical detail. MRI is, however, better than CT for assessing cavernous sinus and early intracranial involvement.

ASPERGILLOSIS

Aspergillosis is the commonest fungal infection. The invasive form frequently originates in one maxillary sinus, producing extensive bone destruction resembling

carcinoma; intracranial extension can also occur. Fungal infections typically contain hyperdense foci on CT and corresponding hypointense areas with a T2-weighted MRI sequence. However, in any form of chronic sinus infection, retained secretions can develop areas of high density on CT.

POLYPS

Polyps are associated with infection, allergy, aspirin sensitivity, asthma and cystic fibrosis. Polyps are

Figure 18.4 *Coronal CT demonstrating an antrochoanal polyp opacifying the maxillary sinus and extending through an expanded ostium into the nasal cavity and bowing the nasal septum. A small polyp is present at the base of the opposite maxillary sinus.*

frequently multiple and expansile, involving the nasal cavities and sinuses and can produce complete opacification of these structures. In such severe cases CT demonstrates opacification with soft-tissue density material in the nasal cavities and sinuses and often marked thinning, or even absence, of the intervening bony septa (Fig. 18.3). The degree of bone loss can occasionally mimic a malignant process. Typical MRI characteristics of polyps are similar to acute infectious mucosal thickening with low to intermediate T1-weighted intensity and T2-weighted hyperintensity. Chronic polyposis produces heterogeneous intensity of the nasal cavities and sinuses even exhibiting areas of signal void, which can be mistaken for air.

Antrochoanal polyps are benign polyps that grow within and usually fill the maxillary sinus before expanding the ostium and extending posteriorly into the nasal cavity towards the nasopharynx (Fig. 18.4). Similar sphenochoanal polyps occasionally occur.

MUCOCELE

Mucoceles are expansile lesions of the sinuses, caused by obstruction of the ostium, usually secondary to infection or, rarely, by tumour or trauma. The ostial obstruction causes an accumulation of secretions within the sinus with absorption of trapped air, thereby creating an opaque sinus. The slow increase in pressure within the sinus produces expansion with bowing and thinning of the bony margins. Mucoceles occur most frequently in the frontal sinuses and with decreasing frequency in the ethmoid, maxillary and sphenoid sinuses. Acute infection produces a **pyocele**, with bone destruction and an associated soft-tissue abscess.

Chronic infection leads to thickening and sclerosis of the expanded bony margins of the sinuses.

A mucocele is shown on CT as an opaque expanded sinus with bony thinning of its walls (Fig. 18.5). MRI demonstrates an opaque, expanded sinus, the contents of which are typically homogeneous and of low to intermediate intensity on T1-weighted and hyperintense on T2-weighted sequences. However, the intensity varies with the relative composition of the contents, and the intensity is frequently either hypo- or hyperintense on both the T1- and T2-weighted sequences.

GRANULOMAS

Wegener's and **midline granulomas** both produce destructive soft-tissue masses involving the nasal cavities and sinuses. **Sarcoidosis** produces irregular mucosal thickening usually confined to the nasal cavities.

BENIGN TUMOURS

Osteomas are benign tumours, usually formed from dense compact bone (ivory osteoma), which commonly occur in the frontal sinus. They are generally an incidental finding unless ostial occlusion produces a mucocele.

Inverted papilloma frequently occurs on the lateral nasal wall and can be expansile and locally invasive, tending to involve the adjacent maxillary and ethmoid sinuses (Fig. 18.6). Local recurrence following excision is not uncommon.

Figure 18.5 *Coronal CT demonstrating an anterior ethmoidal mucocele producing marked bony expansion with thinning but preservation of the lamina papyracea (arrow).*

Figure 18.6 *Coronal CT demonstrating an inverted papilloma originating from the middle turbinate and extending into the maxillary sinus with erosion of the medial wall.*

Figure 18.7 *Axial CT of a squamous cell carcinoma originating within the maxillary sinus but demonstrating early extension into the infratemporal fossa (arrows) with an intact posterior wall.*

MALIGNANT TUMOURS

Squamous cell carcinoma is the commonest malignant tumour to affect the sinuses and most frequently arises in the maxillary sinuses and nasal cavities. Early tumours are radiologically indistinguishable from, and frequently coexist with, inflammatory mucosal thickening. Consequently, on diagnosis there is often a large tumour mass, the radiological characteristics of which are bone destruction and infiltration into adjacent structures, particularly the orbit and infratemporal fossa. Coronal and axial CT are required to assess fully the extent of bone destruction and tumour infiltration. Early infratemporal spread, which can occur without demonstrable bone destruction, is more easily appreciated on axial images (Fig. 18.7). Squamous cell carcinoma often occurs against a background of chronic inflammation and the tumour frequently produces acute inflammatory change secondary to ostial occlusion. The soft-tissue opacification seen with CT is a combination of tumour and inflammation and therefore the actual tumour bulk is overestimated. MRI is frequently able to distinguish tumour from inflammatory change as the inflammation generally appears more hyperintense than tumour on T2-weighted sequences. However, areas of haemorrhage and necrosis can produce heterogeneous foci within the tumour on both T1- and T2-weighted sequences. Tumours usually exhibit diffuse enhancement with intravenous contrast on both CT and MRI as opposed to the peripheral enhancement of acute inflammation.

Adenocarcinoma also appears as a destructive soft-tissue mass with similar MRI characteristics to

Figure 18.8 *Enhanced T1-weighted coronal MRI demonstrating an olfactory neuroblastoma involving the nasal cavity, frontal lobes (with capping cysts), orbits, ethmoid and maxillary sinuses. Note the intermediate signal intensity material in both maxillary sinuses, which exhibits peripheral enhancement (arrows) consistent with secondary acute and chronic inflammatory reaction from ostial obstruction.*

Figure 18.9 *Enhanced T1-weighted sagittal MRI demonstrating a clivus chordoma presenting as a nasopharyngeal mass.*

squamous cell carcinoma, except that adenocarcinoma usually exhibits less marked enhancement. An adenocarcinoma commonly originates within the ethmoid sinuses and frequently extends intracranially.

Non-Hodgkin's lymphoma is the commonest variety of lymphoma to involve the sinuses. Lymphoma generally appears as a more infiltrative rather than a destructive mass and is of intermediate intensity on all MRI sequences.

Olfactory neuroblastoma (or aesthesioneuroblastoma) arises from the olfactory mucosa superiorly within the nasal cavities. The tumour is locally invasive, extending into the adjacent ethmoid sinuses, orbits and anterior cranial fossa and is ideally imaged with MRI (Fig. 18.8).

Other malignancies involving the sinuses and nasal cavities include **primary sarcomas** and **melanoma**, **metastases** and **myeloma**. Infiltration from adjacent salivary gland and dental tumours occurs and some tumours arising from nearby structures may present as nasal masses, including **clivus chordomas** (Fig. 18.9) and **juvenile nasopharyngeal angiofibromas**.

FURTHER READING

Harnsberger, H.R. 1995: *Handbook of head and neck imaging* (2nd edition). St Louis: Mosby.

Gillespie, J.E., Gholkar, A. (eds) 1994: *Magnetic resonance imaging and computed tomography of the head and neck.* London: Chapman & Hall.

Mafee, M.F. (ed.) 1993: Imaging of the paranasal sinuses and oromaxillofacial region. *Radiologic Clinics of North America* **31**(1).

Rao, V.M., Flanders, A.E., Tom, B.M. 1992: *MRI and CT atlas of correlative imaging in otolaryngology.* London: Martin Dunitz.

Rice, D.H. (ed.) 1993: Inflammatory diseases of the sinuses. *Otolaryngologic Clinics of North America* **26**(4).

Som, P.M., Curtin, H.D. (eds) 1996: *Head and neck imaging,* Vol. 1 (3rd edition). St Louis: Mosby.

Valvassori, G.E., Mafee, M.F., Carter, B.L. (eds) 1994: *Imaging of the head and neck.* New York, NY: Thième.

Yousem, D.M. (ed.) 1996: Head and neck imaging. *Neuroimaging Clinics of North America* **6**(2).

19

Ear

IAIN R. COLQUHOUN

Computed tomography (CT) and magnetic resonance imaging (MRI) are the principal radiological investigations for assessing petrous bone pathology. The fine structural detail requires high-resolution CT techniques (HRCT), comprising 1–2 mm thick contiguous sections, ideally in both the axial and coronal planes. MRI has improved soft-tissue resolution, and the development of fast imaging sequences with thinner sections and greater spatial resolution has significantly increased the use of MRI.

ANATOMY

The petrous bone is pyramidal, lying horizontally, the apex directed medially and anteriorly towards the clivus. The upper surface forms the posterior floor of the middle cranial fossa, the posterior surface of the petrous bone forming the anterior border of the posterior cranial fossa with the clivus (Figs 19.1, 19.2).

MIDDLE EAR

The middle ear cavity is divided into three sections. Superiorly is the **epitympanum** containing the head of the malleus and body and short process of the incus. Inferiorly is the **hypotympanum**, the smallest of the three divisions and empty. Between these is the **mesotympanum** containing the handle of the malleus, long process of the incus and the stapes. The lateral wall is formed by the tympanic membrane and above this by a pointed

bony projection, the scutum. The anterior wall is shortened by approximation of the floor and roof and contains the opening for the bony portion of the eustachian tube. The floor is a thin plate of bone separating the middle ear from the jugular foramen posteriorly and the carotid canal anteriorly. The roof is another thin plate of bone, the tegmen tympani, separating the middle ear from the middle cranial fossa dura and extending posteriorly to cover the antrum. The posterior wall is perforated superiorly by an opening into the mastoid antrum – the 'aditus ad antrum' – and blends into the medial wall, the main feature of which is 'the promontory' for the basal turn of the cochlea. Behind and above this is the oval window, closed by the stapes footplate. Above the promontory and oval window is a ridge containing the horizontal portion of the facial nerve canal.

INNER EAR

Deep to the middle ear cavity is the otic capsule formed of dense compact bone. Within this is the labyrinth consisting of the cochlea, vestibule and semicircular canals. The **cochlea** has two and three-quarter turns, the basal turn being the largest and most easily visualized, the middle and apical turns being difficult to separate. The **vestibular** system consists of the **three semicircular canals** and the **vestibule**, the membranous components of which (the saccule and utricle) cannot be separately visualized. The lateral semicircular canal lies near the axial plane, its apex directed laterally; the posterior lies along, and the superior lies across, the long axis of the petrous bone, their apices directed cranially.

Figure 19.1 *Coronal HRCT of normal anatomy. C = basal turn of cochlea; E = stapes articulating in oval window above the promontory; H = hypotympanum; I = incus in epitympanum; M = scutum; P = porus of internal auditory canal; S = semicircular canals; T = tegmen tympani; V = vestibule.*

Figure 19.2 *Coronal HRCT of normal anatomy (2 mm anterior to Fig. 19.1); C = cochlea; M = malleus; V = hairpin turn of facial nerve canal.*

INTERNAL AUDITORY CANAL

The medial end of the internal auditory canal, the porus, is divided into quadrants. Through the anterior two quadrants pass the facial nerve superiorly and the cochlear branch of the eighth nerve inferiorly. The two divisions of the vestibular branch of the eighth pass through the posterior quadrants.

FACIAL NERVE

The facial nerve leaves the pons at the pontomedullary junction and traverses the cerebellopontine angle cistern to the porus. In the internal auditory canal it passes laterally and anteriorly to a point above and lateral to the cochlea, where it is expanded by the geniculate ganglion. It then takes a hairpin turn to run posteriorly through the medial wall of the middle ear cavity, immediately below the lateral semicircular canals, before turning vertically downwards to exit via the stylomastoid foramen.

IMAGING STRATEGIES

HRCT is the method of choice for demonstrating the bony anatomy but the fluid-containing structures of the inner ear, the cochlea, vestibule and semicircular canals are well shown on T2-weighted MRI sequences, appearing hyperintense against the surrounding hypointense bone.

CONGENITAL ABNORMALITIES

Atresia of the external auditory canal is relatively common and may involve the cartilaginous or bony sections. HRCT is essential for assessment of the extent of the atresia and associated anomalies, and for excluding a concomitant primary cholesteatoma of the middle ear. The cochlea may be hypoplastic, as in the Mondini deformity, with an intact basal turn and a common cavity for the middle and apical turns. Anomalies of the semicircular canals most frequently involve the lateral semicircular canal, which is dilated, often in conjunction with the vestibule.

The major congenital **vascular anomalies** relate to variations in position of the internal carotid artery and jugular bulb. An aberrant internal carotid artery passes through the middle ear cavity anterior to the cochlear promontory (Fig. 19.3). Variations in size and position of the jugular bulb can result in it protruding into the middle ear cavity posteriorly. Vascular variations are readily evaluated by HRCT or MRI with flow-sensitive sequences.

OTOSCLEROSIS

Otosclerosis is an idiopathic disease of the labyrinthine capsule with replacement of the normal lamellar bone by initially spongy and later denser bone, and is best assessed by HRCT. Active disease (**otospongiosis**) appears as focal or diffuse areas of reduced density, whereas areas of calcification or sclerosis denote mature disease.

The process most frequently involves the oval window (fenestral), where in the active stage there is

Figure 19.3 *Coronal HRCT demonstrating an aberrant internal carotid artery within the middle ear cavity (arrow).*

Figure 19.4 *Axial HRCT demonstrating bilateral cochlear otosclerosis (arrows).*

apparent widening owing to the surrounding bone resorption. Cochlear otosclerosis may involve the basal turn or be more diffuse, appearing as a zone of reduced density around the labyrinth (Fig. 19.4).

TRAUMA

Temporal bone fractures may be longitudinal (80 per cent), transverse (15 per cent) or mixed (5 per cent). Longitudinal fractures pass through the long axis of the temporal bone, along the external auditory canal and roof of the middle ear to the inner ear (Fig. 19.5), whereas transverse fractures are perpendicular to the long axis. Complications include facial nerve injury (particularly with transverse fractures), CSF fistula, post-traumatic meningoencephaloceles and rarely internal carotid artery aneurysm. Ossicular disruption can occur in conjunction with petrous fractures or in isolation, the incus being most frequently involved. HRCT is ideally suited for assessment of petrous fractures and associated complications.

INFLAMMATORY DISORDERS

Acute otitis media and **acute mastoiditis** are common infections, clinically evident and responsive to antibiotic therapy. Imaging is only required if complications are suspected. Occasionally the infection can extend medially into the petrous apex – **apical petrositis**.

Chronic otitis media and **mastoiditis** are usually the result of eustachian tube dysfunction or secondary to the presence of a cholesteatoma. Evaluation of the extent of disease and degree of bony erosion is best performed with HRCT. The limitation of this technique is the inability to differentiate fluid, inflammatory or fibrous tissue and cholesteatoma, all appearing as non-specific soft-tissue density material.

Malignant otitis externa is an aggressive infection, usually caused by *Pseudomonas aeruginosa*, and frequently seen in elderly diabetics. Infection originates in the external auditory canal and, if untreated, rapidly spreads inferiorly and medially to involve the bone and soft tissues of the skull base; direct spread into the middle ear cavity is rare. Initial radiological assessment is principally by axial HRCT (Figs 19.6, 19.7).

Bell's palsy is the commonest cause of lower motor neurone facial paralysis. Thin section T1-weighted MRI can demonstrate the facial nerve, diffuse linear enhancement of the nerve occurring with Bell's, herpes zoster, postoperative and post-traumatic facial nerve palsies.

Figure 19.5 *Axial HRCT demonstrating bilateral longitudinal petrous bone fractures (arrows). Note extension of the fractures through the sphenoid sinus (arrowheads).*

Figure 19.6 *Malignant otitis externa. Axial CT demonstrating a large soft-tissue mass below the skull base (arrowheads), extending medially from the external auditory canal (arrow).*

Figure 19.8 *Acquired cholesteatoma. Coronal HRCT demonstrating a soft-tissue mass in the epitympanum and mastoid antrum (arrowheads) with early erosion of the scutum (arrow).*

Figure 19.7 *Malignant otitis externa. Axial CT demonstrating bone erosion of the skull base with loss of cortex (arrow). Note the ipsilateral mastoid air cell opacification.*

CHOLESTEATOMA

Cholesteatomas are epidermoids of the petrous bone, composed of keratinizing stratified squamous epithelium that constantly desquamates keratin.

Congenital cholesteatomas, though rare, occur most frequently at the petrous apex or within the middle ear. Lesions at the petrous apex are discussed with cholesterol granulomas. Congenital cholesteatomas of the middle ear are rare, occurring behind an intact ear drum without a history of otitis media, and are difficult to distinguish from acquired lesions.

Acquired cholesteatomas are associated with prior otitis media. They can occur anywhere within the middle ear, but typically originate laterally in the epitympanum, between the scutum and malleus

(Prussak's space). Radiological diagnosis is primarily by direct coronal HRCT with visualization of a soft-tissue mass in the appropriate location and erosion of the scutum and ossicles (Fig. 19.8). With a larger mass occupying the middle ear cavity and extending into the mastoid antrum, differentiation from fluid or granulation tissue is not possible with CT. MRI may be of use, cholesteatomas being low to medium intensity on T1-weighted, and relatively hyperintense on T2-weighted sequences, whereas granulation tissue is less intense on T2-weighted and may enhance with gadolinium. Fluid is more intense on T2-weighted sequences. However, extensive cholesteatomas are usually associated with fluid, granulation tissue and often cholesterol crystals (hyperintense on both T1- and T2-weighted sequences), resulting in a non-specific lesion of heterogeneous intensity. Coronal HRCT will demonstrate local complications including destruction of the medial wall of the middle ear cavity, usually involving the lateral semicircular canal (leading to a labyrinthine fistula) and horizontal segment of the facial nerve, and superior extension into the mastoid antrum with destruction of the tegmen. Contrast-enhanced CT or MRI is essential to exclude the intracranial complications associated with perforation of the tegmen tympani or, more rarely, of the posterior mastoid cortex, namely epidural empyema, or temporal or cerebellar abscess.

CHOLESTEROL CYSTS AND GRANULOMAS

Small cholesterol cysts are frequently seen within the normal petrous apex on MRI. When larger, they are termed giant cholesterol cysts or cholesterol granulomas

Figure 19.9 *Coronal fast spin-echo T2-weighted image through the internal auditory canal clearly demonstrating a small intracanalicular acoustic neuroma (arrow).*

Figure 19.10 *Coronal CT demonstrating a large glomus jugulare tumour (arrowheads), extending into the middle ear (arrow).*

and produce a well-defined expansile and usually destructive mass. The appearances are very similar to those of congenital cholesteatomas of the petrous apex. Differentiation is facilitated by MRI, cholesterol granulomas being hyperintense on both T1- and T2-weighted sequences, whereas congenital cholesteatomas are low to medium intensity on T1-weighted and relatively and relatively hyperintense on T2-weighted sequences.

NEOPLASMS

ACOUSTIC NEUROMA

Acoustic neuromas are the commonest tumours involving the temporal bone and cerebellopontine angle. Approximately 90 per cent arise from the superior division of the vestibular nerve close to the porus. Bilateral acoustic neuromas are found in neurofibromatosis type II. Occasionally vestibular neuromas can arise at the fundus of the internal auditory canal or within the vestibule. Cochlear neuromas are rare, usually arising near the porus, or rarely within the labyrinth.

On both MRI and CT acoustic neuromas usually appear as well-defined masses of homogeneous texture and exhibit marked contrast enhancement. They can contain cystic areas from either necrosis or previous haemorrhage. MRI is the radiological screening test of choice, with the use of thin section axial and coronal T2-weighted images through the internal auditory canal, acoustic neuromas appearing as hypointense masses compared to cerebrospinal fluid (CSF) (Fig. 19.9). If detail is obscured by artefact, usually from CSF flow, post-gadolinium T1-weighted axial and coronal images are necessary.

FACIAL NERVE NEUROMA

Facial nerve neuromas have the same CT and MRI characteristics as acoustic neuromas and mimic them when they occur within the internal auditory canal or

cerebellopontine angle cistern. The commonest site is at the geniculate ganglion where the neuroma produces local erosion of the petrous bone.

PARAGANGLIOMA

Paragangliomas or glomus tumours are highly vascular tumours, usually benign in nature but locally invasive. Glomus tumours of the temporal bone are divided into two groups, tympanicum or jugulare. The tumours originate from glomus cells within the adventitia of the jugular bulb or along the course of the tympanic branch of the glossopharyngeal nerve (Jacobson's nerve) or the auricular branch of the vagus (nerve of Arnold).

Glomus tympanicum tumours arise within the mucosa overlying the cochlear promontory on the medial wall of the middle ear cavity and frequently present with pulsatile tinnitus, from tumour vascularity, or conductive hearing loss from mass effect on the ossicular chain. The tumour is usually visible otoscopically as a reddish-blue pulsatile mass behind an intact tympanic membrane. Radiological examination with coronal and axial HRCT, supplemented by MRI, aims to demonstrate that the tumour is confined to the middle ear cavity, in which case surgical removal is generally straightforward. If the tumour breaches the middle ear cavity it usually extends through the floor into the jugular foramen.

Glomus jugulare tumours originate within the jugular foramen. Presentation depends upon tumour size and pattern of extension. Growth within the jugular foramen leads to palsies of the ninth, tenth and eleventh cranial nerves. Upward extension into the middle ear cavity commonly occurs (Fig. 19.10), producing symptoms similar to those of a glomus tympanicum tumour but there is usually more extensive bone destruction with involvement of the seventh cranial nerve. These tumours also frequently grow superiorly into the posterior cranial fossa and inferiorly into the neck.

HRCT in the axial and coronal planes will show a mass centred on the jugular foramen with varying

Figure 19.11 *Axial CT showing erosion of the jugular foramen (arrows) by a glomus jugulare tumour. Compare with the normally corticated contralateral jugular foramen.*

Figure 19.12 *Coronal MRI clearly demonstrating a small hyperintense glomus jugulare tumour (arrow).*

degrees of erosion and expansion of the foramen. Initially the bone erosion is subtle with slight irregularity and loss of definition of the cortex (Fig. 19.11). Attention to detail is important when the jugular foramina is assessed, as there is marked developmental variation in size and shape, the right foramen being generally the larger.

The full extent of the extraosseous spread is most easily appreciated with MRI. The tumours are hypointense on T1-weighted and hyperintense on T2-weighted sequences (Fig. 19.12) and exhibit marked enhancement. Serpiginous hypointensities present within the tumour represent flow voids from tumour vessels. Where possible, treatment is by surgical excision, the safety and completeness of which is facilitated by preoperative endovascular embolization of the tumour.

CHORDOMA

Chordomas are rare tumours arising from remnants of notochord. Between 35 and 40 per cent occur intracranially, typically within the clivus, but unilateral petrous bone tumours do occur. Chordomas appear as well-defined extra-axial, soft-tissue masses of heterogeneous density, associated with bone destruction, and characteristically contain areas of calcification. On MRI they are heterogeneously hypointense on T1-weighted and markedly hyperintense on T2-weighted images, the heterogeneity probably representing calcification and areas of haemorrhage, as these are very vascular tumours. Marked contrast enhancement with gadolinium usually occurs. Chordomas are predominantly locally invasive, usually presenting with local cranial nerve palsies. Metastases are uncommon.

CARCINOMA

Squamous cell carcinoma of the ear, although rare, is the commonest primary malignant tumour of the ear.

It usually originates from the external auditory canal or middle ear, but localization of the site of origin is rarely possible owing to the marked bony destruction frequently present at diagnosis. Extensive local spread occurs, but metastases are rare.

The degree of bone destruction is best assessed with HRCT, as is bony sclerosis of the adjacent middle cranial fossa, which is frequently associated with this tumour, possibly reflecting previous chronic infection. MRI is more sensitive for demonstrating soft-tissue extension.

PRIMARY BONE TUMOURS

Osteomas can occur within the external auditory canal. **Giant cell tumours** occur at the petrous apex, producing irregular expansion. **Osteosarcomas** and **chondrosarcomas** both produce soft-tissue masses with extensive bone destruction.

METASTASES

The petrous bone can be the site of metastatic deposits, commonly from carcinoma of the breast. The petrous bone may also be involved by myeloma, usually as part of widespread disease, but occasionally as the site of a solitary plasmacytoma. Direct extension of adjacent advanced malignant tumours, particularly nasopharyngeal and parotid carcinomas, can involve the petrous bone.

COMMON DIFFERENTIAL DIAGNOSES

- **Middle ear mass**
  - Cholesteatoma
  - Glomus tumour
  - High jugular bulb
  - Aberrant ICA
  - Seventh nerve neuroma
  - Carcinoma
- **Localized petrous apex destruction**
  - Metastasis
  - Myeloma
  - Chordoma
  - Cholesterol granuloma

- Congenital cholesteatoma
- Nerve sheath tumour
- ICA aneurysm
- **Pulsatile tinnitus**
  - Normal vascular variant
    - ▶ high jugular bulb
    - ▶ aberrant ICA
  - Glomus tumour
  - Dural AV fistula
  - AVM
  - ICA stenosis
- **Jugular foramen tumour**
  - Glomus tumour

- Meningioma
- Nerve sheath tumour
- Metastasis
- Plasmacytoma
- Chondrosarcoma

- **CP angle mass**
  - Acoustic neuroma
  - Meningioma
  - Metastasis
  - Epidermoid
  - Glomus
  - Arachnoid cyst
  - Aneurysm

FURTHER READING

Gillespie, J.E., Gholkar, A. (eds) 1994: *Magnetic resonance imaging and computed tomography of the head and neck*. London: Chapman & Hall.

Harnsberger, H.R. 1995: *Handbook of head and neck imaging* (2nd edition). St Louis: Mosby.

House, J.W. (ed.) 1993: Otosclerosis. *Otolaryngologic Clinics of North America* **26**(3).

Ludman, H., Wright, T. (eds) 1998: *Diseases of the ear* (6th edition). London: Arnold.

Parisier, S.C., Edelstein, D.R. (eds) 1989: Cholesteatoma. *Otolaryngologic Clinics of North America* **22**(5).

Phelps, P.D., Wright, A. 1990: Imaging cholesteatoma. *Clinical Radiology* **41**, 156–62.

Rao, V.M., Flanders, A.E., Tom, B.M. 1992: *MRI and CT atlas of correlative imaging in otolaryngology*. London: Martin Dunitz.

Som, P.M., Curtin, H.D. (eds) 1996: *Head and neck imaging*, Vol. 2 (3rd edition). St. Louis: Mosby.

Swartz, J.D., Faerber, E.N. 1985: Congenital malformations of the external and middle ear: High-resolution CT findings of surgical import. *American Journal of Roentgenology* **144**, 501–6.

Valvassori, G.E., Mafee, M.F., Carter, B.L. (eds) 1994: *Imaging of the head and neck*. New York, NY: Thième.

Virapongse, C., Rothman, S.L.G., Kier, E.L., Sarwar, M. 1982: Computed tomographic anatomy of the temporal bone. *American Journal of Neuroradiology* **3**, 379–89.

Weber, A.L. (ed.) 1994: Imaging of the skull base. *Neuroimaging Clinics of North America* **4**(3).

Yousem, D.M. (ed.) 1996: Head and neck imaging. *Neuroimaging Clinics of North America* **6**(2).

20

Neck

BRIAN K. WIGNALL

IMAGING TECHNIQUES

CONVENTIONAL RADIOGRAPHY

Lateral view of the neck

Excepting suspected vertebral fractures, a lateral view of the neck will suffice for demonstrating most impacted swallowed foreign bodies, and allow initial assessment of laryngeal trauma. Soft-tissue thickening from inflammation or tumour of the larynx, pharynx and thyroid may be demonstrated and any associated airway narrowing identified. A lateral view of the thoracic inlet will indicate intrathoracic extension of a goitre by showing displacement or compression of the trachea.

Chest radiography

A chest radiograph is essential when any primary malignancy is diagnosed to detect metastases in the lungs or mediastinal lymph node enlargement. In addition, malignant lymphadenopathy in the neck can result from a primary bronchial carcinoma. Disease of the larynx and pharynx may cause aspiration pneumonia, which will be demonstrated on a chest radiograph.

BARIUM SWALLOW EXAMINATION

This is an initial investigation of patients with dysphagia and is discussed on page 53.

COMPUTED TOMOGRAPHY (CT)

CT provides cross-sectional images, in which the contrast between different normal soft tissues, as well as between normal soft tissues and areas of pathology, is much greater than on conventional radiography. This contrast difference can be enhanced by means of intravenous contrast agents. Enhancement of blood vessels allows them to be distinguished from other rounded structures, notably enlarged lymph nodes, and displays the vascular anatomy. CT scanning gives excellent detail of bone and other calcified structures. If a tissue diagnosis has not been established, fine-needle aspiration biopsy (FNAB) may be carried out under CT control. The axial images are also used for mapping radiotherapy fields so that the whole tumour is treated. The information from CT can be transferred by computer disk to a CT integrated therapy planning system.

MAGNETIC RESONANCE IMAGING (MRI)

With the use of a variety of pulse sequences, images are obtained, which, compared with CT scanning, have better contrast between the different soft tissues and between normal soft tissues and tumour. This contrast difference is increased by use of intravenous paramagnetic agents, usually gadolinium DTPA. Additionally, the vascular anatomy can be displayed without recourse to contrast agents. With MRI, there are no artefacts from dental amalgam, a common problem with CT scanning of the neck. Thus, except for assessment of bony structures, MRI is a safer and better scanning technique for the neck than CT.

ULTRASOUND

Use of a high-frequency (7.5–10 MHz) linear array transducer will give an excellent display of all but the deepest structures in the neck. It is commonly used to examine the thyroid gland and lymph nodes and to act as a guide to FNAB of any mass detected. The scan can be performed in any plane, is rapid and safe and causes no discomfort.

RADIONUCLIDE SCANNING

This involves an intravenous injection of a suitable radiopharmaceutical, after which the patient is scanned by means of a gamma camera in order to produce images that reveal a pattern of uptake of the radio-nuclide by the various tissues. From this it can be deduced whether these tissues are normal or abnormal.

Investigation of the thyroid and detection of bony metastases are the most common uses of radionuclide scanning in the neck.

CONGENITAL CYSTS OF THE NECK

These arise from duct remnants and often present in adult life owing to enlargement as a result of trauma or infection.

Figure 20.1 *Branchial cleft cyst. CT scan showing the cyst is a low-attenuation mass (M) anterior to sternomastoid (SM). The arrow points to a compressed jugular vein.*

BRANCHIAL CLEFT CYST

This is the most common congenital cyst and usually presents as a smooth fluctuant mass at the angle of the mandible. CT scanning reveals a low-density non-enhancing mass anterior to the sternomastoid muscle and lateral to the carotid sheath. There may be wall thickening or septation, due to infection (Fig. 20.1).

CYSTIC HYGROMA

This arises from lymphoid tissue and has a similar appearance to a branchial cleft cyst but lies posterior to the sternomastoid muscle, i.e. in the posterior triangle of the neck (Fig. 20.2).

Figure 20.2 *Cystic hygroma. Contrast-enhanced CT scan at C6 level shows low-density thin-walled lesion (✻) beneath left sternomastoid muscle (S). Left internal jugular vein (arrows) compressed and displaced medially.*

Figure 20.3 *Thyroglossal duct cyst. Contrast-enhanced CT scan just below hyoid bone shows anterior superficial midline low-density structure (✻).*

(a)   *(b)*

Figure 20.4 *Lipoma. (a) Ultrasound scan. Echogenic lobulated mass (M) lying between the heads of the sternomastoid muscle (SM). (b) CT scan shows very low density mass (M) indicating fat consistency. C = common carotid artery; ✳ = internal jugular vein.*

THYROGLOSSAL DUCT CYST

This can arise at any site along the thyroglossal duct but is usually below the hyoid bone. Most thyroglossal cysts present in childhood and are usually midline in position. The cyst is well demonstrated by CT scanning (Fig. 20.3).

BENIGN TUMOURS OF THE NECK

LIPOMAS

Lipomas occur in the neck and are benign encapsulated lesions. Ultrasound scanning (Fig. 20.4a) reveals a very well-demarcated hyperechoic mass, which will confirm the clinical impression of a lipoma. CT scanning (Fig. 20.4b) shows the mass to be of very low density with an attenuation value of fat, a finding that is diagnostic for lipoma. CT may be preferred by the surgeon since the anatomy is more clearly demonstrated than with ultrasound.

HAEMANGIOMAS

This congenital lesion may occur at any site in the face or neck. Rarely it is very extensive and may involve the oropharynx, causing partial obstruction. Radiographs may show multiple opacities representing phleboliths within the tumour and CT scanning reveals a hypervascular infiltrating mass (Fig. 20.5).

(a)   *(b)*

Figure 20.5 *Cavernous haemangioma in an 11-year-old child. This was present at birth but grew to involve cheeks, oropharynx and right side of neck. (a) Pan-oral view shows multiple ring shadows (arrows) from phleboliths. (b) CT scan of oropharynx shows widespread soft-tissue masses (M) almost occluding the oropharynx. Phleboliths (arrows) again demonstrated.*

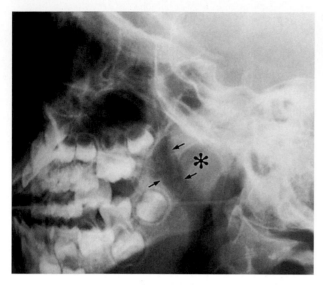

Figure 20.6 *Adenoidal hypertrophy in an 11-year-old child. Note airway narrowing (arrows) by nasopharyngeal mass (٭) posteriorly.*

PHARYNX

INFLAMMATORY DISEASE

Tonsils and adenoids

Hypertrophy of the pharyngeal lymphoid tissue is usually present in childhood and commonly causes symptoms, i.e. mouth breathing and snoring, and, because of eustachian tube obstruction, may result in deafness. A lateral radiograph of the neck (Fig. 20.6) will demonstrate the amount of soft-tissue thickening in the postnasal space and indicate the size of the airway. It is unusual for adenoidal hypertrophy to be symptomatic in adult life. Enlargement of the adenoids can be demonstrated on CT scanning (Fig. 20.7), but a

Figure 20.8 *Tonsillar abscess. CT scan of oropharynx shows bilateral tonsillar enlargement with low-density abscess (٭) in right tonsil.*

biopsy may be required to distinguish hypertrophy from other causes of enlargement such as lymphoma.

Tonsillar enlargement may also be demonstrated but is itself not an indication for radiography. Tonsillar infection, however, may lead to a peritonsillar abscess, the extent of which can be readily assessed by CT scanning (Fig. 20.8). The abscess cavity contains fluid contents, which are of low density, and its wall is thick, with loss of the adjacent fat planes from inflammatory oedema.

Figure 20.7 *Adenoidal hypertrophy in adult. CT scan shows lobulated soft-tissue mass (arrows) in postnasal space.*

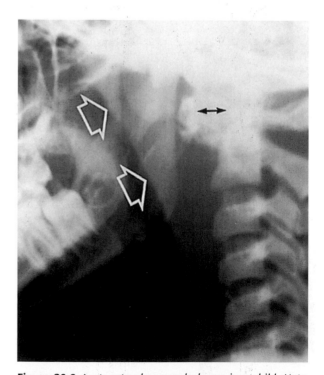

Figure 20.9 *Acute retropharyngeal abscess in a child. Note increased thickness of soft tissues most marked in the nasopharynx (white arrows) and associated atlantoaxial subluxation (arrowheads).*

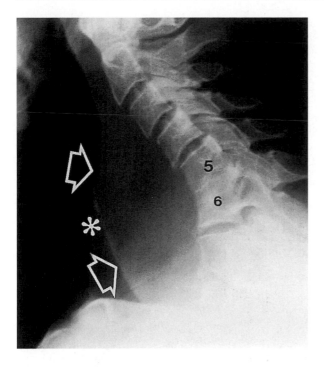

Figure 20.10 *Tuberculous spondylitis causing ankylosis of C5 and C6 vertebral bodies with retropharyngeal abscess (arrows). Note anterior displacement of larynx (✳).*

Retropharyngeal infection

In young children, retropharyngeal infection can lead to abscess formation, the extent of which may be assessed by means of a lateral radiograph of the neck. Infection may spread to the adjacent vertebrae, leading to atlantoaxial subluxation (Fig. 20.9). Conversely, pyogenic or tuberculous infection of the cervical spine may extend to the prevertebral soft tissues, resulting in an abscess (Fig. 20.10).

SWALLOWED FOREIGN BODIES

If there is clinical suspicion of impaction of a foreign body in the pharynx or cervical oesophagus, a lateral radiograph of the neck is indicated. High-density material, such as bones (Fig. 20.11) or metallic objects, will be visible. When the impacted foreign body is not radiopaque, e.g. a plastic dental plate (Fig. 20.12), a barium study will demonstrate it as a filling defect within the lumen of the pharynx or oesophagus.

If perforation of the wall of the pharynx or oesophagus has occurred, resulting haemorrhage or oedema

Figure 20.11 *Swallowed chicken bone. Bone fragment (black arrows) impacted at C7 level. Note thyroid cartilage ossification (✳) and calcified nodule (white arrow) in thyroid gland.*

Figure 20.12 *Impacted radiolucent foreign body. Swallowed broken plastic dental plate. Plain radiograph normal. Barium swallow shows plate as irregular filling defect (arrows) at C7/T1 level.*

(a)   *(b)*

Figure 20.13 *Cricoid cartilage calcification. Dysphagia after swallowing bone. Endoscopy was normal. (a) Linear density (arrow) at C6 level is due to calcification posteriorly in cricoid cartilage. (b) CT scan confirms this.*

causes thickening of the prevertebral soft tissues and may produce surgical emphysema, which may spread into the mediastinum and around the thorax. Abscess formation may develop in the mediastinum. When a perforation is suspected, water-soluble contrast should be used rather than barium because of the risk of barium spreading extraluminally into the soft tissues.

Problems of interpretation of the plain radiograph arise when other opaque structures are present in the neck. These include calcification within lymph nodes and the thyroid gland. Calcification/ossification of the laryngeal cartilages (Fig. 20.13) is commonly incomplete and inhomogeneous. This, as well as the minor laryngeal cartilages, may be mistaken for a swallowed foreign body. It must also be remembered that symptoms may be due to laceration of the mucosa by a foreign body that has not impacted and cannot, therefore, be demonstrated.

PHARYNGEAL DIVERTICULUM (ZENKER'S DIVERTICULUM)

This acquired pulsion diverticulum occurs more commonly in the elderly. A pouch of mucosa protrudes posteriorly through a weakness in the inferior pharyngeal constrictor between its oblique and transverse (cricopharyngeus) portions. Food can accumulate in the pouch, which enlarges, resulting in oesophageal compression causing dysphagia, cough and regurgitation of food eaten hours earlier.

A barium swallow examination (Fig. 20.14) opacifies the diverticulum, which, if large, is directed laterally (usually to the left) as well as posteriorly. It may extend downwards into the mediastinum. Resulting oesophageal compression, as well as any aspiration of barium, is also demonstrated.

Figure 20.14 *Pharyngeal diverticulum. Barium swallow shows posterior diverticulum (✻) at C5 level compressing the pharyngo-oesophageal junction (arrows).*

POSTCRICOID WEB

A web is a thin mucosal membrane that projects at right angles from the anterior aspect of the hypopharynx. Webs may be multiple and, when large, are crescentic. A postcricoid web causes dysphagia and, although often an isolated finding, may be associated with iron-deficiency anaemia and an increased incidence of carcinoma. A barium swallow examination shows very clearly on the lateral view even a small web (Fig. 20.15). As with all barium studies of the pharynx and oesophagus, video recording of the examination allows

Figure 20.15 *Pharyngeal web. Barium swallow reveals thin shelf-like membrane (arrow) projecting anteriorly into hypopharynx at C5/6 level.*

Figure 20.16 *Cervical spondylosis. Large anterior osteophytes (arrows) at C4 to C6 levels causing dysphagia in a patient aged 80 years.*

playback in slow motion for closer scrutiny of the abnormal findings.

CERVICAL SPONDYLOSIS

In the elderly, osteophytes may impinge on the pharynx (Fig. 20.16) but rarely cause dysphagia.

JUVENILE NASOPHARYNGEAL ANGIOFIBROMA

This uncommon, benign, very vascular tumour of adolescent males may cause epistaxis and nasal obstruction. Juvenile nasopharyngeal angiofibroma arises in the sphenopalatine foramen and may spread anteriorly into the nasal cavity, or laterally into the pterygopalatine and infratemporal fossae. Superior extension may occur into the sphenoid, ethmoid or cavernous sinuses and through the medial wall of the middle cranial fossa.

Because biopsy of this vascular tumour is contraindicated, diagnosis is made by imaging techniques, which must also show the extent of the tumour as well as its vascular supply, since therapeutic embolization may be performed prior to surgery. CT scanning with intravenous contrast enhancement (Fig. 20.17) shows the extent of the tumour which appears hyperdense owing to its vascular nature. In addition, CT will demonstrate the characteristic medial pterygoid plate erosion as well

Figure 20.17 *Juvenile nasopharyngeal angiofibroma. Axial CT scan with intravenous contrast. Large enhancing mass (open arrows) obstructs nasopharynx and extends anteriorly into nose mainly on the left side (curved arrow).*

as any infiltration of the skull base with intracranial extension. Angiography demonstrates the marked tumour circulation, which is derived usually from the internal maxillary branch of the external carotid artery.

PHARYNGEAL TUMOURS

Pharyngeal tumours are discussed on page 499.

Figure 20.18 *Epiglottis. Lateral radiograph of neck showing swollen epiglottis (arrow). H = hyoid bone. (Courtesy of Dr Otto Chan, The Royal London Hospital.)*

LARYNX

LARYNGITIS

Inflammatory oedema of the larynx is a cause of dyspnoea and in children is usually the result of viral or bacterial infections (laryngotracheobronchitis). Swallowed irritant liquids or inhaled toxic gases, as well as allergic reactions, may all result in laryngeal oedema. The soft-tissue swelling of the larynx and any associated airway narrowing are readily appreciated on conventional radiography (Fig. 20.18) or CT scanning.

LARYNGEAL TRAUMA

Laryngeal trauma may occur in road traffic accidents and assault cases and also from knife wounds to the neck. Although a hyoid fracture and any surgical emphysema (Fig. 20.19) are usually detectable on conventional radiographs, fractures of the laryngeal cartilages are unlikely to be diagnosed. However, CT scanning clearly demonstrates fractures or dislocations of these cartilages, together with any resulting narrowing of the airway. Untreated cartilage fractures may lead to laryngeal stenosis.

(a)

(b)

Figure 20.19 *Laryngeal trauma. (a) Lateral view of neck with extensive dark streaks (arrows) owing to air in soft tissues. Note laryngeal cartilages (✳) but no fracture seen. (b) Chest radiograph indicates spread of emphysema over right supraclavicular region (large arrow) and into mediastinum (small arrows).*

LARYNGOCELE

An air- or mucus-filled sac may originate in the laryngeal ventricle, probably as a congenital anomaly. The sac can extend upwards and may cause airway obstruc-

Figure 20.20 *Nasopharyngeal carcinoma. CT scan shows right-sided tumour (*) obliterating lateral pharyngeal recess on that side. Loss of adjacent fat planes indicates infiltration of parapharyngeal space. Note normal left lateral pharyngeal recess (arrow).*

tion. An internal laryngocele is one that remains within the thyroid cartilage. If the sac bursts through the thyrohyoid membrane to lie outside the thyroid cartilage, it is termed an external laryngocele. Mixed types occur and laryngoceles may be bilateral. CT scanning will allow a precise diagnosis.

MALIGNANT TUMOURS OF PHARYNX AND LARYNX

Squamous cell carcinomas make up 90 per cent or more of the primary tumours in this region. In most cases, the clinician makes the diagnosis by endoscopy and mucosal biopsy. If it is suspected that the tumour extends deeply, or if enlarged lymph nodes are palpable, then imaging with CT or preferably MRI is necessary. Even if no primary tumour is clinically detected, scanning is required if the following signs or symptoms suspicious of malignancy are present:

- nasal obstruction, discharge or bleeding;
- middle ear symptoms (from eustachian tube obstruction);
- cervical lymphadenopathy;
- cranial nerve defects (from skull-base infiltration).

CT or MRI scanning is necessary in the following situations:

- As part of the **staging of the tumour**, in accordance with the TNM classification system. Scanning reveals:
  - the size and full extent of the tumour
  - associated destruction of bone or cartilage
  - lymph node involvement;
- **Treatment planning**, i.e. surgery or radiotherapy.
- **Follow-up**, to determine the response to treatment and to detect any tumour recurrence.

NASOPHARYNGEAL CARCINOMA

In 50 per cent of patients, the presenting complaint is a mass in the neck from lymphadenopathy. Although the nasopharynx extends from the skull base only to the soft palate inferiorly, axial scans are obtained down to the heads of the clavicles whenever a nasopharyngeal carcinoma is identified, in order to defect any associated lymphadenopathy. Coronal sections are necessary for proper assessment of the skull base.

The tumour usually arises in the region of the lateral pharyngeal recess and commonly extends to the parapharyngeal space (Fig. 20.20) and may obstruct a eustachian tube orifice, resulting in fluid in the middle

(a)

(b)

Figure 20.21 *Lymphadenopathy. MRI using fat-suppression sequence. (a) Reactive: the nodes (n) appear as high signal. V = blood vessels; S = submandibular glands. (b) Malignant: enlarged supraclavicular and mediastinal nodes from breast cancer (arrowed). (Courtesy of Dr Otto Chan, The Royal London Hospital and Dr Wailup Wong, Mount Vernon Hospital, Middlesex.)*

Figure 20.22 *Advanced nasopharyngeal carcinoma. On MRI gadolinium-enhanced T1-weighted coronal scan, a large high-signal tumour mass (T) can be seen filling nasopharynx and extending through skull base and cavernous sinus into left middle cranial fossa (arrow). Note excellent definition of tumour margins.*

ear or mastoid on that side. The tumour may extend intracranially via the foramen lacerum or foramen ovale, and skull-base erosion can occur. Lymphadenopathy is detected in approximately 70 per cent of cases, usually in the upper cervical lymph nodes but, in the minority of cases, extension to the lower cervical nodes occurs.

On T2-weighted MRI images, normal mucosa, tumour and lymph nodes, both reactive or metastatic, are seen as high signal against low-signal muscle. Fat also has a high signal and can obscure a tumour or node, and therefore further imaging is performed using a fat-suppression sequence. Both reactive and malignant lymphadenopathy have a similar appearance on the various sequences (Fig. 20.21).

When a tumour is suspected from these images, a contrast-enhanced MRI scan is required to show the tumour clearly. The tumour margins show a high signal (Fig. 20.22) against the lower signal non-enhancing muscle. Inflammatory oedema does not obscure these margins. In addition, malignant lymph nodes usually show bright outer margins, i.e. peripheral enhancement (Fig. 20.23).

A coronal image is also obtained through the nasopharynx to indicate the extent of the tumour. Coronal images are useful for radiotherapy planning.

CT scanning is an alternative imaging method, although the tumour is less well distinguished from adjacent structures. Contrast enhancement is used in order to increase the density of the tumour tissue and to identify the blood vessels. Malignant lymph nodes are usually over 10 mm in size. The nodes normally show peripheral enhancement but may be seen as low-density masses. Any bone erosion (Fig. 20.24), e.g. of the pterygoid plates, is easily recognized on CT.

OROPHARYNGEAL CARCINOMA

The oropharynx extends from the soft palate inferiorly to the hyoid bone and includes the pharyngeal walls, tonsillar region and base of tongue. The oropharynx is separated from the larynx by the epiglottis and from the hypopharynx by the pharyngo-epiglottic folds.

The patient usually complains of a tonsillar mass, with pain on swallowing, and more than half the

(a)

(b)

Figure 20.23 *Malignant lymph node from nasopharyngeal carcinoma (✳). MRI T1-weighted sagittal scans: (a) pre- and (b) post-gadolinium-enhanced scans. Note ring enhancement (arrow) of suprasternal node on scan (b). (Courtesy of Dr Wailup Wong, Mount Vernon Hospital, Middlesex.)*

Figure 20.24 *Nasopharyngeal carcinoma stage T3 N1. Axial CT scan indicates large tumour (✴) involving left pterygoid muscles and invading left maxillary sinus, with erosion of left pterygoid plates and posterior wall of left maxillary sinus (arrows).*

Figure 20.26 *Carcinoma of tongue. Axial MRI with fat-suppression sequence shows high-signal tumour mass (M) confined to right side of tongue but involving the adjacent tonsillar fossa (arrow). High signal of right submandibular gland (S) is due to inflammation resulting from duct obstruction by tumour. (Courtesy of Dr Otto Chan, The Royal London Hospital.)*

patients have nodal metastases in the internal jugular chain at presentation. The tumour is usually more extensive than clinically apparent, i.e. it commonly spreads to other compartments of the pharynx. The tumour often infiltrates the parapharyngeal space, the prevertebral muscles or around the carotid artery (Fig. 20.25) and may extend into the tongue or larynx. Conversely, a primary carcinoma of the tongue not infrequently spreads to the adjacent tonsillar fossa (Fig. 20.26).

CT scanning identifies the tumour and any associated lymphadenopathy as an enhancing mass displacing tissue planes, and the mass may have a low-density central region from necrosis. It may, however, be impossible to distinguish between malignant and suppurative lymphadenopathy. CT images of the oropharynx are often degraded by streak artefacts from dental amalgam and, because of this and the better demonstration of the soft tissues, MRI is the scanning method of choice for staging oropharyngeal tumours.

HYPOPHARYNGEAL CARCINOMA

The hypopharynx extends from the hyoid bone inferiorly to the cricopharyngeus muscle and includes the piriform sinuses and postcricoid region. The piriform sinuses are situated on either side of the aryepiglottic folds of the larynx and the true vocal cords, and are related laterally to the thyroid cartilage. The postcricoid region joins the oesophagus at the lower border of the cricoid.

Symptoms of squamous cell carcinoma of the hypopharynx include sore throat, dysphagia and otalgia, as well as enlarged cervical lymph nodes. Hoarseness indicates laryngeal invasion. On presentation, the tumour is often advanced (T3 or T4 stage).

The majority of tumours arise in a piriform sinus (Fig. 20.27) and often extend posterolaterally into the soft tissues of the neck and around the carotid artery, and may cause erosion of the thyroid cartilage. Malignant lymphadenopathy is present in 50 per cent of cases, usually at the mandibular angle on the affected side. MRI with contrast enhancement shows well both the extent of the tumour and any lymphadenopathy, but CT scanning is better for displaying cartilage erosion (Fig. 20.28).

Postcricoid carcinoma causes dysphagia. The tumour tends to spread early, either upwards, into the

Figure 20.25 *Carcinoma of tonsil. Enhanced CT scan shows poorly enhancing ill-defined mass (✴) extending posteriorly (arrow) to carotid sheath. Note loss of adjacent fat planes.*

Figure 20.27 *Carcinoma of piriform sinus. CT scan showing large mass (M) obliterating left sinus. Note normal air-filled right pyriform sinus (PS).*

oro- and nasopharynx, or inferiorly into the oeso-phagus. Bilateral internal jugular node involvement is common and the tumour has therefore a poor progno-sis. MRI or CT scanning will demonstrate the extent of the tumour and nodal involvement, but tumour assess-ment is difficult in the postcricoid region because of the normal variation of soft-tissue thickness at this site. A barium swallow examination will aid endoscopy in ascertaining the extent of the mucosal spread of tumour (Fig. 20.29).

LARYNGEAL CARCINOMA

As with pharyngeal malignancy, the diagnosis is made and the mucosal extent of the laryngeal carcinoma is assessed by endoscopy and biopsy. If deeper extension of the tumour is suspected, then MRI or CT scanning of the whole neck is required for staging, prior to therapy, in order to reveal:

- the extent of tumour in the supraglottic or subglot-tic region and any spread to extralaryngeal struc-tures;
- anterior or posterior commissure involvement by glottic tumours;
- cartilage destruction (but assessment is not entirely accurate, owing to normal variation in ossification);
- nodal disease.

CT scanning of the larynx is performed during quiet respiration when the vocal cords are abducted. An enhanced scan with an intravenous injection of contrast medium is also made to identify blood vessels and detect nodal malignancy. MRI gives better soft-tissue contrast and can differentiate the tumour from muscle

(a)

(b)

Figure 20.28 *Carcinoma of piriform sinus. (a) Contrast-enhanced CT scan shows left-sided tumour (T) obliterating left pirIform sinus, and also left lymph node metastasis (N) showing ring enhancement and central necrosis. (b) Recurrence 9 months later with tumour extension (✳) in left side of neck and erosion of thyroid cartilage (arrows) on that side. Note malignant lymphadenopathy (N).*

and fat. Contrast enhancement aids this differentiation and nodal disease is also better identified on postcon-trast images. Coronal images are obtained to verify the origin and extent of glottic and subglottic tumours.

Supraglottic carcinoma

One third of laryngeal tumours arise in the supraglot-tis, which extends from the epiglottis to the false vocal cords and includes the aryepiglottic folds and laryngeal ventricle. Hoarseness is a late symptom and the tumour is usually advanced at presentation; more than 50 per cent of cases have metastases in the internal jugular nodes. Epiglottic tumours (Fig. 20.30) tend to spread to the pre-epiglottic space and tongue base. Carcinoma of

Figure 20.29 *Postcricoid carcinoma. Barium swallow examination showing irregular stricture (arrows) 7 cm long and centred at postcricoid level.*

Figure 20.30 *Supraglottic carcinoma of the larynx. CT scan at level of hyoid bone (H) level reveals tumour (T) of epiglottis extending into right pharyngo-epiglottic fold (arrow).*

the ventricle and false cords may destroy the thyroid cartilage or extend through the true vocal cords to the subglottis.

Glottic carcinoma

Carcinoma of the vocal cords (Fig. 20.31) is the commonest laryngeal tumour and presents early

Figure 20.31 *Carcinoma of left vocal cord. Stage T3 N0 tumour. CT scan showing mass (arrow) extending to anterior commissure but no further, i.e. no spread outside larynx and no erosion of thyroid cartilage.*

because of the associated hoarseness. This, together with slow tumour growth and the sparse lymphatic drainage, accounts for the good prognosis of this malignancy. Thus, most cases are stage I tumours and do not require radiological imaging. Scanning is reserved for more advanced tumours, which may show spread to the anterior commissure and from the anterior commissure to the opposite cord and supra- or subglottic region (Fig. 20.32), possibly with thyroid cartilage destruction. Some tumours spread to the posterior commissure, with cord fixation and erosion of the arytenoid and cricoid cartilages.

Subglottic carcinoma

The subglottis is the region from the under-surface of the true vocal cords to the lower border of cricoid cartilage. Most tumours in this region are extensions from glottic primary tumours and a true subglottic tumour is rare. A subglottic carcinoma usually presents at an advanced stage, and scanning may show spread of the tumour to the vocal cords or extension into the trachea or hypopharynx, with invasion of the cricoid or tracheal cartilages (Fig. 20.33).

LYMPHOMA

Lymphoma usually involves the lymph nodes, tonsils or adenoids but is relatively uncommon elsewhere in the head or neck. The appearances are usually obvious on MRI or CT scans, which show multiple, often bilateral, enlarged, homogeneous lymph nodes (Fig. 20.34). No central necrosis of the nodes is present but, following therapy, necrosis or even calcification can occur. Bone erosion may occur (Fig. 20.35).

(a)

(b)

(c)

Figure 20.32 *Carcinoma of right vocal cord with subglottic extension. (a) CT scan at level of true vocal cords shows large tumour (T) of the right cord, extending across midline both anteriorly and posteriorly (arrows). (b) At cricoid level the scan indicates subglottic tumour (T) extension. (c) MRI coronal scan, fat-suppression sequence shows tumour (✻) and subglottic extension (arrow) very well defined. (Courtesy of Dr Wailup Wong, Mount Vernon Hospital, Middlesex.)*

Figure 20.33 *Subglottic laryngeal carcinoma. Contrast-enhanced CT scan just below level of true vocal cord. Note large tumour (T) almost occluding airway and causing erosion (arrows) of cricoid lamina.*

Figure 20.34 *Non-Hodgkin's lymphoma. CT scan shows multiple bilateral homogeneous enlarged lymph nodes (✻) in the neck. Note dense appearance of thyroid gland (T).*

Because lymphoma presenting in the neck is, in the majority of patients, part of a more widespread disease, CT scanning of the thorax, abdomen and pelvis may also be required for staging. In the less common instances in which lymphoma occurs as a single extra-nodal lesion in the neck, CT or MRI scanning will not differentiate lymphoma from any other primary or secondary malignancy.

MALIGNANT LYMPHADENOPATHY

When nodal malignancy is present in the neck, the patient is usually known to have a primary tumour (Fig. 20.36). Sometimes, there is no clinically obvious primary malignancy. If the involved node lies in the upper half of the neck, i.e. above the cricoid, it is likely that the malignancy has spread from the pharynx,

(a)   (b)

Figure 20.35 *Lymphoma of nasopharynx. (a) CT scan shows large tumour mass (✽) on right side, with obliteration of right lateral pharyngeal recess and parapharyngeal space, and filling infratemporal fossa on that side. Note erosion of right pterygoid plates (arrow). (b) Extensive erosion of skull base (✽) is seen on right side.*

(a)   (b)

Figure 20.36 *Malignant lymphadenopathy: squamous cell carcinoma of oropharynx. CT scan at thyrohyoid level shows large lymph node (a) before and (b) after intravenous contrast enhancement. Note ring enhancement (arrows) and necrotic areas (✽) in enlarged node. Opacified blood vessels are well shown on the enhanced scan (b).*

larynx or parotid glands. Submandibular node involvement is common in squamous carcinoma of the face or oral cavity.

Malignant lymphadenopathy in the lower half of the neck can be the result of carcinoma of the thyroid, oesophagus or breast. However, bronchial carcinoma is the commonest cause of right supraclavicular lymph node enlargement, whereas left supraclavicular lymphadenopathy is more likely to be due to a subdiaphragmatic primary tumour. Lymphoma or metastatic melanoma may involve lymph nodes at any site in the neck (Fig. 20.37).

Although ultrasound can detect nodes as small as 5 mm and can guide a fine-needle aspiration biopsy (Fig. 20.38), contrast-enhanced CT or MRI scanning is a better imaging technique than ultrasound because:

- CT and MRI examine at the same time the likely primary tumour site in the neck. Depending on the clinical presentation, scanning of the thorax and abdomen may also be performed.
- Lymphadenopathy is better demonstrated. Any node with central necrosis, even if less than 10 mm, is considered malignant.

Figure 20.37 *CT scan of malignant lymphadenopathy from melanoma of left forearm. Note several homogeneous enlarged lymph nodes (✱) in left lower cervical group.*

Figure 20.39 *Suppurative lymphadenopathy. CT scan with intravenous contrast at hyoid level. Necrotic nodes with ring enhancement and low-density centres (N). Note thickening of skin and subcutaneous fat (arrows) from inflammatory oedema.*

(a)

(b)

Figure 20.38 *Enlarged lymph node at cricoid level. (a) Ultrasound and (b) CT transverse scans show node (✱) 2.5 cm long, with non-specific appearances. Biopsy indicated squamous cell carcinoma from a nasopharyngeal primary tumour. A = carotid artery; V = internal jugular vein.*

Figure 20.40 *Supraglottic laryngeal cancer at 12 months post-treatment CT scan. Stage T1 N3 tumour treated by left neck dissection and radiotherapy. Scan at thyrohyoid level shows left-sided soft-tissue mass (✱) in laryngeal vestibule, but endoscopic biopsy showed no tumour recurrence. Note thickening of skin and subcutaneous fat (arrows) owing to radiotherapy. Left submandibular gland and sternomastoid muscle have been removed.*

- CT and MRI assess the deep lymph nodes, e.g. the retropharyngeal group, which are not visualized by ultrasound.

Differential diagnosis of lymphadenopathy on CT/MRI

- In reactive lymphadenopathy, i.e. owing to adjacent inflammation, the nodes remain homogeneous and a nearby inflammatory focus may be demonstrated.

(a)   *(b)*

Figure 20.41 *Thrombosis of right internal jugular vein, complicating supraglottic carcinoma. (a) Contrast-enhanced CT scan. Note distended vein with central low density (arrow) representing thrombus within high-density vein wall. (b) Ultrasound scan at same level. Note hyperechoic thrombus totally occluding vein (V). Patent common carotid artery (A) also seen.*

Suppurative lymphadenopathy, i.e. an intranodal abscess (Fig. 20.39), appears exactly similar to a node with carcinomatous involvement. However, the clinical presentation and demonstration of an inflammatory focus should differentiate between the two.

- Tuberculous lymphadenopathy is usually seen as a mass of nodes matted together and may contain areas of calcification. These appearances are unlike those of malignancy.

Post-treatment scanning

Three months after laryngeal surgery, the patient has a baseline MRI at which time all the postsurgical inflammatory changes should have resolved. Later, if there is recurrence of tumour, this is usually obvious clinically or identified by biopsy. The extent of any submucosal spread of recurrent tumour will require a repeat MRI scan (T1-weighted with contrast) to compare with the baseline study. Vascular scar tissue has the same appearance as recurrent tumour. Therefore, in doubtful cases, it is often necessary to repeat this scan again in a further 2 months when any tumour recurrence will be obvious.

During a course of radiotherapy, scanning is performed at regular intervals in order to monitor therapy and repeated after the course of radiotherapy has been completed. A major problem is that irradiation causes a generalized thickening of the soft tissues, with loss of fat planes, because of persisting oedema. This can mask or mimic tumour recurrence on MRI or CT images (Fig. 20.40). MRI scanning of the larynx after radiotherapy is only 50 per cent accurate compared with the results of biopsy.

VENOUS THROMBOSIS

Thrombosis of an internal jugular vein is not uncommon and is usually due to compression of the vein by metastatic lymphadenopathy. Other causes of thrombosis of the internal jugular vein include any obstructing mass in the neck or thoracic inlet, an adjacent inflammatory focus and central venous catheterization.

Ultrasound scanning will show clearly the presence and extent of a thrombus and whether it is totally or only partially occluding the vein. A contrast-enhanced CT scan gives less detailed information but will detect a totally occluded vein and will usually better demonstrate the underlying cause of the thrombosis (Fig. 20.41).

FURTHER READING

Delbalso, A.M. 1990: *Maxillofacial imaging*. Philadelphia: W.B. Saunders.

Gillespie, J.E., Gholkar, A. (eds) 1994: *Magnetic resonance imaging and computed tomography of the head and neck*. London: Chapman & Hall.

Harnsberger, H.R. 1995: *Handbook of head and neck imaging* (2nd edition). St Louis: Mosby.

Hasso, A.N. 1993: *MRI atlas of the head and neck*. London: Martin Dunitz.

Lufkin, R.B., Hanafee, W.N. 1989: *Pocket atlas of head and neck MRI anatomy*. New York: Raven Press.

Mukherji, S.K., Pillsbury, H.R., Castillo, M. 1997: Imaging squamous cell carcinomas of the upper aerodigestive tract: what clinicians need to know. *Radiology* **205**, 629–46.

Shankar, L., Khan, A., Cheuyng, G. 1998: *Head and neck imaging*. New York: McGraw Hill.

Som, P.M., Curtin, H.D. 1995: Lesions of the parapharyngeal space. Role of MRI imaging. *Otolaryngologic Clinics of North America* **28**(3), 515–42.

Som, P.M., Curtin, H.D. (eds) 1996: *Head and neck imaging* (3rd edition). St Louis: Mosby.

Som, P.M., Shapiro, M.D. (eds) 1989: MRI of the head and neck. *Radiologic Clinics of North America* **27**(2).

Vogl, T.J., Balzer, J., Mack, M., Steger, W. 1999: *Differential diagnosis in head and neck imaging*. Stuttgart: Thième.

21

Thyroid and parathyroids

MARTIN L. WASTIE

Thyroid disease is common, although it is not always diagnosed clinically. The main conditions include hyperthyroidism, hypothyroidism and non-toxic goitre, which are all commoner in females than in males. The correct management of thyroid disease depends on an accurate diagnosis.

Hyperthyroidism and hypothyroidism are diagnosed clinically and by the biochemical estimation of the serum levels of tri-iodothyronine (T3), thyroxine (T4) and thyroid-stimulating hormone (TSH). Imaging plays no part in the initial diagnosis of hyper- or hypothyroidism. The important role of imaging in thyroid disease is in the investigation of the thyroid nodule, intrathoracic goitre and thyroid eye disease, and in the management of thyroid cancer.

THYROID

ANATOMY

The lateral lobes of the thyroid measure 5 cm in length and 2.0–2.5 cm in both thickness and width at their widest diameter. The two lateral lobes are joined by an isthmus of variable thickness that crosses the second and third tracheal rings anteriorly. A third lobe, the pyramidal lobe, is sometimes present, arising from the isthmus or adjacent portion of either lobe, more commonly the left. There may be asymmetry in the size of the lateral lobes, with the right lobe normally being larger than the left. The thin capsule of the gland is connected to the pretracheal fascia outside of which lie the sternothyroid muscles. The gland is fixed to the anterior and lateral aspect of the trachea by connective tissue. The carotid arteries and sternocleidomastoid muscles lie lateral to the gland.

IMAGING TECHNIQUES

PLAIN FILMS

A chest radiograph or views of the thoracic inlet may show a soft-tissue mass owing to a goitre in the neck which may be displacing the trachea (Fig. 21.1). An important feature is any compression or narrowing of the trachea. The degree of compression may be judged by assessing the diameter of the trachea on both the frontal and lateral views. The sternoclavicular joints mark the position of the thoracic inlet. Any deviation or compression of the trachea below this level indicates the presence of an intrathoracic or retrosternal goitre. Calcification within a goitre may occur in both benign and malignant tumours, although any obvious coarse calcification is likely to be benign. Displacement and compression of the oesophagus by a goitre may be demonstrated on a barium swallow (Fig. 21.2).

ULTRASOUND

Ultrasound has now become the most important imaging modality for examining the thyroid. It is easily

Figure 21.1 *Goitre. Chest radiograph showing a goitre compressing and narrowing the trachea (arrows).*

Figure 21.2 *Barium swallow showing the oesophagus displaced to the right by a goitre.*

performed by direct contact scanning with a high-frequency (7.5–10 MHz) transducer. The patient lies with the neck extended, and the neck is smeared with jelly to ensure acoustic coupling between the transducer and the skin. Ultrasound gives a good demonstration of the isthmus and the lateral lobes lying adjacent to the air-filled trachea with the carotid artery lying lateral to the gland (Fig. 21.3). The gland has a homogeneous pattern owing to the numerous follicles, and the echo pattern is of higher echogenicity than the adjacent muscles. Images are routinely taken in the axial and sagittal planes. Abnormalities as small as 1 mm in diameter can be detected.

RADIONUCLIDE SCANNING

Scintigraphy has long been the mainstay of thyroid imaging but has to a large extent been replaced by ultrasound scanning, but scintigraphy still has an important role to play. Both ^{99m}Tc-pertechnetate and ^{123}I may be used for imaging. The patient is given an intravenous injection of ^{99m}Tc and scans of the neck taken with a gamma camera 20 minutes later. Alternatively scans can be taken 2 hours after an intravenous injection of ^{123}I.

^{123}I is both trapped and organified by the gland whereas ^{99m}Tc is only trapped. ^{123}I gives less background activity and so results in superior pictures of the thyroid compared to ^{99m}Tc, but ^{123}I is less readily available and more expensive. ^{131}I, because of its high thyroid and body dose, is used only when investigating patients with known thyroid cancer.

Figure 21.3 *Normal ultrasound. The two lobes of the thyroid lie on either side of the trachea (T). The carotid arteries (C) lie lateral to the gland.*

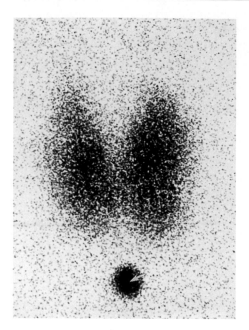

Figure 21.4 *Normal* ^{123}I *scan. The arrow points to a marker on the suprasternal notch.*

Figure 21.5 *Normal CT scan. The enhancing lobes of the thyroid lie on either side of the trachea (T); the carotid arteries are well opacified (arrows). S = sternocleidomastoid muscle.*

A normal thyroid scan shows homogeneous uptake by the two lobes angled towards each other inferiorly and joined by the isthmus (Fig. 21.4). Any asymmetry of the lobes is easy to recognize.

COMPUTED TOMOGRAPHY

CT is used in selected cases such as demonstrating the spread of malignancy in the neck and demonstrating an intrathoracic goitre. The normal thyroid can be seen as a homogeneous structure with higher attenuation than the adjacent soft tissues, the high attenuation being due to the iodine content of the gland. The thyroid enhances quite markedly after intravenous contrast administration (Fig. 21.5).

MAGNETIC RESONANCE IMAGING

MRI also gives an excellent demonstration of the thyroid (Fig. 21.6), and like CT is only used in selected cases. Because of its multiplanar facility, it can readily demonstrate intrathoracic extension of a goitre and its relation to the major vessels.

Figure 21.6 *MRI scan. T1-weighted scan showing colloid nodule (N) in the right lobe of the thyroid. T = trachea. S = sternocleidomastoid muscles; arrows = carotid arteries.*

THYROID NODULES

The finding of a palpable thyroid nodule is a common clinical problem and is by far the commonest indication for imaging the thyroid. Palpable nodules are found in about 4 per cent of the population with 50 per cent thought to be solitary nodules. Nodules are found in 50 per cent of glands *post mortem*, and ultrasound shows a similar number of nodules, although most are not detected clinically. The incidence of malignancy in a single nodule is thought to be about 20–30 per cent, so the problem is how to detect this group and avoid unnecessary surgery on the remainder. Different imaging methods have been advocated using both ultrasound and scintigraphy, whilst recently there has been widespread use of fine-needle aspiration cytology, which many would regard as the preferred investigation.

(a)

(b)

(c)

Figure 21.7 *(a) Solitary nodule. (a) Cyst in right lobe of thyroid; (b) colloid nodule in right lobe showing solid and cystic areas; (c) adenoma appearing as a solid nodule (N) in right lobe.*

The role of imaging is:

- to decide whether a nodule is solitary or multiple;
- to attempt to determine the nature of a solitary nodule;
- to detect a functioning nodule.

ULTRASOUND

This is the best initial imaging investigation. Ultrasound may show that a suspected nodule is not solitary but one of several nodules in a multinodular goitre: in a third of patients with nodules, thought on clinical examination to be solitary, the nodules are shown by imaging to be multiple. The **typical nodule** has the same echo pattern as the rest of the gland and is recognized by a surrounding lower echogenic zone. There may be a low echogenic cystic component in the nodule owing to accumulated colloid, central degeneration or haemorrhage. The incidence of cancer in a multinodular goitre is considerably lower than in a solitary nodule and it has been quoted that 1 per cent or less of multinodular goitres are malignant. However, a dominant swelling in a multinodular goitre may indicate malignancy and should be regarded with greater suspicion.

A solitary lesion may be due to an adenoma, colloid nodule, simple cyst, haemorrhagic or degenerating cyst, focus of inflammation or carcinoma. Ultrasound will go some way to distinguish between these possibilities by showing whether the lesion is solid, cystic or mixed solid and cystic, as well as giving information about the edge of the lesion. Simple **cysts** are rarely malignant. Haemorrhagic cysts may have low level echoes within the cyst. **Mixed solid and cystic lesions** are mostly benign, owing usually to colloid degeneration or degeneration in a follicular adenoma, although cystic degeneration can occur in a carcinoma (Fig. 21.7). Confirmation of the histological nature of the cyst can be obtained by aspiration and cytological examination of the cyst fluid. A problem arises with a **solid lesion** as ultrasound cannot reliably distinguish between a benign and a malignant mass. Adenomas frequently have the same echo pattern as normal thyroid but may show increased or decreased echogenicity. Carcinomas usually show decreased echogenicity compared to the normal thyroid but the echo pattern alone is not a sufficiently reliable indication to tell whether a nodule is benign or malignant. Even a well-defined edge with a surrounding low echogenic zone around the nodule, the so-called 'halo sign', which was originally thought to indicate a benign lesion, can occur with a carcinoma and is not specific for a benign lesion. An irregular edge suggests a malignant lesion but a definitive diagnosis of malignancy can only be made when there is invasion of adjacent structures and if lymph node metastases are present.

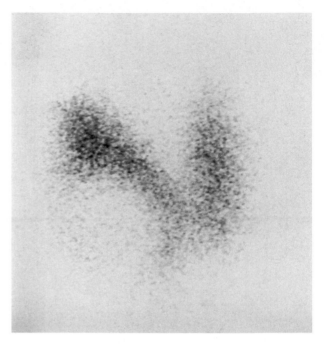

Figure 21.8 *Solitary nodule.* ^{123}I *scan showing a carcinoma as a cold nodule in the right lobe.*

RADIONUCLIDE SCANNING

Traditionally radionuclide scanning has been used to investigate thyroid nodules, although it is now employed much less frequently. The uptake of radioiodine is a reliable index of the rate of secretory activity of the thyroid cells. A **cold nodule** is one that shows reduced uptake of the radionuclide, whilst a hot or functioning nodule shows increased uptake. If the scan shows a solitary cold nodule there is about a 20 per cent probability that the nodule is malignant (Fig. 21.8), but if it is part of a multinodular goitre or if the nodule is hot then the chance of malignancy decreases to a low level (Fig. 21.9). As already mentioned, the probability of malignancy in a multinodular goitre is very much less than for a solitary nodule.

The problem with radionuclide scanning is that, although carcinomas normally show as a cold nodule, cysts, adenomas, colloid nodules and foci of thyroiditis also appear as cold nodules. If all cold nodules were excised on the suspicion of malignancy, then a large number of unnecessary operations would be performed. Ultrasound is often recommended as the next investigation for characterizing the lesion to see whether it is cystic or solid. If a solitary nodule is hot on a radionuclide scan, the likelihood of malignancy is low, since functioning nodules are almost all benign; the probability for malignancy is thought to be about 1 per cent.

Some *functioning nodules* appear **hot** with little or no uptake in the rest of the gland, because the high level of thyroid hormones suppresses the production of TSH by the pituitary, with the result that there is little or no

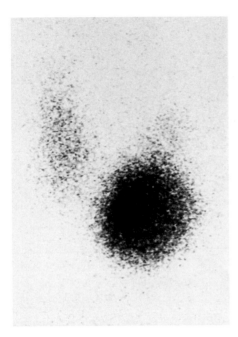

Figure 21.9 *Functioning nodule. ¹²³I scan showing a hot nodule in the left lobe.*

uptake of radionuclide in the normal part of the thyroid gland. A nodule that secretes thyroid hormones independently of TSH control is known as an **autonomous nodule**. There will be no suppression of uptake into the nodule with T3 on a repeat scan. An injection of TSH stimulates uptake into the suppressed part of the gland. Such a nodule is rarely malignant and is known as a **toxic adenoma**. If there are multiple nodules the condition is referred to as a toxic multinodular goitre or **Plummer's disease**.

A hot nodule may rarely be a hypertrophic nodule resulting from **thyroiditis**. Such a nodule is TSH-dependent and will show suppression with T3.

In the uncommon situation of the patient with hyperthyroidism who is found to have a thyroid nodule, a radionuclide scan will indicate if the nodule is hot and functioning and thus responsible for the hyperthyroidism. If the nodule is non-functioning, some other cause such as Graves' disease may be responsible for the hyperthyroidism.

FINE-NEEDLE ASPIRATION

Because of the limitations of both ultrasound and radionuclide scanning, the use of fine-needle aspiration for cytological examination has increased considerably over the past few years. The technique is quick, accurate and easy to perform. A fine needle is passed into the lesion without local anaesthetic and a small amount of material aspirated for smears for cytological examination. The aspiration is often performed without prior imaging, although image-guided aspiration with ultrasound enables the most suspicious lesion to be targeted rather than the most easily palpable mass. When fine-needle aspiration yields non-diagnostic results, a not uncommon occurrence, the aspiration is usually repeated. The use of fine-needle aspiration has resulted in a reduction in the number of surgical operations undertaken.

Many centres advocate fine-needle aspiration as the initial investigation of a thyroid nodule because both solid and cystic lesions require confirmation of the diagnosis.

GOITRE

A goitre is an enlarged thyroid gland that can be due to many causes. Some patients present with hyperthyroidism but many are euthyroid. A clinical history such as iodine deficiency or ingestion of goitrogens may be helpful in making the diagnosis. The age, onset and a family history may suggest Hashimoto's thyroiditis or an enzyme defect. Often the goitre is long-standing, but a recent enlargement should raise the suspicion of malignancy.

SIMPLE GOITRE

Simple goitre may be a diffuse hyperplastic (colloid) goitre or a multinodular goitre. Each is thought to represent different stages of the same pathological process and they are the commonest causes of non-toxic goitre.

In a **diffuse hyperplastic (colloid)** goitre there is diffuse uptake of ^{99m}Tc or ^{123}I, whereas in a **multinodular** goitre the uptake is non-homogeneous with discrete areas of reduced uptake. Both types of goitre may show normal or overall reduced uptake of the radionuclide. Ultrasound in a multinodular goitre will show nodules of varying size which may be solid or have a mixed solid/cystic appearance (Fig. 21.10).

Radiographs of the thoracic inlet show any tracheal displacement or compression. If there is dysphagia, a barium swallow may demonstrate oesophageal compression. Surgery may be required for a goitre causing tracheal or oesophageal compression. Calcification may be seen in the goitre, particularly in long-standing adenomas, though rarely fine dot-like calcification may be seen within a carcinoma.

Certain complications may arise with a goitre:

- There is a danger of respiratory obstruction because of pressure caused by haemorrhage into a thyroid nodule.
- The possibility of malignancy should be considered in a rapidly enlarging goitre.
- Hyperthyroidism may develop in a patient with a long-standing multinodular goitre.

Figure 21.10 *Ultrasound of a multinodular goitre showing marked enlargement of the thyroid which has a nodular appearance. T = trachea.*

INTRATHORACIC (RETROSTERNAL) GOITRE

A colloid or multinodular goitre may extend downwards into the mediastinum to produce a **retrosternal goitre**. Invariably, there is a connection between the cervical and mediastinal components of the gland, which may sometimes only be a fibrous band or vascular pedicle, but this connection is an important diagnostic feature. Usually an intrathoracic goitre is associated with a palpable enlargement of the thyroid in the neck. Most commonly an intrathoracic goitre is situated in the anterior mediastinum in front of the brachiocephalic vessels, but it may occasionally be positioned posteriorly to the trachea. The goitre may be wedged between the oesophagus and trachea, or it may extend posterior to the oesophagus. Intrathoracic goitres may cause symptomatic displacement and/or compression of the trachea and oesophagus, but usually they are discovered on a **chest radiograph** as an asymptomatic mediastinal mass with a well-defined spherical or lobular outline (Fig. 21.11).

(a)

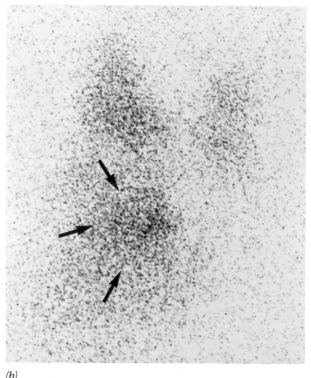

(b)

Figure 21.11 *Intrathoracic goitre. (a) Chest radiograph showing upper right-sided mediastinal mass displacing the trachea to the left. (b) ^{123}I scan showing enlarged thyroid with intrathoracic extension on the right side (arrows).*

(a)   *(b)*

Figure 21.12 *(a) Intrathoracic goitre. CT scan showing a goitre (G) as a mass displacing the trachea to the right. A little calcification is seen within the goitre (arrow). (b) Coronal T1-weighted MRI scan showing a large left-sided goitre (G) extending into the thorax. The patient had had a right hemithyroidectomy for a multinodular goitre 15 years previously.*

Radionuclide scanning demonstrates that the mass is thyroid tissue and a radioactive marker at the sternal notch confirms the intrathoracic location (Fig. 21.11b). [123]I is the agent of choice as the high background activity with ^{99m}Tc prevents satisfactory visualization of an intrathoracic goitre. **CT** shows the characteristic appearance of thyroid tissue, namely high attenuation values and marked enhancement with intravenous contrast. CT and **MRI** show the exact position of the thyroid together with any tracheal, oesophageal or vascular compression (Fig. 21.12).

TOXIC GOITRE

Diffuse toxic goitre (**Graves' disease**) is an autoimmune disorder in which an immunoglobulin produced by intrathyroid lymphocytes stimulates the gland to overactivity through TSH receptors on the thyroid cell membranes. Graves' disease is the commonest cause of hyperthyroidism. Usually the diagnosis is made clinically and with the appropriate thyroid function tests without the need for imaging. A ^{99m}Tc or ^{123}I scan will show uniformly increased uptake, and this test may be useful in certain cases to distinguish between Graves' disease and the hyperthyroidism occurring in thyroiditis. Ultrasound in Graves' disease shows an enlarged gland with a diffuse hypoechoic pattern (Fig. 21.13).

With a toxic nodular goitre (**Plummer's disease**) one or more hot nodules are seen on the radionuclide scan. On ultrasound these nodules appear as solid or have a mixed solid and cystic appearance.

Thyroid eye disease (ophthalmopathy)

In Graves' disease there may be autoimmune reaction affecting the eye muscles in the orbit, which may occur in the absence of clinical or biochemical evidence of

Figure 21.13 *Graves' disease. Ultrasound scan showing a diffusely enlarged gland with a hypoechoic pattern. T = trachea.*

thyroid disease. The topic is further discussed on page 458.

THYROIDITIS

Acute thyroiditis is caused by an acute suppurative infection and imaging plays little part except to determine whether an abscess is present.

Subacute thyroiditis, known as **de Quervain's thyroiditis** or granulomatous thyroiditis, is thought to follow a viral infection. Hyperthyroidism may result because of the release of hormones from the damaged gland. A radionuclide scan may show diffusely reduced uptake or focal areas of decreased uptake in the gland.

Hashimoto's thyroiditis (chronic thyroiditis) is an autoimmune destructive disorder, causing a goitre and hypothyroidism with positive serum thyroid antibodies. Radionuclide scanning reveals a non-homogeneous pattern and there may be hot or cold nodules present, but scanning alone cannot differentiate Hashimoto's disease from subacute thyroiditis and imaging has little part to play in the diagnosis.

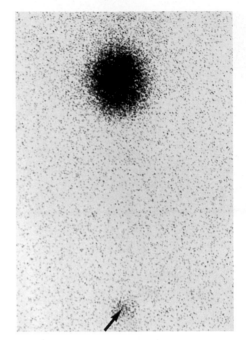

Figure 21.14 *Lingual thyroid. ^{123}I scan showing uptake at the level of the tongue but no uptake in the neck. The arrow indicates a marker on the suprasternal notch.*

ECTOPIC THYROID

The thyroid is normally situated in the neck but thyroid tissue can be found from the base of the tongue to the mediastinum although mediastinal thyroid tissue almost invariably results from downward extension of normally situated thyroid. Failure or incomplete descent from its embryological position at the back of the tongue may result in a **lingual** or **sublingual thyroid**. This possibility must be considered before a mass at the back of the tongue or upper neck is excised,

which could result in the necessity of life-long thyroid replacement. The diagnosis of an ectopic thyroid can be readily made with a radionuclide scan with a marker on the suprasternal notch (Fig. 21.14). Any ectopic thyroid tissue and any normal gland will be readily visualized. A **thyroglossal cyst** arises from remnants of the thyroglossal tract. A thyroglossal cyst can be recognized on CT or MRI as a midline cystic structure between the hyoid bone and the thyroid (Fig. 21.15). The cyst shows no uptake on a radionuclide scan as it contains no functioning thyroid tissue.

(a)

(b)

Figure 21.15 *Thyroglossal cyst. (a) CT scan showing a cyst anteriorly in the neck. (b) T2-weighted MRI scan in another patient showing the cyst as a high-signal area anteriorly in the neck.*

(a)   *(b)*

Figure 21.16 *Carcinoma of the thyroid. (a) ^{131}I scan in patient with follicular carcinoma showing uptake in recurrent tumour in the neck and in lung metastases. (b) Chest radiograph showing fine nodular pattern.*

THYROID CARCINOMA

Thyroid carcinoma may present as a thyroid swelling, but at presentation there may be metastases in the lymph nodes, lungs, liver and bone, which can be further investigated with conventional radiographs, ultrasound, CT or a radionuclide bone scan.

The management and subsequent imaging depend on the histology of the tumour, which is usually classified as papillary, follicular, anaplastic or medullary.

PAPILLARY AND FOLLICULAR CARCINOMA

Papillary and follicular carcinomas are differentiated tumours accounting for 80 per cent of thyroid cancers. As they have some functioning endocrine properties, similar to but less efficient than normal follicles, radionuclide scanning plays a part in their management. The patients often present with a solitary thyroid nodule, which characteristically appears as solid on ultrasound and 'cold' on a radionuclide scan. The diagnosis may also be made by fine-needle aspiration cytology or following partial thyroidectomy to remove the nodule. Treatment for a follicular carcinoma is total thyroidectomy but opinions differ as to the treatment for a papillary carcinoma: some surgeons perform a total thyroidectomy whilst others are content with a partial thyroidectomy. Total thyroidectomy enables the patient to be followed up with ^{131}I scans and further treatment given with a therapeutic dose of ^{131}I if necessary. About 1 month after thyroidectomy a whole-body scan using a

diagnostic dose of 300 MBq ^{131}I is performed to check for complete ablation of the thyroid and to detect metastases which take up the ^{131}I (Fig. 21.16). Physiological uptake of ^{131}I is normally seen in the salivary glands, stomach, colon or bladder. The uptake in metastases is far less than in the thyroid so metastases are detected on a scan only after the thyroid has been ablated either surgically or with a therapeutic dose of ^{131}I. ^{131}I is the radionuclide used for the whole-body scan, since its long half-life of 8 days enables sufficient time to elapse between administration and scanning to allow the ^{131}I to accumulate in any metastases.

If residual tumour is present in the neck or if metastases are demonstrated then a therapeutic dose of ^{131}I can be given and the whole-body scan repeated every 3–6 months; further therapeutic doses of ^{131}I can be given if necessary. Any pathological uptake may be quantified and, if it amounts to over 1 per cent of the administered dose, then a further therapeutic dose of ^{131}I is given. When tumour ablation is complete, a follow-up whole-body ^{131}I scan may be performed annually. Before any ^{131}I whole-body scan is performed, it is essential that the patient stops taking thyroid replacement, to allow TSH levels to rise and stimulate ^{131}I uptake into any metastases. T3 should be stopped at least 10 days and T4 3 weeks before the scan.

ANAPLASTIC CARCINOMA

Anaplastic carcinoma accounts for about 15 per cent of thyroid cancers. It tends to occur in the elderly and has a very poor prognosis. The patients frequently present with lung, liver or bony metastases. This tumour does not concentrate iodine, so radio-iodine scanning or treatment with ^{131}I has no part to play in the management.

MEDULLARY CARCINOMA

This tumour is a neuroendocrine tumour arising from the parafollicular or C cells of the thyroid and accounts for about 5 per cent of thyroid cancers. Involvement of the lymph nodes in the neck commonly occurs. The tumour secretes calcitonin, which can be measured in the blood. The treatment for medullary carcinoma is total thyroidectomy but, as the tumour does not take up iodine, scanning with radio-iodine has no part to play in the management of this tumour. However, other radiopharmaceuticals have been used to localize the primary tumour and any possible metastases. ^{99m}Tc-DMSA-V is the agent of choice, but successful imaging has been performed using Octreoscan, which binds to the somatostatin receptors found on many neuroendocrine tumours.

Medullary carcinoma of the thyroid may be part of the **multiple endocrine neoplasm syndrome** (**MEN 2a syndrome** [**Sipple's syndrome**]) associated with phaeochromocytoma and hyperparathyroidism, either parathyroid hyperplasia or adenoma (see below). Before thyroidectomy for medullary carcinoma is performed, these associated conditions should be excluded by measuring urinary VMA (vanillylmandelic acid) and plasma calcium levels. As the tumour may be inherited as an autosomal dominant condition, any relatives should be screened.

PARATHYROIDS

Imaging in parathyroid disease is usually performed to detect a surgically amenable abnormality causing primary hyperparathyroidism.

ANATOMY

There are normally four parathyroid glands, two upper and two lower, lying on the posterior aspect of the lateral lobes of the thyroid. Each gland measures 5 mm in length, 3 mm in width and 1 mm in thickness. Some patients have five glands and supernumerary glands are reckoned to occur in 6 per cent of adults, probably arising by division of one or more of the parathyroids during development. The inferior glands develop with the thymus from the third branchial pouch. They migrate caudally and usually settle in the lower poles of

the thyroid. Variation in migration results in an ectopic position such as within the thymus, mediastinum or thyroid. The superior glands arise from the fourth branchial pouch; as they migrate little during development, they are more constant in position.

HYPERPARATHYROIDISM

Primary hyperparathyroidism occurs when there is elevated serum parathyroid hormone, usually caused by a parathyroid adenoma (> 80 per cent) and less commonly by parathyroid hyperplasia (10–15 per cent) or carcinoma (3–4 per cent) or, rarely, from ectopic parathyroid hormone produced by a bronchial carcinoma.

Secondary hyperparathyroidism occurs as a response to hypocalcaemia and is most commonly seen in chronic renal failure when the parathyroid glands become hyperplastic. Tertiary hyperparathyroidism occurs when an autonomous adenoma arises following prolonged hypocalcaemia, such as untreated malabsorption or chronic renal failure.

IMAGING TECHNIQUES

Once hyperparathyroidism has been diagnosed, it is generally agreed that surgical removal of the abnormal gland or glands should be performed in symptomatic patients, in asymptomatic patients with high calcium levels, and in younger patients. There is no consensus as to the precise role of localizing tests prior to neck exploration. An experienced surgeon will localize up to 95 per cent of adenomas at the initial operation by identifying and, if necessary, biopsying all four parathyroid glands; 90 per cent of cases of primary hyperthyroidism are due to a single adenoma. It has been shown that preoperative localization does shorten the operating time. Preoperative localization is, however, important in those patients undergoing reoperation, which is invariably technically much more difficult. Initial surgery may be unsuccessful if there is an ectopic gland in the neck or mediastinum, if hyperplasia has not been recognized or if a fifth gland has not been discovered.

Rarely a parathyroid tumour may cause a palpable mass in the neck and may even indent the oesophagus on a barium swallow, but usually parathyroid adenomas are small and impalpable.

RADIONUCLIDE IMAGING

The ^{201}Tl and ^{99m}Tc **subtraction technique** is frequently used and probably should be the initial test to localize

Figure 21.17 *Parathyroid adenoma. Thallium/technetium subtraction scan showing an adenoma of the left inferior parathyroid gland.*

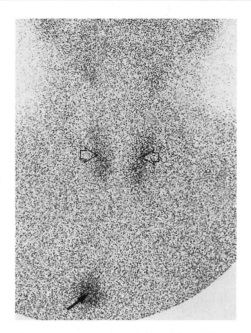

Figure 21.18 *Ectopic parathyroid. Thallium scan showing uptake in a parathyroid adenoma in the mediastinum (arrow). The open arrows point to the lobes of the thyroid.*

a parathyroid abnormality. Thallium given intravenously will be taken up both by the thyroid and by any hyperactive parathyroid tissue that may be present. The thyroid is visualized with ^{99m}Tc and this image is subtracted from the combined thallium image (Fig. 21.17). Normal parathyroid glands are not visualized, so any residual uptake will be in a parathyroid abnormality. The thallium and technetium images are acquired consecutively with a gamma camera and the subsequent subtraction is computer generated. It is important that the patient stays still during the examination so that an accurate subtraction can be performed.

This technique gives good results in localizing adenomas in both normal and ectopic positions (Fig. 21.18), but the results are inferior for the detection of parathyroid hyperplasia in both primary and secondary hyperparathyroidism. False-positive results may occur with coexisting thyroid disease as a thyroid adenoma will trap ^{201}Tl and show reduced uptake with ^{99m}Tc.

An alternative method is to use **^{99m}Tc-sestamibi** and to perform scans after 10 minutes and 2–3 hours. ^{99m}Tc-sestamibi is taken up by both the thyroid and parathyroid but is cleared more rapidly from the thyroid than from any abnormal parathyroid that may be present. A subtraction technique may also be employed using ^{99m}Tc-sestamibi and ^{123}I to visualize the thyroid.

ULTRASOUND

The neck is scanned using a high-frequency 7.5–10 MHz transducer. Normal parathyroid glands

Figure 21.19 *Parathyroid adenoma. Ultrasound scan of the neck showing the adenoma as a hypoechoic mass (M) at the lower pole of the thyroid on the left in the same patient as illustrated in Fig. 21.17. T = trachea.*

Figure 21.20 *Ectopic parathyroid. CT scan showing a mass in the mediastinum (arrow) which proved to be an ectopic parathyroid in a patient with hypercalcaemia who had a previous failed neck exploration.*

cannot usually be identified, but an adenoma can be identified as a mass of low echogenicity, frequently measuring as much as 1 cm in length and usually lying behind the thyroid in the angle between the trachea and oesophagus (Fig. 21.19). Hyperplasia can be recognized when all four glands are enlarged in contradistinction to an adenoma, which involves one or possibly two glands. Ultrasound has difficulty in demonstrating glands in an ectopic position and cannot show a parathyroid gland in the mediastinum.

Neither ultrasound nor radionuclide scanning can reliably demonstrate small adenomas less than 0.3 g in weight.

OTHER TECHNIQUES

CT can localize a parathyroid tumour and its accuracy is largely dependent on the size of the tumour. CT has the advantage that it can locate tumours in the mediastinum (Fig. 21.20). **MRI** gives excellent soft-tissue contrast and can be used to image the neck, thoracic inlet and mediastinum.

Venous sampling involves introducing a catheter into the neck or upper mediastinal veins via the internal jugular vein or from a femoral vein puncture. Parathyroid hormone levels in the blood are measured at various sites to try to localize a hyperactive parathyroid gland. **Arteriography** entails injecting contrast into the carotid or subclavian arteries or their branches to try to demonstrate a parathyroid tumour, which may show a vascular blush. Both venous sampling and arteriography are invasive techniques that are only used when other non-invasive methods have failed to demonstrate any parathyroid abnormality.

MULTIPLE ENDOCRINE NEOPLASIA (MEN)

Hyperparathyroidism may coexist with disorders of other endocrine glands in the various familial MEN syndromes (see box).

MEN type 1
- Parathyroid adenomas or hyperplasia – the commonest endocrine abnormality in this syndrome
- Pancreas, islet cell tumours secreting gastrin (Zollinger–Ellison syndrome), insulin, or more rarely glucagon, somatostatin or vasoactive intestinal peptide
- Pituitary tumours – the commonest being a prolactinoma

MEN type 2A
- Thyroid medullary carcinoma – the commonest abnormality in this syndrome
- Phaeochromocytoma – usually arising within the adrenal medulla and typically bilateral
- Parathyroid adenomas or hyperplasia

MEN type 2B
- Thyroid medullary carcinoma
- Phaeochromocytoma
- Cutaneous ganglioneuromas affecting the gastrointestinal tract, especially the large bowel

---

FURTHER READING

Brown, M.L., Collier, B.D. 1996: *A categorical course in nuclear medicine*. Chicago: Radiological Society of North America.

Fogelman, I., Maisey, M.N., Clarke, S.E.Y. 1994: *An atlas of clinical nuclear medicine* (2nd edition). London: Martin Dunitz.

Franklyn, J., Stewart, P.M. 1998: Diagnosis and treatment of thyroid nodules and goitre. *Journal of the Royal College of Physicians of London* **32**, 6–10.

Franklyn, J., Stewart, P.M. 1998: Multiple endocrine neoplasia. *Journal of the Royal College of Physicians of London* **32**, 98–101.

Maisey, M.N., Britton, K.E., Collier, B.D. 1998: *Clinical nuclear medicine* (3rd edition). London: Chapman & Hall.

Merrick, M.V. 1998: *Essentials of nuclear medicine* (2nd edition). London: Springer Verlag.

Naik, K.S., Bury, R.F. 1998: Imaging the thyroid. *Clinical Radiology* **53**, 630–9.

Nguyen, B.D. 1999: Parathyroid imaging with Tc-99m sestamibi. *Radiographics* **19**, 601–13.

Sharp, P.F., Gemmell, A.G., Smith, F.N. 1998: *Practical nuclear medicine* (2nd edition). Oxford: Oxford University Press.

Breast

A. ROBIN M. WILSON, ANDREW J. EVANS

The investigation and treatment of women with breast problems and best carried out in a coordinated way by a multidisciplinary team. Diagnosis should combine a detailed history, careful clinical examination and, only where clinically indicated, imaging of the breast and fine-needle aspiration cytology or needle core biopsy. Ideally, women with breast problems should have all the necessary investigations carried out at a single clinic visit. This is best achieved in a specialist breast clinic with the resources required to provide rapid access to diagnostic procedures with the surgeon able to consult directly with both the radiologist and the pathologist. This type of clinic will usually be part of a specialist breast unit that has the necessary clinical expertise, infrastructure and support from specialist radiology and pathology services and breast-care nurses.

This chapter outlines the role of imaging in the assessment of patients with breast problems and in screening asymptomatic women for breast cancer.

GENERAL RULES

- Not all women referred with breast problems require imaging; radiological investigations should be used only in circumstances where they are likely to influence management and according to predetermined diagnostic protocols.
- Wherever possible imaging should be carried out before any needle biopsy is performed; needle biopsy may cause a haematoma in the breast that can cause diagnostic confusion on breast ultrasound and mammography.

- Imaging should be carried out under the supervision of a specialist radiologist.

BREAST IMAGING TECHNIQUES

X-RAY MAMMOGRAPHY

Mammography is the most important and most sensitive of the various methods for imaging the breast. It is carried out using a specially designed X-ray unit (Fig. 22.1). Images are produced on X-ray film or digitally recorded on computer disk. Because the breast is made up of soft tissues, the energy of the radiation required to produce an image is considerably less than that required for other X-ray procedures. However, although the radiation dose received by the breast is relatively small, as with all X-ray procedures, mammography should be performed only where it is clinically useful; it should be used judiciously in younger women in whom the breast tissue is potentially more radiosensitive and in whom the sensitivity of mammography for disease is significantly lower.

To obtain a satisfactory mammographic image, the breast must be compressed firmly between the film cassette holder (breast support plate) and a plastic compression paddle (Plate 6, opposite page 358). **Compression** of the breast achieves uniform breast thickness, reduces the radiation dose required and reduces tissue movement, all of which improve image quality. Because the breast must be compressed many women find the examination uncomfortable and a few find it painful; women referred for mammography

Figure 22.1 *A dedicated mammography X-ray unit.*

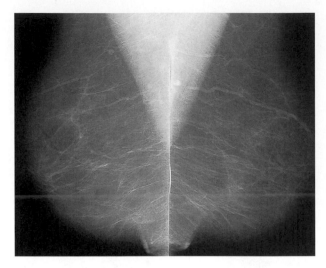

Figure 22.3 *Bilateral mammography showing a fatty background pattern.*

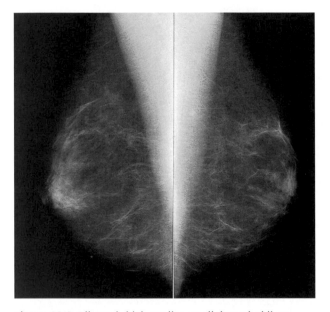

Figure 22.2 *Bilateral, high-quality, mediolateral oblique mammograms.*

Figure 22.4 *Bilateral mammography showing a mixed fatty dense background pattern.*

should be told that the examination may be uncomfortable. This is particularly so for women who have breast tenderness. When there is no urgency for examination in women with cyclical breast pain, it is better to perform mammography in the first half of the menstrual cycle.

The standard mammographic projection is the **mediolateral oblique view**. This single view will image most of the breast tissue and is the view used if only one mammographic view is being obtained. It is performed by placing the film cassette at a 45° angle across the breast. An adequate mediolateral oblique mammogram will demonstrate the pectoral muscle at an angle across the back of the breast with the nipple in profile, the nipple shown at a level at least up to the margin of the lower pectoral muscle and the inframammary angle of the breast clearly demonstrated (Fig. 22.2). Normal

anatomical structures can be easily identified on mammograms: fine linear structures represent the normal stroma (ligaments of Astley Cooper); normal ducts are sometimes large enough to be seen immediately behind the nipple; and veins and arteries are often clearly demonstrated. Normal distal ductal and lobular structures are not demonstrated on mammography. There is great variation in the normal background appearances of breast tissue shown on mammography. Some breasts show a predominantly fatty pattern (Fig. 22.3), some a mixed pattern (Fig. 22.4) and others a dense pattern (Fig. 22.5), all of which are normal. Normal anatomy is more difficult to define in the dense breast and background mammographic density is the main determinant of mammographic sensitivity for cancer. Cancers are easier to see in women with a fatty rather than a dense background pattern.

Figure 22.5 *Bilateral mammography showing a homogeneously dense background pattern. This pattern is commoner in younger women and is associated with a decreased sensitivity for malignancy.*

The companion view to the mediolateral oblique projection is the **craniocaudal view** taken with breast compression applied from above (Plate 7, opposite page 358). In this view a significant proportion of breast tissue is not imaged. As it is the upper inner quadrant of the breast that is often not clearly imaged in the mediolateral oblique view, the craniocaudal projection may be rotated to ensure that this area is included.

A standard mammographic examination of the breast should include mediolateral and craniocaudal views of both breasts and these two views are mandatory for breast screening. Supplementary views, including lateral projections, magnification views and localized paddle compression views, may be performed according to the particular clinical circumstances and as guided by the radiologist.

GALACTOGRAPHY

Galactography is a technique for outlining the duct pattern in the breast by the injection of radiopaque contrast into a duct orifice at the nipple using a small plastic cannula. This procedure is used for further investigation of single duct nipple discharge, which may be a symptom of an underlying carcinoma. However, the cause of single duct nipple discharge is usually benign and galactography is often diagnostically unhelpful. It is now rarely used, as single duct nipple discharge is better managed on the basis of conventional mammographic, clinical and nipple discharge cytological findings.

CYSTOGRAPHY

Cystography is a technique for outlining the inner contours of a breast cyst. After aspiration with a needle, a volume of air equal to the fluid aspirated is injected into the cyst lumen. The air acts as an excellent contrast medium and clearly outlines the internal structure of the cyst. The technique is used when cyst aspiration yields frankly blood-stained fluid, the presence of which may indicate that the cyst wall contains a papilloma or carcinoma. With the increasing use and sophistication of breast ultrasound this procedure is now rarely used; ultrasound is able to demonstrate even a small intramural mass in a cyst.

ULTRASOUND

Ultrasound has been used to image the breast since the early 1970s and is now regarded as a valuable tool in the assessment of both benign and malignant breast problems. Its advantage over mammography is that it can differentiate solid from cystic lesions (Figs 22.6, 22.7) and

Figure 22.6 *Ultrasound of a fibroadenoma showing a well-defined solid mass with a homogeneous internal echo pattern and distal enhancement of the ultrasound beam.*

Figure 22.7 *Ultrasound demonstrating three cysts in close proximity. These are very well-defined abnormalities that have no internal echoes and show distal acoustic enhancement. All these features are characteristic of benign cysts.*

Figure 22.8 *A normal breast ultrasound showing the skin and, beneath it, normal hypoechoic breast tissue with hyperechoic Astley Cooper's ligaments (arrows). Breast ultrasound is particularly useful in differentiating cystic from solid masses.*

Figure 22.9 *Magnetic resonance mammography showing an intracapsular rupture of both silicone implants. The low-signal curvilinear lines (arrows) represent the true implant membrane (Linguini's sign) while the silicone is confined by the fibrous capsule.*

is particularly useful in the mammographically dense breast. **Conventional ultrasound** equipment for breast examination uses higher frequency transducers (7.5–12 MHz) than those used for abdominal ultrasound, which allows better spatial resolution. Ultrasound readily demonstrates normal structures in the breast and shows fat, parenchymal tissue and muscle (Fig. 22.8). It also demonstrates distortions of structure in the breast and oedema.

Colour flow Doppler ultrasound is being increasingly used in the evaluation of breast conditions. Generally, malignant lesions show abnormal Doppler patterns indicative of neovascularity whilst benign lesions do not (Plates 8–10, opposite page 358). Unfortunately many benign and malignant masses show significant overlap in their Doppler signal patterns and distinction between the two is not possible with any certainty using this technique. Colour flow Doppler is also useful for diffuse breast problems, such as prominent clinical thickening where the absence of a Doppler signal makes malignancy unlikely. Ultrasound cannot be used to differentiate definitively benign from malignant solid breast lesions.

Current clinical research into the roles of enhanced Doppler and harmonic imaging in breast disease attempts to assess its ability to select tumours suitable for chemotherapy, to assess response to treatment and to differentiate tumour recurrence from scarring.

Ultrasound is significantly less sensitive for malignancy than X-ray mammography. This is, in part, due to the difficulty of demonstrating microcalcifications and architectural distortion on ultrasound. Ultrasound is particularly insensitive for the detection of ductal carcinoma *in situ*, which is most commonly manifest as microcalcification on mammography. For this reason

mammography is always indicated when there is clinical suspicion of malignancy. It is also inappropriate to use ultrasound as a screening method for breast cancer. The sensitivity of mammography for malignancy increases with age. The normal breast is denser in the younger woman, and this largely explains why breast lesions in young women are more difficult to demonstrate on mammography.

MAGNETIC RESONANCE MAMMOGRAPHY

Magnetic resonance mammography is a technique that requires specialized equipment including a dedicated breast surface coil. It is very sensitive for breast pathology but is non-specific. The exact role of magnetic resonance mammography in the evaluation of patients with breast symptoms is yet to be defined, but it is of value in the assessment of possible multifocal malignancy, in the exclusion of recurrent disease in patients treated with conservation therapy and in the investigation of patients with breast symptoms who have silicone breast implants (Fig. 22.9). Magnetic resonance mammography should not be regarded as a routine investigation in patients with breast problems.

COMPUTED TOMOGRAPHY

CT has no role in the imaging of primary breast disease. However, CT is useful in the evaluation of metastatic disease, particularly in the axilla, and the assessment of metastatic disease of other parts of the body including the brain, chest and abdomen. Again, CT should not be regarded as a routine investigation.

IMAGING WOMEN WITH BREAST IMPLANTS

The presence of silicone implants in the breast inevitably compromises the ability of the radiologist to image the breast. Women who have implants placed for augmentation should be informed by the surgeon beforehand that the presence of implants may interfere with subsequent breast imaging and screening.

Mammography of the augmented or reconstructed breast can be carried out safely. Special displacement techniques can be used to ensure that the majority of the breast tissue itself is imaged but the ability to do so depends on the ratio of the size of the implant to the breast tissue.

Patients with breast implants who present with localized breast symptoms should be first assessed clinically. Needling procedures require special care if a prosthesis is not to be punctured and often aspiration of cysts or fine-needle aspiration cytology/core biopsy of solid structures is best carried out under imaging control. There is no evidence that silicone implants and silicone leakage are associated with increased risk of malignancy and there is a tenuous link with connective tissue disease. Patients in whom implant rupture is suspected usually request further investigation and, in many cases, removal with or without replacement of the prosthesis. Mammography and ultrasound cannot adequately image breast tissue posterior to the implant and in these circumstances the multiplanar imaging capabilities of magnetic resonance mammography are very useful. Magnetic resonance mammography is an excellent technique for identifying rupture of silicone implants (Fig. 22.9).

SENTINEL NODE IMAGING

Staging of the axillary lymph nodes in patients with invasive breast cancer is fundamental to deciding on appropriate treatment; lymph node-negative disease suggests that the disease is confined to the breast and may be managed without systemic therapy. Conventional imaging techniques, including ultrasound, CT and MRI, lack the required sensitivity and specificity for accurate staging, and surgical dissection of the axilla to sample or excise all of the lymph nodes has been required. As this process is associated with significant morbidity, there has been interest in less invasive means of axillary lymph node staging. The first lymph node filtering the lymphatics from the tumour site is known as the sentinel lymph node. The theory is that excision of this node alone should provide accurate assessment of the presence or absence of metastatic spread of tumour beyond the breast.

Injection of dye or ^{99m}Tc-labelled colloid in or around the tumour allows for the sentinel node to be identified. The advantage of the labelled colloid method is that the site of the sentinel node can be identified prior to surgery using a conventional gamma camera. The exact position of the node can then be found using a small hand-held gamma probe and the single sentinel node excised. This node can be removed for histology by surgical or image-guided biopsy and the node stage assessed before final treatment is decided. Initial studies using this technique for axillary node staging are giving promising results.

CLINICAL APPLICATIONS OF BREAST IMAGING

CLINICAL CONTEXT

Imaging of the breast is best undertaken as part of a multidisciplinary assessment. For women with breast symptoms, using imaging as the sole or initial investigation is not recommended. However, mammography is effective on its own for asymptomatic breast cancer screening.

Problems that most commonly result in a referral to a breast clinic are:

- lump in the breast
- pain and tenderness
- family history of breast cancer
- nipple discharge
- nipple eczema
- skin changes
- other miscellaneous symptoms.

ASSESSMENT OF BREAST LUMPS

Whether imaging of a patient with a lump in the breast is required or not and which imaging technique is appropriate depends upon the age of the patient. The primary role of mammography is the exclusion of malignant disease. Although the radiation dose of mammography is relatively low, any test that involves ionizing radiation should be restricted in its use to circumstances where it is likely to be of clinical benefit. It is therefore inappropriate to use mammography where the risk of malignancy is small. Mammography is rarely required in the investigation of women under the age of 35 but should always be performed at any age when there is a strong clinical suspicion of malignancy. Table 22.1 details the criteria, based on triple assessment of clinical examination, imaging and cytology/needle histology, that must be satisfied to make a diagnosis of a benign breast lump, which need not necessarily require surgical excision.

Ultrasound is most useful for further assessment of an abnormality detected on mammography or clinical

Table 22.1 *Benign breast lumps: clinical, imaging and cytological criteria, related to age, required for diagnosis.*

Technique	Age (years)	Findings
Clinical examination	All ages	Smooth and mobile
Imaging		
Not required	< 25	
Ultrasound	25–50	Well-defined with homogeneous internal echo pattern or not identified
Ultrasound	> 50	Well-defined with homogeneous internal echo pattern or not identified
Mammography	> 50	Well-defined mass or not identified
Cytology	All ages	Good yield of benign epithelial cells
or		
Histology	All ages	Benign histology consistent with clinical and imaging findings

examination. Ultrasound is the imaging technique of first choice in women under the age of 35 with localized breast problems confirmed by clinical assessment.

Patients aged under 25 years

A discrete mobile lump in the breast in a patient under the age of 25 is virtually always benign; the vast majority of lumps in women of this age are fibroadenomas; simple cysts are uncommon. Imaging has little to add to the diagnosis or management of a breast lump at this age, unless there is clinical suspicion of malignancy. The conventional management for a fibroadenoma in a young woman is clinical assessment and needle core biopsy or fine-needle aspiration cytology to confirm the benign nature of the lesion. A benign lump does not need to be surgically excised unless it is enlarging or the patient requests its removal. An alternative to surgery for women who choose to have a fibroadenoma removed is by ultrasound-guided vacuum-assisted mammotomy.

Patients aged 25–50 years

After clinical assessment, ultrasound is the examination of first choice in assessment of a lump in a patient in this age group. Mammography is best avoided unless there is suspicion of malignancy. Ultrasound will define the size and nature of the solid lesion in the breast and will also differentiate between a solid and cystic lesion. In this age range, the differential diagnosis of a discrete mobile lump lies between a fibroadenoma and a simple breast cyst. The typical appearances of a fibroadenoma and cyst on ultrasound are shown in Figures 22.6 and 22.7 respectively.

A normal ultrasound examination should not be taken as evidence that no real pathology exists. Some fibroadenomas have appearances very similar to normal breast tissue and are therefore invisible on ultrasound; false-negative ultrasound findings are not uncommon in malignancy particularly with carcinoma *in situ*. If ultrasound examination of a clinically significant abnormality is normal, the patient's management should be based on the clinical and cytological findings.

Patients aged over 50 years

Ultrasound remains the imaging technique of first choice for a discrete palpable mobile lump but, because of the increasing risk of malignancy, mammography should also always be performed in women over 50. As with younger women, core biopsy or fine-needle aspiration is also mandatory.

Imaging the clinically malignant mass

If a mass is clinically malignant, it requires excision irrespective of the imaging and cytological findings. The role of imaging a clinically malignant mass is to define the extent of disease and to screen for malignancy in the contralateral breast. These imaging findings allow the most appropriate treatment to be offered. A clinically small malignant mass may be surrounded by extensive ductal carcinoma *in situ*, which is often impalpable, but which will normally be detected on mammography. In such circumstances it would be inappropriate to offer breast-conserving surgery. Clinical examination has a tendency to overestimate the size of breast carcinomas (Lebourgne's law), whilst size measured by ultrasound and mammography both show better correlation with the actual size of the excised tumour.

Patients presenting with locally advanced breast carcinoma

Mammography is not clinically useful in these circumstances. Breast-conserving surgery cannot be offered and screening the opposite breast for a second carcinoma is unlikely to alter management because of the poor prognosis of the presenting tumour.

Screening women who attend symptomatic breast clinics

Women over 50 years whose symptoms would not normally warrant imaging assessment should undergo screening mammography, assuming they have not already done so within the previous year. In some centres this protocol applies to all women over the age of 40.

ASSESSMENT OF BREAST PAIN AND TENDERNESS

Breast pain is a very common symptom which on its own does not warrant imaging investigation. Pain as the sole symptom or sign of malignancy is rare. Breast pain is best managed by careful clinical history with appropriate medical treatment.

ASSESSMENT OF WOMEN WITH AN INCREASED RISK OF BREAST CANCER

Some women with a family history of breast cancer or who have certain histological abnormalities detected at a previous breast biopsy are known to be at increased risk of developing breast cancer. The exact role of imaging in their management is controversial as there is no current evidence to prove that screening reduces mortality in these groups of patients.

Women with family history of breast cancer

There is no conclusive evidence that mammographic screening of women under 50 years with a family history of breast cancer reduces their mortality from breast cancer. However, if women present with anxiety about their family history, there is general consensus that screening should be offered once their individual risk has been confirmed. This would normally involve counselling by a specially trained clinician or geneticist. No clear protocols for such screening exist but a combination of counselling followed by clinical and mammographic screening and instruction in breast self-examination is frequently provided. Such screening is best provided by a specialist breast clinic under the supervision of a breast clinician. Usually only a premenopausal first-line family history of breast cancer (mother, sister or daughter) is considered significant. Most women over the age of 50 are adequately catered for by routine mammographic screening provided for all women over this age.

Histological risk factors

Certain histological proliferative epithelial abnormalities, such as atypical ductal hyperplasia and lobular neoplasia, are known to be associated with variable increased risk of subsequent breast cancer. In women with a significant histological risk factor the development of breast cancer is highest 10–15 years after the proliferative abnormality has been diagnosed. The increased risk to the individual doubles if there is also a significant family history of breast cancer. Many clinicians recommend regular screening by clinical examination and/or mammography, with professional counselling, for women in this group. Mammography is seldom required more frequently than once a year.

PAGET'S DISEASE OF THE NIPPLE/NIPPLE ECZEMA

Mammography is of limited value in the assessment of patients with Paget's disease of the nipple. The diagnosis can be made by nipple biopsy carried out under local anaesthetic in the clinic. Frequently patients with Paget's disease have no mammographic abnormality and, where an abnormality is present, mammography is not useful in defining the extent or nature of the associated malignancy. Because of this difficulty, both clinically and mammographically, patients with Paget's disease of the nipple are not normally offered breast-conserving surgery. Mammography of the opposite breast is recommended to detect synchronous lesions.

NIPPLE DISCHARGE

Imaging is also of little value in the assessment of patients with multiduct nipple discharge. In most circumstances patients with this symptom do not require investigation other than careful clinical assessment. Occasionally, cytological assessment of the discharge may be considered appropriate.

Single duct nipple discharge is a more significant symptom that does require more detailed investigation including imaging. Conventional mammography is helpful in excluding underlying malignancy, and ultrasound may demonstrate duct ectasia. The surgeon can manage this condition conservatively in the absence of mammographic evidence of malignancy. Large duct papillomas are occasionally visible mammographically and are almost always benign; they require surgical treatment only if symptoms are troublesome.

IMAGING OF METASTATIC BREAST CANCER

Routine investigation of patients with breast cancer at the time of diagnosis to identify metastatic disease is not indicated, as there is a very low yield of true positive results and significant number of false-positive results. Imaging to identify metastatic disease is best reserved for patients who have suggestive symptoms or signs.

SURVEILLANCE AND CHARACTERIZATION OF LOCALLY RECURRENT BREAST CANCER

Follow-up of the treated breast

Where mastectomy has been performed, routine imaging of the mastectomy site or axilla is not helpful; ultrasound is useful in confirming clinical suspicion of recurrence at the mastectomy site. Imaging of suspected

Figure 22.10 *Sagittal magnetic resonance image of the breast after injection of contrast demonstrating enhancing recurrent carcinoma (arrow). (By kind permission of Dr L. Turnbull, Centre for Magnetic Resonance Investigation, Hull Royal Infirmary.)*

Figure 22.11 *A mammogram of a man with breast cancer showing a spiculate mass in the retroareolar region with associated malignant-type calcification.*

axillary recurrence is best performed with either CT or MRI.

In patients treated by lumpectomy (breast conservation), annual routine follow-up mammography is often recommended as part of a combined clinical and imaging follow-up strategy. Mammography will identify 60–80 per cent of recurrence in the breast and in approximately half of these cases the presence of recurrence will not have been apparent clinically. Mammographic surveillance will thus detect recurrent disease at an earlier stage and, in a significant number of patients, this has prognostic significance.

Mammography is particularly effective in detecting recurrent ductal carcinoma *in situ*. The commonest radiological feature of local recurrence is microcalcification, but in the majority of cases microcalcification at the postoperative site is due to fat necrosis or radiotherapy change. If mammographic findings are suspicious of local recurrence, image-guided fine-needle aspiration or core biopsy and magnetic resonance mammography (Fig. 22.10) may be helpful, though some cases will require open diagnostic surgical biopsy. Surgical biopsy must be avoided if at all possible after radiotherapy as wound healing may be delayed. Ultrasound is not effective in screening for recurrence. The risk of recurrence in the treated breast is greatest in the first 10 years after treatment and occurs at a rate of approximately 1 per cent per annum.

Surveillance of the opposite breast

Patients who have developed one breast cancer are at significant increased risk of developing a second primary lesion. For this reason, regular mammography of the opposite breast is recommended, especially in those patients whose first tumour had good prognostic features.

IMAGING OF THE MALE BREAST

Enlargement of the breast or breasts is the most common reason for a male patient to be referred to a breast clinician. Simple obesity is the commonest cause but true gynaecomastia is increasingly common with age. Imaging is rarely necessary as it does not influence clinical management. Breast cancer is rare in men, with less than 1 per cent occurring in males; again imaging is rarely contributory as mastectomy is the standard treatment. Mammography can be performed without difficulty in men. It is usually only required when a strong clinical suspicion of malignancy has not been confirmed by other investigations (Fig. 22.11).

IMAGING FEATURES OF THE COMMON PATHOLOGIES

INVASIVE CARCINOMA

The commonest mammographic manifestation of invasive carcinoma is a spiculate mass often associated with calcification (Figs 22.12, 22.13). Other common appearances of invasive carcinoma are an ill-defined mass, parenchymal distortion and suspicious calcification

Figure 22.12 *A mammogram showing a breast carcinoma. The appearance is of a spiculate mass with associated calcification. Such an appearance has a greater than 90 per cent chance of being due to breast carcinoma.*

Figure 22.13 *Mammogram demonstrating a clinically obvious large carcinoma behind the left nipple. The mass is lobulated, ill-defined and shows subtle spiculation. Enlarged nodes (N) in the left axilla are seen.*

Figure 22.14 *Mammogram showing extensive suspicious calcification and parenchymal distortion owing to an invasive carcinoma with associated ductal carcinoma in situ.*

Figure 22.15 *Breast ultrasound showing typical features of a breast carcinoma (circle): an ill-defined hypoechoic mass with an echogenic halo, an ill-defined internal echo pattern and marked distal attenuation of the ultrasound beam.*

on mammography in some patients. Normal mammography must never be used to exclude carcinoma in patients with significant clinical findings. Carcinomas are seen on ultrasound as hypoechoic, inhomogeneous, ill-defined masses (Fig. 22.15). Other features often seen are an echogenic halo, distal acoustic shadowing and disturbance of the surrounding architecture.

DUCTAL CARCINOMA *IN SITU*

Ductal carcinoma *in situ* (DCIS) has become a more common clinical problem with the widespread introduction of mammographic screening; 15–30 per cent of screen-detected cancer is ductal carcinoma *in situ* compared to only 5 per cent of breast cancer presenting

without a mass (Fig. 22.14). The linear structures seen radiating from spiculate masses and parenchymal distortion represent the inpulling of normal breast structures rather than tumour extending outwards. Up to 10 per cent of clinically apparent carcinomas are not visible on mammography. This is mainly because the tumour is obscured by normal breast tissue, which appears dense

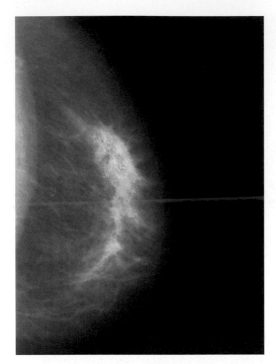

Figure 22.16 *Extensive casting and granular calcifications are demonstrated on mammography in the lateral left breast. The calcifications represent comedo ductal carcinoma in situ, the calcification being formed in necrotic intraductal debris.*

Figure 22.17 *Bilateral mammography showing multiple cysts. These are demonstrated as multiple well-defined masses of varying sizes, which do not show calcification.*

with symptoms. Screen-detected ductal carcinoma *in situ* tends to be impalpable and less extensive than symptomatic ductal carcinoma *in situ*. The most common mammographic feature of ductal carcinoma *in situ* is microcalcification, which is found in around 80–90 per cent of those with a mammographic abnormality. The appearance of the microcalcifications described as characteristic of ductal carcinoma *in situ* is that of granular particles in a ductal distribution, showing a tendency to coalesce to form linear and branching 'casts' with variations in shape, size and density (Fig. 22.16). Such calcifications represent the coalescence of dystrophic calcification formed in necrotic intraluminal debris, and are seen in ductal carcinoma *in situ* of high histological grade. Ductal carcinoma *in situ*, normally of low-grade type, can also manifest as punctate calcification due to calcification in intercellular spaces.

CYSTS

Cysts are demonstrated on mammography as solitary or multiple well-defined masses (Fig. 22.17). They occur most commonly in the 30–50 age group and frequently subside after the menopause. Cysts do not usually present after the menopause unless the patient is on hormone replacement therapy. Cysts are often multiple and bilateral and may be very large. Ultrasound findings

are characteristic with cysts shown as sharply marginated transonic areas with distal acoustic enhancement (see Fig. 22.7).

FIBROADENOMA

Fibroadenomas are also demonstrated on mammography as well-defined masses. They most commonly develop in women under the age of 35, but may present for the first time in older women. They are sometimes multiple and bilateral, but are rarely larger than 3 cm. On mammography, calcification is commonly seen within a fibroadenoma and is often coarse and 'popcorn' in character (Fig. 22.18). On ultrasound a fibroadenoma is typically a well-defined hypoechoic solid mass with a homogeneous internal echo pattern and sharp posterior border, often with distal acoustic enhancement (see Fig. 22.6).

DUCT ECTASIA

Duct ectasia is seen mammographically most commonly as dense, very well-defined linear 'broken needle' or 'pipe-stem' calcification (Fig. 22.19). Occasionally, dilated ducts can be seen as elongated retroareolar soft-tissue structures without calcification.

Figure 22.18 *A mammogram showing a fibroadenoma as a well-defined mass containing coarse popcorn-shaped calcification.*

Figure 22.20 *Ultrasound showing a mixed cystic/solid mass owing to a breast abscess. There is a peripheral solid component and a central cystic component.*

Figure 22.19 *Bilateral mammography showing extensive calcifications diagnostic of duct ectasia.*

Repeated aspiration may be necessary, but it is usually possible to avoid open surgical drainage.

BREAST TRAUMA

On mammography, haematoma in the breast may be shown as an ill-defined mass, spiculate mass or asymmetrical density (Fig. 22.21). On ultrasound, haematomas appear as ill-defined cystic/solid masses with distal acoustic enhancement. Fat necrosis can occur following significant or trivial trauma and following surgery (Fig. 22.22). Acute fat necrosis appears as an ill-defined or spiculate mass and ultrasound can show mass lesions suspicious of malignancy. In time, fat

BREAST ABSCESS

Breast abscesses are normally seen on mammography as ill-defined or spiculate masses. They are usually found in the retroareolar area in women who are breastfeeding but may also occur elsewhere in other patients. The diagnosis is usually suggested by the clinical findings. Ultrasound shows an irregular hypoechoic or transonic mass with distal acoustic enhancement (Fig. 22.20). **Tuberculosis** of the breast is rare and may present as a nodular or ill-defined mass or with diffuse involvement. Abscesses can be successfully treated by aspiration under ultrasound guidance and antibiotic therapy.

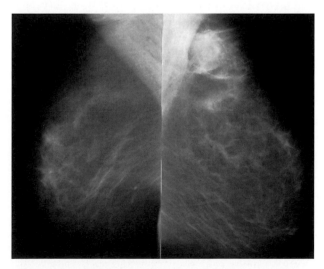

Figure 22.21 *Bilateral mammography showing a large asymmetrical density with associated trabecular thickening in the left axillary tail. This was due to haematoma secondary to a seat-belt injury.*

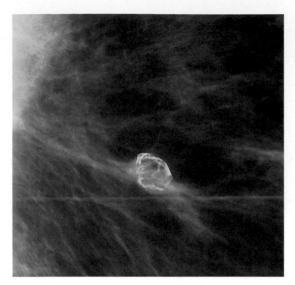

Figure 22.22 *Mammogram demonstrating coarse calcification in an area of architectural distortion. This fat necrosis was secondary to surgery some years before.*

necrosis can calcify; such calcification is usually curvilinear and coarse, but occasionally calcification due to fat necrosis can mimic malignancy.

FIBROCYSTIC CHANGE

Fibrocystic change (the preferred pathological collective term for combinations of benign breast processes including cyst formation, apocrine metaplasia, blunt duct adenosis, sclerosing adenosis and various benign epithelial hyperplasias) is often shown on mammography as areas of asymmetrical density. These asymmetrical densities often contain calcification characterized by multiple, often bilateral, round clusters of punctate calcification. The 'teacup' sign, caused by sedimentation of milk of calcium within small cysts, is often seen. On ultrasound, benign breast change shows as diffuse hyperechoic areas. Small cysts are often seen within these areas.

PHYLLODES TUMOUR

Phyllodes tumours are demonstrated mammographically as large, well-defined, often lobulated masses and are often surprisingly large at presentation. On ultrasound, the typical leaf-like echogenic septations may be seen within a homogeneous well-defined mass (Fig. 22.23). Small, round, hyperechoic foci, rather than septations, are more often seen within the mass. About 5 per cent of phyllodes tumours are malignant, but the distinction from benign tumours cannot be reliably made from their imaging features.

Figure 22.23 *Ultrasound examination of a phyllodes tumour showing a well-defined, hypoechoic solid mass that contains septae.*

ASSESSMENT OF IMPALPABLE LESIONS

IMAGE-GUIDED BREAST BIOPSY AND MARKER LOCALIZATION

The use of mammography for asymptomatic screening and the increasing use of both mammography and ultrasound as part of the assessment of symptomatic breast problems inevitably mean that a significant proportion of breast lesions detected are impalpable and require image-guided biopsy. These techniques require special skills on the part of the radiologist and specialist equipment. The technique of first choice for image-guided biopsy is ultrasound, with X-ray-guided techniques reserved for lesions not seen on ultrasound; ultrasound biopsy is quick, relatively cheap and associated with minimal patient discomfort. Fine-needle aspiration and large-bore needle biopsy under ultrasound guidance are both very accurate techniques and in experienced hands provide a definitive diagnosis in at least 95 per cent of impalpable lesions. Certain lesions cannot be adequately visualized on ultrasound, e.g. areas of architectural distortion and microcalcification, and must be biopsied under X-ray guidance (Fig. 22.24). Stereotactic equipment is more accurate than other X-ray techniques.

Figure 22.24 *Stereotactic check film showing correct positioning of a needle within a cluster of microcalcifications. Two films are taken at an angle of 30° for an accurate localization.*

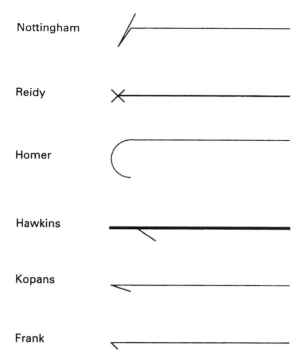

Nottingham	
Reidy	
Homer	
Hawkins	
Kopans	
Frank	

Figure 22.25 *Diagrammatic illustration of some of the various wire markers available for localization of impalpable breast lesions.*

Image-guided biopsy should not be considered in isolation and should be part of multidisciplinary triple assessment (clinical examination, imaging and cytology/histology). If a lesion is considered to be suspicious of malignancy on its imaging appearances then open surgical biopsy should proceed, even if fine-needle aspiration cytology or core biopsy is benign.

IMAGE-GUIDED MARKER LOCALIZATION

Impalpable lesions that require surgical biopsy or excision usually require image-guided localization. Some superficial lesions may be localized by marking the overlying skin, but most lesions require placement of a marker in the breast. A number of different wire devices are available (Fig. 22.25).

Wire markers have the advantage over other techniques:

- They allow very accurate localization (Fig. 22.26).
- They facilitate excision of small specimens for diagnostic biopsies.
- Accurate wide local excision for malignant lesions is obtained.
- The surgeon can choose the best operative approach to achieve the optimal cosmetic result.

SPECIMEN RADIOGRAPHY

Specimen radiography is useful to the surgeon for both palpable and impalpable breast lesions. The specimen radiograph will confirm that an impalpable lesion has been successfully excised (Fig. 22.27) and will also allow

Figure 22.26 *A mammogram performed following insertion of a Nottingham localization wire. The wire is in an ideal position with the lesion transfixed and the 'T' of the wire lying just medially. The radiopaque skin markers represent the site of skin entry of the wire and the position of the lesion closest to the skin.*

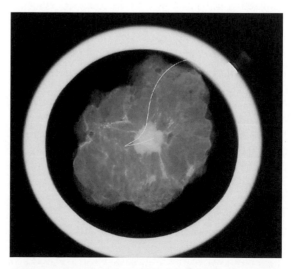

Figure 22.27 *Specimen radiograph showing a spiculate mass in the centre of a therapeutic excision. The lesion appears to be adequately excised with a good clear margin on all sides.*

the surgeon to assess excision margins of palpable abnormalities. When wide local excision for carcinoma is being performed, a specimen radiograph will allow the surgeon to identify a margin that is too close to the lesion and prompt wider excision of this margin. Specimen radiographs are good predictors of inadequate excision but are poor predictors of complete histological excision.

To facilitate re-excision, the specimen must be orientated with respect to the excision bed; this is easily achieved with either radiopaque sutures or surgical staples. Ideally, facilities should be available for carrying out specimen radiographs close to the operating theatre, so that the images are available to the surgeon within a reasonable time. This means that further excision or exploration of the excision cavity, if required, can be carried out by the same operative procedure.

BREAST CANCER SCREENING

Breast cancer remains the commonest cancer worldwide to affect women, and it is particularly common in the western world. As yet there are no known means that can prevent breast cancer. Early detection through breast screening is the best health intervention known to reduce significantly breast cancer mortality. Finding breast cancer when it is small (less than 15 mm) and that has not yet spread to the axillary lymph nodes provides the opportunity for more effective treatment. Screening asymptomatic women for breast cancer by mammography alone has been shown in randomized controlled trials to reduce mortality by around 30 per cent in women between the ages of 50 and 70. Screening of women in this age group is now available in most western countries on either a national population or *ad hoc* decentralized basis. There is now unequivocal evidence that screening provides the best results when two-view mammography is performed every 2 years with the films double-read by two experienced radiologists.

More contentious is screening of women under the age of 50. Although trials have also demonstrated a significant reduction in mortality of around 25 per cent, population screening in this age group is not yet proven to be cost-effective. Screening of younger women has to be carried out more frequently to be effective and is not as widely available. The introduction of digital mammography and computer-aided detection (CAD) may increase sensitivity and specificity sufficiently to allow screening in younger women to be more widely recommended.

Hormone replacement therapy (HRT) is now common in postmenopausal women. HRT is associated with a small increased risk of breast cancer (relative risk 1.7) after 5–7 years. HRT also increases mammographic density in about a third of women and simple cysts and fibroadenomas, which normally regress after the menopause, may continue to grow. These effects are known to reduce the sensitivity of mammography in HRT users by around 7 per cent, and women on HRT are more likely to present with an interval cancer within 1 year of screening.

Effective screening must include comprehensive and effective assessment of screen-detected abnormalities. Assessment is best carried out by a multidisciplinary team following the principles of the 'triple approach', comprising clinical examination, imaging and needle biopsy, to achieve maximum sensitivity and specificity of diagnosis. Surgery is no longer required to diagnose definitively benign breast problems and the great majority of women with cancer are aware of the diagnosis preoperatively and can receive fully informed counselling about their treatment options.

Recent technological advances in imaging and biopsy techniques have significantly improved screening assessment of impalpable lesions. The most significant changes have been the introduction of automated gun core biopsy and vacuum-assisted biopsy devices, prone and upright digital stereotactic equipment and improved breast ultrasound equipment; guided core biopsy with a 14-gauge needle of screen-detected abnormalities provides a preoperative diagnosis of invasive cancers in over 95 per cent of cases. Diagnosing ductal carcinoma *in situ* (DCIS) is more difficult. Although the use of digital stereotactic equipment now means that specimen radiograph confirmation of correct sampling can be obtained in more than 85 per cent of cases, it is common for cores from DCIS lesions to be reported as atypical ductal hyperplasia (ADH) or only suspicious of malignancy. This is because insufficient abnormal ductal tissue has been obtained to enable the pathologist to make a definitive diagnosis. The use of a vacuum-assisted mammotomy device has been shown to increase calcification yield, and decrease ADH core results from DCIS and the need for repeat biopsy.

FURTHER READING

Andersson, I., Janzon, L. 1997: Reduced breast cancer mortality in women under age 50: Updated results from the Malmo mammographic screening program. *JNCI Monograph* **22**, 63–8.

Bjurstam, N., Bjorneld, L., Duffy, S.W. *et al*. 1997: The Gothenburg Breast Screening Trial. First results on mortality, incidence and mode of detection for women ages 39–49 years at randomization. *Cancer* **80**, 2091–9.

Blanks, R.G., Wallis, M.G., Moss, S.M. 1998: A comparison of cancer detection rates achieved by breast cancer screening programmes by number of readers, for one and two view mammography: results from the National Health Service breast screening programme. *Journal of Medical Screening* **5**, 195–201.

Boetes, C., Mus, R.D., Holland, R. *et al*. 1995: Breast tumours: comparative accuracy of MR Imaging relative to mammography and ultrasound for demonstrating extent. *Radiology* **197**, 743–7.

Britton, P.D., Flowers, C.D.R., Freeman *et al*. 1997: Changing to core biopsy in an NHS breast screening unit. *Clinical Radiology* **52**, 764–7.

Burbank, F. 1997: Stereotactic breast biopsy of atypical ductal hyperplasia and ductal carcinoma in situ lesions: improved accuracy with directional, vacuum-assisted biopsy. *Radiology* **202**, 843–7.

Ciatto, S., Rosselli Del Turco, M., Catarzi, S., Morrone, D. 1994: The contribution of ultrasonography to the differential diagnosis of breast cancer. *Neoplasma* **41**, 341–5.

Cyrlak, D., Wong, C.H. 1993: Mammographic changes in post menopausal women undergoing hormone replacement therapy. *American Journal of Roentgenology* **161**, 1177–83.

Ellis, I., Galea, M., Locker, A. *et al*. 1993: Early experience in breast cancer screening: emphasis on development of protocols for triple assessment. *The Breast* **2**, 148–53.

Evans, A.J., Wilson, A.R.M., Blamey, R.W., Elston, C.W., Ellis, I.O., Robertson, J.F.R. 1998: *Atlas of breast disease management: 50 illustrative cases*. London: W.B. Saunders.

Jiang, Y., Nishikawa, R.M., Wolverton, D.E. *et al*. 1996: Malignant and benign clustered microcalcifications: automated feature analysis and classification. *Radiology* **198**, 671–8.

Lister, D., Evans, A.J., Burrell, H.C. *et al*. 1998: The accuracy of breast ultrasound in the evaluation of clinically benign discrete, symptomatic breast lumps. *Clinical Radiology* **53**, 490–2.

Litherland, J.C., Stallard, S., Hole, D., Cordiner, C. 1999: The effect of hormone replacement therapy on the sensitivity of screening mammograms. *Clinical Radiology* **54**, 285–8.

NHSBSP. 1997: *Quality assurance guidelines for radiologists*. Sheffield: NHSBSP Publications.

Nystrom, L., Rutqvist, L., Wall, S. *et al*. 1993: Breast cancer screening with mammography; overview of Swedish randomised trials. *The Lancet* **341**, 973–8.

Parker, S.H., Burbank, F., Jackman, R.J. *et al*. 1994: Percutaneous large-core breast biopsy: a multi-institutional study. *Radiology* **193**, 359–64.

Pauli, R., Hammond, S., Cooke, J., Ansell, J. 1996: Radiographers as film readers in screening mammography: an assessment of competence under test and screening conditions. *British Journal of Radiology* **69**, 10–14.

Philpotts, L.E., Shaheen, N.N.A., Lange, R.C., Lee, C.H. 1999: Comparison of rebiopsy rates after stereotactic core needle biopsy of the breast with 11-gauge vacuum suction probe versus 14-gauge needle and automatic gun. *American Journal of Radiology* **172**, 683–7.

Rosenberg, R.D., Hunt, W.C., Williamson, M.R. *et al*. 1998: Effects of age, breast density, ethnicity, and estrogen replacement therapy on screening mammographic sensitivity and cancer stage at diagnosis: review of 183,134 screening mammograms in Albuqueque, New Mexico. *Radiology* **209**, 511–18.

Sibbering, D., Burrell, H., Evans, A. *et al*. 1995: Mammographic sensitivity in women under 50 presenting symptomatically with breast cancer. *The Breast* **4**, 127–9.

Stavros, A.T., Thickman, D., Rapp, C.L., Dennis, M.A., Parker, S.H., Sisney, G.A. 1995: Solid breast nodules: use of sonography to distinguish between benign ad malignant lesions. *Radiology* **196**, 123–34.

Woodman, C.B.J., Threlfall, A.G., Boggis, C.R.M., Prior, P. 1995: Is the three year breast screening interval too long? Occurrence of interval cancers in NHS breast screening programmes north western region. *British Medical Journal* **310**, 224–6.

Chest

PETER ARMSTRONG

A wide range of intrathoracic diseases can be diagnosed with modern imaging techniques. The first imaging examination is almost invariably a plain chest radiograph and more complex tests may follow. Computed tomography is used increasingly. Techniques such as ultrasound, magnetic resonance imaging, radionuclide examinations and angiography all have specific indications; these are discussed in the appropriate sections of this chapter.

TECHNIQUES

PLAIN CHEST RADIOGRAPHY

The frontal view is the routine plain radiographic projection taken either as a postero-anterior (PA) or anteroposterior (AP) view; the PA view is preferable but may not be practicable in sick patients. A lateral view may be needed as a supplementary view. Routine examinations are exposed on full inspiration with the patient in the upright position (Fig. 23.1).

Mobile X-ray machines are invaluable for taking films on patients who are too sick to move to the X-ray department, but the images may be poor, because the patients cannot stay still or hold their breath during the longer exposure times necessary with mobile machines; also the positioning of the patient is often suboptimal.

Technical evaluation of a film is necessary, since incorrect exposure, poor centring or faulty projection routine may hide or mimic disease. The correctly exposed routine PA chest film shows the lungs well, and the ribs and spine behind the heart can be identified. Unless one can see through the heart and mediastinum, lower-lobe lesions may be completely overlooked. A straight film is one where the medial ends of the clavicles are equidistant from the edges of the thoracic vertebrae. Unless the film is exposed on full inspiration, the heart may appear enlarged and the lung bases may be hazy or show ill-defined densities (Fig. 23.2). Such an appearance may mimic pulmonary oedema, pneumonia or pulmonary infarction. The degree of inspiration is adequate when the dome of the right hemidiaphragm is level with the anterior end of the sixth rib.

Additional plain films of the chest may provide details of lesions seen on routine films or may even enable a previously invisible abnormality to be detected:

- **Oblique views** are useful for demonstrating the chest wall and ribs, particularly fractures, and, occasionally, for showing intrathoracic shadows to better advantage.
- **Lateral decubitus views** are not, as the name suggests, lateral views: they are frontal projections taken with patient lying on one or other side. Their principal use is to demonstrate mobile fluid in the pleural cavities.
- **Expiratory films** are frontal films deliberately exposed on expiration in order to demonstrate diaphragmatic movement and the ability of a lung to deflate, or to detect a pneumothorax which may be more obvious on an expiration than an inspiration film.

(a)

(b)

Figure 23.1 *Routine normal postero-anterior and lateral views of chest. Note that the patient is straight and the films have been exposed on deep inspiration. (a) The heart and mediastinal borders are clearly seen as are the left and right upper surfaces of both hemidiaphragms, except where the aorta passes through the diaphragm. Lung behind the heart can be seen. (b) On the lateral view, the vertebrae appear darker as the eye travels down the spine.*

Figure 23.2 *Chest film in normal patient exposed on expiration. The heart appears enlarged and the lung bases are hazy owing to poor inflation of the lungs. The appearance mimics congestive heart failure or bilateral basal pneumonia.*

- **Lordotic views** provide an alternative, often improved, view of the lung apices by projecting the clavicles above the lung and changing the relationship of ribs to lungs. This allows apical pulmonary lesions to be seen to advantage and makes it possible to distinguish a pulmonary from a bony density.

COMPUTED TOMOGRAPHY

CT provides similar but far superior diagnostic information to plain chest radiography, but is only cost-effective in certain circumstances, particularly to:

- demonstrate enlarged hilar and mediastinal lymph nodes or mediastinal invasion when patients with neoplastic disease, notably lung cancer and lymphoma, are being staged;
- show the presence and extent of mediastinal masses (sometimes it is possible to diagnose the nature of a mass based on shape, precise location and density characteristics);
- diagnose aortic disease (notably dissections and aneurysms) and a variety of mediastinal disorders, such as oesophageal rupture and mediastinitis;
- show the precise shape of a focal intrapulmonary lesion and to detect any calcification or fluid in the lesion, features that may help to decide whether an abnormality is malignant or benign;
- localize an intrathoracic mass prior to biopsy;
- demonstrate the presence of disease when the plain chest radiograph is normal in those cases where the possibility of intrathoracic abnormality is suspected on other grounds, e.g. detecting pulmonary metastases, finding a primary carcinoma in patients whose sputum cytology shows neoplastic cells, and demonstrating thymic tumours in patients with myasthenia gravis;

- elucidate pleural pathology;
- diagnose chest wall disease;
- diagnose airway disease, notably the presence, extent and severity of bronchiectasis, and certain pulmonary parenchymal processes, such as fibrosing alveolitis, using high-resolution CT;
- diagnose moderate-sized and large pulmonary emboli using the technique of CT angiography.

Routine chest CT examinations consist of adjacent 8–10 mm sections through the area of interest. Intravenous contrast medium may be injected when the primary purpose of the examination is to show the mediastinal or hilar structures. The images are usually viewed at two distinct window settings: lung and mediastinal windows. If the CT scan has been performed for bone lesions then bone settings are used.

High-resolution CT (HRCT) uses very thin sections 1–2 mm thick. HRCT of the lungs is a specialized application designed primarily to diagnose bronchiectasis and other airway disorders or to determine the presence, extent and, if possible, the diagnosis in patients with diffuse lung disease, of which fibrosing alveolitis is the commonest.

OTHER TECHNIQUES

Magnetic resonance imaging

MRI of the chest provides similar information to chest CT with respect to pleural, mediastinal or chest wall disorders, but has advantages in certain specific circumstances. The multiplanar imaging capability allows images to be obtained in any desired plane. Coronal, sagittal and oblique planes may provide superior information to images taken in an axial plane, the usual plane for CT. This is particularly true for showing the extent of tumours or lymphadenopathy in the aortopulmonary window, the subcarinal region or the lung apices. Because it is possible to obtain cardiac-gated MR images, the pericardium, myocardium and cardiac chambers can be shown with less degradation from cardiac movement. Also, using surface coils it is possible to obtain very high-resolution MR images of the chest wall and root of neck.

With spin-echo sequences, fast flowing blood produces a signal void. This allows structures such as the aorta, central pulmonary vessels, great veins and cardiac chambers to be imaged without the need for contrast agents. It also allows small masses to be distinguished from blood vessels in areas of complex vascular anatomy such as the hilar regions.

There is no such examination as a routine chest MRI: all chest MRI is tailored to answer specific questions. The most frequently used sequences are T1-weighted, cardiac-gated images, breath-hold images, and magnetic resonance angiography.

Figure 23.3 *Magnetic resonance angiogram of aorta and other arteries. This 3D contrast-enhanced gradient-echo MR image shows the heart, aorta and branches, and central pulmonary arteries. The gadolinium was given by rapid injection into an antecubital vein.*

Magnetic resonance angiography can be performed using a variety of techniques: some depend on the inherently different signal from flowing blood compared to stationary tissues, whereas others rely on contrast enhancement using agents such as intravenous gadolinium chelates (Fig. 22.3).

Radionuclide imaging

The use of radionuclide imaging in diagnosing pulmonary embolic disease is discussed on page 559.

Pulmonary angiography

The pulmonary arteries and veins can be demonstrated by taking serial films following the rapid injection of angiographic contrast media into the pulmonary arterial circulation through a catheter introduced from the groin or antecubital fossa. The catheterization is carried out under fluoroscopic control with continuous electrocardiographic and pressure monitoring by an operator skilled in cardiac catheterization. Pulmonary angiography carries a small but definite risk to the patient. Its major use is to diagnose pulmonary emboli. Occasionally, it is needed to demonstrate congenital vascular anomalies.

CT angiography is best performed using spiral CT. The principle is based on contrast enhancement, using a rapid bolus of contrast agent injected intravenously, with rapid acquisition of a block of CT sections timed to coincide with maximal contrast enhancement. The best images are acquired during a single breath-hold. In the chest, the technique is used predominantly to diagnose pulmonary emboli (*see* Fig. 23.35b) and to demonstrate aortic dissections, aortic aneurysms or other disorders of the larger intrathoracic arteries.

Bronchography

Bronchography involves introducing an iodinated contrast material into the bronchial tree. Nowadays, on the few occasions that bronchography is performed, it is done during bronchoscopsy by injecting the contrast agent via a catheter introduced through a special channel in a bronchoscope. The only remaining indication is for the assessment of selected cases of bronchiectasis. Bronchography has been almost entirely replaced by HRCT.

Fluoroscopy

The image at fluoroscopy is poor compared to that achieved with X-ray film. Fluoroscopy is limited to observing the movement of the diaphragm and shift of the mediastinum caused by air trapping in cases of suspected inhalation of a foreign body.

NORMAL CHEST RADIOGRAPH (Fig. 23.1)

The upper surface of the diaphragm extending from one costophrenic angle to the other should be clearly outlined by aerated lung, except where the mediastinal structures, including the heart, are in contact with the diaphragm. The costophrenic angles are usually sharp, but if the hemidiaphragms are flattened, the angles may become meniscus-shaped, simulating pleural fluid. Failure to see a clear diaphragm outline suggests either pleural or pulmonary disease.

The normal right hemidiaphragm is usually 1–3 cm higher, but may be level with, or even slightly lower than, the left; the midpoint of the right hemidiaphragm is usually level with the anterior end of the sixth rib.

The lateral borders of the heart and mediastinum should be clearly defined between the clavicles and the diaphragm. Any lack of clarity indicates pulmonary or, less often, pleural disease. Above the clavicles the normal mediastinal border may be indistinct. Aortic unfolding often modifies the appearance of the superior

mediastinum and may hide pathology or simulate disease.

On the PA view the centre of the trachea lies midway or slightly to the right of the midpoint between the medial ends of the clavicles. The trachea courses vertically or slightly to the right as it descends into the chest. The position of the heart is variable, making it difficult to diagnose all but the most severe degrees of cardiac displacement. On average, one third of the heart lies to the right of the midline, but the normal range varies from one fifth to one half of the cardiac diameter lying to the right of the midline.

The cardiothoracic ratio is a widely used but crude method of measuring heart size. In normal people the transverse diameter of the heart is usually less than half the internal diameter of the chest. Knowing whether or not the heart has increased in size compared with previous films is often more useful than the cardiothoracic ratio in isolation. It should, however, be realized that the transverse cardiac diameter varies with the phase of respiration and, to a lesser extent, with the cardiac cycle. Thus changes in transverse diameter of less than 1.5 cm should be interpreted with caution.

In children under the age of seven, the thymus may be visible as an anterior mediastinal mass. In babies, the thymus is usually a prominent structure. Its shape is variable, a 'sail' configuration being characteristic, but rounded outlines are frequent and may be mistaken for true mediastinal masses or pulmonary shadowing. As the normal thymus is soft, it does not deform adjacent structures, such as the trachea.

The hilar shadows are produced by the pulmonary arteries and veins. The lower lobe arteries are 9–16 mm in diameter, with parallel walls except where they branch. The hilar lymph nodes cannot be identified as separate shadows, and the walls of the bronchi are thin and contribute little to the image seen on the radiograph. The left hilum is usually slightly higher than the right. Any lobulation of the hilar shadows, or any local expansion or increase in density compared with the opposite side indicates a mass.

The only structures that can be identified within normal lungs are blood vessels, interlobar fissures and the walls of certain larger bronchi seen end-on. The blood vessels show an orderly decrease in diameter as they progress from the hila outward. In the upright patient, equivalent vessels in the upper zones are smaller than in the lower zones; this difference is not seen if the patient is examined supine. The fissures can be seen only if they lie tangential to the X-ray beam. Usually, the minor fissure is the only visible fissure in the frontal projection; it can be identified in over half the population, running from the right hilum to the sixth rib in the axilla. In about 1 per cent of the population, an extra fissure, the so-called azygos fissure, is visible in the frontal view. On the lateral view each major fissure runs obliquely across the chest from the T4 or T5 vertebral body to reach a point on the hemidiaphragm close to the anterior chest wall.

Care should be taken not to confuse chest wall structures, such as pectoral muscles, breasts or costal cartilages, with intrathoracic diseases. In particular, the nipples or any skin lumps may mimic pulmonary nodules, and hair braids or clothing may cause shadows that resemble pulmonary densities. The nipples are usually in the fifth anterior rib space and in general, if one nipple is visible, the other will also be seen.

Finding abnormal pulmonary shadows in the frontal film is usually fairly easy, since it is possible to compare one lung with the other. Detecting shadows on the lateral view may be difficult. A useful rule is that, as the eye travels down the vertebrae towards the diaphragm, each vertebral body should appear more lucent than the one above. Also, but less reliably, the density of the retrocardiac space in most patients is similar to that of the retrosternal space, and the density over the heart shows no abrupt change.

The ribs, sternum, clavicles, scapulae and spine need to be examined for fractures and areas of lysis and sclerosis. The upper cortical line of the ribs is continuous and easy to assess. The inferior cortical line, however, is normally indistinct in the posterior portions of the ribs and its absence should be interpreted as a lytic lesion only with great caution. Each scapula casts

two linear shadows on the lateral view, which can be mistaken for disease or misplaced fissures.

Rib disease may be accompanied by soft-tissue swelling and, not infrequently, the swelling is more obvious than the bone abnormality. Therefore, the outer lung edge should always be reviewed for extrapleural soft-tissue swelling, and the frontal film should be reviewed for ill-defined densities that may lead to the discovery of a rib lesion.

ABNORMAL CHEST RADIOGRAPH

There are many ways of looking at plain chest films. The trained radiologist often uses a problem-oriented approach: the search pattern is varied according to features present on the films, with constant integration of the clinical information. For example, if a nodule representing a possible lung carcinoma is seen, the shape of the nodule itself, other lung lesions and evidence for spread of disease are sought. Those observers with less radiological experience should follow a routine to avoid overlooking important information. One approach is presented here.

The first step in categorizing any abnormality found on plain chest radiography is to decide its location,

(a)

(b)

Figure 23.4 *Silhouette sign. (a) An area of pneumonia in the anterior segment of the left lower lobe has rendered the diaphragm outline lateral to the heart invisible. (b) The same patient after the pneumonia has resolved. The left hemidiaphragm is now clearly visible.*

particularly whether it lies in the lung, pleura, mediastinum, diaphragm or chest wall. Clearly, the differential diagnosis depends on the site of the lesion. Accurate plain film localization frequently requires two views, usually frontal and lateral projections. The location of an abnormality is usually obvious, but, when a lesion is at the boundary between the lung and the chest wall, mediastinum or diaphragm, it may be difficult to decide its site of origin. If the shadow has a broad base with smooth, well-defined convex borders projecting into the lung, it is likely to be pleural, extrapleural or mediastinal in origin (see Fig. 23.69, p. 578).

THE SILHOUETTE SIGN

The information on a chest film is largely dependent on the transradiancy of air in the lung compared with the heart, blood vessels, mediastinum and diaphragm, all of which have a similar density, known as 'soft-tissue density'. An intrathoracic lesion in contact with the heart, mediastinum or diaphragm will cause normal borders to become ill-defined or invisible. This sign, known as the silhouette sign (Figs 23.4, 23.5), may be very helpful in both recognizing and localizing chest disease. The silhouette sign makes it possible to localize a shadow by observing which borders are lost (e.g. loss of the heart border must mean that the shadow lies in the anterior half of the chest). Alternatively, loss of part of the diaphragm outline indicates disease of the pleura or lower lobes.

The silhouette sign also makes it possible, on occasion, to diagnose disorders such as pulmonary consolidation, even when one is uncertain whether an opacity is present. It is a surprising fact that a wedge- or lens-shaped opacity may be very difficult to see because of the way the shadow fades out at its margin, but if such a lesion is in contact with the mediastinum or diaphragm, the normal sharp boundary of these structures is lost.

IMAGING PATTERNS OF LUNG DISEASE

When chest radiographs or CT scans are being viewed, it is helpful to try to categorize the abnormalities into one or more basic patterns in order to limit the differential diagnostic possibilities for lung disease:

PULMONARY SHADOWS

These include:

- pulmonary consolidation or collapse (or a mixture of the two)
- pulmonary oedema
- spherical shadow/lung masses
- line shadows
- widespread small shadows

(a)

(b)

Figure 23.5 *Silhouette sign. (a) PA view. In the lateral view (b), the consolidation of the right middle lobe (arrows) has rendered the adjacent right heart border invisible. (The lobe has also lost volume.)*

PULMONARY CONSOLIDATION

Consolidation and collapse (atelectasis) often coexist. It is, however, convenient to consider these two phenomena separately. The signs of pulmonary consolidation (Fig. 23.5; see also Fig. 23.24, p. 555) are:

- A **shadow with ill-defined borders** except where the disease process contacts a fissure, in which case the shadow has a well-defined edge corresponding to the fissure.
- An **air bronchogram**. If the alveoli are filled with fluid or inflammatory exudate, then air in the bronchi stands out against the background of fluid or exudate in the lung. An opacity containing an air bronchogram is almost always due to either pneumonia or pulmonary oedema.

Consolidation of a whole lobe or the great majority of a lobe (Figs 23.5, 23.6; see also Fig. 23.24, p. 555) is virtually diagnostic of pneumonia or pulmonary oedema.

Patchy consolidation, i.e. one or more patches of ill-defined shadowing up to the size of one or more segments, is usually due to infection, but may occasionally be due to infarction or, even less commonly, to eosinophilic pneumonia or vasculitis. There is no reliable way of telling which of these possibilities is the cause but, in most instances, the clinical and laboratory findings point to one of these options. Another major diagnostic difficulty, particularly on plain chest radiography, is distinguishing widespread patchy consolidation, e.g. due to pneumonia, from pulmonary oedema.

The diagnosis of **cavitation within consolidation** depends on recognizing an air space or an air–fluid level within the consolidation. Patchy consolidation with intervening normal or emphysematous areas of lung can easily be mistaken for cavities, and CT may be helpful to make the distinction. Infectious agents particularly liable to produce cavitation are *Staphylococcus aureus*, *Klebsiella* spp., *Mycobacterium tuberculosis* (Fig. 23.7), anaerobic bacteria and various fungi. Cavitation is occasionally seen in other forms of pulmonary consolidation, e.g. infarction and Wegener's granulomatosis.

PULMONARY COLLAPSE (ATELECTASIS)

Collapse (loss of volume of a lung or lobe) may be due to:

- bronchial obstruction
- fibrosis of a lobe, usually following tuberculosis
- bronchiectasis

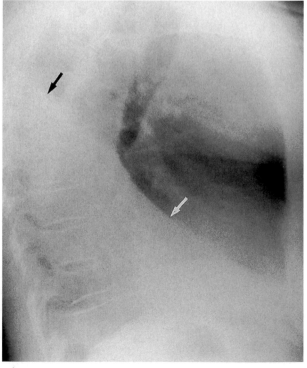

(a)

(b)

Figure 23.6 *Lobar pneumonia. The whole of the right lower lobe is consolidated. The lobar shape is best seen in the lateral view (b) where the opacity is sharply demarcated by the oblique fissure (arrows).*

- pneumothorax
- pleural effusion.

Pulmonary embolism may also lead to minor degrees of loss of volume.

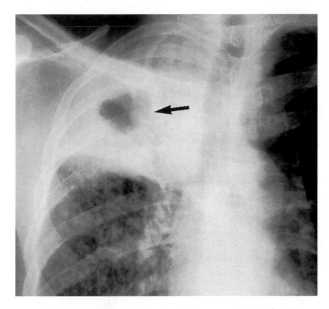

Figure 23.7 *Cavitation (arrow) within consolidation of the right upper lobe in active tuberculosis. The right upper lobe shows extensive consolidation and some loss of volume. Further foci of tuberculous infection are seen in the adjacent lower lobe.*

Collapse from bronchial obstruction

Collapse from bronchial obstruction occurs because no air passes into the lung to replace the air absorbed from the alveoli. Consolidation almost invariably accompanies lobar collapse, so the resulting shadow is usually obvious. The likely causes are:

- **Bronchial wall lesions**
  - usually primary carcinoma
  - rarely, other bronchial tumours such as carcinoid
  - rarely, endobronchial tuberculosis.
- **Intraluminal occlusion**
  - mucus plugging, particularly in postoperative, asthmatic or unconscious patients, or in patients on artificial ventilation
  - inhaled foreign body.
- **Invasion or compression by an adjacent mass**
  - malignant tumour
  - enlarged lymph nodes.

The signs of lobar collapse on plain chest radiography (Figs 23.8–23.11) are the shadow of the collapsed lung tissue, the silhouette sign, and displacement of structures to take up the space normally occupied by the collapsed lobe. The diagnosis of lobar collapse is easy on CT when the opaque lobe of reduced volume is readily identified (Fig. 23.10b).

Occasionally, the lobe becomes so shrunken that, unless the lobe is precisely tangential to the X-ray beam,

(a)

Figure 23.8 *Right upper lobe (RUL) collapse with complete consolidation. Note the opaque RUL with elevation of the horizontal fissure (arrows). The trachea is deviated towards the collapsed lobe. The lobar shape is well shown in both (a) PA and (b) lateral views.*

(b)

Figure 23.9 *Right lower lobe (RLL) collapse. The RLL shows substantial opacity and the oblique fissure (arrows) is pulled downwards and angled so that it can be seen in the frontal view. The trachea is deviated towards the side of the collapse.*

(a)

(b)

Figure 23.10 *Left lower lobe (LLL) collapse. (a) LLL collapse can be much more difficult to diagnose than other collapsed lobes on plain chest radiographs because, as in this case, the collapsed lobe lies entirely behind the heart. The triangular density of the collapsed lobe has a straight linear border (arrow). Note the lack of visibility of the descending aorta and left hemidiaphragm outlines. (b) On CT the collapsed lobe is easy to identify. Note the clear-cut curvilinear anterior margin formed by the backwardly displaced oblique fissure (arrows).*

it may be difficult to see on a plain chest radiograph in one or other projection (Fig. 23.11). The silhouette sign can be very useful in this situation, since the mediastinal and diaphragmatic borders are ill-defined adjacent to the collapsed lobe. The silhouette sign also helps in deciding which lobe is collapsed. Collapse of the anteriorly located lobes (the upper and middle) obliterates portions of the mediastinal and heart outlines, whereas collapse of the lower lobes obscures the outline of the adjacent diaphragm and descending aorta.

When a lobe collapses, the ipsilateral unobstructed lung expands so that the hilum and fissure move towards the collapsed lobe. The hemidiaphragm may become elevated. With collapse of the whole of one lung, the entire hemithorax is opaque and there is substantial mediastinal and tracheal shift (Fig. 23.12).

Collapse from fibrosis or bronchiectasis

When atelectasis is due to lobar fibrosis or bronchiectasis, the lobe usually remains aerated. The signs are, therefore, displacement of structures.

Collapse in association with pleural abnormality

The presence of air or fluid in the pleural cavity allows the lungs to collapse. In pneumothorax, the diagnosis is obvious but, if there is a large pleural effusion with underlying pulmonary collapse, it may be difficult on a chest radiograph to diagnose the presence of collapsed lung. Even if the collapsed lobe is identified, it can be difficult to tell whether the collapse is due to pleural fluid or whether both the collapse and the effusion are due to the same process, e.g. carcinoma of the

(a)

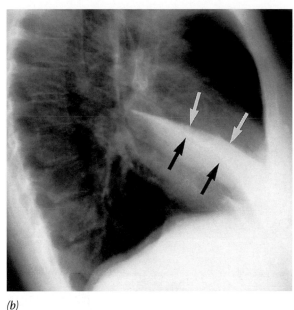

(b)

Figure 23.11 *Severe collapse of the right middle lobe. (a) On the frontal view the opacity of the collapsed lobe is ill-defined and quite difficult to see. Note the lack of clarity of the lower right heart border because of the silhouette sign. (b) The lateral view shows a wedge-shaped density with a clear-cut upper margin owing to the downwardly displaced horizontal fissure (white arrows) and a well-defined lower margin from the upwardly displaced right oblique fissure (black arrows).*

Figure 23.12 *Collapse of the left lung. Both the left upper and left lower lobes are airless and severely collapsed. The whole left hemithorax is opaque with no visible left heart border or left hemidiaphragm. The trachea is greatly displaced towards the side of the opacity.*

Round atelectasis

Round atelectasis is a form of chronic atelectasis that resembles a mass which, particularly on plain films, can be confused with a neoplasm. The process is most frequently associated with asbestos exposure and the features of asbestos-related pleural disease are usually present (see p. 566).

The typical imaging features (Fig. 23.13) are a round, oval or wedge-shaped mass in contact with thickened pleura. The edge is well-defined, albeit often irregular, except where the bronchi and vessels enter the opacity. The bronchovascular structures may visibly converge consequent on the atelectasis and air bronchograms may be visible within the mass. The affected lobe is often recognizably reduced in volume.

PULMONARY OEDEMA

Radiographically, there are two forms of pulmonary oedema – alveolar and interstitial. Since the oedema fluid collects initially in the interstitial compartment of the lungs, patients with alveolar oedema also have interstitial oedema. Alveolar oedema is always acute, whereas interstitial oedema can be acute or chronic. The causes of pulmonary oedema can be divided into:

• those due to circulatory problems, e.g. left ventricular failure, or fluid overload from renal failure or overtransfusion, and

bronchus. At CT it is usually easy to recognize pulmonary collapse despite the presence of a pleural effusion.

(b)

(a)

Figure 23.13 *Round atelectasis in three patients with prior asbestos exposure. (a) Plain chest radiograph showing a posteriorly located mass (arrows) resembling carcinoma of the lung. Note, in addition, the extensive pleural thickening. (b) CT showing a spiculated mass (*) apparently totally surrounded by aerated lung. In fact the mass of round atelectasis was contiguous with a large pleural plaque on the right hemidiaphragm. Note also the typical asbestos-related pleural plaques against the chest wall bilaterally. (c) Lens-shaped round atelectasis (*) based on the anterior chest wall showing distortion of adjacent blood vessels which are pulled into the mass. (Fig. 23.45b shows the pleural plaques in this patient to better advantage.)*

(c)

- non-cardiogenic pulmonary oedema, so-called adult respiratory distress syndrome (ARDS), a topic discussed on p. 561; inhalation of noxious gases; and high-altitude pulmonary oedema.

Alveolar oedema (Fig. 23.14) is almost always bilateral, involving all lobes. The shadowing is greatest close to the hila and fades out peripherally. Sometimes a relatively clear zone is seen around the edges of the lobe and then the resulting radiographic appearance is known as the 'butterfly' or 'bat's wing' pattern. Although the classic description is bilateral symmetry, symmetry is in fact unusual: the oedema often predominates on one side and varies in severity from lobe to lobe. Basal predominance is, however, common.

The differential diagnosis of alveolar pulmonary oedema includes widespread pneumonia, especially aspiration pneumonia, aspiration of gastric contents, inhalation of noxious gases, pulmonary haemorrhage

and alveolar cell carcinoma of the lung. A helpful differential feature is the rapidity with which oedema appears and disappears following treatment. Substantial changes in the severity of air-space shadowing in a 24-hour period strongly suggest pulmonary oedema; resolution within this time scale is pathognomonic.

Interstitial pulmonary oedema causes thickening of the interstitial compartment of the lungs, recognized radiologically (Fig. 23.15) as thickening of the pleural fissures, bronchial wall thickening, lack of clarity of the pulmonary vessels and identifiable septal lines. These signs may be accompanied by cardiac enlargement and evidence of raised pulmonary venous pressure (see p. 597), notably increase in size of the upper zone blood vessels.

When thickened, the interstitial septa are seen as line shadows, known as Kerley A and B lines. The B lines are short, horizontal, 1–2 cm lines at the extreme edge of the lobes, usually best appreciated at the bases. Unlike blood vessels, B lines can be seen to reach the

(a)   *(b)*

Figure 23.14 *Alveolar pulmonary oedema in two patients with acute left ventricular failure. (a) Butterfly pattern – note the relative sparing of the outer portions of both lungs. (b) The more common pattern of mid- and lower-zone, predominant, ill-defined, relatively homogeneous pulmonary shadowing.*

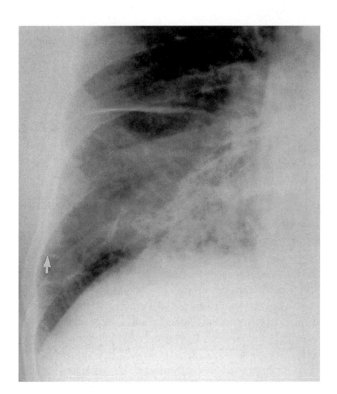

Figure 23.15 *Septal lines (Kerley B lines) from pulmonary oedema. The short horizontal lines (one of which is arrowed) are parallel to one another and reach the pleura. Note the thickening of the horizontal fissure also caused by interstitial oedema.*

pleural edge. A lines are 3–6 cm long and radiate from the hila, mainly the mid and upper zones. They are much thinner than the adjacent blood vessels and show fewer branches. Thickened septal lines are the hallmark

of interstitial pulmonary oedema and obvious septal lines on a plain chest radiograph are seen in few other conditions. As discussed on p. 575, the main differential diagnosis is from lymphangitis carcinomatosa.

Interstitial pulmonary oedema may also be recognized as thickening of the bronchial walls, which is best appreciated where bronchi are seen end-on.

Normal intrapulmonary vessels are moderately well-defined, but, when surrounded by interstitial oedema, they become indistinct. This is a very difficult sign to evaluate. Interstitial oedema also collects subpleurally to produce an extremely useful combination of signs, namely uniform thickening of the fissures together with lamellar fluid collections. Lamellar effusions are vertically oriented, small, well-marginated fluid collections, usually best seen in the costophrenic angles. The term lamellar pleural effusion is a misnomer, since the dense well-defined stripe is due to subpleural pulmonary oedema, not fluid in the pleural cavity.

The pulmonary vascular pattern in patients with pulmonary oedema may or may not show the features of raised pulmonary venous pressure as discussed on p. 597.

SOLITARY PULMONARY NODULE (MASS)

The diagnosis of a solitary spherical shadow in the lung (solitary pulmonary nodule) is a common problem (Fig. 23.16). The usual causes are:

- **bronchial carcinoma** or bronchial carcinoid
- **benign tumour of the lung**, hamartoma being the most common

(a)

(b)

Figure 23.16 *Solitary pulmonary nodule (arrow). (a) The differential diagnosis for this 2 cm rounded, well-defined nodule with no calcification or cavitation and no previous examination with which to compare would be wide (see text). (b) CT scan in different patient showing a 2 cm nodule with an irregular margin with infiltrating edges. The appearances are highly suggestive of bronchial carcinoma; this proved to be the diagnosis in this particular case.*

- **infective granuloma**, tuberculoma being the most common in the UK, fungal granuloma the most frequent in the USA
- **metastasis**
- **lung abscess**, in which the mass will show cavitation.

With the exception of lung abscesses and large bronchial carcinomas, the nodule itself is often asymptomatic, the lesion being first noted on a routine chest film. When a nodule is discovered in a patient who is over 40 and a smoker, bronchial carcinoma becomes the major consideration.

The various possible lesions require totally different forms of management. Hamartomas and granulomas are best left alone, whereas bronchial carcinoma or carcinoid, active tuberculosis and lung abscess require treatment. Curative resection is possible for bronchial carcinoma/carcinoid. Careful observation of the following features may help in making the diagnosis.

Comparison with previous films

Assessing the rate of growth of a spherical lesion by comparing previous examinations is one the most important observations, because lack of change over a period of 18 months is a strong indication of a benign process such as a harmatoma or inactive granuloma. Almost all primary lung cancers double their volume between 1 and 18 months (a 26 per cent increase in diameter corresponds to a doubling in volume).

Calcification

The presence of calcification is the other vital observation, because substantial calcification virtually rules out the diagnosis of a malignant lesion; bronchial carcinoids may, however, show extensive calcification. Calcification is a common finding in hamartomas, tuberculomas and fungal granulomas. In hamartomas the calcification is often of the 'popcorn' type (Fig. 23.17). CT is of great value in detecting calcification and confirming that the calcification is within the lesion, not just projected over it. Uniform calcification can be difficult to recognize on plain chest radiography but is readily diagnosed with CT, and when present carcinoma of the lung can be excluded from the differential diagnosis.

Involvement of the adjacent chest wall

Destruction of the ribs adjacent to a pulmonary mass is virtually diagnostic of invasion by carcinoma. Tumours of the lung apex are particularly liable to invade adjacent bones, the chest wall and the root of the neck (Pancoast's tumour) (Fig. 23.18). CT, MRI or radionuclide bone scan may be indicated to demonstrate invasion.

Figure 23.17 *Hamartoma of the lung. The central 'popcorn' calcification typical of cartilage calcification is diagnostic of hamartoma in this case.*

Figure 23.18 *Pancoast's tumour. The apical bronchial carcinoma is causing opacity of the uppermost portion of the left lung. The left first rib is almost totally destroyed by the tumour. This destruction is difficult to appreciate at first glance but, when the right and left first and second ribs are compared, it is obvious that, apart from a tiny residue of the head of the left first rib, the posterior portion of the rib in question is totally destroyed.*

The shape of the shadow

Primary carcinoma nearly always shows a lobulated, notched or infiltrating outline. Even if only a small portion of the lesion has an ill-defined edge, the diagnosis of primary lung carcinoma should be seriously considered. A markedly infiltrating edge is highly suggestive of bronchial carcinoma (Fig. 23.16b). If the shadow is perfectly spherical and the edge very well-defined the lesion is likely to be a hamartoma, a tuberculoma or a metastasis.

The shape may be obvious from plain films but CT can be used to show the edge of a pulmonary nodule to advantage.

Cavitation

If the centre of the mass undergoes necrosis, it will be possible to see on CT a homogeneous low-attenuation region consistent with fluid density. If enough of the necrotic material is coughed up, air is seen within the mass on CT and plain film. Such air is often accompanied by fluid, in which case an air–fluid level is visible on CT and on erect plain films. The air, which may be difficult to appreciate on plain film, is particularly well seen at CT.

A solitary cavity may be due to the following:

- **Infective lung abscess** (Fig. 23.19a). The most frequent cause of an infective lung abscess is aspiration of food or secretions; such abscesses are usually in the apical (superior) segments of the lower lobes or in the posterior segments of the upper lobes; lung abscesses may also be due to infection beyond an obstructing lesion in the bronchus or beyond infected emboli, particularly in drug addicts.
- **Lung neoplasm** (Fig. 23.19b).
- **Wegener's granulomatosis** (Fig. 23.19c).

It may be difficult or impossible to distinguish lung abscess from other causes of a cavitary mass, including cavitary malignant neoplasm, infarction, and granulomas from collagen vascular disease. Most infective lung abscesses are in the posterior portions of the lung, and caution should be exercised when an anterior cavitary mass is diagnosed as a lung abscess. Non-uniform thickness of cavity walls is an important sign that the lesion is something other than a lung abscess and is probably a lung carcinoma. CT can play a role in determining the thickness and regularity of the cavity wall. Uniformly thin smooth cavity walls are usually benign, whereas a cavity in which any portion of the wall is thicker than 1 cm is usually a malignant neoplasm.

Clinically, it is usually straightforward to distinguish between cavitating neoplasms and infective lung abscesses.

Size

A solitary lesion over 4 cm in diameter that does not contain calcium is nearly always either a primary carcinoma or a lung abscess; rarer causes include hydatid cyst and Wegener's granulomatosis. Lung

(a)

(b)

(c)

Figure 23.19 *Cavitation of rounded lesions owing to (a) bacterial lung abscess (the cavity in this instance is strikingly thin-walled); (b) a lung carcinoma (note the variable thickness of the cavity wall, some portions being notably thick); and (c) Wegener's granulomatosis (both thin- and thick-walled cavities are present on this CT section).*

abscesses and Wegener's lesions of this size virtually always show cavitation, whereas carcinoma may or may not undergo recognizable cavitation.

Other lesions

The rest of the film should be checked carefully after a solitary lung mass has been found. Finding a small pleural effusion or a rib metastasis alters the management of the patient. Alternatively the nodule may not be solitary; multiple pulmonary nodules are likely to be due to metastases.

The role of CT for evaluating a solitary pulmonary nodule

CT is performed in a patient with a solitary pulmonary nodule in order to:

- diagnose the nature of the nodule – the role here is limited since the plain film signs and knowledge of the rate of growth provide adequate information in most cases. CT is better able to detect calcification in a nodule than conventional films and, as mentioned above, extensive calcification of a nodule effectively excludes primary carcinoma of the lung;
- stage the extent of disease in those cases where the nodule is likely to be a primary carcinoma;
- localize accurately the nodule prior to bronchoscopic or percutaneous needle biopsy in cases where localization is difficult from conventional films;
- establish whether or not the nodule is solitary or multiple when the lesion in question is likely to be a metasis. This indication is particularly important when surgical resection of a metastasis is being considered.

MULTIPLE PULMONARY NODULES

Multiple well-defined spherical shadows in the lungs are virtually diagnostic of metastases (Fig. 23.20). Occasionally, such a pattern is seen with abscesses or with granulomatous disorders, such as collagen vascular disease, sarcoidosis and tuberculous or fungal infections.

Figure 23.20 *Pulmonary metastases presenting as multiple pulmonary nodules.*

LINE SHADOWS

Long line shadows, other than normal fissures and the pleural edge of a pneumothorax, are usually due to pleuropulmonary scars from previous infection or infarction. Mostly, these scars reach the pleura and are associated with visible pleural thickening. They are of no significance to the patient. Emphysematous bullae may be bounded and traversed by thin line shadows.

An important cause of line shadows is **septal lines** (Fig. 23.21). They are usually due to pulmonary oedema or lymphangitis carcinomatosa. The pulmonary septa are interlobular connective tissue planes, which are only visible radiologically when thickened. The most readily seen are the so-called **Kerley B lines**: small horizontal lines, never more than 2 cm in length, which are best seen at the periphery of the lung bases. In contrast to the blood vessels, they often reach the edge of the lung. So-called **Kerley A lines** are longer and situated more centrally. They radiate outwards from the hila.

WIDESPREAD SMALL SHADOWS

Nodular and reticular shadows

Plain chest radiographs with widespread small (2–5 mm) pulmonary shadows often present a diagnostic problem. With few exceptions it is only possible to

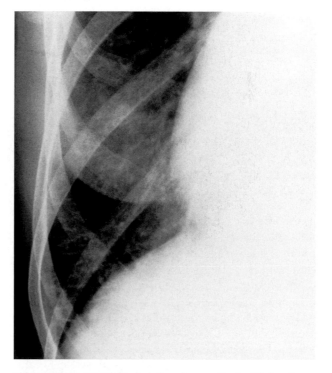

Figure 23.21 *Septal (Kerley) lines in a patient with heart failure. These stacked, short, thin lines, representing thickened interlobular septa, are seen best in the outer centimetre or so of the lungs where the blood vessels are too small to see. They are horizontally oriented and reach the pleura.*

Table 23.1 *Commoner causes of widespread nodular and reticular shadowing*

Diagnosis	Radiographic pattern	Distribution of shadows	Other features which may be seen	High-resolution CT (HRCT)
Miliary tuberculosis	Small nodules of uniform size	Uniform	± Large mediastinal/hilar lymph nodes One or more patches of consolidation	Not necessary
Sarcoidosis	(a) Fine nodular	Uniform	Large hilar and para-tracheal lymph nodes	Shows disease well but adds little of diagnostic value
	(b) Reticulonodular	Often predominant in mid and upper zones	Large hilar and para-tracheal lymph nodes	
Coal-miners' pneumoconiosis	Nodular	Predominant in upper zones	Progressive massive fibrosis in the complicated form of the disease Emphysema	Adds little of diagnostic value
Asbestosis	Fine reticulonodular	Predominant in lower zones	Pleural thickening and/or calcification	Useful for documenting the presence and severity of fibrosis and for showing pleural plaques where the diagnosis of asbestos exposure is in doubt
Fibrosing alveolitis	Reticulonodular	Often radiates from the hila and is predominant in lower zones but may show variety of patterns	Diaphragm often high and indistinct	Characteristically shows peripherally predominant reticulonodular shadowing
Lymphangitis carcinomatosa	Reticulonodular	No predominant pattern	Septal lines Bronchial wall thickening Hilar adenopathy Other signs of carcinoma	The combination of septal lines and interstitial small nodules produces a characteristic pattern
Pulmonary oedema	Ill-defined nodules	May show central predominance with clear zone at periphery of lobes	Cardiac enlargement Left atrial enlargement Septal lines	Not indicated

give a differential diagnosis when faced with such a film. A final diagnosis can rarely be made without an intimate knowledge of the patient's symptoms and clinical signs. HRCT may enable a more confident diagnosis in many cases (see Fig. 23.41, p. 564).

Many descriptive terms have been applied to widespread small pulmonary shadows, notably 'nodular', to signify discrete small round shadows and 'reticular' to describe a net-like pattern of small lines. Often there are both nodular and reticular elements and this appearance is called 'reticulonodular'.

These patterns are due to very small lesions in the lung, no more than 1 or 2 mm in size. Individual lesions of this size are invisible on a chest film. That these very small lesions are seen at all is explained by the phenom-enon of superimposition: when myriads of tiny lesions are present in the lungs, it is inevitable that several are superimposed.

Since such small shadows are only visible when superimposed on one another, it follows that, when very small widespread non-calcified shadows are identi-fied, the lung must be diffusely involved by disease.

How to decide whether or not multiple small pulmonary shadows are present

Often, the greatest problem is to decide whether widespread abnormal shadowing is present at all, since normal blood vessels can also appear as nodules and interconnecting lines. To be confident involves looking carefully at many hundreds of normal films to establish a normal pattern in one's mind. The normal vessel pattern shows a branching system that connects in an orderly way: the vessels are larger centrally and they become smaller as they travel to the periphery. Vessels seen end-on appear as small nodules, but these nodules are no bigger than vessels seen in the immediate vicinity and their number corresponds to the expected number of vessels in that area. There are no visible vessels in the outer centimetre or so of the lung.

The silhouette sign may help when deciding whether widespread small shadows are present, because such shadows often obscure the adjacent vessels and the outline of the heart and diaphragm may be less distinct than normal.

If abnormal shadowing is definitely present and its pattern has been described, the next diagnostic step is to determine the distribution: is the shadowing uniformly distributed, is it more severe in one or other zone, does it extend outward from the hila, or is it more severe in the lung periphery? Other abnormalities on the film should be sought. Once these observations have been made, the differential diagnosis should be considered as shown in Table 23.1.

Inevitably, there will be cases when there is doubt, both clinically and radiographically, whether diffuse lung disease is present. HRCT can then be of considerable help. HRCT can also help define the character and distribution of the abnormal shadowing (Table 23.1 and Fig. 23.22; see also Fig. 22.3).

Multiple ring shadows of 1 cm or larger

Multiple ring shadows larger than 1 cm are virtually diagnostic of bronchiectasis (Fig. 23.23), although Langerhans' histiocytosis, lymphangiomyomatosis and

Figure 23.23 *Bronchiectasis showing multiple overlapping ring shadows representing dilated bronchi.*

multiple superimposed lung cavities can also give this appearance.

Multiple small pulmonary calcifications

Widespread small pulmonary calcifications may occur following tuberculosis, histoplasmosis or chicken-pox pneumonia.

INCREASED TRANSRADIANCY OF THE LUNGS

Localized increase in transradiancy

When one hemithorax appears more transradiant than normal the following causes should considered:

- **emphysema**;
- **compensatory emphysema** (compensatory emphysema occurs when a lobe or a lung is collapsed or has been excised and the remaining lung expands to fill the space);
- **pneumothorax**;
- **reduction in the chest wall soft tissues**, e.g. mastectomy, absence of the pectoralis major;
- **air-trapping due to central obstruction** – most obstructing lesions in a major bronchus lead to lobar collapse; occasionally, particularly with an inhaled foreign body, a check valve mechanism may lead to air-trapping;

Figure 23.22 *Scleroderma. High-resolution CT (HRCT) of the lungs showing changes typical of interstitial pulmonary fibrosis. Note the fine reticular shadowing maximal at the lung periphery.*

- rare causes include **massive pulmonary embolus** and **McLeod's syndrome** (Swyer–James syndrome), a condition that follows severe pneumonia in childhood.

Generalized increase in transradiancy

Generalized increased transradiancy of the lungs is one of the signs of emphysema. This condition is discussed on p. 567.

LUNG DISEASE WITH A NORMAL CHEST RADIOGRAPH

Serious respiratory disease may exist in patients with a normal chest radiograph:

- **Pulmonary emboli without infarction.** The chest radiograph may be normal in patients with pulmonary emboli, even in those with life-threatening emboli.
- **Obstructive airways disease**. Asthma and acute bronchiolitis may produce overinflation of the lungs, but in many cases the chest film is normal. The chest radiograph may be normal or very nearly normal in mild or moderate emphysema. Uncomplicated acute or chronic bronchitis in adults does not produce any radiological signs and many patients with productive cough from bronchiectasis show no plain film abnormality.
- **Infections**. Most patients with acute bacterial pneumonia present with recognizable consolidation, but in other infections, notably *Pneumocystis carinii* pneumonia, visible pulmonary consolidation may only develop after the onset of symptoms. Patients with miliary tuberculosis may initially have a normal chest film.
- **Small lesions**. It is rarely possible to see solitary lung masses or consolidations of less than 1 cm in diameter. Even 2–3 cm lung cancers may be difficult to identify on routine films, if they are partially or wholly hidden behind rib or clavicle shadows, or if they lie behind the heart or diaphragm. Endobronchial lesions, such as carcinoma, cannot usually be diagnosed on routine films unless they cause collapse or consolidation.
- **Diffuse pulmonary disease** may be responsible for breathlessness with substantial alteration in lung function tests before clear-cut abnormalities are evident on plain chest radiography.

SPECIFIC PULMONARY DISEASES

PNEUMONIA

The primary purpose of the chest radiograph in patients with suspected chest infection is to establish whether or not pneumonia is present. Clearly, the chest radiograph cannot replace bacteriological and laboratory information for diagnosing the infective agent. The principal radiographic features of pneumonia are one or more areas of pulmonary consolidation, which may show cavitation and may be accompanied by pleural effusion. The appearance of individual consolidations within the lung varies from a small, ill-defined density to large shadows involving the whole or most of one or more lobes, the pattern depending on the infecting organism and the integrity of the host defences. Where pneumonia lies against a pleural fissure, it has a well-defined edge, but otherwise the margin is hazy. Occasionally, well-defined, rounded consolidation is seen.

Although the term 'segmental consolidation' is used frequently, consolidation conforming precisely to segmental anatomy is rarely seen. Infective consolidation can readily cross segmental boundaries, since there are no anatomical barriers to prevent such spread, but the spread of consolidation is usually held up by the interlobar fissures. Infective consolidation is usually densest in the most dependent portions of a given lobe.

Hospital-acquired pneumonia and pneumonia in the immunocompromised host are highly variable in appearance but certain generalizations can be made regarding the radiographic features of community-acquired pneumonias:

- **Lobar consolidation** or consolidation involving the greater part of one lobe is usually either bacterial (Fig. 23.24) or mycoplasmal (Fig. 23.25) in origin. The usual bacterium responsible is *Streptococcus pneumoniae*; occasionally it is *Klebsiella, Staphylococcus aureus* or *Legionella*. Expansion of the lobe caused by intense exudate is virtually diagnostic of pneumococcal or klebsiella pneumonia.
- **Cavitation** within the consolidation suggests bacterial rather than mycoplasmal pneumonia. The bacterial infections that commonly cause cavitation are tuberculosis (see Fig. 23.7, p. 543), Gram-negative or anaerobic organisms associated with aspiration pneumonia, *Streptococcus pyogenes, Pseudomonas, Staphylococcus aureus, Klebsiella*, or *Escherichia coli*. Neither the number nor the size of the cavities is of diagnostic importance.
- Spherical pneumonia is usually due to pneumococcal infection (Fig. 23.26) or Legionnaire's disease. Spherical pneumonia can be confused radiographically with a lung mass, particularly primary carcinoma. However, spherical pneumonia expands to involve the adjacent lung over the next few hours or days and is associated with obvious clinical features of acute bacterial pneumonia. Also, the edge of at least one portion of spherical pneumonia is ill-defined and air bronchograms are relatively common.
- When widespread, small, ill-defined shadows with or without septal lines (Kerley lines) are due to infection,

(a)

(b)

Figure 23.24 *Pneumonia causing consolidation of the basal segments of the right lower lobe. The superior segment is spared and therefore the upper border of the consolidation is ill-defined in both (a) the PA and (b) the lateral views. The 'lobar' shape of the consolidation is particularly well seen in the lateral view. Note that in the lateral view the lower vertebrae are much whiter than the upper vertebrae. The diagnosis was pneumococcal pneumonia.*

Figure 23.25 *Mycoplasmal pneumonia causing relatively homogeneous consolidation in the left lower lobe.*

Figure 23.26 *Round (spherical) pneumonia which radiologically could be misdiagnosed as a tumour. Note the slightly ill-defined edge. The cause in this case, as in most cases of round pneumonia, was pneumococcal pneumonia.*

the infection is likely to be due to a virus or to *Mycoplasma pneumoniae* (Fig. 23.27). Fungal and tuberculous disease may give a similar appearance.

- Miliary nodulation in the lungs has many causes. When due to infection, the usual responsible organisms are *Mycobacterium tuberculosis* (see Fig. 23.28)

and fungi. The nodules in these infections are well-defined, uniformly distributed and equal in size, usually 2–4 mm in diameter. The nodules are usually present in the first film taken but, if the film is taken early in the course of the disease, it may be normal.

Figure 23.27 *Mycoplasmal pneumonia showing its rarer pattern of interstitial pneumonia. There are bilateral, ill-defined, short, overlapping line shadows resembling pulmonary oedema.*

The entities that most closely resemble miliary infection radiologically are pneumoconiosis and miliary metastases, and the chest radiographic appearances of the three may be totally indistinguishable. The clinical differences are, however, so great that true confusion almost never occurs.

- When hilar adenopathy and pleural effusion accompany pulmonary consolidation, three entities should be seriously considered: carcinoma of the lung, anaerobic bacterial infection, and chronic infection such as tuberculosis and fungal disease.
- Patchy upper lobe consolidation suggests tuberculosis or fungal infection.
- Some pneumonias, notably from anaerobic bacteria or *Staphylococcus aureus*, have a propensity to be associated with empyemas, a topic discussed on p. 579.

Difference between adults and children

It can be difficult to interpret a chest radiograph of an infant or young child with possible pneumonia. The signs of pneumonia are the same regardless of age, but disturbances of aeration such as atelectasis or air-trapping are much more frequent in small children, because the airways in infancy are relatively small and collateral air pathways are less effective. When generalized, as in bronchiolitis, inflammatory narrowing of the smaller airways causes two major radiological signs, irregularity of aeration and generalized hyperinflation. The presence of low flat hemidiaphragms – the best indication of hyperinflation – is often best appreciated on the lateral view.

The question most frequently asked regarding children with suspected chest infection is 'Does this child have bacterial pneumonia?'. If there is no visible consolidation, bacterial infection is unlikely. There are two provisos to this statement. First, the chest radiograph may have been taken too early; in rare instances the consolidation only becomes visible a few hours after the patient first presents with symptoms. Second, the pneumonia may be difficult to identify, if it is hidden behind the heart or mediastinum or is below the levels of the domes of the diaphragm. These areas should therefore be viewed with particular care before the lungs are declared normal.

If there is consolidation on the film, deciding its cause can be a problem since both viral and bacterial pneumonias, as well as atelectasis without pneumonia, may look identical. A large area of consolidation without signs of volume loss usually indicates pneumonia rather than non-infective atelectasis.

Postobstructive pneumonia

Bacterial pneumonia may be secondary to obstruction of a bronchus. In a patient over 35 years of age, the obstruction is likely to be neoplastic, usually carcinoma. Occasionally, the central mass is so large that it deforms the outline of the affected lobe. In children, the common causes of obstruction in a major bronchus are an inhaled foreign body or a mucus plug.

Postobstructive pneumonia is usually confined to one lobe, but if more than one lobe is involved the lobes usually share a common bronchus; for example, the right lower and middle lobes can be involved owing to a lesion in the bronchus intermedius. The lobe almost invariably shows some loss of volume: air bronchograms are rarely visible within the area of consolidation. Typically, the pneumonia does not resolve radiologically on antibiotic therapy, although partial improvement of the radiological appearances is frequently seen.

LUNG ABSCESS

The infectious agents most frequently responsible for lung abscess are *Staphylococcus aureus*, *Klebsiella*, mixed anaerobic organisms, *Mycobacterium tuberculosis* and various fungi. A lung abscess is seen as a spherical

Figure 23.28 *Miliary tuberculosis in a child. Note the innumerable, uniformly distributed, small, nodular shadows.*

Figure 23.29 *Active postprimary pulmonary tuberculosis. There is patchy, moderately well-defined consolidation in the right upper lobe. In this case the left upper lobe appears normal.*

shadow containing central lucency owing to air within the cavity. This air may be difficult to appreciate without CT. The air is often accompanied by fluid, in which case an air–fluid level may be visible on erect films.

PULMONARY TUBERCULOSIS

Pulmonary tuberculosis is often divided into primary and postprimary forms, even though these divisions are not clear-cut. Primary tuberculosis follows the initial infection with *Mycobacterium tuberculosis* and usually occurs in childhood. Postprimary tuberculosis is the usual form seen in adults. It is believed to be a reinfection in a patient who has developed relative immunity.

Primary tuberculosis appears radiographically as an area of consolidation in the lung (Ghon focus) usually in the middle and upper zones, together with enlarged hilar or mediastinal nodes – a combination known as the primary complex. In most cases, whether treated or not, the primary complex heals and may calcify. The disease may progress, giving rise to tuberculous bronchopneumonia, which often cavitates, or miliary tuberculosis, which produces innumerable small pulmonary nodules on the chest radiograph (Fig. 23.28). The nodules are all much the same size, usually well-defined and fairly evenly distributed. Early in the clinical course the chest radiograph may be normal.

Pulmonary involvement in postprimary tuberculosis is usually greatest in the upper portions of the lungs, the apical and posterior segments of the upper lobes (Fig. 23.29), and the superior segments of the lower lobes. Multiple small areas of consolidation are seen initially. As the infection progresses, the consolidations enlarge and frequently cavitate. Extensive bronchial spread may

occur (Fig. 23.30), giving rise to multilobar bronchopneumonia, usually including one or both upper lobes, with cavitation being a frequent phenomenon. Healing occurs with fibrosis and calcification, but signs of healing may be seen despite continuing activity. Occasionally, tuberculosis takes the form of lower or middle-lobe bronchopneumonia and may even resemble lobar pneumonia. As with the primary form, the

Figure 23.30 *Tuberculous bronchopneumonia. Note the very extensive small, but not miliary, shadows. The distribution is not uniform, but is maximal in the left lung, consistent with spread by aspiration from an infected focus.*

(a)

(b)

Figure 23.31 *Tuberculoma in posterior segment of right upper lobe. (a) CT scan displayed at lung windows shows a 1 cm diameter round nodule (arrow) with irregular edges (closely resembling a primary lung carcinoma). (b) Same CT image, but displayed at soft-tissue windows, showing extensive calcification of the nodule. Note that the nodule is the same 'whiteness' as the calcified bone.*

infection may spread via the bloodstream to give rise to miliary tuberculosis.

Pleural effusions are frequent in both primary and postprimary tuberculosis and may be the only manifestation of the disease.

Tuberculoma refers to a tuberculous granuloma in the form of a spherical mass, usually less than 3 cm in diameter (Fig. 23.31). The edge is usually sharply defined and these lesions are often partly calcified. CT may be needed to demonstrate the calcification. Most tuberculomas are inactive but viable tubercle bacilli may be present even in the calcified lesions.

Is the disease active?

The signs of activity are:

- development of new lesions on serial films
- demonstration of cavities.

Lack of change over a period of years is useful evidence against activity, but the change in serial chest films may be subtle, even with active disease. The presence of calcification, whilst it indicates healed disease, does not exclude active disease.

Many routine chest films in asymptomatic patients show evidence of tuberculosis. In a few, the diagnosis of active disease will be readily apparent by the presence of cavities or by comparison with previous films. In the remainder it can be very difficult to decide which patients to investigate further and in which to diagnose old inactive infection. The better defined the shadows and the greater the degree of calcification, the less the likelihood of activity. The presence of ill-defined shadows, even if partially calcified, is suggestive of active disease. However, the decision as to whether the disease

is active is often largely based on the clinical findings and the results of sputum examination for tubercle bacilli.

FUNGAL AND PARASITIC INFECTIONS

The radiological appearances of fungal and parasitic chest infections vary with the particular agent, but a few broad statements can be made:

- Infection of the otherwise normal patient with **histoplasmosis**, **coccidioidomycosis** and **blastomycosis** is encountered chiefly on the continent of North America. The lesions in the lung are very similar and often identical to tuberculosis. Cavitation is a particular feature. Healing by fibrosis and calcification is frequent.
- *Aspergillus fumigatus* affects the lung in three ways: it may colonize a pre-existing cavity forming a fungus ball or mycetoma (see below); it may infect the lung in an immunocompromised patient causing a severe pneumonia (see below); or it may be responsible for allergic bronchopulmonary aspergillosis, a condition discussed on p. 569.
- **Hydatid disease.** Pulmonary infection with *Echinococcus granulosus* may result in cysts in the lung or pleural cavity. These cysts may be solitary or multiple and are seen as spherical shadows with very well-defined borders. Hydatid cysts occasionally rupture to produce complex cavities.

Mycetoma

The fungus *Aspergillus fumigatus* may colonize old tuberculous or other cavities to produce a ball of fungus

(a)

(b)

Figure 23.32 *Mycetoma. CT scans taken in (a) usual supine position and (b) prone position. The mass of the mycetoma is seen lying within an old thin-walled tuberculous cavity (arrow). Note that the mass moves to lie respectively on the posterior wall of the cavity when the patient is supine and on the anterior wall when the patient lies prone. In other words the mycetoma lies in the most dependent portion of the cavity in both positions.*

(mycetoma) lying free within the cavity. Since the fungus ball usually occupies only a portion of the available space, air is seen between the mycetoma and the wall of the cavity (Fig. 23.32). The shape and position of this rim varies with the position of the patient. Cavities containing mycetomas are usually surrounded by evidence of old tuberculous infection, particularly fibrosis and calcification of the adjacent lung. Pleural thickening often develops adjacent to cavities containing mycetomas.

PNEUMONIA IN THE IMMUNOCOMPROMISED HOST

Patients who are immunocompromised are not only more susceptible to pulmonary infection, often with unusual organisms, but the pattern of the resulting pneumonia frequently shows an atypical radiographic appearance. Pneumonia in these patients may be due to the usual pathogens, but often it is due to opportunistic fungi, such as *Candida albicans* and *Aspergillus fumigatus* as well as several of the fungi native to North America, tuberculosis, atypical mycobacteria or *Pneumocystis carinii*.

Pneumonia in immunocompromised patients can be similar in appearance to pneumonia in immunocompetent individuals when the infection is due to standard pathogens. However, when the pneumonia is due to opportunistic organisms, then widespread nonspecific pulmonary shadowing is common. Except for *Pneumocystis carinii* pneumonia it is usually not possible to predict the infecting organism from the chest film. It may not even be possible to say whether the shadowing is due to infection or to such conditions as pulmonary oedema, pulmonary haemorrhage or neoplastic disease.

The predilection of people with AIDS to develop *Pneumocystis carinii* pneumonia means that widespread, uniformly distributed pulmonary shadowing in a patient with AIDS is usually due to this organism (Fig. 23.33), though AIDS patients are also prone to tuberculous infection and the development of extensive Kaposi's sarcoma, both of which can, on occasion, appear similar to *Pneumocystis carinii* pneumonia on plain chest radiography.

PULMONARY EMBOLISM AND INFARCTION

The plain chest radiograph is insensitive for the diagnosis of pulmonary embolism. Indeed, life-threatening pulmonary embolism may occur in patients with normal chest radiographs. Many plain chest radiographic signs are described in pulmonary embolism and infarction, but all are non-specific. It is, therefore, impossible to decide from plain chest radiographs alone whether a patient has or has not had a pulmonary embolus. One of the principal values of the chest radiograph is to exclude clinically similar diseases that may show radiographic abnormalities, e.g. pneumothorax or dissecting aneurysm.

Pulmonary embolism without infarction usually produces no recognizable abnormality. Enlargement of a major arterial trunk at the hilum is a well-known, but very rarely seen, sign. Discoid (linear) atelectasis may be seen, but this phenomenon occurs with numerous disorders and is a reflection of poor diaphragmatic excursion rather than vascular occlusion. Elevation of one hemidiaphragm, a common finding in pulmonary embolism, is non-specific and can be normal.

Pulmonary embolism causing infarction gives rise to consolidation, which tends to be wedge-shaped and

(a)

(b)

Figure 23.33 Pneumocystis carinii *pneumonia. (a) Chest radiograph showing typical, subtle, reasonably uniform, pulmonary shadowing. In this case there is relative sparing of the left lower zone. (b) HRCT showing patchy ground-glass shadowing (shadowing through which the blood vessels can be identified). Visible air bronchograms are typical though non-specific.*

based on the pleura, but many patterns are seen. The consolidation may have a round medial edge (Hampton's hump). This shape is uncommon and, although very suggestive of pulmonary infarction, is also seen with pneumonia. Small ipsilateral pleural effusions are often present in patients with pulmonary infarction.

Since plain film radiology is so non-specific for diagnosing pulmonary embolism, further investigation is often needed.

Radionuclide lung scanning for pulmonary embolism

There are two major types of lung scan, namely perfusion and ventilation scans.

For **perfusion scans**, sometimes called $\dot{Q}$ scans, particulate material such as ^{99m}Tc-labelled macro-aggregates of albumin, with an average particle size of 30 μm, are injected intravenously. These particles become trapped in the pulmonary capillaries and the distribution of radioactivity, when imaged by a gamma camera, accurately reflects blood flow.

For **ventilation scans**, sometimes called $\dot{V}$ scans, the patient inhales a radioactive gas such as xenon-133 or krypton-81m and the distribution of radioactive gas is imaged using a gamma camera. Aerosols labelled with technetium-99m may be used instead of gases.

Interpretation of radionuclide lung scanning

The cardinal sign of pulmonary embolism on radionuclide lung scanning is a perfusion defect. Perfusion defects are usually segmental in shape and extend to the pleural surface. A normal perfusion scan excludes the diagnosis of pulmonary embolism, but the presence of a perfusion defect is non-specific, because many other disease processes can cause focal reduction in blood flow. These include obstructive airways disease (either acute or chronic), pneumonia, atelectasis, pulmonary oedema and vasculitis. Increased specificity for pulmonary embolism can be obtained by adding a ventilation scan to the procedure. The major patterns are:

- **Mismatched ventilation–perfusion defects** ($\dot{V}/\dot{Q}$ mismatches)
  - Perfusion defects in an area with normal ventilation strongly suggest pulmonary embolism without infarction (Fig. 23.34).
  - Perfusion defects which are larger than the corresponding ventilation defects suggest pulmonary infarction. Such cases often show consolidation on plain chest radiograph.
  - There are, however, a number of conditions that can cause perfusion defects without disturbing ventilation and without recognizable abnormality on the chest radiograph, including previous pulmonary emboli, obstruction to pulmonary arteries by vasculitis, neoplasm or inflammation, primary pulmonary arterial hypertension and systemic arterial blood flow to a portion of the lung. This long and varied list highlights the lack of specificity even of mismatched defects.
- **Matched ventilation/perfusion defects** may be seen with pulmonary infarction, pneumonia, pulmonary oedema or airway disease.

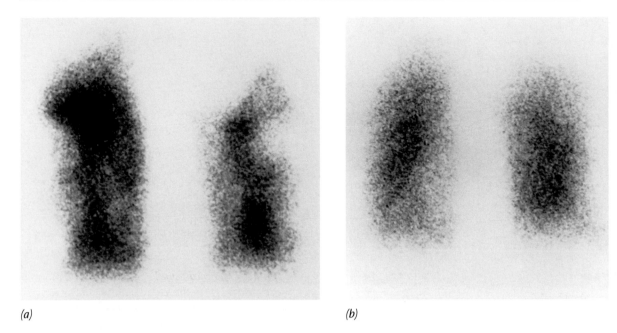

(a)   *(b)*

Figure 23.34 *Ventilation–perfusion (V̇/Q̇) scans in a patient with multiple large pulmonary emboli. (a) The perfusion scan shows multiple, large, segmental-shaped perfusion defects. (b) The ventilation scan shows normal distribution of the inhaled radionuclide.*

Abnormal ventilation–perfusion scan results are expressed in terms that indicate the probability that the diagnosis of pulmonary embolism is correct, but the radionuclide scan findings alone cannot provide a reliable estimate of likelihood without factoring in the clinical probability of pulmonary embolism. Unfortunately, this important concept is often overlooked.

A ventilation–perfusion scan interpreted as low probability, typically a scan with matched ventilation–perfusion defects, is associated with a 10 per cent incidence of pulmonary embolism. The term 'high probability' in general means a likelihood greater than 85 per cent. It is worth noting that, when the diagnosis is clinically likely and there are multiple segmental or larger defects in the presence of a normal ventilation scan, the probability of pulmonary embolism exceeds 90 per cent.

Pulmonary angiography and CT angiography for pulmonary embolism

Pulmonary angiography is the most sensitive and specific available test for pulmonary embolism, but because it is an invasive test the procedure is reserved for those patients who require a precise diagnosis of pulmonary embolism. The diagnostic feature is an intraluminal filling defect within the opacified arterial tree on two or more films (Fig. 23.35a). Occlusion of an artery is less specific and may be seen in a variety of conditions, including previous embolus or occlusion owing to direct involvement by neoplasm or inflammatory disease.

It is possible to obtain high-quality spiral CT images of the pulmonary arterial system using a large bolus of contrast medium (150–200 ml) injected intravenously at a flow rate of 3–5 ml/s. With spiral CT, the opacified pulmonary arterial tree can be imaged on a single breath-hold (Fig. 23.35b). The resolution is sufficient to diagnose emboli in pulmonary arteries down to subsegmental level, but emboli in more distal vessels are more variably identified. The technique, therefore, can diagnose haemodynamically significant emboli, but cannot be used to exclude small peripheral emboli.

ADULT RESPIRATORY DISTRESS SYNDROME (NON-CARDIOGENIC PULMONARY OEDEMA)

Adult respiratory distress syndrome (ARDS) is characterized by unexpected or severe respiratory distress in patients whose lungs were previously normal. There are many precipitating disorders, including hypotension, septic shock, aspiration of gastric contents, haemorrhagic pancreatitis, near drowning, ingestion of drugs, fat embolism, inhalation of toxic fumes and severe trauma. The common feature appears to be increased permeability of the pulmonary capillaries.

Radiologically, the oedema of ARDS is initially identical to cardiogenic alveolar oedema, namely ill-defined pulmonary shadowing in both lungs, maximal close to the hila, fading out towards the periphery of the lobes. Cardiac enlargement and pleural effusions are not features. The pulmonary oedema seen on the chest radiograph may sometimes be identified only a few

(a)

(b)

Figure 23.35 *Pulmonary emboli. (a) Conventional pulmonary angiogram with contrast injected via a catheter in the main pulmonary artery. There are numerous filling defects (arrows) and occluded vessels due to the emboli. (b) CT angiography, performed on a spiral CT scanner, following rapid injection of a large volume of intravenous contrast medium, showing smooth intraluminal filling defects owing to emboli in the right pulmonary artery at the hilum (arrow).*

hours after the onset of hypoxaemia, in contrast to cardiogenic pulmonary oedema, which is visible coincident with the development of hypoxaemia. With time, the patient develops increased lung density involving the whole of both lungs (Fig. 23.36). Such patients invariably require artifical ventilation and are therefore liable to complications of ventilation such as interstitial emphysema, pneumothorax and pneumomediastinum.

SARCOIDOSIS

The radiological manifestations of sarcoidosis are largely confined to the chest. The following are features on plain chest radiograph and CT:

- **Hilar and paratracheal lymphadenopathy**. When hilar lymphadenopathy is present it is almost invariably bilateral and usually symmetrical (Fig 23.37). Mediastinal adenopathy is common and the nodes are large enough to be visible on a plain chest radiograph in about half the patients. The mediastinal lymphadenopathy is most readily recognized in the right paratracheal region. On chest CT (Fig. 33.38), the widespread distribution of the lymphadenopathy is apparent. Unlike lymphoma, the lymph node enlargement is never predominant in the anterior mediastinum.
- **Reticulonodular shadowing in the lungs**. The pattern varies from uniform small nodular shadows,

Figure 23.36 *Adult respiratory distress syndrome. Note the widespread opacity of the lungs. Air bronchograms are visible. The patient is on positive pressure ventilation via an endotracheal tube and a left-sided pneumomediastinum (arrow) has developed.*

Figure 23.37 *Sarcoidosis showing bilateral hilar node enlargement.*

Figure 23.38 *Sarcoidosis. Contrast-enhanced CT showing greatly enlarged lymph nodes at both hila.*

which may clear on steroid therapy, to coarse reticular shadows maximal in the mid and upper zones, which represent gross pulmonary fibrosis (Fig. 23.39). At this stage the pulmonary disease is usually irreversible.

The majority of patients with sarcoidosis of the chest have lymphadenopathy only, which clears without treatment and does not progress to pulmonary involvement. Many are discovered on routine chest radiograph and have no symptoms or signs, though most show non-caseating granulomas on transbronchial biopsy. Some present with iridocyclitis, some with erythema nodosum and fever. A few have, in addition, polyarthritis.

Figure 23.39 *Sarcoidosis showing extensive mid zone predominant pulmonary fibrosis.*

Approximately 10 per cent of patients develop radiographically evident lung involvement; some have visibly enlarged lymph nodes at this stage. Often the lymph nodes get smaller and may return to normal, even though the lung changes persist.

Chest CT (Figs 23.38 and 23.40), which can demonstrate the hilar/mediastinal adenopathy and the lung shadowing to advantage, does not provide useful extra information and is rarely indicated in sarcoidosis.

Figure 23.40 *Sarcoidosis. HRCT showing severe pulmonary involvement. Note that the abnormal densities are maximal in the small perihilar regions. Note also the numerous small nodules, many of which are in lymphatic tissue closely applied to the blood vessels and along the pleura.*

DIFFUSE PULMONARY FIBROSIS

The known causes of diffuse pulmonary fibrosis include: extrinsic alveolitis, collagen vascular disease (including rheumatoid arthritis), drug-induced fibrosis, pneumoconiosis and sarcoidosis, but a substantial proportion of cases are idiopathic in organ. Various names are given to the idiopathic form: idiopathic pulmonary fibrosis, cryptogenic fibrosing alveolitis and usual interstitial pneumonia (UIP).

Idiopathic pulmonary fibrosis (cryptogenic fibrosing alveolitis, UIP)

In cryptogenic fibrosing alveolitis there is thickening of the aveolar walls with fibrosis and desquamation. As the disease progresses, the alveolar walls break down and rounded air spaces develop. At this stage the appearances are known by the descriptive term 'honeycomb lung'. Fibrosing alveolitis causes a restrictive ventilation defect with severe reduction in gas transfer across the alveolar walls.

The radiological features are:

- Hazy shadowing at the lung bases leading to a lack of clarity of the vessel outlines known as 'ground-glass shadowing'. Later, ill-defined nodules with connecting lines become discernible.
- Decreased lung volume, often marked, and circular translucencies are seen producing the pattern known as 'honeycomb lung'. Eventually, the heart and pulmonary arteries enlarge from increasingly severe pulmonary hypertension.

These signs are seen on both plain chest radiographs and HRCT. HRCT is more sensitive for detecting the changes and demonstrates the distribution and severity of disease to advantage (Fig. 23.41). Ground-glass shadowing is particularly well seen with HRCT.

Determining the cause of diffuse pulmonary fibrosis

The distribution of the pulmonary shadowing may give a clue to its aetiology. In idiopathic pulmonary fibrosis, the lung shadowing is often maximal at the bases and at the lung periphery, although it may be fairly uniformly distributed in advanced cases. Scleroderma (see Fig. 23.22, p. 553) and rheumatoid arthritis give an identical picture.

The combination of pulmonary fibrosis with certain other signs may lead to a specific diagnosis:

- Substantial past or present hilar/mediastinal adenopathy suggests sarcoidosis.
- Coexistent conglomerate masses in the mid and

Figure 23.41 *HRCT of interstitial fibrosis of the lungs. The peripherally predominant reticular shadowing is typical of end-stage fibrosing alveolitis, in this case cryptogenic fibrosing alveolitis.*

upper zones are virtually diagnostic of silicosis or coal-miners' pneumoconiosis (see Fig. 23.44, p. 566);
- Coexistent bilateral pleural thickening and calcification are diagnostic of asbestosis.
- Past or present pleural effusions are highly suggestive of rheumatoid arthritis.

COLLAGEN VASCULAR DISEASES

This group of diseases includes rheumatoid arthritis, systemic lupus erythematosus, polyarteritis nodosa, systemic sclerosis, dermatomyositis and Wegner's granulomatosis. Various radiological signs occur in the chest.

Rheumatoid lung

The most common finding is pleural effusion. Pulmonary fibrosis, often indistinguishable from that seen in cryptogenic fibrosing alveolitis, is another important finding.

An interesting feature of pulmonary involvement in rheumatoid arthritis is the development of rounded granulomas in the periphery of the lung, histologically similar to the subcutaneous nodules seen in this disease. These spherical nodules, which may be single or multiple, rarely exceed 3 cm in diameter. Eventually, many cavitate and resolve.

Systemic lupus erythematosus

The chest radiograph is usually normal. The commonest abnormalities are pleural effusion and cardiac enlargement owing to pericardial effusion. Patchy consolidation in the lungs is occasionally seen.

(a)

(b)

Figure 23.42 *Wegener's granulomatosis. (a) Multiple areas of ill-defined consolidation, some very large. (b) Another patient with multiple cavitating pulmonary nodules.*

Scleroderma and dermatomyositis

The cardinal feature is basal reticulonodular shadows from pulmonary fibrosis, similar to that seen in cryptogenic fibrosing alveolitis. Pleural effusion is rare.

Polyarteritis nodosa

Patchy consolidations, which may be fleeting and repetitive, and pleural effusions are occasionally seen in patients with polyarteritis nodosa.

Wegener's granulomatosis

The lungs may show one or more well-defined consolidations or masses, usually in the mid zones, which may cavitate (Fig. 23.42 and see Fig. 23.19c, p. 550). These lesions are often difficult to distinguish from bronchogenic carcinoma, when single, or metastases, when multiple, on radiographic grounds alone.

PNEUMOCONIOSES

The pneumoconioses include a group of conditions caused by the inhalation of a variety of dusts.

Coal-workers' pneumoconiosis and silicosis

Simple pneumoconiosis is due to dust retention in the lungs with minor fibrosis. It is recognized radiologically by many small nodules, initially in the mid and upper zones, eventually involving the whole of the lungs (Fig.

Figure 23.43 *Coal-worker's pneumoconiosis showing widespread small nodular shadows (miliary nodules).*

23.43). Simple pneumoconiosis does not give rise to symptoms and the diagnosis is made on the basis of the chest radiographic appearances.

For reasons that are not entirely clear, progressive massive fibrosis may supervene. It causes homogeneous shadows, which are often ovoid in shape, in the upper halves of the lungs. The shadows may be unilateral or

Figure 23.44 *Progressive massive fibrosis (PMF) in a coal-miner. The bilateral large upper zone masses against a background of widespread small pulmonary nodules (the small nodules are difficult to see in reproduction) are typical PMF in a coal-worker.*

bilateral and there is usually nodular shadowing in the rest of the lungs (Fig. 23.44). Progressive massive fibrosis may be associated with breathlessness and it may result in cor pulmonale.

Asbestos-related disease

Inhalation of asbestos may lead to:

- **Pleural fibrosis and calcification.** Localized plaques of pleural thickening, some of which are calcified, are seen along the lateral chest wall and diaphragm (Fig. 23.45). The plaques, which are a useful pointer to asbestos exposure, are harmless in themselves. Asbestos-related diffuse pleural thickening, however, may cause restriction to breathing.

  The differential diagnosis from post-inflammatory and post-traumatic pleural thickening and calcification is made by noting the extent of the pleural disease: usually, it is bilateral in asbestos-related pleural disease, whereas it is frequently unilateral in the other conditions. If the costophrenic angles are sharp, healed inflammatory disease or old haemothorax is very unlikely, whereas in asbestos-related pleural disease the costophrenic angles may be clear.
- **Interstitial pulmonary fibrosis.** Unlike the pleural plaques, which may be seen following minor exposure to asbestos, pulmonary fibrosis only follows significant exposure. Pulmonary fibrosis in asbestosis is symmetrically bilateral and maximal at the bases, similar to cryptogenic fibrosing alveolitis (Fig. 23.46). The term asbestosis implies pulmonary fibrosis due to asbestos exposure.
- **Round atelectasis.** Round atelectasis (see p. 545) may be present and should not be misinterpreted as a neoplasm.

(a)

(b)

Figure 23.45 *Asbestos-related pleural plaques. (a) Plain chest radiograph showing extensive heavily calcified plaques (arrows). (b) CT showing multiple plaques (arrows point to some of these plaques), three of which have a small amount of dense calcification. (See Figure 23.13c for the round atelectasis in this patient.)*

Figure 23.46 *Asbestosis showing severe pulmonary fibrosis, maximal in both lower lobes. Calcified asbestos-related pleural plaques are also present but difficult to see in reproduction.*

- **The development of malignant neoplasms**. Malignant mesothelioma (see Fig. 23.72, p. 580) and bronchial carcinoma are both seen with far higher frequency in asbestos-exposed patients than in the general population.

AIRWAY DISEASES

Bronchial asthma

The chest radiographic findings in asthma vary with the age of the patient. In children, the lungs may be over-expanded between attacks and show bronchial wall thickening with prominent hilar vasculature. Although adults may show the same signs, they usually have normal chest radiographs. Usually, none of these signs are striking, and the chest radiograph pays no part in the diagnosis of asthma. Its purpose is to diagnose the complications of an attack or to demonstrate a pneumonia that may have precipitated the attack.

During an asthmatic attack, the lungs are often recognizably overexpanded. **Atelectasis** of a whole lobe, or part of one or more lobes, is fairly common (Fig. 23.47). Atelectasis is usually due to retained secretions, but may be due to a pneumonia that precipitated the asthmatic attack. Distinguishing between these two processes can be impossible. In general, the less the loss of volume, the more likely the atelectasis is due to pneumonia, and the greater the loss of volume, the more likely the atelectasis is due to a mucus plug. Tenacious mucus plugs may be a repetitive problem, leading to persistent or recurrent atelectasis. In older children and adults, they may be part of the syndrome of allergic bronchopulmonary aspergillosis.

Pneumothorax is a very rare complication of an asthmatic attack. **Pneumomediastinum** is more

Figure 23.47 *Acute asthma. Multiple patches of atelectasis are evident. There is also a pneumomediastinum.*

common but is, in itself, of no clinical significance to the patient.

Tracheal obstruction from extrinsic compression

Tracheal obstruction is occasionally due to extrinsic compression by a mass or by a congenital vascular anomaly.

When it is due to a mass, the mass is usually large, but may have been asymptomatic up to the time of presentation. Acute obstruction may occur because a critical degree of narrowing has been reached, or it may be precipitated by a sudden increase in the size of the mass following bleeding or infection. The responsible mass usually appears as focal mediastinal widening with displacement or compression of the trachea. It is important to remember that the tracheal narrowing may be visible only in the lateral projection.

Tracheal obstruction from a congenital vascular ring, such as a double aortic arch, is very difficult to diagnose from plain chest films. Since it usually presents in young children in whom the thymus is still large, it is frequently difficult to recognize the aortic arch and to define the tracheal airway. The diagnosis is easily made on barium swallow, where indentations of the barium-filled oesophagus are readily apparent. CT or MRI will show the congenital anomaly in detail.

Chronic obstructive airway disease

Chronic obstructive airway disease is an imprecise, but convenient, term covering several airway disorders: chronic bronchitis, emphysema, bronchiectasis and cystic fibrosis. These disorders may coexist.

Figure 23.48 *Severe panacinar emphysema. The lungs are markedly overinflated with the diaphragm depressed, so that it lies well below the anterior ends of the seventh ribs. The blood vessels, particularly in the mid and upper zones, are significantly attenuated.*

Uncomplicated chronic bronchitis produces no abnormality on plain chest radiographs. Indeed patients may succumb to respiratory failure owing to chronic bronchitis and have normal chest films throughout their course. If the chest film is abnormal, a complication or a coexisting abnormality is present, e.g. emphysema, pneumonia or cor pulmonale. If chronic bronchitis is combined with emphysema or leads to cor pulmonale, the abnormal radiographic signs are the signs of those disorders.

Centrilobular emphysema is not recognizable on plain chest radiographs unless cor pulmonale is present. In panacinar emphysema (Fig. 23.48) the lungs are increased in volume owing to chronic airway obstruction with compliant lungs. The diaphragm is pushed down and appears low (below the seventh anterior rib or the twelfth posterior rib) and flattened. The heart is narrow, partly because the low diaphragm leads to elongation of the heart shadow. The increased lung volume causes widening of the ribs and herniation of the lung behind and in front of the heart.

Attenuation of blood vessels is a more specific sign of emphysema than overinflation of the lung. The reduction in the size and number of the pulmonary vessels can be generalized or localized. In the latter case, the area is labelled a bulla. The margins of bullous areas

can vary greatly: occasionally they are bounded by a sharp line and may resemble a pneumothorax, but more commonly there is an almost imperceptible change to normal lung. Very large bullae may compress the adjacent more normal lung parenchyma.

Chest CT shows the emphysematous changes in the lungs to great advantage. The cardinal signs are diminution in the size and reduction in the number of visible blood vessels in the pulmonary parenchyma. The remaining vessels course through lung parenchyma that is lower in density than normal.

Bronchiectasis

Bronchiectasis is defined as irreversible dilatation of the bronchi, often accompanied by impairment of drainage of bronchial secretions leading to persistent infection.

The conditions that cause bronchiectasis include pulmonary infection in childhood, cystic fibrosis and long-standing bronchial obstruction.

The radiological features are:

- Visibly dilated bronchi may be seen as tubular or ring shadows. If filled with fluid, the dilated bronchi are either opaque or contain air–fluid levels. Since these fluid levels are very short they have to be looked for very carefully.
- Persistent consolidation, often containing dilated bronchi.
- Loss of volume of the affected lobe or lobes is almost invariable.

A proportion of patients with symptomatic bronchiectasis have normal plain chest films.

Computed tomography has now replaced bronchography as the method of determining the presence of bronchiectasis, where this is in doubt, and the extent of disease. HRCT is employed in order to obtain high-resolution images (Fig. 23.49). On HRCT the dilated, thick-walled bronchi are individually identified. A

Figure 23.49 *HRCT of lungs showing bilateral lower lobe bronchiectasis. There are numerous greatly dilated bronchi (arrows), many of which have thick walls.*

Figure 23.50 *Cystic fibrosis. Typical plain chest radiograph showing bronchial wall thickening (arrows), predominant in the upper zones, and overinflated lungs.*

Figure 23.51 *Allergic bronchopulmonary aspergilliosis. Numerous, centrally predominant areas of atelectasis are seen. Arrows point to a dilated fluid/mucus-filled bronchus.*

useful rule is that the bronchi should normally be approximately the same diameter as their accompanying artery and that their walls should be thin. Loss of volume is very readily seen at CT, because the position of the hila and fissures is clearly demonstrated.

Cystic fibrosis

In cystic fibrosis the small airways become blocked and secondary infections supervene.

The chest radiograph and CT findings are (Fig. 23.50):

- small ill-defined consolidations, maximal in the upper zones, some of which show cavitation;
- bronchial wall thickening and the signs of bronchiectasis, both usually maximal in the upper zones.
- evidence of airway obstruction; the diaphragm is low and flat and the heart is narrow and vertical, until cor pulmonale develops when cardiac enlargement may occur.

MRI has been advocated as a method of follow-up, because of the lack of radiation for young patients who require frequent imaging. The signs at MRI are the same as for CT.

Allergic bronchopulmonary aspergillosis

Allergic bronchopulmonary aspergillosis is first encountered in older children and younger adults, though many have a long-standing history of asthma. The fungus in mucus plugs damages the walls of relatively proximal bronchi. The mechanism of the inflammatory damage is a localized allergic reaction. The result is obstruction, often transient, and localized dilatation of the affected bronchi. The manifestations on plain film (Fig. 23.51) and CT include:

- large-volume lungs due to long-standing severe asthma;
- transient collapse/consolidation of portions of the lung;
- visualization of the bronchi from mucus plugging forming a cast of the bronchi;
- a nearly unique form of bronchiectasis with dilatation of proximal bronchi leading to non-obstructed normal appearing distal bronchi;
- on CT, particularly HRCT, patchy ground-glass shadowing seen from uneven aeration of the lung parenchyma, in which the normal lung may show ground-glass opacity in comparison to the overinflated lung supplied by obstructed bronchi.

RESPIRATORY DISTRESS IN THE NEWBORN

There are many causes of respiratory distress in the first few days of life. Abnormalities are visible on the chest radiograph in the majority; only four conditions are discussed here.

Hyaline membrane disease

Hyaline membrane disease is one of the commonest abnormalities. It is a disease of the premature infant and

Figure 23.52 *Hyaline membrane disease in a neonate. There are uniform granular shadows in the lungs, so numerous that they cause visible bronchograms. Note the normal diaphragm position.*

Figure 23.53 *Neonatal pulmonary haemorrhage showing very extensive consolidations similar to hyaline membrane disease.*

is due to deficiency of surfactant in the lungs. Consequently the alveoli collapse, so preventing gas exchange. The chest radiographic appearance is one of the most important criteria in making the diagnosis.

The basic signs are widespread very small pulmonary opacities and visible air bronchograms (Fig. 23.52). The air bronchograms are visible because the bronchi are surrounded by airless alveoli. The changes are nearly always uniform in distribution. In the milder forms, the nodules are small and the air bronchograms may be the most obvious and easily recognized sign. In the more severe forms, the pulmonary opacities become more obvious and may be confluent; the lungs then appear almost opaque, except for air bronchograms.

Pulmonary haemorrhage

Pulmonary haemorrhage gives a similar radiographic appearance to hyaline membrane disease (Fig. 23.53).

Meconium aspiration (Fig. 23.54)

Here the pulmonary shadowing is usually patchy and distinctly streaky. Air bronchograms are not an obvious feature. The diaphragm is often lower than normal, owing to airway obstruction associated with sticky meconium in the bronchi.

Transient tachypnoea of the newborn

This condition resembles mild or moderate hyaline membrane disease clinically, but radiologically (Fig.

Figure 23.54 *Neonatal meconium aspiration showing streaky pulmonary shadowing and, most importantly for diagnosis, overinflation of the lungs, as shown by the low flat hemidiaphragms.*

23.55) the lungs appear overinflated, the widespread pulmonary opacity is more streaky, closely resembling pulmonary oedema, and pleural effusions are common.

Complications of therapy

In addition to establishing the initial diagnosis in neonates with various causes of respiratory distress, the

Figure 23.55 *Transient tachypnoea of the newborn shadowing ill-defined patchy shadowing radiating from the hila, together with bilateral pleural effusions and overinflated lungs.*

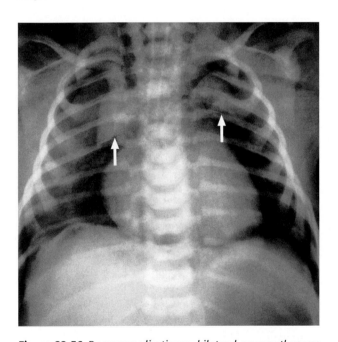

Figure 23.56 *Pneumomediastinum, bilateral pneumothoraces and pneumoperitoneum in a patient on positive pressure ventilation for hyaline membrane disease. The air lifting the lobes of the thymus (arrows) away from the other mediastinal structures is diagnostic of pneumomediastinum.*

plain chest film is vital in detecting complications of therapy. These include lobar collapse, pneumomediastinum (Fig. 23.56) and pneumothorax. Pneumothorax may be difficult to recognize as the films are often taken with the baby supine, and the air may collect in an unusual position.

Figure 23.57 *Radiation fibrosis. The dense opacity within the lung adjacent to the right hilum and upper mediastinum has a geometric shape in this case conforming to the rectangular radiation field. Note the fibrotic contraction, which has caused the trachea to shift towards the fibrotic area.*

RADIATION PNEUMONITIS AND FIBROSIS

The response of normal lung to radiation varies from patient to patient. Initially, there is no radiological change, but within a few weeks ill-defined, small shadows, indistinguishable from infective consolidation, are seen in the radiation field. If the inflammatory change progresses to fibrosis, there is dense, coarse shadowing, which may be sharply demarcated from the normal lung in a geometric fashion, conforming to the field of radiation rather than the lobar boundaries of the lung (Fig. 23.57). There is loss of volume of the fibrosed areas and extensive pleural thickening is often seen.

INHALED FOREIGN BODIES

Metallic foreign bodies in the bronchial tree are usually readily visualized and localized radiographically. Teeth fragments, however, may be difficult to recognize. Most foreign bodies, e.g. nuts, sweets and small plastic objects, are not radiopaque. The radiographic signs are, therefore, those of the effects of the foreign body on the lungs, namely the signs of major airway obstruction. In children, the obstruction is usually of the ball-valve type, and evidence of air trapping is the commonest

(a)

(b)

Figure 23.58 *Bronchial carcinoma causing right upper lobe collapse and a right hilar mass. (a) The chest radiograph shows right upper lobe collapse. (The arrows point to the greatly elevated horizontal fissure.) (b) The mass of tumour at the right hilum is best seen at CT (solid arrow). The greatly collapsed right upper lobe is seen as sliver of tissue plastered against the mediastinum anteriorly (open arrows).*

sign. A minority show atelectasis or postobstructive pneumonia. A significant proportion of children with a proven foreign body in the trachea or bronchi have normal plain chest radiographs.

Air trapping is rarely severe enough to be appreciated on standard films taken on full inspiration. The sign is always more obvious on expiration. Indeed, the inspiratory film may be completely normal in cases when the diagnosis is obvious on expiration. The signs of air trapping are increased radiolucency of the affected lung with a decrease in the size of the vessels within that lung, together with the signs of increased or fixed volume, flat hemidiaphragm and mediastinal shift to the opposite side.

Chest fluoroscopy is the most sensitive radiographic technique for detecting an inhaled foreign body in a bronchus and is abnormal in over 90 per cent of cases. The changing volume and density of normally aerated lung contrasts sharply with the fixed volume and unchanging density of lung with air-trapping. This differential aeration of different portions of the lung is not, of course, visible with tracheal foreign bodies, and they can be more difficult to diagnose.

INHALATION OF NOXIOUS GASES AND SMOKE

The initial radiological finding seen in the lungs following inhalation of a variety of toxic gases (including carbon monoxide, nitrogen dioxide, sulphur dioxide, ammonia, and chlorine) is pulmonary oedema within 4 to 24 hours of the injury.

Smoke inhalation may also produce a pattern, soon after injury, resembling pulmonary oedema, but this may not develop for up to 96 hours after exposure. Other patterns seen with smoke inhalation include focal pulmonary collapse and/or consolidation or irregular patchy consolidation. The average time of appearance of these abnormalities is 24 to 36 hours after injury. It is important to realize that there is no correlation between the chest radiography findings and the degree of hypoxaemia or carboxyhaemoglobinaemia. Significant hypoxaemia and carboxyhaemoglobinaemia can exist within a film that remains normal throughout the patient's hospital stay.

HYDROCARBON PNEUMONIA

Patients who ingest petroleum distillates, such as paraffin, frequently develop patchy consolidations at the lung bases. The severity of the pulmonary change is related to the volume ingested. The pulmonary consolidations usually appear within an hour of ingestion. They resolve slowly, taking up to 2 weeks or more to clear, and their resolution usually lags well behind the clinical improvement. Pneumatoceles may develop, as may pleural effusion.

CARCINOMA OF THE BRONCHUS

The majority of bronchial carcinomas arise in larger bronchi at, or close to, the hilum. These tumours are

Figure 23.59 *Peripheral bronchial carcinoma presenting as a 4 cm diameter lobulated mass in the right upper lobe.*

Figure 23.60 *Squamous cell carcinoma of the lung. CT scan showing a strikingly thin-walled cavitating tumour. A little fluid is seen lying in the dependent portion of the cavity (arrows).*

usually confirmed or excluded by bronchoscopy and transbronchial biopsy. The remainder arise peripherally and their investigation can be more problematic.

Signs of a central tumour

The tumour itself may present as a hilar mass and the effects of obstruction by the tumour may be seen: usually a combination of collapse and consolidation (Fig. 23.58).

Signs of a peripheral tumour

A peripheral primary carcinoma usually presents as a rounded shadow with an irregular border showing lobulated, notched or infiltrating edges (Fig. 23.59). Cavitation may be seen within the mass. Peripheral squamous cell carcinomas show a particular tendency for cavitation (Fig. 23.60). The walls of the cavity are classically thick and irregular, but thin-walled smooth cavities due to carcinoma do occur. On very rare occasions primary lung carcinomas may show calcification on computed tomography.

Signs of spread of bronchial carcinoma

The signs of spread of bronchial carcinoma may be visible on plain chest radiography. Computed tomography has made a major contribution to the staging of lung cancer, because CT may show mediastinal lymph node enlargement or direct invasion of the mediastinum that is invisible or questionable on the plain chest film – information that may save the patient an unnecessary thoracotomy. MRI is used only to solve specific problems following CT. Positron emission tomography,

usually abbreviated to PET, is only available in a few centres. It is proving highly accurate for diagnosing and excluding intrathoracic lymph node metastases from bronchial carcinoma (see Fig. 1.4, p. 5).

The following signs should be looked for on plain radiographs, CT and MRI:

- **Hilar and mediastinal lymph node enlargement** from lymphatic spread of tumour. Only greatly enlarged lymph nodes can be recognized on plain chest radiographs. The sites in which nodes are most readily identified are at the hilum and in the right paratracheal area. CT (Fig. 23.61) has the ability to

Figure 23.61 *Bronchial carcinoma with metastases to mediastinal lymph nodes. The large primary bronchial carcinoma in the right upper lobe has metastasized to mediastinal lymph nodes lying between the superior vena cava (S) and the right main bronchus (white arrow). The black arrow points to the largest of the enlarged nodes.*

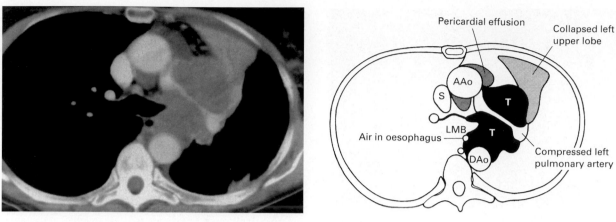

Figure 23.62 *Extensive mediastinal invasion by a left hilar bronchial carcinoma (T). Contrast-enhanced CT scan showing the tumour surrounding, invading and narrowing the main and left pulmonary arteries and the descending aorta. The tumour obstructing the left upper lobe bronchus has caused left upper lobe collapse. AAo = ascending aorta; DAo = descending aorta = LMB = left main bronchus; S = superior vena cava.*

Figure 23.63 *Extensive mediastinal invasion by a left hilar bronchial carcinoma shown by coronal MRI scan. Note the tumour extending into the aortopulmonary window and lying medial to the aortic arch. The mediastinal fat is bright white (tinted areas in the diagram).*

show all enlarged nodes, even those only mildly enlarged, in any site in the mediastinum and hila. However, enlargement of lymph nodes does not necessarily mean metastatic involvement, since reactive hyperplasia to the tumour or associated infection can be responsible for nodal enlargement as can pre-existing disease, such as granulomatous infection, sarcoidosis or pneumoconiosis. In practice, the role of CT is to decide which patients are unsuitable for surgery and which patients need mediastinoscopy or mediastinotomy prior to thoracotomy, and to show the surgeon which nodes to biopsy preoperatively. Nodes below 1 cm in diame-

ter can be considered as normal in size and need not be biopsied prior to thoracotomy. Nodes above 1 cm in diameter should be biopsied prior to surgical resection of the primary tumour, though it should be borne in mind that nodes of 2 cm or greater in the lymphatic drainage of a bronchial carcinoma almost invariably contain metastatic neoplasm. MRI, in general, has no advantages over CT for demonstrating mediastinal lymph node enlargement.

- **Pleural effusion**, particularly if bloody, in a patient with lung cancer is usually due to malignant involvement of the pleura. If so, the tumour is classified as a T4 tumour and is considered unsuitable for surgi-

Figure 23.64 *Chest wall invasion by a peripheral bronchial carcinoma. The tumour has invaded the adjacent rib (arrow).*

Figure 23.65 *Right-sided lymphangitis carcinomatosa, which developed in someone who presented with a hilar mass (see Fig. 23.74).*

Figure 23.66 *Lymphangitis carcinomatosa. HRCT showing thickening and nodularity of the interlobular septa of the lung. The arrow points to one septum, which shows the abnormality particularly well.*

cal resection. Pleural effusion may also be secondary to associated infection of the lung or coincidental, as in heart failure. Pleural aspiration and biopsy are, therefore, indicated.

- **Invasion of the mediastinum**. On plain films the signs of mediastinal invasion are widening of the mediastinal shadow; elevation of one or other hemidiaphragm may indicate involvement of the phrenic nerve by tumour. Mediastinal widening can be difficult to evaluate, particularly in older people with aortic unfolding.

  CT and, in selected cases, MRI are better methods than plain films for assessing mediastinal invasion by tumour, because the neoplasm and the mediastinal structures can be directly visualized (Figs 23.61–23.63). Note, however, that it can be very difficult to decide whether the degree of invasion is sufficient to make the tumour inoperable. The visible tumour mass may show contact with the mediastinal pleura and yet be confined to the lung at thoracotomy. Similarly, tumours that have clearly invaded the mediastinal fat and show contact with such vital structures as the aorta, trachea or oesophagus, may still be resectable at thoracotomy.

- **Invasion of the chest wall**. Destruction of a rib immediately adjacent to a pulmonary shadow indicates chest wall invasion. Recognizing rib destruction can be difficult unless a conscious effort is made to look at the ribs directly. Oblique views may be helpful in detecting bone destruction. CT can demonstrate chest wall invasion to advantage (Fig. 23.64) and may show soft-tissue invasion even when the bone is not visibly eroded. Imaging techniques, however, even CT and MRI, may not always be reliable for diagnosing chest wall invasion, and local chest wall pain remains the most important feature indicating that the tumour has crossed the pleura.

  Invasion of the root of the neck by so-called **Pancoast's tumours** (**superior sulcus tumours**) may be difficult to diagnose by CT. MRI, because of its multiplanar imaging capability, is particularly useful for showing the full extent of such tumours.

- **Lymphangitis carcinomatosa**. Lymphangitis carcinomatosa can be due to spread from abdominal, breast and other extrathoracic cancers as well as from carcinoma of the lung. The lymphatic vessels become grossly distended and the lungs become oedematous. When bilateral, the signs on plain film radiography can be identical to those seen in interstitial pulmonary oedema (septal lines, loss of vessel clarity and peribronchial thickening) but, if the heart is normal in size and there is hilar adenopathy and/or lobar consolidation, or if the changes are unilateral, the diagnosis of lymphangitis carcinomatosa deserves serious consideration (Fig. 23.65). The clinical story is very helpful because, if the changes are due to pulmonary oedema, the patient usually complains of sudden onset of breathlessness, whereas a patient with lymphangitis carcinomatosa gives a story of slowly increasing dyspnoea over the preceding weeks or months. CT, particularly HRCT, has proved very valuable in demonstrating lymphangitis carcinomatosa, because the appearances, in the correct clinical circumstances, are highly specific (Fig. 23.66). The cardinal signs are non-uniform thickening of the interlobular septa with thickening of the bronchovascular bundles in the centre of the pulmonary lobules.

- **Haematogenous metastases**. Distant metastases may be seen in the lungs, bones, liver and adrenals.

PULMONARY METASTASES

The hallmark of blood-borne metastases to the lungs on imaging studies is one or more discrete pulmonary nodules, maximal in the outer portions of the lungs. Metastases vary in size from microscopic to many centimetres in diameter, are usually multiple, and have well or moderately well-defined outlines. On occasion, particularly when they are due to metastatic adenocarcinoma or if the metastases have bled into the surrounding lung, they show irregular or ill-defined edges. Cavitation is seen from time to time, particularly with metastatic squamous cell carcinomas.

Detectable calcification in metastases is very unusual, except in metastases from sarcomas, notably osteosarcoma and chondrosarcoma, in which the calcification is part of the tumour matrix just as it is in the primary tumour.

Miliary nodulation, a pattern of innumerable tiny nodules resembling miliary tuberculosis, is occasionally encountered but is decidedly rare. Miliary metastases are most likely to be due to thyroid or renal carcinomas. A pattern of lymphangitis carcinomatosa is seen with metastases from a variety of primary tumours, the commonest being lung and breast.

The standard initial test for the detection of pulmonary metastases is the plain chest radiograph. As with primary lung tumours, metastases have to be almost a centimetre in diameter or larger to be visible on plain chest radiographs or conventional tomograms. CT, particularly spiral (helical) CT, is currently the most sensitive technique available for the detection of pulmonary metastases and can detect metastases as small as 3 mm in diameter. There is, however, a disadvantage attached to the excellent sensitivity of CT. Some small nodules are benign processes, such as tuberculomas or fungal granulomas. This is a major diagnostic problem in those parts of the world where tuberculosis and fungal infections are common.

Currently, MRI plays no part in diagnosing pulmonary metastases. CT is only used in selected cases, for example in:

- patients with a normal chest radiograph in whom the presence of pulmonary metastases is likely and would significantly alter patient management, e.g. osteosarcoma;
- patients who are being considered for surgical resection of known pulmonary metastases;
- distinguishing solitary from multiple pulmonary nodules where the diagnostic dilemma is metastasis versus new primary bronchial carcinoma.

THE PLEURA

PLEURAL EFFUSION

Fluid in the pleural cavity has the same appearance on plain chest radiographs regardless of whether the fluid is a transudate, pus or blood. With rare exceptions this is also true even for CT and MRI, though ultrasound may show numerous echoes within the fluid when it is due to pus. Fluid that is free to move collects in the most dependent portions of the pleural cavities, which clearly varies with the position of the patient.

CT and MRI examinations are routinely conducted with the patient in the supine position, whereas ultrasound examination is carried out with the patient in any position that seems desirable to the operator. Position becomes a very important issue when deciding where to place a thoracentesis needle or chest tube, as the fluid may well be in a different position at the time of the procedure than when the imaging was performed.

The main causes for pleural effusion are:

- **Infection**. Pleural effusions from pneumonia are on the whole small, and the pneumonia is usually the dominant feature on the chest film. Large loculated effusions in association with pneumonia often indicate empyema formation. In some cases of tuberculosis, the effusion is the only visible abnormality and the effusion may be large. Subphrenic abscess nearly always produces a pleural effusion. Pleural empyemas are discussed on p. 579.
- **Malignancy**. Effusions are seen with pleural metastases, but it is unusual to see the pleural deposits themselves on plain chest radiographs. Malignant

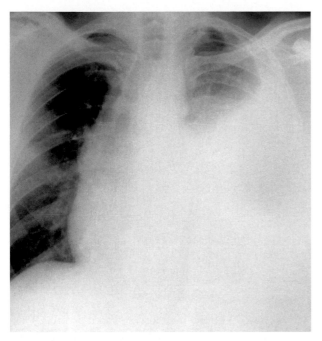

Figure 23.67 *Large left pleural effusion. Note the tracheal and mediastinal shift to the opposite side and the homogeneous opacity of the pleural fluid. The opacity can be seen running up the side of the chest wall to extend over the lung apex, a feature typical of large pleural effusions.*

Figure 23.68 *Massive left pleural effusion leading to total opacity of the left hemithorax. The distinction from left lung consolidation or left lung collapse is made by noting the displacement of the trachea away from the side of the opacity. (See Fig. 23.12 for illustration of complete left lung collapse.)*

effusions are frequently large. If the effusion is due to bronchogenic carcinoma, other signs of tumour are usually evident.

- **Cardiac failure**. Small bilateral pleural effusions are frequently seen in acute left ventricular failure. Larger pleural effusions may be present in long-standing congestive cardiac failure. The effusions are usually bilateral, often larger on the right than on the left. Other evidence of cardiac failure is usually present.
- **Pulmonary infarction** can cause effusions which are usually small and accompanied by a lung shadow due to the pulmonary infarct itself.
- **Collagen vascular diseases, nephrotic syndrome, renal failure, ascites and Mieg's syndrome** can give rise to pleural effusions, which are usually bilateral
- **Pleural haemorrhage** from trauma, aortic dissection or aneurysm, ruptured bulla, pleural metastasis or endometriosis.

On plain chest radiographs, pleural fluid casts a homogeneous shadow. Free pleural effusions assume a variety of shapes, the commonest of which is similar to the shape that would be seen if a large balloon were pressed down into a container of water. The water would be forced around the outer surface of the balloon up the sides of the container. Similarly, in most pleural effusions some fluid is seen running up the side of the lungs (Fig. 23.67) and into the fissures. With large effusions, fluid may be seen extending over the lung

apex. The smooth edge between lung and pleural fluid can often be recognized on an adequately penetrated film, provided the underlying lung is aerated. In the upright position, all the fluid may lie in a subpulmonary location, and the upper border of the fluid may assume a shape similar to the normal hemidiaphragm.

Free pleural effusions have a different appearance on supine compared to upright examinations. In the supine position, the posteriorly layered fluid causes an ill-defined increase in density of the hemithorax and the hemidiaphragm outline is often indistinct. Fluid may be seen over the lung apex, forming a well-demarcated band of density. With large effusions this band of density extends around the outer edge of the whole lung and the entire hemithorax is clearly denser than normal.

Up to 300 ml of pleural fluid may be difficult or impossible to see on standard PA and lateral chest films. If there is doubt about the presence or the amount of fluid, a lateral decubitus view can be of great help. The fluid, if free to move, settles along the dependent lateral chest wall where it can be recognized.

Very large effusions with little underlying pulmonary collapse displace the mediastinum and trachea to the opposite side (Fig. 23.68). Pulmonary collapse is seen in association with larger pleural effusions: the pleural effusion and the pulmonary collapse can both be due to the same basic process, e.g. pneumonia or carcinoma of the lung, or the effusion may have caused compression and collapse of the underlying lung. If the trachea is displaced to the side of the effusion, there must be substantial collapse of the lung, more than could be accounted for by compression collapse alone.

Loculated pleural effusions occur whenever the movement of pleural fluid within the pleural cavity is prevented by pleural adhesions. Loculation occurs in many types of effusions, but is a particular feature of empyema. The loculations may be anywhere in the pleural cavity, including the fissures. Loculated fluid collections cause oval, lens-shaped or rounded expansions of the pleura and may be confused with pulmonary consolidation or lung abscess. These misdiagnoses can be avoided by recognizing the clearly defined curved border of a pleural-based density (Fig. 23.69). Often, one or more interfaces with the lung are not tangential to the X-ray beam, and the density, therefore, fades off with an imperceptible border. On a lateral view, a loculated effusion within the oblique or horizontal fissure is clearly lens-shaped and lies within the known position of one of the fissures.

It may be difficult to tell from plain chest radiographs whether an opacity at a lung base is due to pleural effusion or whether it is due to pulmonary consolidation or collapse. When both pleural fluid and lower lobe collapse are present together, it can be particularly difficult to decide the size of the pleural fluid component. The shadow of pleural fluid is usually higher laterally than medially, is homogeneous in density and lies outside the lung, being bounded by a sharp concave interface with the lung. Where the effusion runs into a fissure, both sides of the fissure are visible. The trachea and mediastinum are either central or are pushed to the opposite side. Conversely, with consolidation or collapse, the shape of the shadow conforms to that of a lobe or segment, an air bronchogram may be present and, where the consolidation abuts a fissure, the fissure is seen as an edge with only one side being visible. With consolidation or collapse, the trachea and mediastinum are either central or pulled towards the side of the shadow.

Computed tomography of pleural effusion

The basic signs of pleural effusion on CT are similar to those on plain film, with the additional information that the density of pleural fluid is homogeneous and, characteristically, pleural fluid is of lower density than most soft tissues (Fig. 23.70), being in the range expected for water, namely −10 to +10 Hounsfield units (HU). Distinguishing between pleural effusion and lobar collapse is very easy with CT, but CT is only occasionally needed because the lateral decubitus plain film is a simpler method. At CT, the density of the collapsed lobe is usually appreciably greater than that of the pleural effusion, even more so if intravenous contrast enhancement is used. Also, air within the bronchi can often be traced into the compressed lung. The MRI features are essentially the same as for CT.

(a)

(b)

Figure 23.69 *Comparison of loculated pleural fluid and an intrapulmonary lung abscess. (a) The asterisk is in the centre of a loculated pleural fluid collection lying against the left chest wall. Note the flat base on the parietal pleura and the smoothly curved edge gently fusing with the chest wall pleura. The arrows point to a lung abscess in the left lower lobe. The abscess is round and has a less well-defined interface with surrounding lung. (b) Another loculated fluid collection is present in the upper portion of the left oblique fissure. This collection is best seen in the lateral projection as a lens-shaped opacity, sometimes called an interlobar effusion (arrows).*

Figure 23.70 *Pleural effusion on CT scan. Note the shape of the opacity, conforming to the shape of the pleural cavity, the smooth interface with lung and a CT density lower than muscle. (The measured density was in the range expected for water.)*

Surprisingly, it is sometimes difficult to say at CT whether fluid is pleural effusion or ascites. The distinction is made by noting the relationship of the fluid to the diaphragm. Pleural fluid collects outside the diaphragmatic dome and can be seen posterior to the portion of diaphragm that covers the bare area of the liver.

Ultrasound of pleural effusion

Ultrasound examination can be very useful for investigating pleural effusion. At ultrasound, pleural fluid can be recognized as a transonic area between the lung and

Figure 23.71 *Empyema. CT scan shows a lens-shaped, loculated fluid collection in the right pleural cavity. Note the thickened pleura (horizontal arrows) and the air–fluid level (vertical arrows). There are multiple bubbles of gas trapped in the empyema. Enlarged right hilar nodes are also present.*

the chest wall or diaphragm. Since the diaphragm is so well seen there is no confusion with ascites. When pleural fluid loculates against the chest wall, it is possible to place the ultrasound probe directly over the fluid collection, show its size and extent, and determine the best site for needle or chest tube placement.

PARAPNEUMONIC PLEURAL EFFUSIONS AND EMPYEMA

There is no generally accepted definition that distinguishes an uncomplicated parapneumonic pleural effusion from an empyema. The factors used to make the distinction centre on the protein levels and white blood cell count of the pleural fluid.

The diagnosis of parapneumonic effusion and empyema depends on recognizing fluid in the pleural cavity and performing thoracentesis to analyse the fluid. Because empyemas are so protein-rich, there is a strong tendency for the pleural fluid to loculate and, therefore, ultrasound or CT may be required to appreciate the size and precise position of the pleural fluid collection.

The distinction between lung abscess and loculated pleural fluid has important therapeutic consequences. Empyema requires early tube drainage, whereas adequate antibiotic therapy obviates the need for drainage in most cases of lung abscess. The distinction on conventional radiographs can be difficult. The inner margin of the empyema, like all loculated fluid collections, is sharply defined with a curved smooth interface with the adjacent lung when tangential to the X-ray beam.

Computed tomography can be very valuable in deciding between empyema (Fig. 23.71) and a peripherally positioned lung abscess in those cases when the plain chest radiographic or ultrasound features are ambiguous. The distinguishing features at CT are:

- Empyemas, unless very large, are basically **lenticular in shape**. The angle formed at the interface with the chest wall is obtuse or tapering. Lung abscesses, on the other hand, tend to be spherical and show acute angles at their margins with the chest wall.
- The **walls** of an empyema are formed by thickened visceral and parietal pleura. This thickened pleura is of uniform thickness, enhances following intravenous contrast injection and has a smooth inner and outer wall, enclosing the empyema fluid. The wall of a lung abscess is irregular in thickness and has an irregular inner and outer margin. It may contain multiple dots of air and, on occasion, may even show distorted air bronchograms.

PRIMARY PLEURAL TUMOURS

Primary pleural tumours, namely localized fibrous tumour of the pleura and diffuse malignant mesothelioma, are relatively uncommon.

Localized fibrous tumour of the pleura

Localized fibrous tumour of the pleura has been given a variety of names, including pleural fibroma and benign mesothelioma. These tumours are mostly benign though some are locally invasive. Unlike malignant mesothelioma, the localized tumour is not related to asbestos exposure.

On plain chest radiography, the usual finding is a slow-growing, rounded or oval, often lobulated, homogeneous mass in contact with a pleural surface. The lesions vary in size from less than 1 cm to 30 cm diameter, but are usually 7 cm or more at initial presentation.

On CT and MRI, the lesions are well marginated, based on a pleural surface, and show acute angles at their margins. In other words they grow outwards from a relatively narrow base or pedicle. Smaller lesions show uniform soft-tissue density, and enhance after intravenous contrast injection, whereas a substantial proportion of the larger lesions show the CT or MRI features of central necrosis.

Malignant mesothelioma

Malignant mesothelioma is a rare tumour except in patients exposed to asbestos. The imaging features are similar on plain chest radiographs, CT and MRI, but the extent of the tumour and any accompanying pleural fluid is shown with greater accuracy by CT and MRI than by plain radiography.

The imaging findings typically consist of extensive nodular thickening of the pleura (Fig. 23.72), which may conglomerate to form a circumferential lobular sheet of soft-tissue density encasing the lung. A useful distin-

Figure 23.72 *Malignant mesothelioma in a patient with previous asbestos exposure. The sheet of tumour masses in the pleura surrounding the right lung is well demonstrated. Note the calcified pleural plaques in both the right and left pleural cavities (the arrow points to one of the partially calcified asbestos-related pleural plaques in the left pleural cavity).*

guishing feature from benign postinflammatory pleural thickening is that mesothelioma may show substantial involvement of the mediastinal pleura, whereas benign pleural thickening rarely does so. The tumour often runs into the fissures. Sometimes the accompanying pleural effusion is very large and, if it obscures the pleural masses, the chest radiographic appearances may be indistinguishable from other causes of pleural effusion. At CT (and MRI scanning), the soft-tissue density of the tumour tissue can be readily distinguished from the adjacent pleural effusion, but the nodules may on occasion be so tiny that they are unrecognizable, and the only imaging feature in these cases is a pleural effusion.

Chest wall invasion, bone destruction and direct extension to the pericardium and other mediastinal structures, involvement of mediastinal lymph nodes and invasion through the diaphragm into the upper abdomen are all best seen on CT (or MRI). Since many malignant mesotheliomas are secondary to asbestos exposure, asbestos-related pleural plaques may be seen in either pleural cavity.

Very occasionally malignant mesothelioma may take the form of a focal mass similar to localized fibrous tumour of the pleura.

PLEURAL THICKENING

Pleural thickening can be due to fibrosis following previous pleural effusion or haemorrhage, asbestos exposure or, on occasion, pleural neoplasm. It may be impossible to distinguish pleural fluid from pleural fibrosis on conventional radiographic projections. Comparison with previous films may be necessary to show that the pleural shadow is not changing and is, therefore, likely to be fibrosis. Alternatively, the problem can be tackled by taking a lateral decubitus view, in which free fluid changes its appearance as it falls to lie along the lateral chest wall, whereas pleural thickening or loculated fluid is unaltered in appearance.

The distinction between pleural fluid and soft-tissue thickening, such as fibrosis or neoplasm, is readily made at CT because most pleural fluid shows a CT density of −10 to +10 HU whereas fibrosis/neoplasm shows a density similar to muscle (30–50 HU). The distinction is particularly easy with ultrasound because fluid and solid have such different ultrasonic characteristics. Pleural fibrosis usually produces a smooth edge to the pleural echoes, whereas pleural tumours produce lobulated pleural masses typical of neoplasm. Asbestos-related pleural plaques are flat, sharply demarcated and usually show minimal, if any, lobulation.

PLEURAL CALCIFICATION

Irregular plaques of calcium may be seen with or without accompanying pleural thickening. When unilateral and focal they are likely to be due to either an old empyema, usually tuberculous, or an old haemothorax. Bilateral, patchy pleural calcification is often related to asbestos exposure. Sometimes no cause for pleural calcification can be found.

PLEURAL METASTASES AND MALIGNANT PLEURAL EFFUSION

Metastases to the pleura can originate from almost any primary tumour, but the lung appears to be the most frequent primary site, followed by breast, pancreas, stomach and ovary.

Usually the findings on plain chest radiograph, CT, MRI and ultrasound are those of free or loculated pleural effusion without any specific features to the effusion itself. There may be recognizable tumour nodules in the pleura on CT, MRI, ultrasound or even, occasionally, chest radiographs.

PNEUMOTHORAX

The diagnosis of pneumothorax depends on recognizing the line of the pleura separated by air from the chest wall, mediastinum or diaphragm with no vessels beyond this line (Fig. 23.73). Lack of vessel shadows alone is insufficient evidence on which to make the diagnosis, since there may be few or no visible vessels in emphysematous bullae. There is often no appreciable increase in

the density of the collapsed lung beneath the pneumothorax unless the pneumothorax is very large.

The detection of a small pneumothorax can be very difficult. It is easy to confuse the pleural edge with the cortex of normal ribs and a skin fold can, on occasion, be confused with a pneumothorax. Sometimes a pneumothorax is more obvious on a film taken in expiration.

With tension pneumothorax, there is mediastinal shift, and the hemidiaphragm is often flattened. It is worth noting that tension pneumothoraces are almost invariably large because the underlying lung collapses owing to increased pressure in the pleural space.

Causes of pneumothorax

Pneumothorax is associated with many underlying disorders of the lung including emphysema, trauma, certain forms of pulmonary fibrosis, tuberculosis and rarely metastases.

The majority, however, occur in young people who have no recognizable lung disease but who burst small blebs or bullae at the periphery of their lungs, the bleb or bulla rarely being recognizable on plain film.

Hydropneumothorax, haemopneumothorax and pyopneumothorax

In most cases of pneumothorax, whatever the cause, some fluid is present in the pleural cavity. In spontaneous pneumothorax the fluid is often bloody but the amount is small.

Fluid in the pleural cavity, whether it be a pleural effusion, blood or pus, assumes a different shape in the presence of pneumothorax. The diagnostic feature is an air–fluid level which extends across the hemithorax.

PULMONARY HILA

Enlargement of the hila presents two main diagnostic questions. Firstly, is the enlarged hilum due entirely to large blood vessels or caused by a mass? Secondly, if a hilar mass is present, what is its nature? The chief possibilities for a hilar mass are enlarged lymph nodes, a bronchial carcinoma or a combination of the two (Fig. 23.74).

It is usually possible to decide on plain chest radiographs whether hilar enlargement is due to large pulmonary arteries by appreciating the branching nature of the shadows and the fact that vascular enlargement is usually bilateral and accompanied by enlargement of the main pulmonary artery and heart. On occasion, it is necessary to perform contrast-enhanced CT, which will differentiate between enlarged pulmonary arteries and adenopathy.

MRI is the single best technique for elucidating hilar enlargement. It is, however, rarely required because

Figure 23.73 *Pneumothorax. The lung edge can be identified (arrows) with a large air collection between the partially collapsed right lung and the right chest wall.*

Figure 23.74 *Hilar mass. The right hilum is substantially larger than the left hilum and shows a lobular outline. The cause in this case was a bronchial carcinoma at the right hilum together with enlargement of the adjacent lymph nodes. Two years later (see Fig. 23.65) the patient developed right-sided lymphangitis carcinomatosa.*

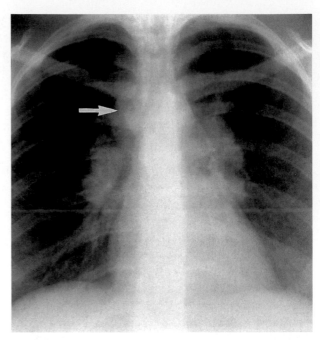

Figure 23.75 *Bilateral hilar lymph node enlargement in sarcoidosis. Note the symmetrical enlargement, the lobular outline of the hila and the enlargement of nodes in the right paratracheal area (arrow).*

plain films and CT usually give the necessary information. The advantage of MRI is that there is very little signal from the hilar structures in normal individuals using the usual spin-echo sequences, because there is no signal from fast-flowing blood in the major hilar vessels and no signal from the air within the bronchi. Thus, any hilar mass stands out clearly against the low-signal background.

HILAR LYMPH NODE ENLARGEMENT

Usually more than one lymph node is enlarged, so the hilum appears lobulated in outline on plain films.

- **Unilateral enlargement** of hilar lymph nodes may be due to:
  - metastases from carcinoma of the bronchus, in which case the primary tumour is often visible; metastases from other sites are rare;
  - malignant lymphoma;
  - infections, particularly tuberculosis and histoplasmosis in endemic areas. Hilar adenopathy is occasionally seen accompanying acute bacterial infection. Tuberculosis is the commonest cause of unilateral hilar adenopathy in children.
- **Bilateral enlargement** of hilar nodes occurs in:
  - sarcoidosis (Fig. 23.75), which is far and away the commonest cause. The diagnosis is almost certain

if the hilar enlargement is symmetrical and if the patient is asymptomatic, or has either erythema nodosum or iridocyclitis. Simultaneous enlargement of mediastinal lymph nodes is common and lung changes are sometimes visible;
  - malignant lymphoma;
  - tuberculosis; the African and Asian races show this form of the disease but it is rare in Caucasians;
  - fungus disease, which is a rare cause of hilar enlargement.

THE MEDIASTINUM

CT AND MRI OF THE NORMAL MEDIASTINUM

The appearances at four levels of the thorax are illustrated in Fig. 23.76. The mediastinal structures are surrounded by fat. Important features to note are:

- The bulk of the mediastinum is due to the heart and blood vessels. Blood vessels are easy to recognize as tubular structures retaining a near constant diameter on several adjacent sections. For CT they can be opacified by intravenous contrast medium (in some centres such opacification is used almost routinely). On standard MRI spin-echo sequences, the lumina of the larger mediastinal blood vessels are seen as signal void due to fast-flowing blood.

(a)

(b)

(c)

(d)

(e)

Figure 23.76 *Normal mediastinum. (a)–(d) Contrast-enhanced CT scans at the four levels shown in (e). A catheter is present in the left innominate vein. AoA = aortic arch; AAo = ascending aorta; AzV = azygos vein; DAo = descending aorta; IA = innominate artery; LIV = left innominate vein; LCA = left carotid artery; LPA = left pulmonary artery; LSA = left subclavian artery; MPA = main pulmonary artery; Oe = oesophagus; RIV = right innominate vein; RPA = right pulmonary artery; SVC = superior vena cava; T = trachea; Th = thymus.*

- The only other normal structures of appreciable size are the thymus, oesophagus, trachea and bronchi. The thymus is the most difficult to assess because it is so variable in size.
- Normal lymph nodes are small, usually less than 6 mm in short-axis diameter, but 10 mm is regarded as the maximum.

MEDIASTINAL MASSES

Mediastinal masses are usually classified according to their position in the mediastinum; so the first step in diagnosis is to establish the likely anatomical origin using frontal and lateral radiographs supplemented, when necessary, by CT or MRI.

Plain chest films in mediastinal masses

The presence of a mediastinal mass is often first observed on plain chest radiography. The following general points are helpful when deciding the next steps in the diagnostic process.

- **Goitre**. Intrathoracic thyroid masses are the most frequent cause of a mediastinal mass. The characteristic feature is that the mass extends from the superior mediastinum into the neck and almost invariably compresses or displaces the trachea.
- **Lymphadenopathy** is the next most frequent cause of a mediastinal swelling. Lymphadenopathy may occur in any of the mediastinal compartments. It is often possible to diagnose enlarged lymph nodes from their multiplicity and their lobulated outlines.
- **Neurogenic tumours** are by far the commonest posterior mediastinal masses. They frequently cause pressure deformity of the adjacent ribs and thoracic spine.
- Certain tumours, such as **thymomas** and **teratomas/germ-cell tumours**, are, for practical purposes, confined to the anterior mediastinum.
- **Calcification** occurs in many conditions but almost never in malignant lymphadenopathy. Occasionally, the calcification is characteristic in appearance, e.g. in aneurysms of the aorta.
- A mediastinal mass due to a **hiatus hernia** is usually easy to diagnose on plain films because it often contains air and may have an air–fluid level, best seen on the lateral view. A film taken after a mouthful of barium has been swallowed will confirm the diagnosis of hiatus hernia.
- Most masses in the **right cardiophrenic angle** anteriorly are benign, e.g. large fat pads, benign pericardial cysts or hernias through the foramen of Morgagni. However, neoplastic involvement of lymph nodes should be considered in patients with known lymphoma or breast carcinoma.

Computed tomography of mediastinal masses

CT is usually the best method of assessing mediastinal abnormalities when problems remain unanswered from the plain chest radiographs.

- Abnormalities can be localized accurately. Knowledge of the precise shape, position, size and multiplicity of masses frequently narrows the differential diagnosis. For instance, contiguity of the mass with the thyroid in the neck suggests a goitre and multiple oval-shaped masses suggest lymphadenopathy.
- Occasionally, the density of the abnormality reveals its nature:
  - Fat can be recognized as such. This is useful for distinguishing tumours from large cardiophrenic

angle fat pads or unusual fat collections. Cystic teratomas (dermoid cysts) may contain recognizable fat.
- Thyroid tissue characteristically has a higher density than muscle both before and after contrast enhancement.
- Intravenous contrast enhancement permits ready differentiation of aneurysms and anomalous blood vessels from other masses.
- Calcification is more readily seen at CT than on plain radiographs. For practical purposes, the presence of calcification in a mass excludes untreated malignant neoplastic adenopathy.
- Cysts containing clear fluid, e.g. pericardial cysts and some bronchogenic cysts, can be diagnosed based on a CT number close to water (0 HU) provided the mass has smooth thin walls and a smooth outline.

Magnetic resonance imaging of mediastinal masses

MRI gives similar information to CT regarding most mediastinal masses but, because it is a more complex and more expensive examination, it is rarely indicated. MRI does, however, have certain specific advantages. For example:

- Aneurysms and vascular anomalies are readily demonstrable without the need for contrast medium.
- The degree of intraspinal extension of a neurogenic tumour can be assessed without the need either for multiple imaging examinations or for contrast opacification of the spinal subarachnoid space.
- In some instances, the ability to image in coronal, sagittal or oblique planes may show anatomical relationships that are difficult to demonstrate with CT. This information may help with surgical planning and, on rare occasions, may be of diagnostic value.

INTRATHORACIC THYROID MASSES

Intrathoracic thyroid masses are usually benign multinodular colloid goitres or adenomas, but may occasionally be carcinomas. They are almost invariably downward extensions of thyroid masses that originate in the neck and descend into the mediastinum; the continuity between the mediastinal mass and the thyroid gland in the neck is, therefore, an important diagnostic feature both on conventional films and at CT or MRI (Fig. 23.77).

On plain films, intrathoracic thyroid masses usually have a well-defined outline which may be lobular. Many displace and narrow the trachea; occasionally the narrowing is substantial. The pattern of displacement of the trachea depends on the location of the mass, which is

(a)

(b)

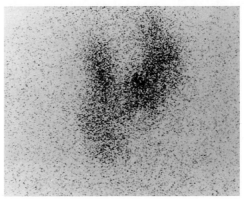

(c)

Figure 23.77 *Intrathoracic multinodular colloid goitre. (a) Note the mass (arrows) to either side of the trachea and contiguity of the mass with the neck. The trachea is deformed and narrowed by the goitre. (b) Contrast-enhanced CT scan of same patient showing a mass of almost the same density as the adjacent enhanced blood vessels. Typical small calcifications are seen within the goitre. (c) Radionuclide scan (iodine-123) showing that the intrathoracic mass concentrates the radionuclide, confirming the diagnosis of a thyroid mass.*

usually predominantly anterior or lateral to the trachea, but is posterior to it in as many as a quarter of cases.

CT demonstrates the shape, size and position of the mass which can be followed to the thyroid gland in the neck. A useful sign indicating a thyroid origin is the relatively high attenuation value of thyroid tissue compared to that of the adjacent muscles on both pre- and postcontrast CT images. The attenuation of the normal thyroid tissue within a goitre is the same as thyroid tissue in the neck.

Calcification, which is better seen at CT than on plain film, is a common finding that further helps differential diagnosis from other causes of mediastinal mass. Rounded, focal, low-density areas, more easily visible on the postcontrast films, are all common.

It is not possible to distinguish definitively between a benign and malignant mass at CT (or MRI) unless the tumour has clearly spread beyond the thyroid gland. If such spread is unequivocal, then the mass should be considered malignant. Multiple masses lying within the thyroid gland suggest a benign multinodular goitre.

Radionuclide imaging of the thyroid using radio-iodine shows some functioning thyroid tissue in almost all intrathoracic goitres (Fig. 23.77c). Radionuclide

imaging is very sensitive and specific for determining the thyroid nature of an intrathoracic mass. CT is, however, a useful initial test, because it provides more information should the mass turn out to be something other than thyroid, and is almost as specific for diagnosing a thyroid origin.

PARATHYROID MASSES

Hyperparathyroidism may be due to parathyroid adenomas that arise in ectopic parathyroid glands in the mediastinum, usually in or near the thymus. Parathyroid adenomas are often less than 2 cm in diameter. When larger than 1.5 cm they can usually be recognized at CT, but smaller lesions may be difficult to distinguish from thymic remnants or lymph nodes. Mediastinal parathyroid glands also can be demonstrated by radionuclide imaging (see above) and by MRI.

THYMIC MASSES

The size of the normal thymus varies dramatically from person to person below the age of 15; therefore size alone is an unreliable guide to pathology in younger

(a)   (b)

Figure 23.78 *Thymoma. (a) Plain film showing the smooth, well-defined mass (arrows) projecting from the left side of the mediastinum. (b) Contrast-enhanced CT scan in the same patient showing the thymoma (arrows). In this case there is variable contrast enhancement in different parts of the tumour.*

patients. In adults, the transverse diameter of each lobe is 1 cm or less. The normal thymus conforms to the shape of the adjacent great vessels on CT and MRI, whereas a thymic mass does not mould to structures such as the aorta. Also, a mass gives rise to a focal asymmetrical swelling.

The most common thymic tumour in adults is thymoma. Other tumours include thymolipoma, malignant lymphoma (notably Hodgkin's disease), thymic carcinoid (which may secrete ACTH and consequently may be responsible for Cushing's syndrome), germ cell tumours or teratomas, and thymic carcinoma.

Thymoma

Thymomas vary in size from very small to larger than 20 cm in diameter. The tumour may be contained within a capsule or may penetrate the capsule, eventually invading the mediastinum. It is the presence or absence of spread beyond the capsule rather than the histological appearance that determines whether a tumour is labelled benign or malignant (invasive) by the pathologist.

Most patients with non-invasive thymoma have no clinical symptoms from the tumour itself. Thymomas are, however, associated with a large variety of auto-immune diseases, most notably myasthenia gravis: approximately 35–40 per cent of patients with thymoma have myasthenia gravis and the incidence of thymoma in patients with myasthenia gravis is approximately 10–15 per cent. A variety of other conditions have a recognized association with thymoma, including haematological cytopenia, notably pure red cell aplasia and hypogammaglobulinaemia.

Only the larger tumours are visible on plain film (Fig. 23.78). Most thymomas are anterior to the ascending aorta above the right ventricular outflow tract. A few are situated in the lower third of the mediastinum. Thymomas are usually spherical or have lobulated borders.

Thymic tumours are best seen with CT: thymomas are usually of homogeneous density and enhance either patchily or uniformly (Fig. 23.78). Punctate, curvilinear or ring-like calcification is frequent in both benign and invasive thymomas.

The diagnosis of thymoma depends on identifying a focal swelling rather than applying specific measurements. Before the age of 20, diagnosing a small thymoma can be difficult because the normal gland is variable in size and, in myasthenia gravis, the associated hyperplasia may lead to a bulky gland. Fortunately thymoma is so infrequent in children that the potentially difficult problem of finding a thymoma in a child with myasthenia gravis rarely arises.

Invasive thymomas invade the mediastinal fat and eventually spread to the pericardium and pleura; they may spread via the pleura and may give rise to 'drop metastases' to non-contiguous pleural locations. Blood-borne metastases are rare. Until mediastinal or pleural invasion has occurred, it is not possible to distinguish benign from invasive thymoma even with CT.

Thymic cysts

Thymic cysts are usually simple cysts, some of which may be congenital in origin, within an otherwise normal or hyperplastic gland. Simple thymic cysts may be unilocular or multilocular. They are most frequently encountered in

Figure 23.79 *Thymic cyst. Contrast-enhanced CT scan showing a lobular-shaped, fluid density mass (arrows) centred on the thymus.*

Figure 23.80 *Benign cystic teratoma of mediastinum. Contrast-enhanced CT scan showing a large oval-shaped anterior mass containing a combination of densities: fluid, fat (arrow) and enhancing septa.*

children and are usually asymptomatic. Thymic cysts may also be found within thymomas, lymphoma or thymic germ-cell tumours, or may be due to radiotherapy.

On plain film, simple thymic cysts are indistinguishable from other non-lobulated thymic masses, notably thymoma. CT and MRI may demonstrate the presence of pure fluid within the cyst (Fig. 23.79), but thymic cysts may be of higher CT density, depending on the nature of the fluid, and be misdiagnosed as solid.

Thymic hyperplasia

Thymic hyperplasia is rarely recognizable on any imaging modality. CT and MRI may show enlargement of both lobes of an otherwise normally shaped gland with density/signal compatible with normal thymus.

The thymus may atrophy rapidly in response to stress or to therapy with steroids and antineoplastic drugs. The gland usually grows back to its original size upon recovery or cessation of treatment. In the phenomenon known as rebound thymic hyperplasia, the gland grows back to become larger than normal.

When rebound thymic hyperplasia is seen in patients previously treated for a malignant neoplasm, there may be difficulty in distinguishing thymic involvement by neoplasm from thymic rebound. The diagnosis depends on the absence of clinical or other features indicating recurrence of tumour in a patient with a reason for thymic rebound. Helpful features on CT are that the gland, though enlarged, has normal density, retains a normal shape with a smooth outline, conforms to the shape of adjacent structures and is symmetrical in shape.

Teratoma and germ-cell tumours of the mediastinum

Benign cystic teratomas usually produce a well-defined, rounded or lobulated mass in the anterior mediastinum. Most teratomas project mainly to one side of the midline; sometimes markedly so. Calcification, ossification or even teeth may be visible on plain chest radiograph and, occasionally, sufficient fat is present to be detectable radiographically.

CT and MRI show the shape and contents of the mass to advantage (Fig. 23.80). Fat and fluid contents are readily identified. The combination of a large anterior mediastinal mass that is wholly or predominantly cystic, together with a well-defined wall, is highly suggestive of the diagnosis of benign cystic teratoma. The presence of teeth or unequivocal fat within the mass is pathognomonic.

The plain film findings of **malignant germ-cell tumours** are similar to benign teratomas except that the mass is often lobular in outline, fat density is not noted and calcification is a rare finding. Unlike benign teratoma, the malignant forms grow rapidly, and metastases may be seen in the lungs, bones or pleura. CT and MRI show an asymmetrical mass, which may have a lobular outline. The adjacent mediastinal fat planes may be obliterated and extensive local invasion may be identified. The tumours show either homogeneous soft-tissue density or multiple areas of contrast enhancement interspersed with rounded areas of decreased attenuation owing to necrosis and haemorrhage. Rarely, coarse tumour calcification may be seen.

MEDIASTINAL CYSTS

Most mediastinal cysts are developmental in origin. The usual entities included in this category are bronchogenic (bronchial) cysts, oesophageal duplication cysts, neurenteric cysts and pericardial cysts. The distinction between these cysts is not always clear cut. On rare occasions, a pancreatic pseudocyst extends into the posterior mediastinum.

(a)

(b)

Figure 23.81 *Neural tumour in the posterior mediastinum. (a) Plain film showing a smooth, round, right paravertebral mass (arrow). (b) Contrast-enhanced CT scan showing the precise location of the tumour (arrow). The small cross is a cursor used to measure density. In this case the measured density was in the low soft-tissue range.*

On plain film all these cysts are usually predominantly spherical or oval in shape. Most bronchogenic cysts are in intimate contact with a major airway, whereas oesophageal cysts contact the oesophagus, pericardial cysts contact the pericardium and neurenteric cysts lie between the oesophagus and the spine. A characteristic of neurenteric cysts is an associated vertebral anomaly. CT and MRI show a thin or thick-walled cyst containing fluid, but the fluid content may be difficult to diagnose if previous haemorrhage has occurred.

INTRATHORACIC NEURAL TUMOURS

Intrathoracic neural tumours can be divided into nerve sheath tumours, ganglion cell tumours and paragangliomas (e.g. phaeochromocytoma).

Nerve sheath tumours comprise schwannomas (neurilemmomas), neurofibromas and their malignant counterparts. All are more common in patients with neurofibromatosis. Nerve sheath tumours arise predominantly from either the intercostal or the sympathetic nerves; some arise from the phrenic or vagus nerves. Many arise close to the spine and may extend through the neural exit foramina into the spinal canal (the so-called 'dumb-bell tumour').

The **ganglion cell tumours** form a spectrum, with neuroblastoma at the malignant end and ganglioneuroma at the benign end, ganglioneuroblastoma being an intermediate form. Neuroblastoma and ganglioneuroblastoma are essentially tumours of childhood.

Ganglioneuroma shows a wider and more even age distribution, ranging from 1 to 50 years.

Nerve sheath and ganglion cell tumours appear as well-defined masses with a smooth or lobulated outline. When they are localized, it is not possible to distinguish benign from malignant tumours. The tumours may be almost any size; some are very large, occupying most of a hemithorax. Except for vagal and phrenic nerve tumours, and the occasional neuroblastoma, neural tumours are situated in the posterior mediastinum (Fig. 23.81). An important diagnostic feature is pressure deformity and displacement of the adjacent ribs and vertebrae, and the intervertebral foramina may appear widened.

On CT, many neural tumours have mixed density, including low-attenuation regions. Being vascular lesions, they enhance on images taken after the administration of intravascular contrast medium. Calcification is a feature of ganglion cell tumours. One great advantage of CT is the superior demonstration of spinal and intraspinal involvement compared to plain films, with the use of CT myelography, if necessary. MRI is even better than CT at demonstrating or excluding intraspinal involvement because it shows the tumour, its effect on the adjacent vertebrae and intraspinal involvement, without the need for contrast injections into the subarachnoid space.

Less than 2 per cent of **phaeochromocytomas** occur in the chest. When encountered, they are found in the posterior mediastinum or adjacent to the heart and pericardium, particularly in the wall of the left atrium or the interatrial septum. They form rounded soft-tissue

Figure 23.82 *Pneumomediastinum following a severe attack of asthma. The streaky air throughout the mediastinum has displaced the mediastinal pleura laterally (arrows).*

masses which are usually extremely vascular and, therefore, enhance brightly at CT after administration of intravenous contrast material. Radionuclide MIBG (*meta*-iodobenzylguanidine) and somatostatin receptor scintigraphy are good methods of identifying extra-adrenal phaeochromocytomas.

On MRI, phaeochromocytomas show signal intensity similar to muscle on T1-weighted images and very high signal intensity on T2-weighted images. MRI is particularly useful for demonstrating intracardiac phaeochromocytomas.

THORACIC AORTIC ANEURYSMS

This subject is discussed on page 652.

OESOPHAGEAL RUPTURE

This subject is discussed on page 63.

PNEUMOMEDIASTINUM

Air in the mediastinum indicates a tear in the oesophagus or an air leak from the bronchi, which may be spontaneous or follow trauma.

Pneumomediastinum may be a clinically unimportant finding, e.g. when it is due to air leak from a small bronchus during an attack of asthma, or it may indicate serious underlying pathology, e.g. rupture of a major bronchus following a road traffic accident, or a ruptured/perforated oesophagus following a severe bout

of vomiting (Booerhaeve's syndrome) or endoscopy.

Spontaneous leakage of air from the bronchial tree is most commonly seen in patients with asthma or following severe vomiting, when air tracks through the interstitial tissues of the lung into the mediastinum after rupture of a small airway. Pneumomediastinum on plain film and CT is seen as fine streaks of transradiancy within the mediastinum, often extending upwards into the neck (Fig. 23.82).

THE DIAPHRAGM

The position of the diaphragm may reflect disease. Both domes may be pulled up by bilateral pulmonary disease or pushed up by abdominal distension. Unilateral elevation of a hemidiaphragm occurs with loss of volume of the ipsilateral lung or abdominal pathology, such as an abdominal mass or a subphrenic abscess. It is important to realize that a minor or moderate elevation of a hemidiaphragm is a relatively common incidental finding of no significance. The cause of a substantially elevated hemidiaphragm should be sought from the clinical features or from chest or abdominal films. It should always be borne in mind that subpulmonary effusion may mimic elevation of one or both hemidiaphragms. Marked elevation of one hemidiaphragm with no other visible abnormality suggests either paralysis or eventration.

Paralysis of the diaphragm results from disorders of the phrenic nerves, e.g. invasion by carcinoma of the bronchus. The signs are elevation of one hemidiaphragm which on fluoroscopy or ultrasound shows paradoxical movement, i.e. it moves upwards on inspiration.

Eventration of the diaphragm is a congenital condition in which the diaphragm lacks muscle and becomes a thin membranous sheet. Except in the neonatal period it is almost always an incidental finding and does not cause symptoms. When the whole of one hemidiaphragm is involved, almost invariably the left, that hemidiaphragm is markedly elevated. On fluoroscopy or ultrasound, the hemidiaphragm may remain fixed during inspiration and expiration but, when more severely involved, it moves paradoxically and cannot be distinguished from paralysis. The eventration may only involve part of one hemidiaphragm, resulting in a smooth 'hump'.

Traumatic rupture of the diaphragm is discussed on page 591.

THE CHEST WALL

The chest wall should be examined for evidence of soft-tissue swelling or rib abnormality. Because ribs are curved

(a)   *(b)*

Figure 24.3 *(a) Localized view of a pulmonary arteriogram showing the pattern of normal pulmonary arteries in the right lower zone. (b) Follow-through venous phase showing the pulmonary veins. The veins have a more horizontal course than the arteries.*

(a)   *(b)*

Figure 24.4 *(a) Normal erect adult chest radiograph showing dominant vascular distribution to the lower zones. (b) Erect adult chest radiograph showing pulmonary venous hypertension. The upper zone vessels are prominent and the lower zone vessels are diminished. There is also cardiomegaly.*

escape into the pulmonary air spaces and may be insufficient to distend the lymphatic channels. Thus the fluid itself is not be visible on the chest radiograph (as pulmonary oedema or interstitial lines), but the fluid shift has a profound effect on the compliance of the lower lungs, causing them to be 'stiff' or less compliant.

As a result there is redistribution of flow to the upper zones of the lungs seen as an equalization of size of the upper and lower pulmonary vessels without loss of clarity in their contour and without the presence of frank pulmonary oedema. These features can he said to be the earliest manifestation of left heart failure on the

Figure 24.5 *Erect adult chest radiograph showing marked perihilar alveolar pulmonary oedema in a classic pattern.*

chest radiograph. When the condition is more advanced there is a further discrepancy in size, the upper zone vessels becoming larger and the lower zone vessels becoming abnormally attenuated (Fig. 24.4b). As the loss of fluid into the lung tissues increases or becomes chronic, the lymphatic channels become distended as excess fluid is drained away. Other signs of accumulating pulmonary fluid are thickening of the horizontal (frontal view) or oblique (lateral view) pleural fissures, and possible the development of pleural effusions. If the accumulation of fluid in the extravascular compartment cannot be drained away sufficiently fast by the lymphatics, it extends into the air spaces to give alveolar oedema. The enlargement of lymphatic channels and the development of alveolar oedema both obscure the outlines of the pulmonary vessels.

The pattern seen in a particular patient depends on both the severity and the duration of the left heart failure. In acute-onset left heart failure owing to myocardial infarction, there may be rapid transit of small amounts of fluid to the air spaces to give the characteristic sudden-onset alveolar pulmonary oedema in a very breathless patient (Fig. 24.5). In contrast, patients with long-standing mitral valve disease may have severely elevated pulmonary venous pressures and exhibit prominent lymphatic channels both basally (Kerley B lines, Fig. 24.6) and radiating towards the hila (Kerley A lines), but they may have no evidence of intra-alveolar fluid and may not be significantly breathless.

In many cases of persistent left heart failure there are consequent effects on the right heart causing combined heart failure (**congestive heart failure**). This has an effect on the heart chambers but the vascular effects of **right heart failure** on the chest radiograph are much more subtle, applying as they do to the systemic veins. Right heart failure may be identified by the distension

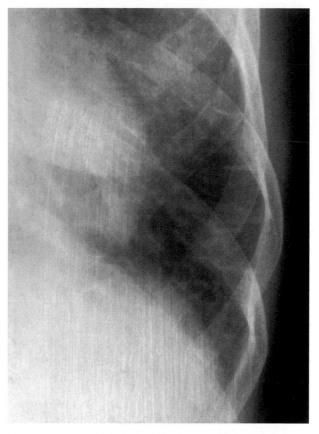

Figure 24.6 *Localized view of the lower zone of an erect adult chest radiograph with left heart failure showing pulmonary lymphatic channels as short horizontal lines (Kerley B lines).*

of the azygos vein as it passes over the right main bronchus. In some cases there is enlargement of the upper mediastinum owing to engorgement of the superior systemic veins.

Pulmonary arterial hypertension

In addition to pulmonary vascular disease secondary to pulmonary pathology, pulmonary artery pressure can be raised by:

- effects secondary to pulmonary venous hypertension;
- pathology of the pulmonary arterial tree (embolic or primary in origin);
- effects secondary to increased flow (long-standing left-to-right shunt).

The characteristic sign on the chest radiograph is 'pruning' of the pulmonary arterial tree. The term pruning refers essentially to a more rapid than normal decrease in size of the pulmonary artery branches. In advanced cases there is marked dilatation of the central arteries with small vessels in the mid third of the lungs (Fig. 24.7), but in many cases the appearances are more

Figure 24.7 *Chest radiograph showing a severe case of pulmonary arterial hypertension in a patient with an atrial septal defect and a reversed shunt (Eisenmenger's syndrome). The main pulmonary artery and hilar pulmonary arteries are grossly enlarged but the peripheral vessels are relatively attenuated.*

Figure 24.8 *Chest radiograph in an adult with untreated atrial septal defect and a large left-to-right shunt. The pulmonary arteries are prominent centrally and peripherally (pulmonary plethora).*

subtle and can be detected by inappropriate differences in size between central and peripheral arteries, even if the central arteries are not much enlarged. In most cases of pulmonary arterial hypertension there is equalization of size of upper and lower zone vessels.

Plethora and oligaemia

Plethora and oligaemia of the lungs are most common in paediatric practice, but it is not unusual for the first presentation of an adult with congenital heart disease to be a consequence of a chest radiography diagnosis. Plethora (uniformly increased vessel size implying increased flow) and oligaemia (uniformly decreased vessel size implying decreased flow) can be detected by an experienced observer, but there are no precise measurements. In cases of plethora the central and peripheral arteries are all large (Fig. 24.8). Once suspicion is raised, it is necessary to investigate further to avoid missing a treatable lesion and echocardiography will frequently be the next investigation of choice.

Uneven patterns

Patchy pulmonary disease can lead to patchy alteration of pulmonary compliance and consequent uneven distribution of the pulmonary vascular pattern. In these circumstances it can be extremely difficult to diagnose the haemodynamic problems described above.

In some cases of complex congenital heart disease, such as pulmonary atresia, abnormal collateral vessels may supply the lungs and, as a consequence, the pulmonary vascular pattern can be very disorganized.

Cardiac calcification and implants

Valvular calcification

The two main causes of valvular calcification are degenerative and rheumatic. Normal valves are subject to degeneration in the elderly, which is most commonly seen in the annulus of the mitral valve and to a lesser extent in the annulus of the aortic valve. Mitral annulus calcification is often seen as a large radius calcific crescent surrounding the position of the mitral valve, particularly in females of 70 or more years of age (Fig. 24.9). These deposits of calcification rarely cause significant valve dysfunction, even with very dense calcification, although they may produce mild flow disturbance and a heart murmur.

The degenerative process in valves is accelerated in the presence of an underlying abnormality, the most common of which is the bicuspid aortic valve. The presence of a calcified aortic valve in a middle-aged patient is most likely due to a degenerative bicuspid aortic valve (strictly speaking a congenital condition) and heavy calcification in such a valve is almost always related to significant stenosis (Fig. 24.10).

Rheumatic heart disease is now much less common in western countries, but it is still the most frequent cause of calcification of the mitral leaflets themselves, usually associated with stenosis. In any case of doubt about the site of calcification, a brief fluoroscopic study of the movement of the calcification will reveal its nature, although other investigations such as echocardiography will generally provide the answer.

Figure 24.9 *Lateral chest radiograph showing mitral annular calcification (arrowed).*

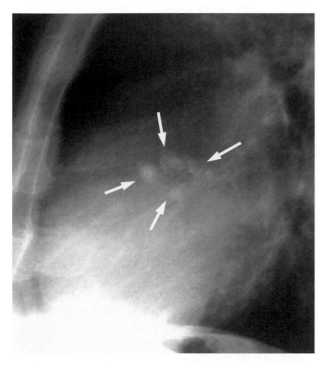

Figure 24.10 *Lateral chest radiograph showing aortic valve calcification (arrowed).*

Calcification of implanted bioprosthetic valves is quite often seen but its nature is usually obvious from the surrounding metallic valve ring. Calcification is also seen following various surgical repairs that use implants such as Dacron or bovine pericardium.

Figure 24.11 *Lateral chest radiograph showing coronary artery calcification (arrowed).*

Coronary artery calcification

Calcification of coronary arteries is common in the elderly and in patients over 70 years of age it carries little significance, usually being related to degenerative changes in the arterial wall. In younger patients, however, calcified coronary arteries are related to calcification of atheromatous plaque and are of prognostic significance. Proximal left coronary artery calcification is often seen on a frontal chest radiograph just to the left of the spine but it is often more clearly visualized on the lateral film (Fig. 24.11).

Myocardial and pericardial calcification

Myocardial calcification is quite commonly seen in the wall of a left ventricular aneurysm (Fig. 24.12). Rarer causes include collagen disorders (Ehler–Danlos syndrome) and chronic renal disease. In patients with healed tuberculous pericarditis, there is often extensive sheet-like pericardial calcification, which can produce restrictive haemodynamic symptoms (Fig. 24.13). Other rare causes of calcification in the heart include chronic abscess formation, tumours, haematomas and false aneurysms.

Medical implants

Permanent pacing systems are common and well recognized on chest radiographs but it is important to check a number of features. In newly implanted systems a pneumothorax should always be excluded and a normal route of the electrode wires to the heart should be confirmed. In routine follow-up films it is important to confirm the consistency of the position of both the

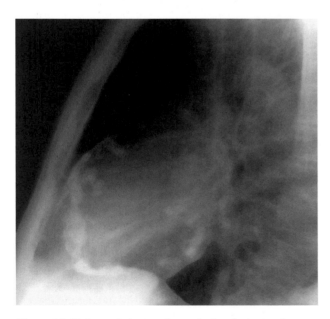

Figure 24.12 *Localized view of the cardiac apex in a chest radiograph showing a calcified left ventricular aneurysm.*

Figure 24.13 *Lateral chest radiograph showing extensive pericardial calcification owing to healed tuberculous pericarditis.*

Figure 24.14 *Chest radiograph showing a permanent pacing system implanted on the right side and two old non-functional leads on the left which could not be removed.*

be detected. Non-specialists will not be familiar with all types of pacemaker electrodes but dual-lead (two electrode wires) systems are now common, one leading to the right atrium and one to the right ventricle. In patients with renewed systems, the old unremovable wires can sometimes be seen in addition to the current system (Fig. 24.14). Implantable defibrillators are now more frequently used which resemble large bulky pacing systems.

The other common medically implanted device is the intracoronary stent, a small tubular stainless steel mesh, used in conjunction with a coronary angioplasty procedure. They are difficult to see, but are normally identifiable lying along the line of the relevant artery. Sometimes long stents or multiple stents are implanted. The patency of the stent cannot be determined from the chest radiograph. It is exceedingly rare for stents to displace once they are satisfactorily deployed.

A variety of other devices is seen from time to time, most commonly after intervention for treatment of a congenital heart lesion. Commonly used devices are for closure of patent ductus arteriosus (coils or umbrella devices), and atrial septal defect (a number of different devices are in use). Stents are sometimes implanted in stenotic pulmonary arteries.

Surgical implants

Prosthetic heart valves are the most obvious radiopaque implant and these are usually easy to see unless they lie over the spine on an underpenetrated film. Almost always there is some metal in the construction (even for bioprostheses), but the design varies widely. Mechanical valves are increasingly of the bileaflet type and in

generator (the 'box') and the electrode in order to detect movement, either displacement of the intracardiac electrode or movement or rotation of the generator itself ('pacemaker twiddler syndrome'). Breaks in the electrode wire are hard to see but can occasionally

(a)

(b)

Figure 24.15 *Chest radiograph showing (a) a prosthetic mitral valve implant, (b) a prosthetic aortic valve implant.*

such cases the leaflet movement can be assessed on fluoroscopy if necessary. The position of the valves clearly corresponds with the site of the native valves and it is usually straightforward to distinguish aortic from mitral prostheses, often by the architecture of the valve struts and the implied direction of flow (Fig. 24.15). Some mitral and tricuspid valve repairs leave a supportive metallic ring round the valve annulus.

The most common cardiac surgical procedure is coronary artery bypass grafting, usually performed by median sternotomy with sternal closure achieved using multiple stainless steel wires. The coronary surgery often involves the use of small stainless steel clips, particularly when arterial grafts are used. The presence of such clips high in the left anterior mediastinum usually indicates the use of a left internal mammary artery graft.

In the immediate postoperative period there are many radiopaque objects visible on the chest radiograph. Pericardial drains are usually employed together with one or more chest drains if the pleural cavity has been opened. There is usually a nasogastric tube and in the first few hours an endotracheal tube is present. Fine epicardial pacing electrodes are often employed, being removed after a few days, along with external electrocardiographic electrodes and wires. Occasionally an intra-aortic balloon pump is seen. Routine reporting of such films requires confident knowledge of these devices.

CORONARY ARTERY DISEASE (CAD)

In general, CAD is taken to mean atheromatous disease with plaque formation and partial or complete occlusion of coronary arteries as well as all the sequelae of this process. There are, however, other disease processes that affect the coronary arteries, for example arteritis, congenital variants, trauma and so forth, but these are rare and are not normally considered under the term 'coronary artery disease'. The term 'ischaemic heart disease' is frequently used interchangeably with 'coronary artery disease' but it has a slightly different meaning. A plaque of atheroma may not have developed sufficiently to give rise to any myocardial ischaemia yet 'coronary artery disease' is still present. Alternatively, a coronary embolus or spasm could give an 'ischaemic heart disease' syndrome without there being any actual atheromatous disease of the coronary arteries themselves. The term 'coronary artery disease' in this chapter is thus used to indicate the atheromatous disease process of the coronary arteries.

In developed western countries, CAD is the largest single cause of mortality and accounts for a higher number of hospital admissions than any other single condition. There have been very great improvements in diagnosis and treatment of the disease in the last two or three decades, resulting in effective but expensive improvements in management that have contributed to an important decline in morbidity and mortality. The high prevalence of the disease together with the relatively expensive costs of management means that CAD is a major financial cost for any healthcare system.

MYOCARDIAL INFARCTION

Coronary arteries are 'end arteries' which supply individual territory and sudden occlusion of a major vessel leads to acute ischaemia, which, if sufficiently profound, leads to tissue infarction. The occlusion is almost always based on a plaque of atheroma that has become 'unstable', exposing its contents to the bloodstream and stimulating acute thrombus formation.

Chest radiographic appearances in acute myocardial infarction

In small or uncomplicated infarcts the chest radiograph may remain normal, although even in these situations careful inspection of a good film will often show signs of pulmonary venous hypertension or mild loss of clarity of the pulmonary vessels owing to a mild degree of pulmonary oedema. In more severe cases there is obvious alveolar pulmonary oedema, usually in a central zone around the hilar regions, but in the most severe cases involving most of the lung fields. The changes can arise very rapidly and can also resolve rapidly after diuretic treatment. In patients with a previous history of pulmonary oedema or heart failure, the heart is of normal size and shape. In patients with previous damage to the left ventricle, from either infarction or cardiomyopathy, the heart may be enlarged at the time of infarction.

Early complications of myocardial infarction

A number of important radiologically detectable complications can occur in the first few days following the infarct. In cases of a large full-thickness infarct there is risk of rupture of the heart wall, which occurs most commonly from 2 to 8 days post-onset of the infarction. The consequences depend on the site of rupture. If the rupture is in the free wall, there can be massive extravasation into the pericardial cavity with sudden death but, if the leak is slower, it can cause haemopericardium and possible tamponade. Sometimes the acute rupture remains undetected and a false aneurysm is diagnosed at a later stage. If the left ventricular wall ruptures through the interventricular septum, there will be a postinfarct ventricular septal defect, also a very serious complication. If the necrosis involves a papillary muscle, there may be disruption with concomitant severe mitral regurgitation. These different complications are all life-threatening and usually associated with an abrupt change in clinical condition. The chest radiograph is usually non-specific in these situations,

partly because the patient is very ill and may not be fit enough for an erect film, and also because the signs of increased heart size and pulmonary oedema are present in several of the conditions. Occasionally pulmonary plethora may suggest the diagnosis of a ventricular septal defect.

Rapid definitive diagnosis is required and echocardiography (with Doppler studies) is usually the investigation of choice, enabling both the structural abnormality and the haemodynamic consequences to be detected. Angiography is generally required only as a preoperative assessment of the coronary arteries, and other imaging tests such as CT or MRI can occasionally be useful but are generally not employed in the acute situation.

Intracardiac thrombus is more common than might be expected and early echocardiography can often show thrombus at the site of infarction. The thrombus usually disperses rapidly without consequence, but occasionally the thrombus becomes organized and may lead to systemic embolization. Echocardiography is not usually employed routinely in the early stage postinfarction.

Pericardial effusion in the first few days is potentially more serious but a small effusion in an otherwise stable patient is not uncommon.

Late complications of myocardial infarction

The healing process following infarction inevitably leads to some degree of myocardial fibrosis. In the case of a large full-thickness myocardial infarction, the development of a thin-walled fibrous aneurysm is not uncommon. It may take several weeks to develop and may show as a prominent bulge in the left heart border (Fig. 24.16) or as more generalized cardiomegaly. In some cases there is gradual development of calcification in the aneurysm wall or sometimes within laminated thrombus lying in the aneurysm sac. The chest radiograph does not always demonstrate a left ventricular aneurysm because a diffuse sac or a posterior or inferior position may not distort the left heart border. A lateral film may sometimes reveal a posterior aneurysm.

If the infarct is small or diffuse in nature, the resulting fibrotic damage does not lead to an aneurysm and may sometimes be hard to detect by any technique. In the case of a series of small or even subclinical infarctions a dilated left ventricle with impaired function may result (ischaemic cardiomyopathy). This may be seen as an enlarged left ventricle on the chest radiograph, possibly with associated signs of heart failure.

Left ventricular dilatation, regardless of cause, may lead to dilatation of the mitral valve annulus and distortion of the architecture of the mitral valve apparatus. Mild or moderate mitral regurgitation is thus a common consequence of ischaemic left ventricular damage.

Figure 24.16 *Chest radiograph showing a prominent bulge at the cardiac apex owing to a large left ventricular aneurysm.*

In most cases of moderate or severe myocardial infarction, it is becoming normal practice to carry out echocardiography at around 6 weeks, to evaluate the degree of regional or generalized ventricular damage in order to guide future management, particularly the use of drug therapy to optimize cardiac function.

A postinfarct inflammatory reaction (Dressler's syndrome) can occur at around 6 weeks postinfarction with symptoms of pericarditis and a small or moderate-sized pericardial effusion.

ANGINA PECTORIS

This very common condition consists of chest pain but occasionally dyspnoea, related to inadequate perfusion of the myocardium owing to diseased coronary arteries. The classic condition of 'stable angina' is one where crushing chest, arm or throat pain is brought on by increased exertion and relieved by rest. This condition may remain unchanged in severity for months or years, but it may also progress rapidly. If the symptoms become worse over a few days and are stimulated by lesser amounts of exertion or even come on at rest the condition is called 'unstable angina'. This change is usually related to instability of the atheromatous plaque and build-up of thrombus in the vessel, and there is increased risk of myocardial infarction. All angina needs investigation and treatment but 'unstable angina' requires urgent hospital treatment.

Investigation of angina pectoris

In the absence of pre-existing disease, the chest radiograph in patients with angina is normal except that in some patients coronary calcification is visible. The presence of cardiomegaly indicates some form of pre-existing left ventricular or valvular disease.

The usual initial approach to investigation of angina is more functional than structural. It is usually carried out with some form of stress test, usually exercise but sometimes pharmacological stress, to detect abnormalities that are absent at rest but are revealed by the stress. The electrocardiogram (ECG) taken during exercise is the commonest screening tool for patients with angina but sometimes it is supplemented with stress perfusion radionuclide scanning or stress echocardiography. Both these techniques add functional and regional information to the basic ECG data.

Radionuclide perfusion scanning is usually performed in diagnostically doubtful or difficult cases or on those in whom revascularization is planned but the site of ischaemia is not clear. The traditional radiopharmaceutical has been thallium-201, but technetium-99m-labelled agents such as sestamibi are gradually taking its place. Imaging is performed after stress and at rest, with emission tomography now being the usual image acquisition technique. Techniques and protocols vary considerably and local factors determine the precise methodology. The perfusion scan is most helpful when there is a clear-cut region of reversible ischaemia that contrasts with normal perfusion elsewhere. Reversible ischaemia is recognized as an area of reduced uptake on the exercise scan with normal redistribution of the radionuclide on the rest scan (Plate 11, opposite page 358). Diffuse ischaemia is less easy to diagnose as there will be uniformly reduced uptake of isotope throughout the myocardium.

Stress echocardiography is a specialist technique that has been shown to be very sensitive in detecting abnormally contracting segments that function normally at rest. The technique demands high-quality imaging techniques preferably coupled with digital cine-loop recording, to allow rest and stress function to be compared simultaneously.

Coronary angiography

In the majority of patients with a clear clinical history and a positive exercise ECG the next investigation is coronary angiography. The technical aspects are listed in Box 24.1. This is an invasive investigation that is performed on hundreds of thousands of patients worldwide every year. Coronary angiography is presently the only technique for analysing the detailed coronary anatomy and pathology sufficiently accurately to allow planning of treatment by surgery or angioplasty (Fig. 24.17). The individual branching of the coronary arterial

Box 24.1 Technical aspects of coronary angiography

- **Preparation**
  - Full explanation and informed consent is required
  - Nil by mouth 4–6 hours before procedure
  - Prior chest radiograph and electrocardiogram
  - Intravenous access required
  - Premedication is optional
- **Catheter technique**
  - Usually percutaneous femoral technique using 6 French preshaped catheters (usually Judkin's shapes)
  - Percutaneous radial or brachial approach is useful if difficult femoral access
  - Brachial cutdown techniques (Sones' catheter) infrequently used
  - Day patient procedure is possible
- **Haemodynamic assessment**
  - Left ventricular (LV) angiography usually performed additionally (not essential if LV data otherwise determined) – demonstration of LV function and any mitral regurgitation
  - If LV angiogram is performed LV pressures can be measured – end-diastolic pressure indirectly reflects LV function
- **Imaging equipment**
  - High-quality digital imaging and archiving preferable, cine film also acceptable
  - Focal spot 0.6 mm, individual exposure times 1–5 ms, acquisition at 12.5 or 25 images per second
  - Multiangular projections are necessary, all oblique and up to 40° cranial and caudal angulation required
  - Biplane acquisition optional
- **Contrast medium**
  - Non-ionic medium is preferable, 320–350 mg/ml iodine
  - Typical left coronary artery 6-8 ml hand injection per view
  - Typical right coronary artery 2–5 ml hand injection per view
  - LV angiogram 30–40 ml at 10–15 ml/s pump injection
- **Views**
  - Left coronary typically 5 views, right coronary typically 3 views
  - Flexible selection of projections must include clear views of all major branches and bifurcations – anatomy varies with individual patients
  - LV angiograms usually 30–40° right anterior oblique view
- **Safety requirements**
  - Specialist training essential for operator and supporting staff
  - High-volume department (500+ cases annually) is likely to be safer
  - Patient has ECG and arterial pressure monitoring throughout
  - Full resuscitation equipment immediately available
  - Full radiation safety precautions employed
- **Complications**
  - Mortality rate should be substantially below 0.1 per cent for total caseload
  - Arrhythmias generally transient and usually induced by catheter manipulation
  - Anatomical damage by the catheter tip in the coronary ostium is rare but serious
  - Detection of significant left main-stem disease raises risk of major complication
  - There is always a small risk of stroke from aortic catheter manipulation
  - Local arterial complications as for other arterial catheter techniques

tree and the distribution of the branches is very variable, but there is a typical pattern with common variations. The angiographic technique should of course assess the pathology of the vessels and the atheromatous lesions, but firstly the angiogram should be used to establish the underlying anatomical pattern, because appropriate revascularization depends on precise anatomical knowledge of the site of lesions.

The posterior descending artery (PDA) most frequently arises from the right coronary artery but in 5 per cent of cases it arises from the circumflex branch of the left coronary artery (left dominant system). In a further 5–10 per cent of cases there is 'balanced' dominance with a contribution to the blood supply of the inferior septum coming from both right and left coronary arteries. In some patients the left anterior descending coronary artery (LAD) continues into the posterior interventricular groove. In many patients this vessel is longer or shorter than average with consequent variations in distribution of the blood supply.

(a)

(b)

Figure 24.17 *(a) Selective left coronary angiogram in the cranially angulated left anterior oblique position. The catheter tip is engaged in the left main stem (LMS); there is a long moderate stenosis in the left anterior descending artery (LAD) and a severe short stenosis in the circumflex artery (Cx). (b) Selective right coronary angiogram in the left anterior oblique position in a different patient showing a moderate short stenosis in the mid vessel (arrowed).*

Usually the size of the PDA is in inverse proportion to the LAD.

Coronary arteriography is an essential prerequisite of coronary artery bypass grafting (CABG), and is frequently required in the follow-up of symptomatic patients following CABG. It is also an integral part of interventional techniques.

INTERVENTIONAL CORONARY ARTERY PROCEDURES

The fundamental interventional coronary artery procedure is percutaneous transluminal coronary angioplasty (PTCA). The basis of the technique (Box 24.2) is the use of a low-profile semicompliant balloon to disrupt plaque and displace the material into the wall of the artery, usually with accompanying disruption of some layers of the vessel wall.

The clinical indications for coronary angioplasty are very similar to those for CABG, stable angina and unstable angina being the commonest. All patients offered coronary angioplasty should normally be potential surgical candidates. There are, however, exceptions; some patients are too ill or too frail (poor left ventricular function, renal failure or other coexisting disease) to be candidates for cardiac surgery, but they may still benefit from revascularization using PTCA. Patients with an acute myocardial infarct of less than 4 hours' duration may be suitable for 'primary coronary angioplasty' or 'rescue coronary angioplasty' (coronary angioplasty following failed thrombolysis). Patients with a recent infarct and continuing angina may also be

Box 24.2 Technical requirements for PTCA

- A catheter laboratory with high-resolution imaging (preferably digital, with reference image and quantitative angiography capability)
- A well-trained team capable of monitoring patient condition and treating any complications including major cardiovascular events
- A full range of angioplasty hardware including guide catheters, guidewires, balloons and stents
- Appropriate adjunctive technologies including pharmacological agents
- Access to a cardiac surgical team, either in the same building or at least within close reach in the event of a major emergency

treated by coronary angioplasty. In symptomatic patients with previous CABG, angioplasty of the graft or native vessel is sometimes more appropriate than repeat surgery.

Certain lesions are less suitable than others for coronary angioplasty. Chronic occlusions may be difficult or impossible to cross with the guidewire and certainly have a much lower success rate. Lesions in the left mainstem are usually contraindicated for coronary angioplasty because complication occurring here can be catastrophic, although some have been successfully treated by coronary angioplasty. Bifurcation lesions, distal lesions and lesions in very tortuous vessels can all be difficult to treat. In general, however, the technology of catheters, wires, balloons and stents is improving rapidly, which allows increasingly complex lesions to be treated.

(a)

(b)

(c)

(d)

Figure 24.18 *Percutaneous transluminal coronary angioplasty. Critical stenosis in the right coronary artery prior to PTCA shown on (a) left anterior oblique and (b) right anterior oblique views. The stent is deployed on an inflated balloon (c) and the fully reconstituted lumen is shown in orthogonal views (d) and (e).*

(e)

Successful coronary angioplasty is dependent on the combination of appropriate skill and experience with the best available technology. It is thus essential to state that the technique must only be undertaken by someone with the appropriate level of skill and training.

An essential step in PTCA is the acquisition of high-quality images of the lesion(s). The imaging needs to be of a sufficiently high quality to judge not only the severity of the lesion(s) and the state of the distal arteries but also the morphology of the lesion and its relationship with the main vessel and important branches. Important factors to be assessed are the curvature, tortuosity and size of the artery and the anatomy and orientation of the proximal vessel, the ostium and the aortic root.

Coronary angioplasty is performed under local anaesthesia and most procedures are performed from the femoral artery by direct puncture. The brachial (cut-down) and radial routes can also be used. The procedure uses a co-axial approach with a guide catheter positioned at the coronary ostium and a balloon passing through the guide catheter and over a low-profile steerable guidewire (usually diameter 0.014 inches (0.356 mm)). The guide catheter is normally 6 French in size but occasionally a larger catheter is required. The tip of the guide catheter must engage atraumatically in the ostium and must afford sufficient back-up to support the advancing devices in the coronary artery. Appropriate selection of the guide catheter and its correct deployment are two of the most important determinants of a successful outcome.

The patient is normally heparinized and will have been pretreated with aspirin and with additional antiplatelet agents (ticlopidine or clopidrogel). The guidewire can then be advanced and manipulated through the lesion. The uninflated low-profile balloon is tracked along the wire to the lesion and through it (Fig. 24.18). The lower the balloon profile, the easier it is to cross very severe stenoses. In the case of complete occlusions, it may be possible to cross with a simple wire technique, but frequently other more complex techniques with stronger wire and more support may be needed.

The early use of stents was for 'bail-out' situations, where an arterial intima was damaged by balloon inflation and led to flow restriction and ischaemia. The stent was used to re-establish the vessel lumen and this approach is still occasionally required. It is, however, common to deploy a stent if the balloon dilatation is judged as 'suboptimal' or if an initial assessment of the lesion suggests that the plaque is too large or complex for simple balloon treatment only and requires 'elective' stenting. The decision to stent is somewhat subjective and there is still much debate about the precise indications but stenting is now regarded as an integral part of many procedures. In major centres, 50–90 per cent of treated lesions will be stented.

Table 24.3 *Adjunctive techniques and therapies in PTCA*

Technique/Application	Comments
Stent Widespread use (50–90 per cent of treated lesions) Can be used for 'elective', 'suboptimal' or 'bailout' indications Studies show lower early and late restenosis rates than for balloon alone Less suited to small vessels (2.5 mm or below)	Use of stents substantially increases costs of PTCA
Intracoronary ultrasound Low-profile transducer tracking along coronary guidewire Diagnostic application to assess lesion or vessel wall prior to dilatation Assessment of treatment including checking of adequate stent deployment	Expensive, useful in selected cases
Rotablator High-speed rotational burr tracking along coronary guidewire	Expensive but in selected cases it is useful for long concentric lesions
Atherectomy Various devices are available to resect and remove bulky plaque	Expensive Needs larger guide catheter
Brachytherapy Intracoronary radiation therapy is in its early stages of development, and its aim is to reduce to prevent restenosis	As yet unproven
New antiplatelet agents (GP IIb/IIIa receptor blockers, e.g. abciximab) HIghly active in preventing and dispersing actively forming thrombus at the site of PTCA; superior to anticoagulation or thrombolysis for this application Suitable for 'unstable' or complex situations	Expensive but very effective in selected cases

Unexpanded stents are now increasingly low in profile and there is a trend towards 'direct' or *de novo* stenting without predilatation.

Once the dilatation is complete, with or without a stent, it is important to confirm a good result. There must be no impairment of flow, there must be no threatening occlusive lesion and the patient must not exhibit signs or symptoms of continuing ischaemia. At this stage the guidewire and catheter can be removed. Anticoagulation must be allowed to wear off and

Table 24.4 *Aetiology of heart valve disease*

Clinical setting	Valve lesions
Rheumatic Although the low incidence of rheumatic fever has much reduced the incidence of rheumatic heart valve disease in western countries, there are still a significant number of cases; this is still an important disease entity to recognize	Mitral valve is most commonly affected with stenosis being much more common than regurgitation; advanced cases will have combined stenosis and regurgitation The aortic valve is less commonly affected and in a minority of cases there is tricuspid involvement
Degenerative An ageing population has made degenerative valve disease much more common Many degenerative lesions are mild or trivial in severity but some will produce major problems	Degeneration of congenital bicuspid aortic valves is the commonest cause of calcific aortic stenosis Mitral valve prolapse and rupture of mitral chordae can produced severe regurgitation Mitral annular thickening can be very marked with only minor haemodynamic effects Sclerosis of the aortic valve will often produce a heart murmur which is not of haemodynamic importance
Infective Infective endocarditis is a complex and increasing problem A high index of suspicion and early echocardiographic diagnosis is necessary – transoesophageal echo study has now become very important	All valves can be affected A pre-existing lesion on a valve, even if minor, may raise the risk of infection Aortic and mitral valves are most commonly affected Prosthetic heart valves are particularly prone to infection
Functional Abnormality of the supporting tissues of a valve can lead to malfunction even if the leaflets themselves are normal	A dilated and impaired left ventricle is almost always accompanied by some mitral regurgitation owing to annular dilatation and possibly also from papillary muscle dysfunction
Metabolic Connective-tissue disorders are important causes of weakening valves and supporting tissues Some rare metabolic diseases can distort valve tissues	Marfan's syndrome is the commonest connective-tissue disorder, predominantly involving the aortic valve and root Metastatic carcinoid syndrome is a rare metabolic cause of right heart valve lesions

catheter withdrawal must be delayed for 4–6 hours, unless the vessel puncture is closed with a closure device. Most patients will be fully mobile within 12 hours of the procedure and are often discharged within 24 hours.

Much technical development is ongoing in this field and there are many adjunctive techniques (Table 24.3) and therapies. Some are still under evaluation and many are expensive.

VALVULAR HEART DISEASE

Heart valve disease is classified functionally as well as by aetiology (Table 24.4). The functional diagnosis of valve disease requires both the identification of the abnormality and its severity. Both these aspects, qualitative and quantitative, are essential for full evaluation of a valve lesion.

A stenotic valve has a restricted orifice size that creates abnormal pressure drop across the valve during the flow period. The term 'sclerosis' is used to describe a condition of thickening of valve leaflets or annulus, which may cause abnormal appearances with some flow disturbance, but which does not produce significant measurable flow restriction.

Quantitation of **valve stenosis** is usually described in terms of a 'gradient' (mmHg), which describes the pressure difference across the valve. Mean and peak pressure gradients can both be of clinical value. In some cases it is more appropriate to express the severity of the stenosis in terms of the cross-sectional area of the valve orifice. Quantitation of valve stenosis has traditionally required catheter-based techniques, but Doppler echocardiography has now superseded invasive methods in the routine evaluation of most such lesions.

Valve regurgitation (sometimes termed 'incompetence' or 'insufficiency') occurs when there is a significant leak back through a valve during the phase of the cardiac cycle when the leaflets should be fully closed. Current Doppler techniques have now shown that very small amounts of regurgitation are detectable in many normal valves, and this phenomenon must be distinguished from pathological regurgitation. As with stenosis, quantitation of regurgitation is necessary, but this is more difficult and very few techniques allow accurate

Figure 24.19 *Mitral stenosis. There is prominence of the left atrial appendage, a double shadow near the right heart border and prominence of the upper zone vessels.*

volumetric calculation of the regurgitant fraction. A semiquantitative approach is generally used, either descriptively using the terms mild, moderate or severe, or on a numerical 5-point scale.

MITRAL STENOSIS

Mitral stenosis is virtually always due to chronic rheumatic heart disease. The chest radiographic features (Fig. 24.19) are listed in Box 24.3.

Echocardiography

Classic appearances are seen on echocardiography, which is now essential in the diagnosis and management of the condition.

Two-dimensional imaging shows thickened leaflets, most marked at their margins, with doming movement of the valve leaflets during diastole (Fig. 24.20). In good quality images it may be possible to see the size of the stenotic orifice itself. There may be high echo levels due to calcification. The subvalvar apparatus may also be thickened. Left atrial enlargement is usual and may be very marked, exceeding 10 cm in extreme cases. Thrombus may be present in the atrium or atrial appendage. In pure mitral stenosis the left ventricle remains small. The right-sided chambers are enlarged.

M-mode recording reflects all the same features and the tracing of the leaflet movements is classic, showing

Box 24.3 *Chest radiograph features of mitral stenosis*

- **Heart size**
  - In many cases of pure mitral stenosis there is little or no cardiomegaly
  - In long-standing severe cases there can be very marked cardiomegaly
- **Heart shape**
  - Left atrial enlargement is the key feature
  - Prominent left atrial appendage (an early sign)
  - Increased size and density of left atrial shadow
  - Double shadow of right heart border
  - Widening of cardinal angle
  - Left ventricular contour not increased
  - Right atrium and ventricle also enlarged
- **Lung fields**
  - Pulmonary venous hypertension (an early sign)
  - Interstitial oedema
  - Prominent lymphatic channels in advanced cases (Kerley lines)
  - Pleural effusions in advanced cases
- **Great arteries**
  - Aortic knuckle normal or small
  - Main pulmonary artery may be enlarged
- **Calcification**
  - Mitral leaflet calcification indicates advanced disease (often better seen on the lateral film)
  - Mitral annulus calcification is not relevant
  - Advanced cases may have calcified left atrial wall or left atrial thrombus
- **Implants and postsurgical appearances**
  - Sternal wires and metallic ring indicate valve prosthesis
  - Left-sided rib rejection and sutures suggest surgical commissurotomy

loss of the normal opposite movement of the leaflet, which now moves in a parallel way owing to the commissural tethering. The trace often reveals loss of atrial contraction owing to the common presence of atrial fibrillation. Doppler studies (continuous wave, pulsed or colour flow mapping) are complex but can contribute substantially to the quantitation of severity of the lesion by calculating the pressure gradient across the mitral valve and will show flow accelerating through the narrow orifice. Mitral regurgitation can be detected if present.

Cardiac catheter and angiography

If good quality echocardiography studies are available, cardiac catheterization should be reserved for preoperative investigation. Pressure measurement across the valve is usually estimated by comparing the pulmonary artery wedge pressure (an indirect measure of left atrial

Figure 24.20 *Parasternal long axis echo view showing a stenotic doming mitral valve open in diastole, between the left atrium (LA) and the left ventricle (LV). The arrow points to the stenotic orifice.*

Figure 24.21 *Cine-recording of Inoue balloon inflation in the mitral orifice during percutaneous mitral valve commissurotomy. The 'waist' of the balloon is designed to align with the valve orifice.*

pressure) with the left ventricular diastolic pressure using right and left heart catheter techniques. Left ventricular angiography shows a doming movement of the mitral valve with a restricted inflow bolus and a slow filling pattern. It also shows the presence of any mitral regurgitation. Although the procedure is used to confirm the haemodynamic features, the major requirement for catheterization is for the investigation of the coronary arteries to detect any coexisting coronary problems that may affect the conduct of surgery.

Interventional treatment

Catheter-based balloon mitral commissurotomy is the treatment of choice in carefully selected cases with pure mitral stenosis, preservation of flexible valve leaflets and no left atrial thrombus. The principle is essentially similar to the technique of surgical commissurotomy and is very effective in appropriate cases. It is a specialized technique that involves a femoral venous approach and puncture of the interatrial septum to allow antegrade passage of the balloon through the mitral orifice. The Inoue balloon is specifically designed for the procedure, the balloon having a central waist that allows correct positioning for inflation (Fig. 24.21). A balloon diameter of 28–30 mm is typically used. In all such procedures there is a risk of a complication or a poor result and so surgical backing should be available, although this is rarely required. Transoesophageal echocardiography is a very important tool in the assessment of these patients.

MITRAL REGURGITATION

Mitral regurgitation is associated with chronic rheumatic heart disease in a minority of cases but is much more commonly due to degenerative changes. In some cases of degeneration and thickening, the 'floppy mitral valve syndrome' can lead to important disease in early adult life. Mitral valve prolapse and rupture of valve chordae can both cause severe valve regurgitation, although mild degrees of prolapse may not cause regurgitation. Dilatation and impairment of the left ventricle are often associated with 'functional' regurgitation, usually mild in degree. Infective endocarditis, usually affecting a previously abnormal valve, is an important cause of mitral regurgitation that requires early diagnosis. The chest radiographic features of mitral regurgitation are listed in Box 24.4.

Echocardiography

Echocardiography is once again the key diagnostic investigation with complex or uncertain cases requiring transoesophageal echocardiography (TOE). The morphology of the valve is usually well seen and the site and degree of prolapse in either leaflet are normally

Box 24.4 *Chest radiographic features of mitral regurgitation*

- **Heart size**
  - There is no cardiomegaly with mild regurgitation
  - Long-standing moderate and severe cases are generally associated with significant cardiomegaly
  - Acute-onset regurgitation may not show cardiomegaly
- **Heart shape**
  - Combined left atrial and left ventricular enlargement is the key feature
  - Right atrium and ventricle also enlarged
- **Lung fields**
  - Pulmonary venous hypertension (an early sign)
  - Interstitial oedema
  - Prominent lymphatic channels in advanced cases (Kerley lines)
  - Pleural effusions in advanced cases
- **Great arteries**
  - Aortic knuckle normal or small
  - Main pulmonary artery may be enlarged
- **Calcification**
  - Mitral leaflet not calcified in degenerative causes
  - Mitral annulus calcification not relevant
- **Implants and postsurgical appearances**
  - Sternal wires and metallic ring indicate valve prosthesis
  - Incomplete metallic valve ring may indicate valve repair

Box 24.5 *Chest radiographic features of aortic stenosis*

- **Heart size**
  - In many cases of pure aortic stenosis there is little or no cardiomegaly
  - There will be cardiomegaly only when the left ventricle has failed, usually late in the disease
- **Heart shape**
  - Left ventricular contour is not increased in most cases
  - Right atrium and ventricle not enlarged in most cases
- **Lung fields**
  - Signs of heart failure are only seen in advanced cases with left ventricular failure
- **Great arteries**
  - Aortic knuckle normal but the ascending aorta (right heart border) is often prominent due to post-stenotic dilatation
  - Main pulmonary artery not enlarged
- **Calcification**
  - Aortic leaflet calcification indicates advanced disease (often better seen on the lateral film)
- **Implants and postsurgical appearances**
  - Sternal wires and metallic ring indicate valve prosthesis

clear. In cases of endocarditis, vegetations on the valve leaflets and abscess formation in the valve annulus are both detectable, although TOE is required to identify smaller vegetations. Associated enlargements of the left atrium and left ventricle are both seen.

Doppler studies are essential for assessing the degree of regurgitation and colour flow studies are very valuable (see Plate 12, opposite page 358). This assessment can still be difficult even with the best skills and equipment because judgement of severity depends on various semiquantitative aspects of the regurgitant jet (colour flow mapping) and the secondary effects on the left ventricle.

Cardiac catheter and angiography

If good quality echocardiography studies are available, cardiac catheterization should be reserved for preoperative investigation. Left ventricular angiography can show the presence of any mitral regurgitation. Although catheterization is used to confirm the haemodynamic features, the major requirement is for the investigation of the coronary arteries to detect any coexisting coronary problems that may affect the conduct of surgery. There is no catheter-based interventional treatment for mitral regurgitation.

AORTIC STENOSIS

Aortic stenosis is occasionally due to chronic rheumatic heart disease, usually in association with mitral stenosis, but is most commonly due to degeneration of a congenitally bicuspid aortic valve. The chest radiographic features are listed in Box 24.5.

Echocardiography

Echocardiography can clearly demonstrate the diagnosis, showing thickening and restriction of movement of the valve leaflets with increased echo return and acoustic shadowing suggesting calcification. In most well-compensated cases the left ventricle contracts well, but often shows hypertrophy of the wall. Doppler studies in most cases allow measurement of the peak velocity of flow through the narrow valve orifice which can be used to calculate the pressure drop or 'gradient' (Fig. 24.22). More sophisticated calculations can be used to estimate the valve orifice area.

In late or advanced cases there is left ventricular failure with consequent dilatation and impairment of left ventricular function. Under these circumstances the right heart chambers may also be affected.

The majority of cases of aortic stenosis from a degenerative bicuspid valve have little or no associated

Figure 24.22 *Continuous wave Doppler trace, using atypical transducer position, showing high-velocity systolic flow away from the transducer (below the baseline) of over 4 m/s. This indicates severe aortic stenosis. The diastolic flow above the baseline indicates coexisting aortic regurgitation.*

Figure 24.23 *Chest radiograph showing a prominent increased curvature to the left heart border owing to left ventricular enlargement caused by chronic severe aortic regurgitation.*

regurgitation, but in rheumatic aortic disease the pattern is usually mixed.

Cardiac catheterization and angiography

In some cases where Doppler studies have been difficult or inconclusive, it is necessary to measure the pressure drop across the valve using catheter techniques. As with other valve lesions, in the majority of cases catheterization is required only as a preoperative investigation to confirm the diagnosis and check the coronary arteries.

Limited success has been achieved with interventional treatment of aortic stenosis. It is technically feasible to dilate the stenotic orifice with a large balloon, but it is not usually possible to relieve the stenosis fully and there is rapid return of the stenosis over a few months. The technique is reserved for a few patients where palliative treatment is needed or where the condition can be alleviated sufficiently to allow subsequent surgery.

AORTIC REGURGITATION

Aortic regurgitation is occasionally due to chronic rheumatic heart disease, usually in association with mitral valve disease, but is most commonly due to degeneration of a congenitally bicuspid aortic valve or to dilatation of the aortic root caused by connective-tissue disease such as Marfan's syndrome. In the presence of a healthy left ventricle, pure aortic regurgitation can be well tolerated for many years. Infective endocarditis is a common complication in patients with abnormal aortic valves and destruction of valve leaflets or annulus can lead to severe regurgitation. The chest radiographic features of aortic regurgitation (Fig. 24.23) are listed in Box 24.6.

Box 24.6 *Chest radiographic features of aortic regurgitation*

- **Heart size**
  - In mild cases of pure aortic regurgitation there is little or no cardiomegaly
  - There is usually cardiomegaly in all cases of moderate or severe regurgitation
- **Heart shape**
  - Left ventricular contour enlargement is the most prominent feature in most cases, the cardiac apex being displaced inferiorly and laterally
  - Right atrium and ventricle not enlarged
- **Lung fields**
  - Signs of heart failure are only seen in advanced cases with left ventricular failure
- **Great arteries**
  - Aortic knuckle normal but the ascending aorta (right heart border) is often prominent owing to aortic root enlargement or aneurysm
  - The thoracic aorta may be abnormal owing to underlying aortic disease, e.g. Marfan's syndrome
  - Main pulmonary artery not enlarged
- **Calcification**
  - Aortic leaflet calcification is rare unless there is coexisting aortic stenosis
- **Implants and postsurgical appearances**
  - Sternal wires and metallic ring indicate valve prosthesis

Figure 24.24 *Parasternal long axis echocardiogram showing prominent vegetations attached to the aortic valve leaflets (arrows). There is also a small posterior pericardial effusion.*

Figure 24.25 *Chest radiograph showing marked right atrial enlargement owing to chronic severe tricuspid regurgitation.*

Echocardiography

Echocardiography is an essential diagnostic and management technique. The morphology of the aortic valve leaflets can be inspected and the anatomy of the aortic root itself can be evaluated.

Associated abnormalities such as vegetations (Fig. 24.24) or abscess formation can be detected. Doppler studies of the left ventricle and aortic arch can be used to evaluate the severity of the regurgitation. The left ventricular function should always be evaluated and it is commonplace to use echocardiography to monitor the left ventricular function over a period of years, to detect any signs of decompensation that would trigger the decision for surgery.

Sectional imaging

CT and MIRI are not usually necessary in the evaluation of heart valve disease, but in the case of aortic valve disease, and particularly aortic regurgitation, it may be necessary to evaluate the anatomy of the thoracic aorta in detail to aid surgical planning. Sectional techniques are often helpful here as echocardiography is less well suited to the assessment of the aorta beyond the aortic root itself owing to difficulties with achieving adequate echocardiographic windows.

Cardiac catheter and angiography

As with most other valve lesions a catheter is required only as a preoperative investigation to confirm the diagnosis and check the coronary arteries. Angiographic assessment of aortic regurgitation with an aortogram is only semiquantitative and usually offers little more than the echo study. Anatomical assessment of the ascending aorta is usually better achieved with sectional imaging.

TRICUSPID VALVE DISEASE

The tricuspid valve is rarely the main cause of a haemodynamic cardiac problem, but it is frequently affected by secondary changes accompanying left-sided heart disease. The commonest primary problem affecting the tricuspid valve is **infective endocarditis**, often associated with intravenous drug abuse, but the condition is still rare. In the case of a severely damaged valve, the volume overload produces marked right atrial enlargement and sometimes right ventricular enlargement (Fig. 24.25). Damage to the tricuspid valve by the metabolites of metastatic carcinoid disease can cause tricuspid valve damage.

In contrast, many conditions affecting the mitral and aortic valves and the left ventricle can cause pulmonary venous hypertension which in turn can lead to right heart dilatation and consequent mild tricuspid regurgitation. This is rarely clinically important in comparison to the primary condition, but is often demonstrated on Doppler studies. The velocity of the tricuspid regurgitant jet can be used to estimate right-sided heart pressures.

Tricuspid valve disease is usually diagnosed by echocardiography and other techniques are rarely required.

PROSTHETIC VALVE DISEASE

There is an increasing number of patients in the population who have a prosthetic heart valve, and it is essential to monitor the satisfactory function of these valves. Prosthetic valves are of two main types: mechanical and biological. Mechanical valves are normally of the bileaflet tilting disc design, but older valves of the single tilting disc or ball-and-cage design are still seen. Biological valves are most commonly made of porcine tissue mounted on a metallic support, but homograft (human) aortic valve tissue is sometimes used. Mechanical valves generally function well for a longer period, in many cases exceeding 20 years, but lifetime anticoagulation is required. Mechanical valves tend to be used in younger patients. Biological valves last less well, a minority lasting over 10 years, but they require less or no anticoagulation and are often used in older patients.

The valve-supporting mechanism is almost always visible on the plain chest radiograph, and it is important to check the consistency of position of the valve on serial films. Fluoroscopy can be useful to check valve movements and, with care, it can be used to evaluate the movement of mechanical valve leaflets. Echocardiography is generally used for serial monitoring of the function of these valves, which can be difficult because the images are degraded by the metallic valve components. In addition the flow patterns through the prosthetic valve are never normal, even when the valve is functioning well. Assessment of prosthetic valve function requires specialist skills.

Early failure of all types of prosthesis is most commonly due to infection. Late failure of biological valves is due to tissue changes, restricting either the opening of the leaflets or tearing of the prosthetic tissue. Late malfunction of mechanical valves is rare but there is always a risk of valve thrombosis, especially if anticoagulant control has been suboptimal.

HEART MUSCLE DISEASE

Coronary artery disease is the commonest cause of heart muscle impairment but there are many other causes of heart muscle disease and this group of conditions is termed the cardiomyopathies. There are three main types of cardiomyopathy: dilated, hypertrophic and restrictive.

DILATED CARDIOMYOPATHY

This condition is characterized by global dilatation of the left ventricle accompanied by poor systolic function and a reduced ejection fraction. There is often mild or occasionally moderate functional mitral regurgitation. The causes are listed in Box 24.7.

The chest radiograph may be normal in mild cases but in most there will be global cardiomegaly, sometimes quite marked. Pulmonary changes of heart

Box 24.7 *Common causes of dilated cardiomyopathy*

- Idiopathic (no cause found)
- Ischaemic
- Postinfection
  - viral myocarditis
    - cytomegalovirus
    - Coxsackievirus B
  - Chagas' disease (South America)
- Inflammatory and infiltrative
  - amyloidosis
  - arrhythmogenic right ventricular cardiomyopathy
  - endomyocardial fibrosis
  - sarcoidosis
  - rheumatic carditis
  - thalassaemia – iron deposition
- Toxic
  - drugs
  - alcohol
- Nutritional
- Inherited
  - muscular dystrophy

failure may be present if there is decompensation, but quite often, in patients on heart failure treatment who have adjusted their lifestyle, there may be relatively few pulmonary abnormalities.

Echocardiography demonstrates left ventricular function (Fig. 24.26) and is an important technique in the monitoring and management of the condition. MRI scanning is able to achieve sophisticated evaluation of left ventricular function and is increasingly used in this

Figure 24.26 *M-mode echocardiogram showing a markedly dilated and thin-walled left ventricle in a patient with a severely dilated cardiomyopathy. Inset image shows the corresponding two-dimensional scan. Diastolic left ventricular diameter is markedly increased at 8.1 cm, and the systolic diameter is 7.3 cm.*

Figure 24.27 *M-mode echocardiogram showing markedly thickened interventricular septum (arrowed) which is over 4 cm in thickness, compared to the free wall which is 1.0 cm in thickness.*

trophy of the myocardium, particularly of the interventricular septum. The pattern can be quite varied with the hypertrophy being present elsewhere in the left ventricle and sometimes in the right ventricle. The condition is usually associated with a normal chest radiograph and the diagnosis is made on echocardiography (Fig. 24.27).

Echocardiographic features of hypertrophic cardiomyopathy include:

- asymmetrical septal hypertrophy, septal to free wall ratio over 1.5:1;
- hypertrophy sometimes affecting different regions of the left or right ventricle;
- systolic anterior motion of the mitral valve;
- dynamic left ventricular outflow tract obstruction;
- small left ventricular cavity sometimes obliterated in late systole;
- possible early closure of the aortic valve.

These features are variably expressed and symptoms are also variable.

condition. Left ventricular blood pool nuclear medicine studies are sometimes employed to assess left ventricular function. Angiography has little part to play in the diagnosis and management of the condition unless radical surgery such as heart transplantation is planned. Under these circumstances full haemodynamic cardiac evaluation and coronary arteriography are required.

HYPERTROPHIC CARDIOMYOPATHY

Hypertrophic cardiomyopathy is a classically recognized syndrome with a variable spectrum of features. There is a basic underlying abnormality of the heart muscle fibres, and the condition is manifest as abnormal hyper-

RESTRICTIVE CARDIOMYOPATHY

Restrictive cardiomyopathy is relatively rare and is not easy to diagnose with certainty. Filling of the left ventricle is impaired by heart muscle disease and consequently systolic function and left ventricular reserve are reduced. In some cases the condition is associated with clear-cut pathology, such as infiltration in amyloid disease, endomyocardial fibrosis or coexisting hypertrophic cardiomyopathy, but in the majority of cases there is no obvious cause. The main feature on echocardiography is disproportionate left atrial enlargement with no apparent cause.

(a)

(b)

Figure 24.28 *A patient with widespread sarcomatous metastases. (a) There is a pleural mass (P) with an associated pleural effusion (Pl) and an associated pericardial effusion (Pe). (b) The same case showing an intracardiac metastasis in the left ventricle (LV).*

(a)

(b)

Figure 24.29 *(a) Two-dimensional echocardiogram taken from the subcostal window showing a moderate-sized pericardial effusion. (b) Apical four-chamber view in the same patient. Asterisks indicate the effusion.*

TUMOURS OF THE HEART

Primary tumours of the heart are rare and three-quarters are benign. Of the benign tumours the commonest are myxomas (50 per cent) and lipomas (10 per cent). Haemangiomas, fibromas, rhabdomyomas and teratomas are all rare. A quarter of all primary cardiac tumours are malignant, of which haemangiosarcomas are the most common. Secondary involvement of the heart by malignant tumours is much more common but usually occurs late in the malignant process. Secondary cardiac tumours in the pericardium arise from the bronchus, breast and stomach and from methotheliomas. Intramyocardial or intracavity secondary deposits more commonly arise from renal carcinoma, lymphoma and melanoma.

Cardiac tumours may be imaged by a variety of techniques including echocardiography (Fig. 24.28), MRI and angiography, depending on their site and size. Transoesophageal echocardiography is often the most elegant technique for showing the site and size of tumours.

MYXOMA

Myxomas are the commonest primary cardiac tumour. In about 90 per cent of cases they occur in the left atrium. The condition presents in a variety of ways but has a classic echocardiographic appearance, with a tumour usually arising from the interatrial septum showing a soft and mobile texture, with a tendency to prolapse into the mitral orifice during diastole. The tumour has a high risk of fragmentation and embolization, and recognition of the diagnosis should lead to immediate cardiac surgical referral.

PERICARDIAL DISEASE

The normal heart is surrounded by the thin layers of parietal and visceral pericardium, and little is normally seen of these structures on most imaging techniques. MRI perhaps best demonstrates the thin normal pericardium outlined by adjacent fat layers. Pericardial disease can be divided into those that cause pericardial effusion and those that cause thickening or other abnormality of the pericardium itself

PERICARDIAL EFFUSION

Pericardial effusion is sometimes seen as cardiomegaly on the chest radiograph, but this is only evident with moderate or large effusions. Echocardiography is the most practical technique for diagnosing all types of pericardial effusion (Fig. 24.29). Many effusions are asymptomatic but rapid accumulation of fluid or a restrictive pericardial sac will lead to pericardial tamponade. Pericardial tamponade causes impaired venous return to the heart and consequently restricts cardiac output. In this situation there is evidence of compressed right-sided cardiac chambers and impaired filling patterns on the Doppler study. In pericardial tamponade urgent drainage of the fluid is required; this is best achieved under ultrasound guidance, which allows an appropriate needle position to reach the most easily accessible part of the collection. Drainage is usually achieved with an indwelling catheter inserted over a guidewire which can be left in position for a few days if necessary (Fig. 24.30).

There are very many causes of pericardial effusion, the commonest of which are congestive heart failure, postviral infection, malignant effusion and post-

(a)

(b)

Figure 24.30 *(a) Chest radiograph of a patient with a moderate-sized pericardial effusion. (b) Same patient a few days later after drainage of the effusion.*

myocardial infarction syndrome. Haemopericardium, often indistinguishable from other types of pericardial effusion, can be due to recent cardiac surgery or in association with aortic root dissection and rarely cardiac trauma. Rarer causes of pericardial effusion include uraemia and collagen diseases, but quite frequently no cause will be found.

PERICARDIAL THICKENING AND INFILTRATION

Pericardial thickening and infiltration are usually the consequence of chronic inflammation or infection. Chronic tuberculous pericarditis can lead to remarkable thickening and rigidity of the pericardium, which can sometimes become heavily calcified. In symptomatic cases it may need surgical removal. Many malignant tumours can infiltrate the pericardium but few can be resected.

CONGENITAL HEART DISEASE IN THE OLDER CHILD AND ADULT

There are increasing numbers of patients with congenital heart disease who survive beyond adolescence having had surgical or interventional therapy. A few only present later in life with signs or symptoms of congenital heart disease. Many of these patients have complex problems and require management in specialist centres. They may, however, present to general

departments. It is, therefore, important that radiologists are able to assist in the management, by recognizing the condition either on first presentation or when interpreting follow-up examinations.

The chest radiograph is a key investigation in the recognition of these conditions. Most forms of congenital heart disease in the older child and adult require specialist follow-up, which involves the use of many imaging techniques, notably echocardiography and MRI. MRI is particularly useful in larger patients and when complex anatomy has to be demonstrated in detail.

Chest radiographic signs suggesting presence of congenital heart disease are listed in Box 24.8.

A few conditions can be diagnosed directly from the chest radiograph.

ATRIAL SEPTAL DEFECT

This condition can present at any age, depending on the size of the defect, the degree of shunting and the pulmonary vascular physiology. The left-to-right shunt occurs at atrial level and leads to enlargement of the right atrium and the right ventricle, with the left ventricle remaining small. The increased flow in the pulmonary artery is seen on the chest radiograph as a prominent pulmonary trunk with pulmonary plethora (see Fig. 24.8, p. 600). The diagnosis is made by echocardiography which can reveal that the defect is either a simple secundum defect in the centre of the interatrial septum or a more complex primum defect near the atrioventricular valves. The latter is associated with abnormality of the mitral and tricuspid valves and

Box 24.8 *Chest radiographic signs of congenital heart disease*

- **Features of abnormal situs**
  - Abnormal heart position, e.g. dextrocardia
  - Abnormal abdominal situs, e.g. liver on the left
  - Bronchial situs (Fig. 24.31)
  - Right aortic arch (Fig. 24.32) may be a feature of congenital heart disease, but in most cases the anomaly is not associated with a cardiac anomaly
- **Abnormal heart shape**
  - Unusually prominent main pulmonary artery
  - Unusually small main pulmonary artery
  - Abnormal contour of the left heart border (inability to recognize aorta, PA, LV)
  - Indistinct aortic knuckle
  - Chamber enlargement
- **Abnormal pulmonary vascularity**
  - Pulmonary plethora (large vessels in all lung zones)
  - Pulmonary oligaemia (small vessels in all lung zones)
  - Patchy or unusual vascular pattern indicating abnormal vessels or surgical shunt
- **Evidence of previous surgery or intervention**
  - Sternal wires or surgical clips
  - Rib deformities due to thoracotomy
  - Abnormal diaphragm position
  - Implants, e.g. prosthetic valves, coils, occlusion devices, pacemakers
  - Sudden change in cardiac contour on sequential films

Figure 24.31 *Localized penetrated view showing normal bronchial situs. The right main bronchus is shorter, wider and more vertically orientated than the left. Upper margins of main bronchi are arrowed.*

can be part of a more extensive syndrome (atrioventricular septal defect). In some cases of ostium primum there is a cleft mitral valve with mitral regurgitation and left heart failure. These cases usually present in childhood.

In patients with significant shunts the defect usually needs closure. This is traditionally a surgical procedure, but recently closure devices have been introduced to close the more simple defects. These devices are visible on the chest radiograph.

VENTRICULAR SEPTAL DEFECT (VSD)

This condition usually presents in childhood but in rare cases first presents in adults. Typically there is a large left atrium and a large left ventricle. The chest radiograph shows moderate cardiomegaly with moderate enlargement of the pulmonary trunk and pulmonary plethora. If the defect is restrictive with a high-pressure jet across it, the haemodynamic consequences may be small and the chest radiograph may be normal. In the case of a large VSD detected in adult-

hood, there is likely to be pulmonary vascular damage and pulmonary hypertension with large central pulmonary arteries and attenuated peripheral vessels. If there has been a high-pressure shunt for many years, the ensuing pulmonary hypertension will lead to a decrease in left-to-right shunting and plethora. This can ultimately lead to reversal of the shunt and cyanosis owing to right-to-left shunting across the defect – so-called **Eisenmenger's syndrome**. In any patient with a left-to-right shunt, a decrease in heart size and diminution in pulmonary vascularity must be seen as the possible onset of Eisenmenger's syndrome.

TETRALOGY OF FALLOT

This condition usually presents in childhood but will occasionally present in late childhood or adulthood, The defect comprises a large subaortic VSD with overriding of the aorta onto the right ventricle. There will be additional pulmonary stenosis. The condition is very variable, depending mainly on the severity of the pulmonary stenosis. Typically, the chest radiograph will

Figure 24.32 *Chest radiograph showing an isolated right-sided aortic arch.*

show moderate cardiomegaly with a somewhat upturned apex, a small pulmonary trunk, pulmonary oligaemia and, in 25 per cent of cases, a right-sided aortic arch. There may well be signs of previous surgery, such as thoracotomy, for a systemic-to-pulmonary shunt. If a right ventricular outflow patch has been placed, the pulmonary trunk may be surprisingly large. The pulmonary vascularity may have a rather complex and disorganizd pattern if there are prominent aortopulmonary collateral vessels.

PULMONARY STENOSIS

On the chest radiograph, pulmonary valvular stenosis causes post-stenotic dilatation of the main pulmonary artery and the left pulmonary artery. There is no simple relationship with the degree of dilatation and the haemodynamic severity of the valvular stenosis. When the condition is first discovered in adulthood, the size of the other pulmonary vessels is normal and the diameter of the heart is usually normal.

PATENT DUCTUS ARTERIOSUS (PDA)

A small defect will sometimes be detected late in life, but large defects usually lead to obvious symptoms in childhood. There is little to distinguish the PDA from a VSD on the chest radiograph except that the aorta may be more prominent than usual and the normal clear line of the descending aorta may be lost. PDA closure devices are increasingly common and can sometimes be visible on the plain film.

COMPLEX LESIONS

Many complex lesions can be seen in adult patients. The non-cardiac radiologist will not be expected to make specific diagnoses but cardiomegaly, unusual cardiac contours, abnormal pulmonary vascularity, signs of previous surgery and metallic implants should all raise the suspicion of congenital cardiac lesions. Further evaluation requires specialist consultation and investigation.

FURTHER READING

Elliott, L.P. (ed.) 1991: *Cardiac imaging in infants, children and adults.* Philadelphia: J. B. Lippincott.

Kilner, P.J. 1998: Imaging of adults with congenital heart disease. In Lima, J. (ed.), *Diagnostic imaging in clinical cardiology.* London: Martin Dunitz.

Marcus, M.L., Schelbert, H.R., Skortoil, D.J., Wolf, G.L. (eds) 1991: *Cardiac imaging – a companion to Braunwald's heart disease.* Philadelphia: W.B. Saunders.

Roobottom, C., Wilde, P. 1996: Heart and pulmonary circulation. In Whitehouse, G.H., Worthington, B.S. (eds), *Techniques in diagnostic imaging.* Oxford: Blackwell Science.

Underwood, R., Firmin, D. (eds) 1991: *Magnetic resonance of the cardiovascular system.* Oxford: Blackwell Science.

Wilde, P. (ed.) 1993: *Cardiac ultrasound.* Edinburgh: Churchill Livingstone.

Wilde, P., Hartnell, G.G. 1995: Cardiac imaging; Acquired heart disease; Congenital heart disease; Cardiac tumours; Implants; Pericardium; and Interventional techniques. In Sutton, D. Young, J.W.R. (eds), *A concise textbook of clinical imaging.* St Louis, MO: Mosby.

Arteries and lymphatics

ROGER H.S. GREGSON

Arteriography is an invasive radiological procedure that involves the injection of a radiopaque liquid into an artery resulting in the production of exquisite diagnostic information. Modern diagnostic arteriography owes its widespread development to Seldinger, a Swedish radiologist, who described the technique of percutaneous catheterization of the femoral artery in 1953. The unrivalled position of arteriography has been eroded over the last 20 years by the introduction of non-invasive imaging techniques, such as ultrasound, radionuclide studies, computed tomography (CT) and magnetic resonance imaging (MRI). Today arteriography is undergoing a renaissance owing to the development of therapeutic interventional vascular techniques, many of which were originally pioneered by Dotter, an American radiologist.

ARTERIAL CATHETERIZATION

EQUIPMENT

The requirements for the percutaneous catheterization of an artery are a needle, a guidewire and a catheter.

Needles

The needle is used to produce a direct percutaneous channel into the artery. There are two types of arterial puncture needle in common usage – a one-piece disposable needle with a sharp bevelled tip and a two-piece disposable needle with an outer cannula and an inner stylette. Most needles are 18–20 gauge in size and 6–10 cm in length. A guidewire is passed through the needle or cannula into the lumen of the artery.

Guidewires

The guidewire is initially used to carry the catheter through the skin and subcutaneous soft tissues into the artery and then to carry the catheter through the arterial system itself. There are many types of guidewire, but they all have a single basic design – a short, soft, flexible tip at one end, which is relatively atraumatic to the arterial intima; a long, firm, flexible wire in the middle; and a short stiffer rigid tip at the other end, onto which the catheter is threaded. Most guidewires are coated with Teflon to reduce friction, are 0.035–0.038 inches in diameter and 100–150 cm in length. The flexible tip is either straight or J-shaped with a radius of curvature between 1.5 and 15 mm. A guidewire with a straight tip is suitable for a non-diseased vessel, whereas a guidewire with a 3 mm J-shaped tip is best in an atheromatous vessel.

There are also a variety of specialist guidewires:

- smaller calibre guidewires with diameters of 0.014–0.025 inches for thinner catheters;
- fixed core heavy duty guidewires for added stiffness;
- movable core guidewires for variable stiffness and shape;

- extra long guidewires with lengths of 200–260 cm for catheter exchanges to avoid losing the position of the catheter in the arterial system;
- steerable guidewires for difficult manipulations in tortuous or stenosed vessels;
- hydrophilic coated guidewires for interventional vascular techniques;
- guidewires with a central lumen for injections.

Catheters

The catheter is used to inject the contrast medium at a precise site within the arterial system. There are also many types of angiographic catheter, but again they all have a single basic design – a tapered tip with an end hole or an end hole and side holes at a specially shaped end, a length of flexible tubing in the middle and a flattened hub at the other end with a locking connection, through which contrast medium or heparinized saline is injected. Most catheters are made of polyethylene or polyurethane but some are made of Teflon or nylon. They are usually 4–7F in size and 60–100 cm in length. The shape of the tip of the catheter is designed for use in a particular artery. A straight catheter with an end hole and multiple side holes is used for abdominal aortography, but a pig-tail catheter with an end hole and multiple side holes is used for cardiac chamber angiography, thoracic and abdominal aortography, because a pig-tail catheter is more stable in position during an injection of contrast medium. Single or double curve catheters with an end hole or an end hole and two side holes are used for selective arteriography, such as the cobra and side-winder catheters for mesenteric and renal arteriography and the mani and headhunter catheters for carotid and subclavian arteriography.

There are also specialist catheters mainly used for interventional vascular techniques:

- balloon catheters for angioplasty;
- co-axial catheters for embolization and thrombolysis;
- 2–3F microcatheters for superselective arteriography;
- 8–12F macrocatheters for embolectomy and stent insertion.

Dilators and vascular sheaths

A **dilator** is used to produce a tunnel through the subcutaneous soft tissues and arterial wall prior to the insertion of the catheter over the guidewire, to prevent damage to the tip of the catheter in patients with scar tissue at the site of arterial puncture, in patients with heavily calcified vessel walls and in obese patients. Most dilators are made of Teflon with a smooth tapered tip and are usually 4–12F in size.

A dilator can also be used with an introducer **vascular sheath** which reduces trauma to the arterial wall in patients requiring multiple catheter exchanges. Most introducer sheaths have a very thin wall and a haemostatic valve.

Contrast media

The new non-ionic contrast media such as iopamidol (Niopam), iohexol (Omnipaque) and iopramide (Ultravist) have become the media of choice for angiography. These contrast media have a low osmolality (290 mOsm/kg water), which is only two to three times that of plasma, in comparison to the high osmolality of the ionic contrast media, which is five to seven times that of plasma. The non-ionic contrast media do, however, have a higher viscosity than the ionic contrast media, but this can be reduced by warming them to body temperature before injection.

A contrast medium containing 340–370 mg iodine/ml is used for conventional film aortography and a contrast medium containing 300 mg iodine/ml is used for conventional film arteriography. However, for intra-arterial angiography. However, for intra-arterial angiography with a digital subtraction technique, a less concentrated contrast medium containing 150–300 mg iodine/ml is suitable, although for intravenous digital subtraction angiography, a contrast medium containing 340–370 mg iodine/ml is required, because of the dilution that occurs in the vascular system.

The contrast medium is injected through the catheter by a pressure injector for thoracic and abdominal aortography and pulmonary, mesenteric, renal and pelvic arteriography, but is injected by hand for carotid, coronary and superselective arteriography. The volume of contrast medium used during an examination should not exceed 4–5 ml/kg body weight.

TECHNIQUE

Arteriography is generally performed as an inpatient procedure, but is also being done as either a day case or an outpatient procedure in increasing numbers.

Patient care

A 12–24 hour hospital admission is ideal for patients undergoing arteriography and allows the radiologist the opportunity of visiting the patient before the procedure in order to explain the technique and its risks, obtain informed consent and examine the proposed puncture site, which is usually the femoral artery in the groin. Patients with a history of a previous hypersensitivity reaction to intravascular contrast media require corticosteroid cover for the procedure or an alternative imaging study, and oral anticoagulant therapy should be withdrawn at least 3 days before the procedure so that the INR is less than 1.4. Preangiographic investigations include the haemoglobin level, platelet count, urea and electrolytes, and clotting studies, but other investigations such as ECG, blood sugar, sickle test and hepatitis antigen are occasionally needed.

The patient requires a groin shave and must not eat any solid food for 6 hours before the procedure, but can continue with free oral fluids to within 2 hours of coming to the angiography suite.

Arteriography is usually done under local anaesthetic in adults, but a general anaesthetic is required for babies and children and some long complex vascular interventional procedures, such as embolization. A premedication of 10 mg temazepam orally, 10 mg papaveretum (Omnopon) intramuscularly and 12.5 mg prochlorperazine (Stemetil) intramuscularly is useful in the majority of adults 1 hour before the procedure. Antibiotic cover is also occasionally needed.

After the procedure the patient requires 6–12 hours of bed rest and regular observation of the puncture site, the pulse and blood pressure checked every 15 minutes for 1 hour, hourly for 4 hours and then 4-hourly to 12 hours. The hospital admission also allows the radiologist to visit the patient after the procedure to check for complications and discuss the results and proposed management.

Contraindications to arteriography

There are no absolute contraindications to arteriography, but relative contraindications include a previous hypersensitivity reaction to contrast media, severe hypertension with a diastolic blood pressure over 120 mmHg, anticoagulant treatment, a bleeding diathesis, severe anaemia with a haemoglobin level less than 8 g/dl and pregnancy.

Arteriography also carries more risk in patients with cardiac failure, respiratory failure, renal failure, hepatic failure, thyrotoxicosis and dehydration, and requires great care in children and elderly patients.

Catheterization of the femoral artery in the groin may be contraindicated by the presence of an occlusion or an aneurysm of the common femoral artery, a synthetic graft and scar formation or infection in the soft tissues overlying the artery. Marked obesity can also make the procedure rather difficult.

Femoral arterial catheterization

The common femoral artery is the best vessel to use for percutaneous arterial catheterization, because it is a larger superficial vessel, which allows access to the whole arterial tree.

The artery is catheterized in the groin under local anaesthetic with sterile conditions in the following stages:

1. The artery is palpated in the right or left groin and 5–10 ml of 1 per cent lidocaine is injected into the skin and soft tissues around the artery at the point of maximum pulsation below the inguinal ligament, but not necessarily in the skin crease in the groin because it is variable in position.

2. A 19-gauge thin-wall one-piece needle is introduced into the artery at an angle of 30–45° with one hand while the artery is held in position by the index and middle fingers of the other hand. The needle is advanced through both the anterior and posterior walls of the artery in Seldinger's original description, but today the needle is often just advanced through the anterior wall of the vessel.

3. A 0.035 inch guidewire with a 3 mm J-shaped tip is advanced through the tip of the needle and up into the abdominal aorta, once a good backflow of arterial blood has been obtained.

4. The needle is withdrawn over the guidewire, while compression is applied to the groin by the fingers of one hand.

5. A 5F catheter (or dilator and introducer vascular sheath) is advanced over the guidewire and into the artery, while compression is still maintained.

6. The guidewire is removed leaving the catheter within the arterial tree. The catheter is flushed with heparinized saline containing 5000 units of heparin/litre and positioned for arteriography.

7. The catheter is removed at the end of the procedure and compression is again applied at the arterial puncture site for 5–10 min to prevent the formation of a haematoma.

Some bruising in the groin often becomes apparent a few days later in the majority of patients.

This technique is described as a retrograde catheterization of the common femoral artery with passage of the guidewire and catheter into the iliac arteries and abdominal aorta, but it is also possible to catheterize the common femoral artery in an antegrade direction with passage of the guidewire and catheter into the superficial femoral and popliteal arteries for the purpose of angioplasty.

Other arterial catheterization sites

In the majority of patients at least one of the femoral pulses is present. When there is only one weak femoral pulse, it is still possible to catheterize the common femoral artery using fluoroscopy to localize any arterial calcification or using ultrasound to visualize the artery directly.

When both femoral pulses are absent, it is advisable to use other arteries for catheterization or direct needle puncture. The axillary or brachial artery and even the radial artery can be catheterized in either arm using an identical technique to that already described for femoral arterial catheterization. A puncture site in the right arm gives access to the thoracic aorta and the carotid and coronary arteries, whereas the left arm gives access to the abdominal aorta and the distal part of the arterial tree.

Direct needle puncture of the upper or lower abdominal aorta, so-called translumbar aortography, is now only occasionally performed, because it inevitably results in a significant retroperitoneal haematoma and is often done under general anaesthetic.

Direct needle puncture of the carotid or subclavian arteries is no longer performed, but direct needle puncture of the femoral artery can be very useful in a scarred groin when it is difficult to catheterize the artery because of the fibrous tissue.

An arteriotomy of the brachial artery in the catheter suite is still used for coronary arteriography as an alternative to the transfemoral route. An arteriotomy of the artery in theatre is useful in combined vascular surgical and interventional radiological procedures.

Venous catheterization

The femoral vein can be catheterized in the groin using an identical technique to that already described for femoral arterial catheterization. Femoral vein catheterization gives access to the pulmonary arteries.

The technique of intravenous digital subtraction angiography is used to produce images of the arteries following a central venous injection of contrast medium into the superior vena cava or right atrium, despite the dilution of the contrast medium that occurs. The procedure is usually performed after catheterization of the median basilic or cephalic veins in the cubital fossa of either arm, but can also be done following catheterization of the femoral vein.

COMPLICATIONS OF ARTERIOGRAPHY

Arteriography carries a small degree of risk to the patient. Because of the high-quality diagnostic information that is produced, the benefits of arteriography are invariably much greater than the risks and therefore outweigh the morbidity and mortality of the procedure, which are both extremely low. Not all problems that develop after an arteriogram are necessarily caused by the procedure; many of the patients undergoing arteriography have generalized vascular disease or multiple medical problems.

Contrast medium reactions (see p. 4)

A fatal reaction is commoner after an intravenous than an intra-arterial injection. Patients who have had a previous major reaction to contrast media and require further angiography should be covered by corticosteroid treatment or should undergo an imaging procedure that does not require contrast media such as duplex ultrasound or magnetic resonance angiography.

Figure 25.1 *Femoral arteriography showing a subintimal dissection in the whole of the right external iliac artery (arrows) produced by a straight guidewire.*

Adverse reactions to other drugs

Reactions to drugs used during angiography are rare but include complications related to the premedication, the local anaesthetic and any drug given during the procedure. Intravenous diazepam can produce a respiratory arrest in an elderly patient, lidocaine can produce convulsions and cardiac dysrhythmias and glyceryl trinitrate can produce hypotension.

Arterial puncture site complications

Complications at the arterial puncture site occur in about 5 per cent of patients undergoing arteriography and include haemorrhage, haematoma, arterial spasm, subintimal dissection (Fig. 25.1), thrombosis, perivascular extravasation of contrast medium, false aneurysms, arteriovenous fistula, nerve trauma and local sepsis. However, only 0.2 per cent of these complications require surgical treatment.

Haemorrhage from the puncture site with external bleeding or the formation of a subcutaneous haematoma is the commonest complication of arterial catheterization. It is more likely to occur with poor angiographic technique, in hypertensive patients and in patients with clotting disorders. Some bruising in the groin a few days after the procedure is normal. The formation of a false aneurysm is uncommon and the development of an arteriovenous fistula is rare. Subintimal dissection and local arterial spasm at the puncture site are not usually clinically significant, but can produce thrombosis, which is also an uncommon complication. It is more likely to occur with poor angiographic technique, in atheromatous vessels and in patients with thrombotic tendencies.

Perivascular extravasation of contrast medium produces pain at the arterial puncture site. Nerve trauma is rare but is most likely to occur with trans-axillary arteriography. Local sepsis at the puncture site is also rare.

Complications within the arterial system

Complications owing to the catheter being within the arterial system occur in about 0.5 per cent of patients and include:

- embolization (Fig. 25.2)
- subintimal dissection
- arterial spasm
- thrombosis
- perforation of the arterial wall
- vasovagal reactions
- subacute bacterial endocarditis
- septicaemia
- guidewire or catheter fracture
- organ infarction.

However, only 0.1 per cent of these complications require surgical treatment.

Distal embolization into the arterial tree is caused by dislodging an atheromatous plaque from the arterial wall or by stripping thrombus off the guidewire or catheter, but is an uncommon complication. Embolization is more likely to occur with poor angiographic technique and the absence of heparin in the flushing solution. Embolization of cholesterol crystals or air can be fatal. Guidewire or catheter fracture is rare.

Thrombosis within the arterial system is also uncommon. It is usually caused by subintimal dissection or arterial spasm and is more likely to occur with poor angiographic technique, in atheromatous vessels and in patients having angioplasty. Perforation of the arterial wall by the catheter or guidewire is rare.

Subacute bacterial endocarditis is commoner after cardiac angiography and septicaemia is more likely to occur with long procedure times, but both are rare complications. Vasovagal reactions also occur during arteriography and pyrogenic reactions can occur after the procedure.

Damage or infarction of specific organs is rare, but is usually caused by subintimal dissection during

Figure 25.2 *Femoral arteriography showing a distal embolus in the left tibioperoneal trunk (arrow) produced by a large catheter.*

selective arteriography or embolization during aortography or arteriography. Renal function can deteriorate following renal arteriography, myocardial infarction is likely to occur after dissection of the left or right coronary artery and leg ischaemia is likely to develop after a popliteal artery embolus.

Arteriography is best performed by the transfemoral route because the overall complication rate is 1.7 per cent, with a mortality rate of 0.03 per cent. This is significantly lower than for transaxillary arteriography, which has an overall complication rate of 3.3 per cent and a mortality rate of 0.09 per cent. Translumbar aortography has an overall complication rate of 2.9 per cent and a mortality rate of 0.05 per cent.

RADIOLOGICAL INVESTIGATION OF ARTERIAL DISEASE

The investigation of the patient with vascular disease obviously begins with a good history and thorough clinical examination and includes a number of laboratory tests, in addition to the pre-angiographic investigations, such as thombophilia screen, and blood cholesterol and serum fibrinogen estimation. The radiological imaging techniques available include:

- plain films
- ultrasound
- arteriography
- computed tomography
- magnetic resonance imaging
- radionuclide imaging
- other imaging techniques.

PLAIN FILMS

Plain films are of limited value in the investigation of arterial disease, because the arteries have a similar radiographic density to the surrounding soft tissues and therefore cannot be seen. The demonstration of calcification in the arterial wall, however, indicates the presence of arterial disease. Intimal calcification has an irregular amorphous pattern in atherosclerotic vessels and is common in elderly patients. It is diagnostic of an aneurysm when there is a curvilinear element to the calcification (Fig. 25.3). Calcification in the media has a regular tubular pattern in atherosclerotic vessels and is seen in patients with diabetes mellitus, characteristi-

cally in the tibial and foot vessels. This type of vascular calcification also occurs in hyperparathyroidism.

The presence of a soft-tissue mass can be due to a true or false aneurysm or an arteriovenous malformation, which can also produce pressure erosion of adjacent bones. Phleboliths in an unusual site are diagnostic of an arteriovenous malformation.

ULTRASOUND

Ultrasound is an extremely useful imaging modality in the investigation of arterial disease, because it is a non-invasive technique that does not use ionizing radiation and is therefore safe. Real-time ultrasound produces an anatomical image of a blood vessel, whereas duplex ultrasound combines pulsed Doppler with an image of a blood vessel to produce a physiological image by colour coding the blood flow. This is called colour flow mapping, with the flow of blood away from the transducer conventionally coded red and the flow of blood towards the transducer coded blue.

Real-time ultrasound is mainly used to assess the size, extent and rate of growth of an abdominal aortic aneurysm (Fig. 25.4) or any other peripheral aneurysm, and has been used in screening studies. Ultrasound is also used in the follow-up of aortic grafts, to measure the size of ectatic arteries and in the investigation of a pulsating mass in the neck, groin, axilla or popliteal fossa, to see whether the mass is a true or false aneurysm or a soft-tissue mass simply transmitting the arterial pulsation. Real-time ultrasound is also occasionally used to aid the vascular radiologist in performing an arterial or venous puncture, by actually visualizing the needle tip passing through the soft tissues to enter the blood vessel.

Figure 25.3 *Lateral radiograph of the knee showing calcification in an aneurysm of the popliteal artery (arrows).*

Figure 25.4 *Ultrasound scan showing a large infrarenal aneurysm of the lower abdominal aorta measuring 8 cm in diameter and containing thrombus (*).*

Duplex ultrasound is mainly used to detect and assess the severity of stenoses in the peripheral arteries and femoropopliteal grafts, and stenoses in the extra-cranial carotid arteries in the neck (Plate 13, opposite page 358) and the renal and mesenteric arteries in the abdomen. Duplex ultrasound is also used to see whether the tibial arteries are patent in the calf before a femorodistal graft, and to assess the patency of the long saphenous vein before the by-pass is performed.

Doppler ultrasound is helpful in those cases of suspected testicular torsion when differentiation from acute epididymo-orchitis is difficult. Testicular torsion results in diminished or absent blood flow in the testis, whereas epididymo-orchitis produces hypervascularity of the affected testis.

ARTERIOGRAPHY

Arteriography is still the most useful imaging modality in the investigation of arterial disease, but it requires the use of a large volume of contrast medium (100–250 ml) and is an X-ray imaging technique, which therefore results in a radiation dose to the patient.

The commonest indications for arteriography are:

- peripheral vascular disease
- ischaemic heart disease
- cerebrovascular disease.

Femoral arteriography, coronary arteriography and carotid arteriography account for well over 90 per cent of the workload of most angiographic units, but arteriography is also indicated in:

- the investigation of the ischaemic arm;
- the investigation of renovascular hypertension and mesenteric ischaemia;
- the assessment of abdominal aortic and other aneurysms;
- the staging of both primary and secondary malignant tumours;
- the localization of the site of bleeding from any organ system;
- the investigation of pulmonary emboli;
- the investigation of trauma;
- the assessment of arteriovenous malformations.

There are three slightly different methods of producing the arterial images:

- conventional arteriography
- intra-arterial digital subtraction angiography
- intravenous digital subtraction angiography.

The advantage of intravenous digital subtraction angiography over either conventional arteriography or its intra-arterial counterpart is that it is an outpatient procedure. The disadvantages of intravenous digital subtraction angiography are that the total volume and iodine load of the contrast medium are greater than for a similar conventional arteriographic procedure and the image quality is less than for a similar arterial digital subtraction technique. The procedure is also, in essence, a right-heart catheter and for optimal images it is necessary to inject the contrast medium through a catheter in the superior vena cava.

Conventional arteriography is the classic form of arteriography in which the arterial images are recorded directly on radiographic film. Conventional arteriography has the best spatial resolution and is therefore used when high-definition images of the arteries are required as in coronary arteriography, intracerebral arteriography and arteriography involving analysis of the finest vessels, such as tumour vascularity and angiodysplasia. The conventional arteriogram image can be visually enhanced by the manual process of photographic subtraction, which highlights the arterial image by removing from the arteriogram film the unwanted images of bone, soft tissue and gas-filled structures, with the use of a mask film. The mask is obtained by producing a film with a reverse image to that normally seen on a radiograph (i.e. black bones instead of white bones) from the initial film of the angiographic series, which has no contrast medium in the arteries. The mask film is exactly superimposed on one of the later films from the angiographic series, which will therefore have contrast medium in the arteries. This is quite easy to do as long as there has been no movement of the patient between the two films. The effect is that the unwanted images of bone, soft tissue and gas-filled structures are cancelled out from an optical viewpoint by different densities on the two films (i.e. white bones cancelled by black bones). The subtraction film is obtained from these two exactly superimposed films and results in a reverse image of the arteries (i.e. black arteries instead of white arteries).

Intra-arterial digital subtraction angiography is the modern form of arteriography and all new angiographic units now have this facility, which uses a computer to produce an electronic subtraction of the arterial image by a similar process to manual photographic subtraction just described. The images are initially recorded by an image intensifier coupled to a television camera. This analogue data is then digitized and the mask image is subtracted from the subsequent arterial images and displayed. These images can be manipulated by computer processing, before being recorded on radiographic film. Once again it is very important that no movement occurs during the angiographic series. Digital subtraction angiography therefore quires cooperative patients who do not move and are able to hold their breath. Examinations of the abdomen are done after an intravenous injection of 20 mg hyoscine butylbromide (Buscopan) to prevent peristaltic movement, examinations of the neck are done without swallowing and examinations of the chest can be done with ECG gating to eliminate the effects of cardiac pulsation. The advantages of intra-arterial digital subtraction angiography over conventional arteriography include reductions in:

- the volume and iodine concentration of the contrast medium used for each angiographic series, which is beneficial in reducing side-effects;
- the total volume and iodine load of the contrast medium used for the whole examination, which is beneficial in children and patients with impaired cardiac and renal function;
- the length of the procedure due to rapid acquisition of each angiographic series, which is likely to reduce complications;
- the diameter of the catheters used, 3–4F, which facilitates day case and outpatient procedures;
- the amount of radiographic film used;

and also the ability to:

- use carbon dioxide gas as a contrast medium in patients with a previous hypersensitivity reaction to intravascular contrast medium, although the spatial resolution with carbon dioxide is lower than when conventional contrast agents are used;
- produce measurements such as the grade of stenosis in an artery and the cardiac output.

Intra-arterial digital subtraction angiography is being increasingly used for all types of arteriography but is particularly useful in interventional vascular procedures, such as embolization and angioplasty, and paediatric arteriography.

Intravenous digital subtraction angiography results in the production of arterial images following an intravenous injection of contrast medium. The images are produced in exactly the same way as for intra-arterial digital subtraction angiography but a delay is required before the angiographic series is obtained, as the contrast medium has to travel from the superior vena cava, inferior vena cava or right atrium, through the lungs and left side of the heart, before reaching the arteries. The contrast medium has been diluted in the blood by this stage but, because of the high-contrast resolution of a digital subtraction system, an acceptable arterial image is produced, if the cardiac output is normal.

Intravenous digital subtraction angiography is used for:

- screening for carotid and renal artery disease;
- follow-up peripheral angiography after a by-pass graft or angioplasty;
- thoracic outlet syndrome and aortic disease in young patients;

- angiography in older patients with no femoral pulses;
- venography in patients with venous occlusion in the pelvic veins, inferior vena cava, subclavian and brachiocephalic veins and superior vena cava.

COMPUTED TOMOGRAPHY

CT is also a useful imaging modality in the investigation of arterial disease, but requires the use of large volumes of contrast medium (100–150 ml) and is a digital X-ray imaging technique with a significant radiation dose to the patient. The recent introduction of slip ring technology for CT (spiral or helical CT) allows a volume of tissue 10–50 cm in length to be scanned very rapidly in 10–25 s. Images of tissue slices of any thickness from 1 to 10 mm thick can then be produced. The advantages of spiral CT over conventional CT for demonstrating arterial disease are the improved contrast enhancement that is produced with a smaller volume of contrast medium (50–100 ml) and the very high-quality reconstructed images that can be obtained.

CT is mainly used for:

- confirming the diagnosis and indicating the type of a dissecting thoracic aortic aneurysm;
- assessing the size and extent of an abdominal aortic aneurysm and its relationship to the renal and iliac arteries (see Fig. 1.13, p. 11);
- assessing the size and extent of a thoracic aortic aneurysm;
- confirming the diagnosis of a ruptured thoracic aorta;
- confirming the diagnosis of a leaking abdominal aortic aneurysm;
- the follow-up of aortic graft complications;
- the investigation of a pulsating mass in the neck or groin;
- the investigation of carotid, renal and mesenteric artery disease.

MAGNETIC RESONANCE IMAGING

MRI is a very useful imaging modality in the investigation of arterial disease that is becoming more widely available. It is a non-invasive technique that does not use ionizing radiation.

MRI using a T1-weighted spin-echo sequence with cardiac gating is used for:

- diagnosing and indicating the type of a dissecting thoracic aortic aneurysm;
- showing the location and severity of a coarctation of the aorta;
- assessing the size and extent of a thoracic or abdominal aortic aneurysm.

Figure 25.5 *Magnetic resonance angiography showing normal renal arteries with an accessory artery to the right kidney on this 3D time-of-flight study.*

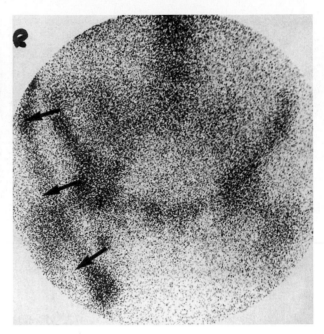

Figure 25.6 *Radionuclide study using indium-labelled white blood cells showing isotope activity in an infected right axillofemoral Dacron graft (arrows). Normal uptake is seen in the bone marrow in the lumbar spine and pelvis.*

Magnetic resonance angiography, with the use of fast-gradient echo sequences, such as the time of flight and phase contrast techniques, is used for showing the location and severity of stenoses and occlusions in peripheral vascular disease, and for confirming the diagnosis of carotid artery disease, renal artery stenosis and mesenteric ischaemia (Fig. 25.5).

In T1-weighted spin-echo sequences, flowing blood produces a signal void and therefore appears black, but in fast-gradient echo sequences flowing blood produces a high signal and therefore appears white. The main advantages of MRI over CT as regards arterial disease are the multiplanar imaging capability, which includes axial, coronal, sagittal and oblique image planes, and the lack of requirement for any contrast medium. However, the paramagnetic agent gadolinium-DTPA, when injected intravenously, can be used to increase the signal intensity of flowing blood to produce high-quality arterial images.

RADIONUCLIDE IMAGING

Radionuclide studies are a useful imaging modality in the investigation of specific problems in arterial disease but involve the use of ionizing radiation.

The diagnosis of an infected arterial graft can most easily be confirmed with a radiolabelled white cell scan (Fig. 25.6). The site of active bleeding from the gastrointestinal tract can be located with ^{99m}Tc-labelled red cells or ^{99m}Tc-labelled colloid. A radionuclide scan is an adjunct to arteriography.

OTHER TECHNIQUES

Intravascular ultrasound is performed by introducing a catheter with a crystal transducer mounted at its tip into the arterial system through a vascular sheath. It produces radial ultrasound images of the arterial wall and is at present used as a research tool to study atheromatous plaque morphology before and after angioplasty. **Angioscopy** is also performed by introducing an angioscope catheter, containing optical fibres, into the arterial system through a vascular sheath. The field of view is continually obscured by blood, which has to be flushed away. Angioscopy does, however, produce spectacular visualization of the normal arterial wall, arterial graft, atheroma, thrombus and blood-flow patterns.

NEOPLASTIC DISEASE

Arteriography is useful in the management of tumours, but its diagnostic role has been significantly reduced by the non-invasive imaging modalities, such as ultrasound, CT, radionuclide studies and MRI, which are used for diagnosis and staging, often in conjunction with needle biopsy under ultrasound or CT guidance. The indications for arteriography include both the diagnosis and localization of primary tumours, pre-operative assessment of primary and secondary tumours, and therapeutic intervention.

Arteriography can be used to distinguish between an atypical benign cyst, an abscess, and a cystic or necrotic tumour, because a pathological circulation may be

Figure 25.7 *Coeliac arteriography showing a large hypervascular tumour in the body and tail of the pancreas (arrows) due to a VIPoma.*

demonstrated in the wall of the tumour but not the cyst. Arteriography can also localize a small endocrine tumour that has not been demonstrated by non-invasive imaging modalities, but is known to be present because of positive biochemical tests. An insulinoma or a glucagonoma in the pancreas and an ectopic parathyroid adenoma in the mediastinum all tend to be hypervascular and, therefore, demonstrable by arteriography (Fig. 25.7).

In the preoperative assessment of patients with primary or secondary hepatic tumours and ampullary tumours in the head of the pancreas, arteriography is used to map out the vascular anatomy and to identify encasement of the vessels that would make the tumour inoperable. Arteriography is also occasionally used to demonstrate the blood vessels supplying very large intra-abdominal tumours and soft-tissue tumours in the limbs.

Embolization is used to prevent bleeding from an inoperable renal or bladder tumour, to devascularize primary tumours prior to surgery such as an angiofibroma in the nasopharynx or an intracranial meningioma, and to ablate the function of hepatic metastases from a carcinoid tumour. Arteriography is also useful in positioning a catheter in the main feeding artery to a tumour for intra-arterial chemotherapy.

Ultrasound of tumour vasculature has been found to be useful in the context of a number of different tumours, notably hepatocellular carcinoma, not only for diagnosis but also for treatment guidance and assessment of response. Peritumoral and intratumoral vessels with pulsatile flow are considered typical of hepatocellular carcinoma. Because of its sensitivity to slow flow and angle independence, power Doppler is more sensitive than colour Doppler for the demonstration of flow within tumour vessels in hepatocellular

carcinoma. The use of intravascular ultrasound contrast agents can improve visualization still further.

HAEMORRHAGE

Arteriography can be extremely useful in localizing the site of bleeding from the gastrointestinal tract, the urinary tract and the respiratory tract, and occasionally in patients following severe trauma.

Acute gastrointestinal haemorrhage presents clinically with haematemesis, melaena, rectal bleeding and hypovolaemic shock. The initial investigations are endoscopy, which has a diagnostic accuracy of 90 per cent, and flexible sigmoidoscopy/colonoscopy, which has a diagnostic accuracy of 50–90 per cent. Arteriography is indicated in patients who continue to bleed severely, particularly when the initial investigations have failed to demonstrate the site of the bleeding. Arteriography has a diagnostic accuracy of 50–75 per cent, but this approaches 90 per cent if the procedure is performed while the patient is actively bleeding. Arteriography demonstrates active bleeding when the rate of blood loss exceeds 0.5–1 ml/min, but radionuclide studies using either ^{99m}Tc-labelled colloid or ^{99m}Tc-labelled red cells are more sensitive and can detect active bleeding when the rate of blood loss is as low as 0.1–0.5 ml/min. Radionuclide studies have a diagnostic accuracy of 30–90 per cent and can be used prior to arteriography.

In acute upper gastrointestinal haemorrhage, arteriography may show extravasation of contrast medium onto the gastroduodenal mucosa from a gastric or duodenal ulcer, gastro-oesophageal varices, a false aneurysm in pancreatitis or the nipple-like projection of an aortoenteric fistula. In acute lower gastrointestinal leiomyoma, a small intestinal arteriovenous malformation, caecal angiodysplasia, or extravasation of contrast medium onto the colonic mucosa from a colonic diverticulum (Fig. 25.8) or ulcer.

Bleeding from erosive gastritis or a colonic diverticulum can be controlled by an intra-arterial infusion of vasopressin, which produces vasoconstriction, and bleeding from a peptic ulcer, or a false aneurysm within the pancreas or liver can be treated by embolization with sponge foam fragments and steel coils. Tumours, arteriovenous malformations and an aortoenteric fistula are treated surgically. A small intestinal arteriovenous malformation can be very difficult to locate during a laparotomy but, if an angiographic catheter is selectively placed in its feeding artery before surgery, an injection of either methylene blue or fluorescein through the catheter will visualize the abnormal loop of small intestine during the operation. Arteriography is also useful in the investigation of both chronic and obscure gastrointestinal haemorrhage, because it may show a vascular abnormality as the cause of the anaemia or recurrent bleeding.

Figure 25.8 *Superior mesenteric arteriography showing active bleeding from a branch of the right colic (arrow) artery into a diverticulum in the ascending colon (*).*

Renal arteriography is indicated in patients with severe haematuria following a renal biopsy. The arteriography may show a false aneurysm or an arteriocaliceal fistula which can be treated by embolization with steel coils or a detachable balloon. Renal arteriography is also indicated in patients with recurrent haematuria who have a normal intravenous urogram and cystoscopy, because an arteriovenous malformation may be present within the kidney. Embolization is used to control haematuria in patients with an inoperable renal or bladder tumour.

Bronchial arteriography is indicated in patients with chronic fibrotic lung diseases, such as tuberculosis, bronchiectasis and cystic fibrosis, who have severe haemoptysis. Arteriography shows hypertrophied bronchial arteries with extravasation of the contrast medium into the bronchial tree and the haemoptysis can be treated by embolization with sponge foam fragments.

TRAUMA

Blunt trauma, such as soft-tissue injury or bone fracture, and penetrating trauma, such as gunshot and

stab wounds as well as iatrogenic needle injuries, can all produce damage to the vascular system. Arteriography may be required to characterize the acute vascular injury, but it should not delay resuscitation or treatment of the patient. Arteriography is also occasionally used to assess the blood supply to a limb in the patient who requires orthopaedic surgery, but may be compromised by peripheral vascular disease.

The types of arterial injury that can occur in acute trauma include:

- arterial spasm;
- extrinsic compression and displacement of the artery from a haematoma;
- narrowing of the artery from an intramural bleed;
- intimal damage to the artery with or without occlusion;
- partial tears or complete transection of the artery with the formation of a false aneurysm or an arteriovenous fistula.

Blunt trauma to the chest, in the form of a rapid deceleration injury during a road traffic accident or an air crash, produces a partial tear in the arch of the aorta distal to the origin of the left subclavian artery with the formation of a false aneurysm in the survivors. An aneurysm is usually apparent on a chest radiograph as widening of the mediastinum, but occasionally presents years later as a mediastinal mass. Care must be taken when portable films are interpreted, as magnification factors may result in a widened mediastinum. Urgent CT and aortography confirm the diagnosis of a false aneurysm. Chest injury may also damage any of the large arteries or veins in the mediastinum.

Blunt trauma to the abdomen fractures solid organs, such as the spleen and tears the blood vessels in the mesentery, producing haemorrhage and haematoma formation, whereas penetrating trauma to the liver and kidney from a stab wound or biopsy produces a false aneurysm or arteriovenous fistula as well. Both of these can be treated by embolization with steel coils or detachable balloons. Embolization is particularly important and may be life-saving in patients with pelvic fractures (Fig. 25.9), where partial tears in the internal iliac arteries or their branches can produce massive haemorrhage that not be controlled by external fixation of the fractures.

Arteriography is rarely required in patients with long bone fractures in the upper or lower limbs, unless the limb is ischaemic, and even this may resolve with reduction of the fracture. The ischaemia may be due to arterial spasm or occlusion. Stab wounds or other penetrating injuries to the limbs produce a false aneurysm or arteriovenous fistula, whereas gunshot wounds produce arterial occlusion and occasionally embolization of bullet fragments within the vascular

Figure 25.9 *Pelvic arteriography showing a large false aneurysm of the left internal iliac artery in a patient with fractures of the pelvis sustained in a road traffic accident.*

Figure 25.10 *Femoral arteriography showing an arteriovenous malformation in the lower thigh supplied by hypertrophied branches of the right superficial femoral artery and draining into the long saphenous vein.*

system. Vascular spasm and mycotic aneurysms may occur following arterial injuries in drug abuse.

VASCULAR MALFORMATIONS

Congenital vascular malformations are a type of benign vascular tumour consisting of a collection of abnormal blood vessels, which do not have the normal anatomical pattern of development with blood passing from an artery through arterioles, capillaries and venules to a vein. Vascular malformations can be classified according to their angiographic characteristics into a high-flow arteriovenous malformation and a low-flow capillary venous malformation or venous haemangioma.

Clinically, **arteriovenous malformations** present in children and young adult patients as a pulsatile soft-tissue mass with a bruit in the head and neck or in one of the limbs. Arteriovenous malformations may be complicated by cutaneous ulceration and haemorrhage, limb hypertrophy or even cardiac failure. Arteriovenous malformations can also occur in any internal organ and tend to present with bleeding; but pulmonary arteriovenous malformations are usually seen as an incidental finding on a chest radiograph. **Pulmonary arteriovenous malformations** occur in the **Osler–Rendu–Weber syndrome**. Presentation may be as a cerebral abscess when infected material is shunted through the lungs and not filtered by the pulmonary capillaries.

Arteriography of arteriovenous malformations shows a single or several hypertrophied tortuous feeding arteries, a network of abnormal vessels with arteriovenous shunting and aneurysm formation, and enlarged draining veins filling in the arterial phase of the study (Fig. 25.10). Arteriovenous malformations can be treated by either surgery or embolization with polyvinyl alcohol particles, sponge foam fragments or steel coils.

Capillary venous malformations present clinically in children and young adult patients as non-pulsatile swellings in the head and neck or limbs; they are easily compressed and fill when gravity dependent. They may be complicated by pain and thrombosis. Capillary venous malformations can also occur in any internal organ and are usually seen as an incidental finding on an arteriogram. Capillary venous malformations occur in the **Klippel–Trenaunay** and **Parkes–Weber syndromes**. Arteriography of capillary venous malformations shows a normal artery and either venous pooling or enlarged veins in the venous phase of the study. Direct puncture venography is more useful in delineating the venous side of the malformation, but MRI demonstrates both the blood vessel and soft-tissue

Figure 25.11 *Axial T1-weighted MRI scan (in same patient as in Fig. 25.10) showing that the arteriovenous malformation (arrows) does not involve the muscles in the thigh.*

components and is therefore the most useful investigation. Capillary venous malformations are difficult to treat surgically, because they are often more extensive than demonstrated clinically but are well shown on MRI (Fig. 25.11). They tend to recur and do not respond to embolization.

PERIPHERAL VASCULAR DISEASE

THE ISCHAEMIC LEG

Patients with chronic ischaemia of the lower limb present with symptoms ranging from intermittent claudication and rest pain to ischaemic ulceration and gangrene; they have reduced or absent pulses below the stenosis or occlusion, whereas patients with an acutely ischaemic leg present with severe pain, altered sensation, loss of motor power and a cold leg. They also have no pulses below the occlusion.

The assessment of these patients includes clinical investigations such as relevant blood tests, urine analysis and ECG, tests in the vascular laboratory such as Doppler arterial pressure measurements, plethysmography and treadmill testing, together with radiological investigations such as duplex ultrasound, MRI and arteriography.

Arteriography is the best method of imaging the lower limb arteries with digital subtraction enhancing visualization of the tibial arteries and even the vessels in the foot can be well visualized. Arteriography is usually performed via catheterization of the femoral artery, as long as one of the femoral pulses is present in the groin.

If neither of the femoral pulses is present in the groins, as in patients with the Leriche syndrome, in which there is aortoiliac occlusive disease and impotence, the arteriography can be performed by catheterization of the brachial or axillary artery or by catheterizing an arm vein and using intravenous digital subtraction angiography (Fig. 25.12). Translumbar aortography is now rarely performed, because of the inevitable retroperitoneal bleeding that occurs on withdrawal of the needle from the aorta.

Femoral arteriography may show various patterns of atheromatous disease with stenoses or thrombotic occlusions in the aortoiliac segment, the superficial femoral artery, the popliteal artery and distal vessels, or combinations of these patterns in one or both legs. Ectatic arteries with slow flow and unsuspected aneurysms in the lower abdominal aorta and iliac arteries, as well as the common femoral and popliteal arteries, may also be demonstrated. Embolic occlusions are also occasionally demonstrated. The popliteal entrapment syndrome, which is due to medial displacement and extrinsic compression of the popliteal artery by the medial head of the gastrocnemius muscle, cystic adventitial disease of the popliteal artery and an arteritis, such as Buerger's disease, are causes of peripheral vascular disease.

Significant stenoses of over 50 per cent in lower limb arteries, short chronic occlusions up to 5–7 cm in length in the iliac arteries and long chronic occlusions up to 10–15 cm in length in the superficial femoral and popliteal arteries are suitable for treatment by percutaneous transluminal angioplasty. Longer occlusions in the lower limb arteries can be treated by angioplasty, but really require a surgical bypass with either a synthetic or vein graft; the choice of graft material depends upon the site. Short or long acute occlusions can be treated by either surgical embolectomy or thrombolysis.

In many institutions, **duplex** and **colour Doppler ultrasound** have become the first-line investigations in peripheral vascular disease. In the lower limb, the principal vessels are all visible from the groin down to the foot. The iliac arteries are more difficult to examine because of overlying bowel but, if direct visualization of the iliac arteries is not possible, the flow pattern in the common femoral artery is a good indicator of the state of the inflow vessels to the leg. The waveform in the common femoral artery is bi- or triphasic, with rapid acceleration at the start of systole and cessation of flow in late diastole. Proximal disease may produce turbulence or damping of the velocity waveform.

An arterial occlusion is identified by the absence of flow in the affected segment when the vessel is examined with colour Doppler. Care must be taken to ensure that the occlusion is genuine and not due to artefact such as inappropriate equipment settings or calcification in the vessel wall. Demonstration of echogenic material within the lumen or collateral vessels at the margins of an

(a)

(b)

Figure 25.12 *Intravenous digital subtraction angiography showing (a) an infrarenal occlusion of the lower abdominal aorta (arrow) extending into the iliac arteries and (b) patent common, superficial and deep femoral arteries filling through collateral vessels.*

occluded segment helps to avoid these pitfalls (Plate 14, opposite p. 358). Arterial stenoses can be identified with colour Doppler by the reduction in apparent lumen and, more importantly, by the colour change that occurs due to the elevated flow velocity (Plate 15, opposite p. 358). In order for a given flow rate to be maintained the flow velocity must increase within the stenosis to compensate for the reduction in cross-sectional area. The amount of narrowing can be estimated from measurements of velocity immediately above and within the lesion. As a rough guide, a two-fold velocity increase indicates moderate narrowing of approximately 50 per cent diameter reduction. A four-fold velocity increase indicates a more significant lesion of about 75 per cent diameter reduction. The velocity waveform recorded beyond a significant stenosis will be very damped (Plate 14c, opposite p. 000).

SURGICAL GRAFTS

There are two types of surgical graft material – **synthetic grafts** with either Dacron or polytetrafluoroethylene and **vein grafts** using either *in situ* or reversed saphenous vein, or processed human umbilical vein. Radiological imaging techniques play a central role in the management of patients who have had a surgical bypass graft.

All patients who have undergone either a femoropopliteal or a femorodistal vein bypass should enter a graft surveillance programme consisting of duplex ultrasound examinations at intervals of 1 month, 3 months, 6 months, 1 year and 2 years after the surgery, in order to look for the development of stenoses which can lead to graft failure, at the proximal or distal anastomoses or within the graft itself (Plate 15, opposite p. 358).

Immediate graft failure, within the first month, is usually due to a technical complication during the operation, but can be due to unsuitable patient selection. Early graft failure, within the first year, is usually due to graft stenosis, and late graft failure, after the first year, is commonly due to progression of distal disease and occasionally due to development of proximal disease.

Duplex ultrasound will also detect arteriovenous fistulae in the *in situ* vein graft (Plate 16, opposite page 358) and false aneurysms at the proximal or distal anastomoses of the synthetic grafts. Subsequent angiography may also be required and this can be performed either by intravenous digital subtraction angiography (Fig. 25.13) or by arteriography via the contralateral femoral artery. It is, however, possible to perform arteriography by direct puncture of the graft itself, if this provides the most suitable or only vascular access.

Graft stenoses can be treated by either vein patch or balloon angioplasty, and graft arteriovenous fistulae can be treated by either ligation or embolization. Occluded vein and synthetic grafts can be salvaged with thrombolysis, but false aneurysms usually require surgery.

Figure 25.13 *Intravenous digital subtraction angiography showing a false aneurysm at the proximal anastomosis of an axillofemoral Dacron graft with compression of the right brachial artery.*

Radionuclide studies using radiolabelled white cells can be used to confirm the diagnosis of an infected graft and CT can be used in the assessment of false aneurysms within the abdomen and pelvis.

THE ISCHAEMIC ARM

Patients with an acutely ischaemic arm present with severe pain, altered sensation and loss of motor power, and have no pulses below the occlusion as in the lower limb, but patients with chronic ischaemic of the upper limb can present with either Raynaud's phenomenon in the fingers or pain in the arm. The assessment of these patients is similar to that in the lower limbs, but once again **arteriography** remains the best method of imaging the upper limb arteries.

The arteriography can be performed either as an arch aortogram with selective subclavian arteriography, or as intravenous digital subtraction angiography. Selective brachial arteriography is required to demonstrate the arteries in the hand. Subclavian arteriography may show embolic occlusions (Fig. 25.14), or stenoses, thrombotic occlusions due to atheromatous disease, vasculitis or radiotherapy. Aneurysms and a thoracic outlet syndrome, which is due to extrinsic compression of the subclavian artery by a cervical rib or fibrous band as it passes over the first rib, can also be demonstrated.

Significant stenoses of over 50 per cent and short chronic occlusions in the subclavian, axillary or brachial arteries are suitable for treatment by **angioplasty**, but longer occlusions require a surgical bypass. Acute occlu-

Figure 25.14 *Brachial arteriography showing an embolus in the right brachial artery (arrow).*

sions are usually treated by embolectomy, but can be treated by thrombolysis.

THERAPEUTIC EMBOLIZATION

Vascular embolization is a therapeutic radiological procedure that involves the injection of embolic material through a catheter selectively positioned in a blood vessel to produce thrombus, which results in the deliberate occlusion of that blood vessel or vascular bed.

Embolization requires an experienced and skilled vascular radiologist to position the catheter and inject the embolic material safely using high-quality angiographic apparatus, preferably with a digital subtraction facility. Close monitoring of the patient's pulse rate, blood pressure and peripheral oxygen saturation is required, and clotting abnormalities should be corrected. Bladder catheterization is also advised as the procedure is frequently protracted. Embolization is used as an alternative method of treatment to surgery and tends to carry less risk, because it is performed percutaneously under local anaesthetic in many cases. It can, however, be a time-consuming procedure, lasting several hours. The ideal embolic material should be:

- thrombogenic, but not toxic
- able to produce a permanent occlusion
- easy to inject through a catheter
- available in wide range of sizes and shapes
- sterile
- radiopaque.

Many different solid and liquid agents have been used for embolization, but none is absolutely ideal, although the ones used most commonly include:

- gelatin sponge fragments
- polyvinyl alcohol particles
- spiral metal coils
- detachable balloons
- hypertonic dextrose solution
- absolute ethyl alcohol
- tissue adhesives, such as bucrylate.

These embolic agents can be used either on their own or in combination cocktails that should include antibiotics. Gelatin sponge has to be cut into small 1–2 mm fragments which are then suspended in contrast medium before injection because it is not radiopaque. Gelatin sponge fragments only produce a temporary occlusion with recanalization of the artery occurring within a few weeks. Polyvinyl alcohol particles are available in a range of sizes from 100 to 250, 250 to 500 and 500 to 1000 µm, and also have to be suspended in contrast medium before injection because they are not radiopaque. Polyvinyl alcohol particles do, however, produce a permanent occulsion of small arteries.

Metal coils made of steel or tungsten are available in a range of sizes with the diameter of the spiral from 1 to 200 mm. The steel coils are radiopaque and often have silk, wool or synthetic fibrils attached to them to increase their thrombogenicity. They are pushed through the catheter by a guidewire, and produce permanent occlusion of large arteries. Detachable balloons made of latex or silicone are available in 1 and 2 mm sizes with the diameter of the inflated balloon reaching up to 4 or 8 mm. The balloon is filled with contrast medium before detachment from its microcatheter and this produces a permanent occlusion of aneurysms and arteriovenous fistulae.

Hypertonic dextrose solution, absolute alcohol and bucrylate all permeate into the smallest arterial branches because they are liquids and, although they are very effective at producing a permanent occlusion, they are also more likely to reach critical vessels close to the target organ. Hypertonic 50 per cent dextrose solution and absolute alcohol can be mixed with contrast medium to make then radiopaque, but bucrylate is mixed with either tantalum powder or ethiodol to make it radiopaque, and this also prolongs its polymerization time.

The indications for arterial embolization include the treatment of:

- acute haemorrhage
- tumours
- arteriovenous malformations
- hypersplenism
- priapism.

The indications for venous embolization include the treatment of:

- gastro-oesophageal varices
- testicular varicoceles
- some adrenal tumours.

Embolization is used in the management of patients who are bleeding, but are unfit for surgery or in whom the surgery would be difficult. Active bleeding from the stomach, duodenum or rectum can be stopped by embolizing the left gastric, gastroduodenal or superior rectal arteries with very little risk of infarction because of the good collateral supply to these organs, unless there has been previous surgery. However, this risk of infarction is much greater in the small intestine and colon, where embolization is relatively contraindicated.

A false aneurysm within the liver or kidney following either penetrating trauma or a biopsy can be treated by selectively embolizing a branch of the hepatic or renal artery. A false aneurysm within the pancreas following recurrent pancreatitis can be treated by embolizing the gastroduodenal artery. Intractable haematuria from a inoperable renal tumour or a bladder tumour previously treated with radiotherapy can be treated by embolizing the renal arteries or both internal iliac arteries. Embolization has also been used to control haemoptysis from chronic fibrotic lung disease, epistaxis, vaginal bleeding and internal haemorrhage from a pelvic fracture (Fig. 25.15).

Embolization is used in the management of patients with neoplastic disease to control bleeding from the tumour as already described, and to devascularize a tumour prior to surgery, such as an intracranial meningioma, a nasopharyngeal angiofibroma or a malignant bone tumour. Embolization of the liver is useful in ablating the function of hepatic metastases from carcinoid tumours, insulinomas and glucagonomas, reducing the size of the liver in patients with painful hepatomegaly from metastases and controlling haemobilia from metastases. Hepatic artery embolization is, however, contraindicated if the hepatic portal vein is occluded.

Congenital arteriovenous malformations, particularly those with a large arterial component, are best treated by embolization. Traumatic arteriovenous fistulae and false aneurysms are also suitable for treatment.

Embolization of the splenic artery can be used in patients with hypersplenism, who are a poor surgical

Figure 25.15 *Intravenous digital subtraction angiography showing no filling of the false aneurysm of the left internal iliac artery following embolization (in same patient as in Fig. 25.9).*

risk owing to their clotting abnormalities. The internal pudendal artery is embolized in patients with priapism where medical treatment has failed.

Embolization of the gonadal vein can be used to manage patients with infertility, who have a testicular varicocele and embolization of the adrenal vein has been performed in patients to ablate a functioning adrenal tumour.

The complications of embolization include those of arteriography and the use of contrast media as well as accidental embolization of an adjacent critical normal organ, abscess formation in the infarcted tissue, renal failure and death. A postembolization syndrome of pain, fever and leucocytosis also develops within a few days of the procedure owing to tissue necrosis. An embolic agent, such as a steel coil or a detachable balloon misplaced within the vascular system, can be retrieved with a snare.

PERCUTANEOUS TRANSLUMINAL ANGIOPLASTY

Vascular dilatation or angioplasty is a therapeutic radiological procedure, which involves the inflation of a balloon catheter positioned at the site of a stenosis or an occlusion in a blood vessel to increase blood flow through the vessel and improve perfusion to a limb or organ. Angioplasty requires an experienced and skilled vascular radiologist to cross the stenosis or recanalize the occlusion and inflate/deflate the balloon safely.

High-quality angiographic apparatus should be used, preferably with a digital subtraction facility. Angioplasty is the commonest vascular interventional procedure and is an alternative method of treatment to a surgical bypass graft, but carries less risk because it is performed percutaneously under local anaesthetic. However, it can also be used to treat patients whose symptoms are not severe enough to merit reconstructive surgery and in patients to prevent amputation. It is also used in combination with a surgical bypass graft to improve the inflow or outflow in the adjacent arteries.

The indications for angioplasty include:

- peripheral vascular disease of the lower or upper limbs with stenoses or short occlusions in the peripheral arteries;
- ischaemic heart disease with stenosis in the coronary arteries;
- hypertension or chronic renal failure with renal or transplant artery stenosis;
- mesenteric and even carotid artery stenosis.

The technique, which can be performed in conjunction with a diagnostic arteriogram or as a separate procedure, is really quite simple in theory, but can be more complex to perform in practice. The contraindications to angioplasty in patients with peripheral vascular disease are the presence of fresh thrombus, which should be treated by thrombolysis, an aortic occlusion and long occlusions in the iliac, femoral, popliteal and tibial arteries.

The ideal lesion for angioplasty is a short, smooth, central stenosis in a large artery, such as the iliac artery, with normal distal arteries, although most patients tend to have more generalized vascular disease with stenoses and occlusions in several arteries (Fig. 25.16).

After catheterization of the femoral artery, a guidewire and catheter are gently used to cross the stenosis or recanalize the occlusion; the artery is then dilated up to the size of the adjacent vessel by a suitable balloon. This is then deflated again and, if the blood flow has been improved, the balloon catheter is removed. The process can be repeated several times if there is a residual stenosis. Patients undergoing angioplasty should be started on an antiplatelet drug such as aspirin or dipyridamole about 24 hours before the procedure and this should be continued after a successful procedure for at least 3–6 months and possibly forever. During the angioplasty, patients should receive 3000–5000 units of heparin intra-arterially. The success of the procedure is based on eliminating the pressure gradient across a stenosis and producing a good angiographic result with no residual stenosis at arteriography. Endovascular ultrasound and angioscopy have been used to assess the effectiveness of angioplasty. Iliac artery stenoses and short iliac artery occlusions up to 5–7 cm in length are usually approached from below

(a)　　　　　　　　　　　　　　　　　　　　(b)

Figure 25.16 *Iliac arteriography showing (a) a 50 per cent stenosis of the left common iliac artery (arrow) before angioplasty and (b) the result 2 years after angioplasty.*

following a retrograde catheterization of the ipsilateral common femoral artery, but can be approached from above following a retrograde catheterization of the contralateral common femoral artery and crossing of the aortic bifurcation, or following catheterization of the axillary or brachial artery. Stenoses in the internal iliac, common femoral, proximal superficial and deep femoral arteries are best approached across the aortic bifurcation, but stenoses or short occlusions up to 10–15 cm in length in the distal superficial femoral and popliteal arteries are usually approached from above, following an antegrade catheterization of the ipsilateral common or proximal superficial femoral arteries; they can be approached from below following catheterization of the ipsilateral popliteal artery. Stenoses in the lower abdominal aorta and stenoses or short occlusions up to 5 cm in length in the tibial arteries are also suitable for angioplasty.

Coronary, renal, mesenteric, subclavian and carotid artery stenoses are usually approached from below following a retrograde catheterization of the femoral artery, but can be approached from above following catheterization of the axillary or brachial artery.

Before angioplasty a pressure gradient of over 20 mmHg at rest across an iliac artery stenosis or occlusion is significant but, if it is only 10 mmHg at rest, a vasodilator such as papaverine, tolazoline or glyceryl trinitrate should be injected through the catheter. An increase in the pressure gradient to over 20 mmHg indicates that the stenosis is significant and requires angioplasty. Following angioplasty the ideal result is no gradient at all, but a residual gradient of below 10 mmHg is often acceptable. Pressure monitoring across femoral and popliteal artery stenoses and occlusions is not accurate in an antegrade direction and angiography is therefore used to monitor the procedure. Following angioplasty the ideal result is no residual stenosis, but a slight narrowing of the arterial lumen up to 25 per cent of its diameter is often acceptable.

The complications of angioplasty are the same as the complications of arteriography and can therefore occur at the arterial puncture site, at the angioplasty site, distal to the site of the angioplasty and in the systemic circulation. The complications at the puncture site are:

- haemorrhage and haematoma formation
- thrombosis
- false aneurysm formation
- nerve trauma
- local infection.

The complications at the site of the angioplasty include arterial subintimal dissection, which is not usually significant with angioplasty performed in a retrograde direction, as the flow of blood tends to close the flap; it can be significant in the antegrade direction as the flow of blood tends to open the flap and lead to thrombus formation. Perforation of the artery within an occlusion is not usually significant, but rupture of an iliac or renal artery produces significant haemorrhage, which can be life-threatening.

Complications distal to the site of angioplasty are arterial spasm and distal embolization of atheromatous or thrombotic debris. Systemic complications include:

- vasovagal reaction
- hypotension
- cardiac arrythmias
- myocardial infarction
- cerebrovascular accident
- cholesterol crystal embolization
- renal failure
- septicaemia
- death.

Re-stenosis occurs more frequently after coronary and renal artery angioplasty than following iliac, femoral or popliteal artery angioplasty. Recurrent stenosis can be treated by angioplasty or with an arterial stent. Acute reocclusion at the site of the angioplasty is an indication for thrombolysis, but chronic reocclusion can be treated by repeat angioplasty. The initial technical success for iliac artery angioplasty is 90–95 per cent for stenoses and 80–90 per cent for occlusions with a patency rate of 50–90 per cent at 5 years, whereas the initial technical success for femoral and popliteal angioplasty is 85–95 per cent for stenoses, 60–90 per cent for occlusions and 20–70 per cent patency rate at 5 years.

OTHER TECHNIQUES FOR TREATING ARTERIAL OBSTRUCTION

There are a number of a new techniques or devices that have been developed either to assist or to replace balloon angioplasty, but these tend to be expensive and should therefore produce either a higher initial technical success rate or a better long-term patency rate to be of any real clinical value.

Most of these new devices are used to recanalize complete occlusions in the femoral and popliteal arteries, which then still require balloon angioplasty of the recanalized channel. The **Rotational Transluminal Angioplasty Catheter System** (ROTACS) is a low-speed rotating mechanical device, which rotates at about 100 rpm and produces recanalization in about 80 per cent of cases. The **Kensey catheter** is a high-speed rotating mechanical device, which rotates at speeds up to 10 000 rpm and produces recanalization in up to 90 per cent of occlusions where a guidewire and catheter system has previously been unsuccessful. Long-term patency is 50–70 per cent at 2 years. The **Rotablator** is a very high-speed rotating mechanical device, rotating at over 100 000 rpm and is used over a guidewire. It produces a recanalization in over 90 per cent of cases, but tends to produce peripheral emboli. Long-term patency is only 25–40 per cent at 2 years. **Laser-assisted angioplasty** using continuous or pulsed wave lasers and direct laser energy, hybrid or hot-tip probes produces recanalization in up to 90 per cent of cases with a high risk of arterial perforation of about 20 per cent. Long-term patency is 60–70 per cent at 2 years.

The **Transluminal Endarterectomy Catheter** (TEC) is used over a guidewire for either stenoses or occlusions. The atheroma is aspirated through the catheter to produce a recanalization in about 80 per cent of cases. Long-term patency is compromised by a high re-stenosis rate of 25–40 per cent. The **Simpson atherectomy catheter** is used over a guidewire for eccentric stenoses. The atheroma is collected in a small chamber, which limits its use in occlusions.

Vascular stents are used for intraluminal mechanical arterial support to prevent an acute occlusion or improve long-term patency in the iliac arteries. The indications for their use include acute occlusion from an initimal flap after angioplasty, residual stenosis after angioplasty, and following the successful recanalization of an occlusion in the iliac arteries (Fig. 25.17). Types include the flexible Wallstent, the Strecker stent and the rigid Palmaz stent. Long-term patency is 80–95 per cent at 2 years. The Gianturco Z stent is used in the treatment of superior vena caval obstruction and has been used in the endovascular stenting of abdominal aortic aneurysms. Dacron-covered stents have been used successfully in the treatment of selected cases of infrarenal abdominal aortic aneurysms. Similarly, aorto-caval fistulae can be treated with endoluminal stents.

THROMBOLYSIS

Thrombolysis is a new technique that can be used in the treatment of the acutely ischaemic leg or arm and may well be the most effective form of treatment for patients with a critically ischaemic limb, because the results of reconstructive vascular surgery are poor in these patients who have a mortality rate of 15–50 per cent and an amputation rate of 20–60 per cent. Embolectomy, however, produces a limb salvage rate of 95 per cent with a mortality rate of about 12 per cent, but most of the acute occlusions are caused by thrombus from underlying atherosclerotic disease.

The indications or intra-arterial thrombolytic therapy include:

- distal arterial thrombosis or embolus involving the popliteal artery with extension into the tibial arteries;
- proximal arterial thrombosis of the iliac, femoral and popliteal arteries (Fig. 25.18);
- thrombosis of a vein or a synthetic graft;
- thrombosis at the site of a recent angioplasty;
- proximal or distal arterial thrombosis in a patient at risk from vascular surgery.

The indications for vascular surgery include:

- proximal arterial embolus involving the aortic bifurcation, the iliac and the femoral arteries;

(a)

(b)

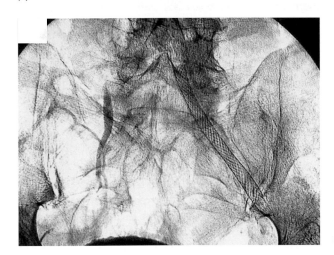

(c)

Figure 25.17 *Vascular stent. Iliac arteriography in a patient with an occlusion of the left common iliac artery. (a) A guidewire has been introduced across the occlusion and angioplasty subsequently performed. (b) The result after angioplasty and insertion of a vascular stent. (c) The vascular Wallstent (Schneider) in place extending from the aortic bifurcation to the external iliac artery.*

- proximal arterial thrombosis of the iliac and femoral arteries, if there is insufficient time for intra-arterial thrombolysis to work in a severely ischaemic leg;
- thrombosis of a synthetic or vein graft.

The contraindications to thrombolysis are:

- recent bleeding from any site;
- a stroke within the last three months;
- recent major surgery or trauma;
- coagulation defect;
- potential bleeding site.

Thrombolysis is performed following diagnostic arteriography with the tip of the catheter positioned in the occlusion either across the aortic bifurcation for proximal occlusions or following an ipsilateral antegrade catheterization for distal occlusions.

With the low-dose infusion technique that uses 5000 units streptokinase/h, 50 000 units urokinase/h or 0.5 mg recombinant tissue plasminogen activator/h, the catheter can be advanced as the thrombus lyses. Lysis is monitored by arteriography and any underlying stenosis revealed requires immediate angioplasty. With the high-dose infusion or bolus technique that uses 20 000 units streptokinase/h, 240 000 units urokinase/h or 10 mg recombinant tissue plasminogen activator/h, the time taken for the thrombus to lyse falls from 25–40 to 6–18 h. A new development of these accelerated thrombolytic regimens is pulse spray pharmacomechanical thrombolysis. This involves injecting 0.2 ml of fluid every 30 s into the thrombus through multiple slits in the catheter and results in a lysis time of about 90 min.

The complications of thrombolysis include:

- groin haematoma and haemorrhage from the puncture site;
- distal embolization of thrombus;
- gastrointestinal and retroperitoneal haemorrhage;

Figure 25.18 *Femoral arteriography showing (a) an occlusion of the right superficial femoral artery; (b) during lysis of the thrombus; (c) after lysis, revealing 50–75 per cent stenoses; (d) the result after angioplasty.*

- acute renal failure owing to the release of myoglobin from necrotic muscle;
- cerebrovascular accident;
- death.

Intra-arterial thrombolysis results in limb salvage in 70–80 per cent of patients with a critically ischaemic limb, with an amputation rate of 5–10 per cent and a mortality rate of about 10 per cent. Thrombolysis has also been used in the treatment of renal artery occlusions, superior vena caval obstruction and deep vein thrombosis. Small amounts of fresh thrombus can be aspirated through a catheter with a large internal luminal diameter and large amounts of fresh thrombus can be removed by a rotating mechanical device or disintegrated with an ultrasonic prove.

LYMPHATICS

LYMPHOGRAPHY

Lymphography is an invasive radiological procedure, involving the injection of contrast medium into a lymphatic to give diagnostic information about not only the lymphatics but also the lymph nodes. Lymphography has been largely replaced by various non-invasive radiological imaging techniques, but is still used in the investigation of patients with lymphoedema and lymphatic leaks, and the demonstration of diseased lymph nodes. An advantage of lymphography is that it can demonstrate metastatic disease or lymphoma in normal-sized glands, but its disadvantage is that many

Figure 25.19 *Lymphography showing abnormal enlarged iliac lymph nodes infiltrated by non-Hodgkin's lymphoma.*

nodal groups in the abdomen and pelvis, such as the internal iliac and mesenteric lymph nodes, are not demonstrated at all by the technique.

Lymphography only demonstrates the retroperitoneal and some pelvic and inguinal lymph nodes. It may show focal deposits typically in metastatic disease or diffusely enlarged glands with abnormal internal architecture as in lymphoma (Fig. 25.19). The appearances are, however, not specific for malignant disease, as fibrolipomatosis produces a focal deposit in the inguinal nodes in elderly patients, and reactive hyperplasia produces diffusely enlarged glands.

Technique

Lymphography is performed as an in- or outpatient procedure and involves the cannulation of a lymphatic in the foot; this procedure is quite difficult, because these vessels are very small and lymph is a colourless fluid. In order to identify the lymphatics, a non-toxic dye, such as Patent Blue Violet, is injected subcutaneously into the first and second web spaces between the toes on both feet. The dye is taken up into the lymphatics within 10–20 minutes, which then become visible through the skin.

The subcutaneous tissues on the dorsum of the foot are infiltrated with local anaesthetic and an incision is made in the skin. A lymphatic vessel, which now appears blue in colour, is then very carefully dissected free from the surrounding tissues and cannulated with a 27- or 30-gauge lymphography needle attached to soft, fine, plastic tubing with a hub at the other end. The needle is tied in position with black silk and the tubing is secured to the skin of the foot. About 1–2 ml of a non-ionic contrast medium is injected slowly by hand in order to check for leaks and then 6–8 ml of Lipiodol Ultra Fluid is injected by a pump over 1 hour.

Figure 25.20 *Lymphogram showing normal lymphatic vessels and femoral lymph nodes in the lymphatic phase of the study.*

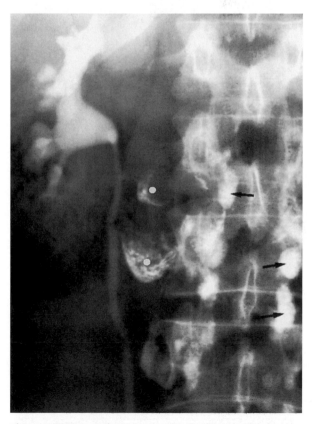

Figure 25.21 *Lymphogram showing both normal (arrows) and abnormal enlarged para-aortic lymph nodes (circles) in the nodal phase of the study, owing to metastatic deposits from testicular teratoma.*

Figure 25.22 *Lymphogram showing lymphatic hypoplasia with only one lymphatic vessel visualized instead of the normal five vessels.*

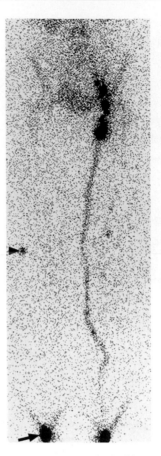

Figure 25.23 *Radionuclide study using* ^{99m}*Tc-labelled antimony colloid in a patient with a swollen right leg due to lymphatic aplasia with no lymphatics visualized and no filling of the pelvic lymph nodes. Isotope remains at the injection site in the foot (arrow). Normal lymphatics are present in the left leg. A marker is placed at the level of the knee (arrow head).*

In the investigation of **nodal disease** in the abdomen and pelvis, contrast medium is injected into both feet until it reaches the level of the sacroiliac joints. In the investigation of lymphoedema water-soluble contrast medium can be used instead of the oily Lipiodol and this may be sufficient to examine only the swollen leg. The patient should be warned that skin and urine will become blue in colour for 24–48 h. Lymphography can be performed in the arm by cannulating a lymphatic on the dorsum of the hand.

In patients with **lymphoedema**, radiographs are taken of the lower and upper leg (or arm) at the end of the procedure to show the lymphatics, but in the investigation of patients with suspected nodal disease, radiographs are taken of the abdomen and pelvis at the end of the procedure to show the lymphatic phase (Fig. 25.20), and then repeated the next day in association with an intravenous urogram to show the nodal phase (Fig. 25.21) of the investigation. Chest radiographs taken at the end of the procedure show the thoracic duct and, if repeated the next day, oil emboli in the lungs. The oily Lipiodol will remain in the opacified lymph nodes for up to a year.

The contraindications to lymphography include:

- soft-tissue infection in the foot;
- venous thrombosis in the leg;
- previous hypersensitivity reaction to contrast media;
- right-to-left cardiac shunts;
- pulmonary arteriovenous malformations;
- severe chest disease with compromised lung function;
- radiotherapy to the lungs.

Complications include:

- leg pains during the infusion of the contrast medium;
- mild symptoms such as headache, nausea and pyrexia the following day;
- pulmonary oil emboli which reduce lung function for 24–48 h;
- hypersensitivity reactions to the local anaesthetic, dye and contrast media;
- blue skin on the feet lasting several weeks.

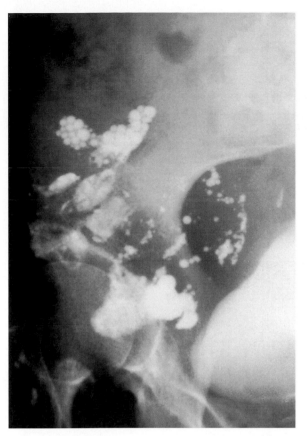

Figure 25.24 *Lymphogram showing globules of oily contrast in a large lymphocele in the pelvis following a hysterectomy for uterine carcinoma. (Contrast given for an intravenous urogram is present in the urinary bladder.)*

LYMPHOEDEMA

Lymphoedema can be either congenital or acquired in origin and is one of the few remaining indications for lymphography. **Congenital lymphoedema** is due to aplasia, hypoplasia or hyperplasia of the lymphatics in the leg and these can be distinguished by lymphography. In aplasia there are no lymphatic vessels found in the foot, which becomes rapidly stained blue from dermal backflow of the dye. In hypoplasia there are only one or two lymphatic vessels in the leg (Fig. 25.22) instead of the usual five, and in hyperplasia there are numerous dilated lymphatic vessels in the leg. Lymphatic hypoplasia is the cause of the swollen leg in 87 per cent of patients with congenital lymphoedema. **Acquired lymphoedema** may be secondary to neoplastic disease or the surgery or radiotherapy associated with it, chronic infections such as filariasis and trauma.

Lymphatic flow can be assessed in patients with lymphoedema by lymphoscintigraphy using ^{99m}Tc-labelled antimony colloid and imaging with a gamma camera. The labelled colloid is injected into the web spaces between the second and third toes and is rapidly taken up into the lymphatic system so that the lymphatics in the legs and the pelvic lymph nodes are visualized within 1 hour. In lymphoedema the usual pattern is for no lymphatics to be demonstrated (Fig. 25.23).

LYMPHATIC LEAKS AND COLLECTIONS

A **lymphocele** is a localized collection of lymph which usually occurs after pelvic lymph node dissection for neoplastic disease, but occasionally after renal transplantation, vascular reconstructive surgery and trauma. Ultrasound and CT both show a localized fluid collection in the pelvis that can be drained using image guidance. Lymphography will demonstrate a lymphocele or a cystic lymphangioma as a localized collection of oily Lipiodol in the pelvis or leg (Fig. 25.24) and lymphoscintigraphy can also demonstrate a lymphocele or lymphangioma.

A **chylous pleural effusion, chylous ascites** and **chyluria** are the remaining indications for lymphography, to demonstrate the site of the leak and the cause of the obstruction. A chylothorax and chylous ascites are usually congenital in children and due to neoplastic and chronic inflammatory disease, surgery or trauma in adults. Chyluria is usually due to filariasis and is caused by a communication between the obstructed lymphatics and the pelvicalyceal system. Lymphovenous communications also occur in lymphatics obstructed by neoplastic or chronic inflammatory disease.

FURTHER READING

Abrams, H.L. (ed.) 1977: *Angiography.* Boston: Little Brown.

Ansell, G., Wilkins, R.A. (eds) 1996: *Complications in diagnostic radiology.* Oxford: Blackwell.

Belli, A.M. (ed.) 1994: *Interventional radiology of the peripheral vascular system.* Sevenoaks: Edward Arnold.

Earnshaw, J.J., Gregson, R.H.S. (eds) 1994: *Practical peripheral arterial thrombolysis.* Oxford: Butterworth-Heinemann.

Hessel, S.J., Adams, D.F., Abrams, H.L. 1981: Complications of angiography. *Radiology* **138**, 273–81.

Hillman, B.J., Newll, J.D. (eds) 1985: Digital radiography. *Radiologic Clinics of North America* **23**(2).

Johnsrude, I.S., Jackson, D.C., Dunnick, N.R. 1987: *A practical approach to angiography.* Boston: Little Brown.

Kadir, S. 1986: *Diagnostic angiography.* Philadelphia: W.B. Saunders.

Koolpe, H.A. (ed.) 1986: Vascular imaging: angiography and the new modalities. *Radiologic Clinics of North America* **24**(3).

Kremkau, F.W. 1997: *Diagnostic ultrasound: principles and instruments.* Philadelphia: W.B. Saunders.

Melany, M.L., Grant, E.G. 1997: Clinical experience with sonographic contrast agents. *Seminars in Ultrasound CT & MR* **18**, 3–12.

Murphy, K.J., Rubin, J.M. 1997: Power Doppler: it's a good thing. *Seminars in Ultrasound CT & MR* **18**, 13–21.

Reuter, S.R., Redman, H.C. 1977: *Gastrointestinal angiography*. Philadelphia: W.B. Saunders.

Rubin, J.M. Bude, R.O., Carson, P.L., Bree, R.L., Alder, R.S. 1994: Power Doppler US: a potentionally useful alternative to mean frequency-based colour Doppler US. *Radiology* **190**, 853–6.

Seldinger, S. 1953: Catheter replacement of needle in percutaneous arteriography: a new technique. *Acta Radiologica* **39**, 368–76.

Taylor, K.J.W., Burns, P.N., Wells, P.N.T. (eds) 1995: *Clinical application of Doppler ultrasound*. New York: Raven.

Thrush, A., Hartshorne, T. 1999: *Peripheral vascular ultrasound*. London: Churchill Livingstone.

Whitehouse, G.H., Worthington, B.S. (eds) 1996: *Techniques in diagnostic imaging* Oxford: Blackwell.

Zweibel, W.J. (ed). 1992: *Introduction to vascular ultrasonography*. Philadelphia: W.B. Saunders.

Aorta

SIMON C. WHITAKER

ANATOMY

The **ascending aorta** begins at the aortic valve, at the level of T8. It is about 5 cm long and 3–3.5 cm in diameter. There are three recesses, the sinuses of Valsalva, in the aortic root, which accommodate the aortic valve leaflets. The right coronary artery arises from the anterior sinus and the left coronary from the left posterior sinus. Spiral section of the truncus arteriosus during fetal development results in the formation of the ascending aorta and the pulmonary trunk, which spiral around each other in the anterior mediastinum. The aortic valve lies posterior and to the right of the pulmonary valve. The right atrium lies to the right of the aortic root and the left atrium posteriorly. The ascending aorta passes briefly to the right of the midline, where the superior vena cava lies first posteriorly and then to its right, before passing back towards the left, anterior to the trachea, to become the aortic arch at about the level of T4. The pulmonary artery winds posteriorly around the left side of the ascending aorta, so that the pulmonary artery bifurcation lies posterior and to the left of the aorta. The right main pulmonary artery continues this spiral path by passing behind the ascending aorta and superior vena cava to reach the right hilum.

The **aortic arch** gives rise to three major branches which are the right brachiocephalic artery (which divides into the right common carotid and subclavian arteries), the left common carotid and the left subclavian artery (Fig. 26.1). This order of branching is found in 70 per cent of the population. Other variations include a common origin for the right brachiocephalic and the left common carotid arteries (13 per cent), origin of the left common carotid artery from the right

Figure 26.1 *Arch aortogram showing the normal branching anatomy of the thoracic aorta. The branches are, in order, the right brachiocephalic artery (B), the left carotid artery (LC) and the left subclavian artery (LS). AA = ascending thoracic aorta; DA = descending thoracic aorta; RC = right common carotid artery; I = internal carotid arteries; V = vertebral arteries; RS = right subclavian artery.*

brachiocephalic artery (9 per cent), and right and left brachiocephalic arteries (less than 1 per cent). Rarely (in less than 1 per cent), the right subclavian artery arises as the most distal aortic branch, passing to the right side behind the oesophagus.

The descending **thoracic aorta** commences at the aortic isthmus, at about the level of T4. From this level, the aorta descends along the left anterolateral aspects of the thoracic vertebral bodies towards the aortic hiatus in the diaphragm, at the level of T11. Mild, asymptomatic narrowing at the aortic isthmus may persist into adult life. Symptomatic stenosis is known as coarctation (see below). A localized bulge of the aorta just beyond the isthmus, known as a ductus diverticulum (see Fig. 26.10b, p. 653), may be seen in up to 33 per cent of patients. The oesophagus runs along the anterior surface of the descending thoracic aorta as it passes posterior to the left pulmonary artery, the left main bronchus, the left pulmonary veins and the posterior aspect of the heart. The descending aorta is related to the vertebral column along its medial aspect and to pleura and lung laterally and posteriorly. The descending thoracic aorta has both intercostal and bronchial branches. The third to eleventh intercostal arteries arise from the descending aorta posteriorly. Only nine pairs of intercostal arteries arise from the aorta, because the first and second intercostal arteries derive their supply from the subclavian artery via the costocervical trunk and superior intercostal artery. The artery of Adamkiewicz is an important vessel that feeds the lower portion of the anterior spinal artery. It arises from a lower intercostal or lumbar artery (more commonly on the left) at a variable level from T6 to L2. Paraplegia is a recognized risk of the repair of thoracic and, to a lesser degree, abdominal aortic aneurysms because of compromise to this vessel. The upper intercostal vessels may also give small branches to the anterior spinal artery. The bronchial arteries, usually one or two on each side, arise from the anterior aspect of the descending thoracic aorta at about the level of T5 and T6. The descending aorta is approximately 30 cm in length and 2.5 cm in diameter.

The **abdominal aorta** continues from the level of the aortic hiatus in the diaphragm to the aortic bifurcation at the level of L4, where it divides into right and left common iliac arteries. It has important branches, which supply the abdominal viscera. Anteriorly it gives rise to the small inferior phrenic arteries, the coeliac artery (which divides into common hepatic, splenic and left gastric branches), the superior mesenteric and the inferior mesenteric arteries. The renal arteries arise from the lateral aspects of the aorta at about the level of L2. The gonadal arteries arise anteriorly a short distance below this level. Posteriorly arise the paired lumbar arteries and, close to the bifurcation, the median sacral artery. Anteriorly, the aorta is crossed by the left renal vein and the third part of the duodenum (which pass between it and the superior mesenteric artery). The pancreas and the splenic vein also cross over the aorta but are separated from it by the superior

mesenteric artery. Inferiorly, the aorta is crossed by the root of the mesentery. The inferior vena cava is closely applied to the right side of the aorta. Posteriorly, the abdominal aorta is in close proximity to the lumbar vertebrae throughout its length. The abdominal aorta is usually 2.0–2.3 cm in diameter.

METHODS OF IMAGING THE AORTA

Various methods are available for imaging the aorta.

PLAIN RADIOGRAPHS

Radiological investigation of aortic disease should always include posteroanterior and lateral radiographs of the chest. The thoracic aorta is well shown on plain films because of its proximity to lung. Calcification and dilatation of the aorta are readily demonstrated. An abnormal contour of the aorta may be a valuable clue in conditions such as blunt trauma to the chest, coarctation and aortic aneurysm. Associated pathology may be visible, such as mediastinal widening, displacement of mediastinal structures, pleural effusion, left ventricular hypertrophy or cardiac failure.

ULTRASOUND

Echocardiography is useful for the examination of the aortic valve and the aortic root, but has poor ability to demonstrate the ascending aorta or the aortic arch, because of the interposed ribs and lungs. Glimpses of the arch may be seen in some patients from a supraclavicular view, and of the descending aorta from a posterior intercostal view. **Transoesophageal echocardiography** addresses these problems by placing the ultrasound transducer in close proximity to the aorta. Biplane or multiplane probes with frequencies of 5–7 MHz are used and can provide high-resolution, real-time images of most of the thoracic aorta, with the exception of part of the distal ascending aorta, which is always invisible because of interposition of the trachea. It is possible to perform transoesophageal eachocardiography at the patient's bedside. It is, however, an invasive procedure that requires a skilled operator, and is inappropriate in some clinical contexts, such as severe facial or cervical trauma.

Abdominal ultrasound of the abdominal aorta is a simple examination that is readily available. It is the usual method for confirmation and measurement of abdominal aortic aneurysm. The aorta is imaged in axial, sagittal or coronal planes using probes with frequencies in the range of 3–4 MHz. Examination of

(a)

(b)

Figure 26.2 *Three-dimensional contrast-enhanced magnetic angiography of the abdominal aorta: (a) anterior view; (b) lateral view. In this case there is an enormous aneurysm of the upper abdominal aorta (A), just above the level of the coeliac artery (C). R = renal arteries; I = common iliac arteries; L = lumbar arteries; S = superior mesenteric artery. (By courtesy of Dr C.N. Ludman, University Hospital Nottingham.)*

the abdominal aorta should also include an assessment of the kidneys (for hydronephrosis) and of the iliac arteries (for iliac aneurysms). Ultrasound is not reliable for the detection of some aortic pathology, particularly retroperitoneal haemorrhage (in the context of ruptured aortic aneurysm) and luminal conditions such as aortic dissection. Doppler ultrasound of the abdominal aorta is difficult because it is deeply placed and therefore difficult to image with angled probe. Both grey-scale and Doppler ultrasound of the abdominal aorta may be significantly limited in obese patients and by bowel gas.

Intravascular ultrasound produces high-resolution axial images of the aorta. The probe consists of a high-frequency rotating transducer mounted at the tip of an arterial catheter, introduced through a sheath in the common femoral artery. The abdominal and descending aorta are readily examined with this technique but the ascending aorta is not well shown. The examination is invasive and usually performed in conjunction with aortography to clarify equivocal findings or to guide complex interventions, such as the placement of endovascular stent-grafts. The cost of the transducers (which are for one-time use only) is a limitation to the use of this modality.

COMPUTED TOMOGRAPHY

Computed tomography (CT) is an excellent method for visualization of any segment of the aorta as well as its major branches. It is quick, minimally invasive and well tolerated. Anaesthetized patients can usually be accommodated without difficulty, making CT especially useful in the context of severe trauma. Intravenous contrast is required in most cases, however, so it is less suitable for patients with impaired renal function or contrast sensitivity. **Spiral CT** is particularly valuable for vascular imaging for it allows rapid acquisition of image data during the time frame of a single breath-hold. This ensures maximal enhancement of blood vessels and minimal movement artefact. The data may be subsequently reformatted in a variety of ways for two- or three-dimensional viewing (see Fig. 1.13, p. 11).

MAGNETIC RESONANCE IMAGING

Magnetic resonance imaging (MRI) can be used to image the aorta and its branches, with or without the use of intravenous paramagnetic contrast agents. Non-enhanced techniques include simple black-blood, spin-echo T1-weighted sequences, bright blood gradient-recalled-echo (GRE) sequences, time-of-flight magnetic resonance angiography (MRA) and phase contrast MRA. Phase contrast techniques allow flow velocity and volume measurements to be made. Studies of the thoracic aorta usually require cardiac gating to compensate for cardiac motion. This increases the acquisition time and is also difficult in those patients with cardiac arrhythmias. Flow-dependent techniques show reduced vessel-background contrast in low-flow states, and difficulty may be encountered in visualization of vessels that run in the plane of the image owing to progressive saturation and signal loss. With refinements of hardware and sequence design, much faster image acquisition is possible with cardiac gated, segmented k-space GRE techniques. These can produce multiple frames of a cine sequence during a single breath-hold and are likely to be especially valuable for cardiac imaging.

Three-dimensional contrast MRA techniques overcome most of the difficulties encountered with the non-contrast-enhanced methods. Gadolinium, bound to a chelator, is the usual contrast agent as it has a good safety profile and produces excellent signal enhancement. Following intravenous injection, such agents ultimately equilibrate between the circulating blood and the extra-cellular fluid; however, for the first few minutes they will be largely contained within the blood volume. This produces selective enhancement of the delivering vein first, then of the right side of the heart and the pulmonary tree, the arterial tree, and finally all arterial and venous structures as recirculation occurs. The thoracic or abdominal aorta can be imaged within the time frame of a single breath-hold and without the need for cardiac gating. Because the technique is not flow-dependent, the problems of slow-flow artefacts and signal loss within in-plane vessels are eliminated. The data, which is acquired as a three-dimensional block, can be viewed as two-dimensional sections or as three-dimensional reconstructions that can be oriented to any desired viewpoint (Fig. 26.2). Subtraction techniques can also be used to increase the vessel-background contrast.

MRI is contraindicated in patients who have cardiac pacemakers, ferromagnetic intracranial surgical clips or metallic intraocular foreign bodies. The presence of metallic implants (e.g. orthopaedic prostheses, vascular stents) may severely degrade images in their vicinity because of signal loss.

AORTOGRAPHY

For many years, intra-arterial aortography, with either cut-film or digital subtraction angiography, has been the definitive method of aortic imaging. Even now, with modern CT and MRA techniques, it still plays a central role in both diagnostic and interventional radiology of the aorta. Intravenous digital subtraction angiography (IV-DSA) has been used extensively for aortic imaging, but it is still an invasive technique very dependent upon cardiac output and easily affected by patient movement. In many circumstances, diagnostically superior images can now be obtained with MRA or CT.

THORACIC AORTA

ANOMALIES OF THE AORTIC ARCH

Right-sided aortic arch occurs as an isolated anomaly in 0.1 per cent of the population (Fig. 26.3). The pattern of branching of the major vessels follows one of two patterns. The order of origin of the major branches from the arch is unchanged, so that the left subclavian artery is the last branch. This vessel then passes to the left behind the oesophagus. By comparison, the mirror-image right-sided aortic arch has as its first branch the left brachiocephalic, followed by the right common carotid and finally the right subclavian artery. This pattern has strong association with cyanotic congenital heart disease, particularly truncus arteriosus, tetralogy of Fallot and tricuspid atresia.

Rarely, a **double aortic arch** may exist.

Pseudocoarctation is a congenital deformity of the aorta, which shows elongation of the distal part of the arch. There is no significant pressure gradient and the features of brachiofemoral blood pressure discrepancy and rib notching, seen in true coarctation, are absent. On the posteroanterior chest radiograph there appear to be two aortic knuckles whereas, on the lateral view, the arch is M-shaped. The condition is associated with other congenital anomalies such as bicuspid aortic valve.

COARCTATION

Coarctation refers to congenital narrowing of the thoracic aorta in the region of the isthmus and is present in 5–8 per cent of all congenital heart defects. It is usually classified into **pre-** and **postductal types**, depending upon the position of the stenosis relative to the ductus arteriosus. The condition is more common in males and has important associations with bicuspid aortic valve and with aneurysms of the circle of Willis. In severe cases, cardiac failure may occur in the neo-natal period, but most patients are asymptomatic at the time of detection. Symptoms are usually related to cardiac failure, bacterial endocarditis, aortic dissection or intracranial haemorrhage from a ruptured aneurysm.

Figure 26.3 *Chest radiograph showing a right-sided aortic arch (arrows).*

Clinical features include a cardiac murmur, hypertension and a systolic blood pressure difference between the arms and legs. Early detection and repair of coarctation in childhood is important because of its association with premature cardiovascular disease in the adult.

The **chest radiograph** may show a dimple in the lateral aspect of the aortic arch at the site of the coarct and, in severe cases, there may be evidence of cardiac failure. The classic radiological sign of coarctation is notching of the ribs (Fig. 26.4) owing to erosion of the inferior surfaces of the ribs by the pulsation of enlarged and tortuous intercostal arteries. These, in tandem with the subclavian and internal mammary arteries, act as collateral supply to the aorta below the coarctation. Rib notching is not usually seen until the patient is about 10 years old and normally affects the fourth to eighth ribs bilaterally.

Most patients will require treatment, preceded by detailed radiological assessment of the site and severity of the coarctation. **Aortography** with measurement of the pressure gradient across the coarctation has long been the principal investigation for this purpose (Fig. 26.5) but non-invasive assessment with MRI is becoming more widely accepted as the method of choice. Gadolinium contrast-enhanced **MRA** can provide excellent detail regarding the site and extent of the stenosis (Fig. 26.6), and phase-contrast MRA can provide functional information in the form of velocity measurements within the jet caused by the coarct. Cranial MRA, to look for aneurysms of the circle of Willis, may also be performed at the same time. Echocardiography should be undertaken in all patients to look for bicuspid aortic valve

Interventional radiology. There is controversy regarding the optimum treatment for coarctation.

Figure 26.4 *Coarctation. The chest radiograph shows the classic erosion of undersurfaces of the ribs due to pulsation of enlarged, tortuous intercostal arteries (arrows).*

Figure 26.5 *Arch aortogram showing the site of the coarctation (arrow).*

Percutaneous balloon dilatation and dilatation combined with insertion of a metal stent are alternatives to conventional surgical repair.

Figure 26.6 *Three-dimensional contrast-enhanced MR angiogram. The coarctation (straight arrow) is sited just beyond the enlarged left subclavian artery (S). Large collaterals have formed (curved arrows) which communicate with the intercostal arteries beyond the coarct. PA = pulmonary artery; Ao = ascending aorta.*

THORACIC AORTIC ANEURYSM

A quarter of aortic aneurysms occur above the diaphragm; 70 per cent of thoracic aneurysms are due to atherosclerosis, 15 per cent are traumatic and the rest are due to rare conditions such as syphilis, mycotic aneurysms, Marfan's disease and Takayasu's arteritis.

True aneurysms result from local or diffuse weakening of the aortic wall due to degeneration of medial elastic fibres, and are bounded by the aortic intima. **False aneurysms** are usually secondary to trauma and are due to a breach in one or more layers of the aortic wall. They are bounded by adventitia, perivascular connective tissue or haematoma. Aneurysms may be saccular or fusiform in shape, saccular aneurysms having the greater risk of rupture.

Degenerative (atherosclerotic) aneurysm

Atherosclerosis is now the commonest cause of aortic aneurysm. Atherosclerotic aneurysms are more common in the abdominal aorta than in the thorax but may occur at the aortic arch or in the descending thoracic aorta. They are more common in males, with increasing age and in patients with hypertension. The

Figure 26.7 *Thoracic aortic aneurysm. (a) Chest radiograph showing dilatation of the descending portion of the thoracic aorta (arrows).*

presence of a thoracic aneurysm is usually evident on the chest radiograph (Fig. 26.7). CT or MRI is used to demonstrate the size and extent of the aneurysmal sac in patients in whom repair is considered (Fig. 26.8).

Traumatic aneurysm

Thoracic aortic injury occurs as a result of a blunt, decelerating injury to the chest, usually from a road traffic accident. The damage to the aorta is generally

Figure 26.8 *CT scan of the same patient as in Fig. 26.7, confirming aneurysmal dilatation of the thoracic aorta (AN). Compare the diameter of the aorta at this site with that of the ascending aorta (A).*

considered to be due to a differential deceleration of fixed and non-fixed parts of the thoracic aorta, but momentary crushing of the aortic arch between sternum and thoracic spine may also play a part. The type of trauma sustained by the patient is a valuable clue to the possibility of aortic injury. There is focal disruption of one or more layers of the aortic wall. In 90 per cent this occurs at the site of the ligamentum arteriosum, but occasionally the aorta at the level of the aortic valve or pericardial reflection is involved. The result in 85 per cent of cases is death at the scene of the accident with only 15 per cent surviving to reach hospital. In this latter group the adventitia may still be intact, but the majority will still die from delayed rupture, if the aortic injury is not detected and repaired.

The **chest radiograph** is rarely normal in cases of aortic injury. The radiographic signs that may be present are non-specific and indicate mediastinal haematoma, usually owing to associated injury of smaller mediastinal vessels. Signs of aortic rupture include superior mediastinal widening, left apical pleural shadowing, downward displacement of the left main bronchus, tracheal displacement to the right, nasogastric tube displacement, widening of the paraspinal soft tissues and loss of contour of the descending aorta (Fig. 26.9). There may also be evidence of pleural effusion (haemothorax). Fractures of the first or second ribs or of the upper thoracic spine indicate severe thoracic trauma in which aortic injury becomes more probable.

(a)

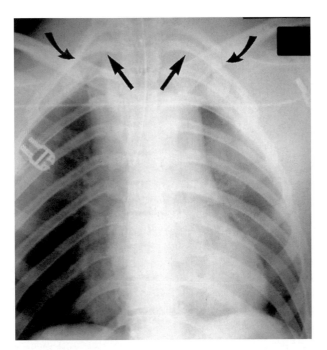

Figure 26.9 *Traumatic rupture of thoracic aorta. The chest radiograph shows bilateral first rib fractures (curved arrows), an indication of severe thoracic trauma. The mediastinum is widened and there are bilateral apical pleural caps owing to haematoma (arrows).*

(b)

Figure 26.10 *Arch aortography for suspected aortic injury in separate patients. (a) Classic appearance of aortic injury owing to blunt, decelerating trauma to the chest, which occurred in a motor vehicle accident. A false aneurysm of the descending aorta (A) is present just beyond the origin of the left subclavian artery (S). The edge of the torn intima is clearly visible (curved arrow). (b) Rupture of the right brachiocephalic artery (curved arrow). The aortic arch itself is intact. A ductus diverticulum (straight arrows) is visible which is a common normal variant.*

The definitive diagnosis of aortic injury is made with contrast-enhanced spiral CT or arch aortography, one of which should be performed without delay whenever the condition is suspected. Only 15 per cent of such examinations are likely to be positive but the low yield is justified by the poor prognosis should the diagnosis be missed.

Spiral CT is performed with overlapping axial images produced at 2–4 mm intervals. From these, oblique sections or three-dimensional images are constructed as appropriate. Direct signs of aortic injury include intimal flaps, thrombus or debris within the aortic lumen, deformity of the aortic contour and tapering of the aortic lumen (pseudo-coarctation). Mediastinal haematoma alone is an indirect sign, which has a high sensitivity but a low specificity for aortic injury.

Arch aortography should include at least two orthogonal views, usually the left and right anterior oblique projections. The usual angiographic finding is the presence of a false aneurysm just distal to the left subclavian artery (Fig. 26.10a) but transverse lucencies representing intimal edges or extravasation of contrast may also be seen.

Transoesophageal echocardiography (TOE) may be helpful in some cases as it can be performed at the bedside. Unfortunately the sensitivity and specificity of TOE in various reports have been disappointing, making it unsuitable as a routine method of investigation. The examination requires a skilled operator and, even then, parts of the thoracic aorta may not be visible. The complication rate of TOE is of the order of 2.9 per cent and it is not suitable for patients with significant facial or cervical injury.

The imaging method that is used will in each case depend upon the local facilities and expertise as well as the nature and extent of other injuries that may be present. Spiral CT is less invasive than angiography and allows the evaluation of non-vascular structures in the chest and other regions of the body at the same examination. However, angiography is still regarded as the standard of reference for the depiction of subtle aortic damage and injury to branch vessels (Fig. 26.10b). The appropriate use of CT can reduce the number of negative aortograms in patients with chest trauma by excluding those who do not have mediastinal haematoma. Angiography should be undertaken if CT shows mediastinal haematoma without definitive evidence of aortic injury.

Interventional radiology

Surgery for thoracic aortic disease is a major undertaking. There is growing interest in endovascular techniques of the repair for both degenerative and traumatic false aneurysms of the thoracic aorta. An endograft is deployed in the thoracic aorta under fluoroscopic guidance using a tubular delivery system advanced through a femoral arteriotomy. Displacement of the partly open graft during deployment, as a result of the large forces exerted on it during systole, is a potential hazard. The deployment sequence of newer systems is very rapid to allow fixation of the graft during diastole. Paraplegia is a risk of both surgical and endovascular methods of repair.

Mycotic aneurysm

These are due to focal destruction of the aortic wall by bacterial infection. The normal aorta is relatively resistant to infection and pre-existing aortic disease, such as atherosclerosis, is usually present. Conditions that predispose to mycotic aneurysms are bacterial endocarditis, intravenous drug abuse, coarctation and local trauma to the vessel (e.g. catheter-related). Infection may also arise from direct spread of an adjacent focus. The commonest sites for mycotic aneurysms in the thoracic aorta are at the sinuses of Valsalva and the ascending aorta. Because the mural destruction is focal, such aneurysms are usually saccular in shape. They may enlarge rapidly and their presence may be suggested by the rapid appearance of aneurysmal dilatation of the aorta between successive chest radiographs (Fig. 26.11). The diagnosis is readily confirmed by CT. Prompt surgical repair is essential because of the very high risk of rupture.

Syphilitic aneurysm

Cardiovascular syphilis is part of the spectrum of tertiary syphilis and is caused by an obliterative endarteritis of the vasa vasorum leading to necrotic changes in the aortic media. Typically, this results in fusiform dilatation of the ascending aorta, which also shows a fine line of calcification within its wall. Dilatation of the aortic valve ring may give rise to aortic regurgitation. With modern methods of treatment of syphilis, this is now a rare cause of thoracic aneurysm.

Marfan's syndrome

This is an inherited autosomal dominant condition in which production of collagen is defective. Cystic medial degeneration in the aorta in patients with Marfan's syndrome leads to widening of the aortic root and valve ring with accompanying aortic insufficiency. This condition also predisposes to aortic dissection (see below). Other hereditary disorders such as Ehlers–Danlos syndrome and homocystinuria may also affect the thoracic aorta.

AORTIC DISSECTION

Aortic dissection occurs when a breech in the intima allows blood under arterial pressure to form an intramural

(a)

(b)

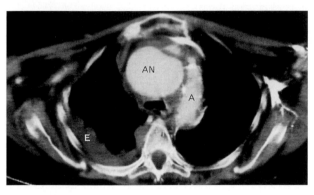

(c)

Figure 26.11 *Mycotic aortic aneurysm. Two chest radiographs (a, b) performed two weeks apart in this patient with salmonella septicaemia show rapid development of mediastinal widening. (c) Contrast-enhanced CT shows the mycotic aneurysm of the aortic arch. The aortic arch (A) is displaced to the left by a large aneurysm sac (AN) arising from the right lateral aspect of the ascending aorta. There is also a right pleural effusion (E), representing some leakage from the aneurysm.*

channel or haematoma. In most cases there is pre-existing degenerative disease of the media owing to atherosclerosis or cystic medial necrosis. Dissection is more commonly seen in male patients over the age of 50. Hypertension, trauma, Marfan's and Ehlers–Danlos syndromes, coarctation, pregnancy, and bicuspid aortic valve and aortic valve surgery all predispose to aortic dissection. The intramural track may burst through the adventitia into the pericardial sac, mediastinum or pleural space, or back through the intima to re-enter the aortic lumen at another site. The dissection may also extend into (and possibly occlude) branches of the aorta, such as the major branches in the chest, the mesenteric and renal arteries in the abdomen, or the iliac arteries.

Aortic dissection may be classified according to two schemes. The first reported was that of DeBakey who proposed three categories:

- type I affecting both ascending and descending aorta;

- type II affecting the aorta proximal to the ligamentum arteriosum only;
- type III affecting the aorta distal to the ligamentum arteriosum only.

In 1970, Dailey and colleagues proposed the simpler Stanford classification of type A (involving the ascending aorta – DeBakey types I and II) and type B (confined to the descending aorta – DeBakey type III). This reflects the usual management strategy of surgical management for type A dissections and conservative management for those of type B.

The presentation of aortic dissection is sudden onset of chest and interscapular back pain and collapse. Other clinical features are determined by adventitial rupture (which may be fatal) or aortic branch occlusion. Involvement of branches of the aortic arch may lead to a blood pressure difference between the arms. Unless the dissection track has involved and occluded one of

(a)   *(b)*

Figure 26.12 *Stanford type B dissection of the thoracic aorta in different patients. (a) CT showing a thin line traversing the descending thoracic aorta (arrows), which is the dissection flap, separating the true and false lumina. (b) Spiral CT with oblique coronal reconstruction clearly showing the true (T) and false (F) lumina. PA = pulmonary artery; LA = left atrium.*

the coronary artery ostia, the ECG is normal. The initial radiological examination is the chest radiograph.

The **chest radiograph** may show evidence of mediastinal haematoma in the form of mediastinal widening (50–70 per cent), left pleural effusion, left apical pleural cap, displacement of the trachea to the right and loss of definition of the aortic arch. Intimal calcification, if present, may be seen to be displaced into the aortic lumen. Confirmation of the diagnosis made by echocardiography, angiography, contrast-enhanced CT or MRI.

Two-dimensional echocardiography is quick, non-invasive and sensitive for dissections that involve the aortic root. The dissection flap is shown within the aortic lumen together with other important features, such as dilatation of the valve ring, aortic regurgitation or pericardial effusion. More distal dissections will not be visible unless biplane **transoesophageal echocardiography** is used. With this technique, the ultrasound probe is introduced into the oesophagus and is therefore in close proximity to the heart and great vessels. The accuracy of diagnosis that can be achieved is comparable to CT with the advantages that additional information, such as the presence of aortic regurgitation, is gained, and that the examination can take place at the bedside.

In most centres, **contrast-enhanced CT** will be the method of diagnosis. This must be performed with care to avoid false-negative studies. Adequate opacification of the aorta is essential and various methods have been described to achieve this. The usual technique is to inject a large volume of contrast (100–150 ml of

300–340 mg/ml iodine) via a cannula in the antecubital vein, while axial scans are performed from just above the arch to the level of the diaphragm. Spiral CT is particularly useful in aortic dissection as the entire thorax may be scanned in one breath-hold with greater and more uniform contrast enhancement of the aortic lumen.

Aortic dissection is shown as a thin band traversing the aortic lumen when the true and false channels are both patent (Fig. 26.12). The dissection flap may be quite thin and easily confused with linear artefacts that are commonly present. Where any doubt exists, a repeat scan concentrating at the level in question should be performed for clarification. If the false lumen has thrombosed, the dissection is seen as a non-opacified crescent around the edge of the true lumen (Fig. 26.13). This appearance should not be confused with a crescentic artefact which may be seen in the ascending aorta on spiral CT images (Fig. 26.14). The presence of mediastinal haematoma, pleural or pericardial effusion may also be visible. If a dissection of the descending aorta is found, the scan can be continued into the abdomen to look for renal and mesenteric involvement.

For many years, **arch aortography** has been the mainstay of diagnosis, but is now superseded by CT for the initial assessment. The intimal flap may be visible as a thin radiolucent line within the aortic lumen, or there may be distortion of the true lumen by a thrombosed false channel. It is also possible to identify aortic regurgitation and involvement of aortic branches. There are a number of potential diagnostic pitfalls and the examination must be performed carefully by an experienced operator.

Figure 26.13 *Dissection of the thoracic aorta: in this case there is thrombosis of the false lumen, which is seen as a non-enhanced crescent of thrombus at the periphery of the aortic lumen (F). This feature is well demonstrated in the ascending aorta, indicating a Stanford type A dissection. The dissection also continues into the descending aorta (arrows). P = pulmonary artery; T = true lumen. (By courtesy of Dr I. Davidson, University Hospital Nottingham.)*

Figure 26.14 *Spiral CT artefacts that simulate aortic dissection. Movement of the ascending aorta during data acquisition can produce crescents (straight arrows) and linear defects at the lumen edge (curved arrows). In this case examination of adjacent slices (which were normal) confirmed that both features were artefacts.*

MRI is also an excellent modality for imaging the thoracic aorta. Conventional T1-weighted, cardiac gated spin-echo images provide good detail but are time-consuming. Segmented k-space techniques or 3D contrast-enhanced MRA also provide excellent image quality within the time frame of a single breath-hold.

Interventional radiology

In some cases the false lumen of an aortic dissection is a blind ending sac, which compromises the true lumen to the extent that ischaemic symptoms, such as renal failure, mesenteric ischaemia or spinal cord ischaemia, occur. In this circumstance, clinical improvement may be obtained by deliberately creating a hole in the dissection flap by interventional techniques, a procedure known as **fenestration**. Once such a communication is established, it can be enlarged with balloon dilatation or stenting.

INFLAMMATORY DISEASE

Takayasu's disease is a form of autoimmune vasculitis that may affect the thoracic aorta, abdominal aorta, aortic branches or the pulmonary arteries in various combinations. Females are affected eight times more commonly than men. It has a worldwide distribution but is commonest in young oriental females. Fibrosis and degeneration of elastic fibres in the media occur together with thickening of the adventitia and intima. Symptoms commence in adolescence with fevers, malaise, pain and fatigue. Bruits may be audible and hypertension or cardiac failure may occur. The chest radiograph is usually unhelpful but may show rib notching or aortic calcification (Fig. 26.15). Angiography shows various combinations of stenoses of the aorta or its branches and saccular or fusiform dilatation of the aorta, usually of its ascending portion.

ABDOMINAL AORTA

ABDOMINAL AORTIC ANEURYSM

Abdominal aortic aneurysm may be asymptomatic or present as an acute abdomen following rupture. Occasionally, an abdominal aortic aneurysm may produce emboli to the legs, resulting in lower limb ischaemia. The incidence of asymptomatic abdominal

(a)   (b)

Figure 26.15 *Takayasu's arteritis. (a) Chest radiograph of a 45-year-old female patient showing calcification of both ascending (straight arrows) and descending (curved arrows) thoracic aorta. (b) Contrast-enhanced MRA of the upper abdominal aorta showing an irregular stenosis at the level of the renal arteries (arrow). C = coeliac axis; S = superior mesenteric artery.*

aortic aneurysms greater than 4 cm in diameter in the 55–75 year age group is 2–3 per cent. Ruptured aneurysm has a mortality rate of 75–95 per cent and accounts for some 10 000 deaths per year in England and Wales. The likelihood of aneurysm rupture increases as the aneurysm increases in size, and surgery is usually planned once the aneurysm diameter exceeds 5.5 cm.

Conventional surgical aneurysm repair is a major undertaking, which, in specialist units, has a mortality rate of between 1 and 7 per cent. This figure can be significantly higher in non-specialist units. Techniques for endovascular repair of abdominal aortic aneurysms are now available. Over half of patients with abdominal aortic aneurysm have coronary artery disease and serious, potentially fatal complications of surgery are usually cardiovascular in nature, precipitated by the tremendous change in haemodynamics that occurs with aortic clamping and unclamping.

Some 5–15 per cent of abdominal aneurysms are **inflammatory aneurysms**. These are characterized by the accumulation of fibrotic inflammatory tissue around the outside of the aneurysm wall. The inflammatory tissue is glistening and pearly white in external appearance and shows lymphocytic infiltration micro-

scopically. Fibrosis and adhesions may lead to complications such as renal hydronephrosis. The aetiology of the inflammatory aneurysm is uncertain but it appears to be an immune response, possibly to atheromatous material in the aortic wall. Open surgical repair is more difficult for inflammatory aneurysms, and is associated with an increased morbidity and mortality in this condition. Abdominal aortic aneurysms are frequently associated with aneurysms elsewhere, particularly the iliac and popliteal arteries and the thoracic aorta.

An **aneurysm** may be detected on a **plain abdominal radiograph** as a soft-tissue density with a thin peripheral rim of calcium (Fig. 26.16). Aneurysms may also be detected or assessed at ultrasound, CT or angiography.

Ultrasound is used for the initial diagnosis and measurement of abdominal aortic aneurysms (Fig. 26.17a). Aneurysms that are not large enough to warrant repair may be monitored by serial ultrasound examinations. Associated complications such as hydronephrosis should be identified together with potential risk factors for surgery, such as inflammatory change or the presence of a horseshoe kidney. When aneurysmal dilatation of the aorta is detected, a search should be also made for aneurysms of the iliac, femoral and popliteal arteries.

Figure 26.16 *Aortic aneurysm. Plain abdominal radiograph showing calcification in the walls of aortic and left iliac artery aneurysms.*

Abdominal aortic aneurysms are readily demonstrated with **CT** (Fig. 26.17b), and the examination is largely unaffected by patient obesity or excessive bowel gas, which makes ultrasound examination difficult. Inflammatory aneurysms are characterized by a rind of soft-tissue density around their lateral and anterior aspects (Fig. 26.18) and they may be associated with hydronephrosis. Aortic diameter is, of course, easily measured but the real power of this modality lies in the ability of spiral CT to demonstrate the three-dimensional anatomy of the aneurysm neck, the aneurysm itself and the iliac arteries in a single examination. This information is becoming increasingly important with the advent of endovascular techniques of aneurysm repair, for both case selection and procedure planning.

Aortic aneurysms may be identified on the initial frames of a femoral **angiogram** performed for lower limb ischaemia. The lumen may be obviously widened (Fig. 26.19), but the angiogram does not give a true impression of the external diameter of the aneurysm because of the variable amount of mural thrombus that may be present. Indeed, the aorta may look almost normal in calibre, the clue to the presence of an aneurysm being the thin rim of calcification that marks the true site of the aortic wall. Angiography should be performed with care

(a)

(b)

Figure 26.17 *Abdominal aortic aneurysm (a) Ultrasound. The arrows indicate the lateral extent of the aneurysm. (b) Intravenous contrast-enhanced CT in the same patient. T = thrombus lining the aneurysm sac; L = patent aortic lumen; I = inferior vena cava; V = vertebral body.*

when an aneurysm is present to avoid dislodging thrombus from the aneurysm sac. Angiography is not usually required prior to conventional surgical repair but often performed prior to endovascular repair.

Ruptured abdominal aortic aneurysm

This presents with acute onset of abdominal and back pain together with collapse. The plain abdominal radiograph will often show characteristic curvilinear

Figure 26.18 *Inflammatory aortic aneurysm. The wall of the aortic aneurysm (A) shows marked thickening (arrows).*

Figure 26.20 *Ruptured aortic aneurysm. In this example, the CT scan shows a large haematoma (H) adjacent to the aortic aneurysm (A).*

Figure 26.19 *Angiography of aortic aneurysm. The contrast shows the lumen only. There is a large amount of thrombus lining the wall, and the true diameter of the aneurysm can only be inferred from the thin line of calcification in the aneurysm wall (arrows).*

calcification in the aneurysm wall, and the psoas muscle outlines may be obscured by retroperitoneal haematoma. The mortality from this condition is high and most patients will die before they reach hospital. The best

chance of survival lies with urgent repair. When an abdominal aneurysm is palpable and the clinical picture is consistent with rupture, further preoperative investigation is usually unnecessary and serves only to delay surgery. Ultrasound is helpful when there is doubt about the diagnosis of aortic aneurysm, for instance in an obese patient. Ultrasound can also detect large retroperitoneal haematomas (and thereby confirm rupture) but does not do so reliably. CT should be employed if there is doubt about the diagnosis of aneurysm rupture (Fig. 26.20).

Interventional radiology

Various techniques for minimally invasive, endovascular aneurysm repair are now available in which a tubular delivery system is used to place an endovascular graft within the aorta using femoral arteriotomies for access. The endograft is constructed from a metal framework which supports a fabric or membranous graft. The endograft can be straight (aorto-uni-iliac) or bifurcated (aorto-bi-iliac) (Fig. 26.21). Correct sizing of the prosthesis for each patient is critical to the success of these procedures and requires careful preoperative assessment of the size and shape of the abdominal aorta and iliac arteries with spiral CT or MRI. For this reason, endovascular aneurysm repair is usually an elective procedure, but there are a growing number of reports of the successful use of this technique for the repair of ruptured aortic aneurysms, for which the mortality rate from open repair is still in the region of 50 per cent.

ATHEROMATOUS DISEASE

Atheromatous disease or occlusion may occur in the abdominal aorta just as in any part of the arterial

(a)

Figure 26.21 *Endovascular aneurysm repair. (a) The prosthesis. A number of different types are now available. The device shown (Zenith Endograft, Cook, Bloomington, USA) consists of synthetic graft material supported by a skeleton of Gianturco metal stents. (b) CT angiography performed after endovascular aneurysm repair, showing the prosthesis in place. In this design, the topmost Gianturco stent is uncovered and is placed above the renal arteries. The wall of the aneurysm is clearly visible because of calcification.*

(b)

system. Symptomatic patients with infrarenal aortic stenosis tend to be female, presenting at a younger age than those with peripheral disease, and they are often heavy smokers. Symptoms include intermittent claudication affecting the buttocks and both legs, impotence in the male, emboli to the feet with gangrenous changes (blue toe syndrome) or severe, critical ischaemia of the lower extremities. Neurological deficit, such as muscle weakness, sensory loss or absent tendon reflexes, may also be found in severe cases. In the absence of both femoral pulses, non-invasive imaging of the aorta should be used first.

Abdominal ultrasound is essential whenever aortoiliac disease is suspected, to look for an unsuspected aortic aneurysm. The abdominal aorta is not ideally suited to **Doppler ultrasound** because of its deep location and, for this reason, Doppler studies may be difficult or impossible in larger patients or in the presence of excessive bowel gas. Despite this drawback, it is possible to identify and differentiate aortoiliac stenosis or occlusion in some patients with Doppler ultrasound. In addition, the presence of significant disease can be confirmed from the flow pattern in the external iliac and common femoral arteries.

Angiography (Fig. 26.22a) or **intravenous digital subtraction angiography** will show the extent of disease and differentiate stenosis from occlusion. **MRA** is proving to be an excellent, non-invasive alternative to IV-DSA. Similarly, **spiral CT** is also capable of producing high-quality images of the lower abdominal aorta, but uses ionizing radiation and requires intravenous contrast.

Interventional radiology

Infrarenal aortic occlusion is usually treated with surgical repair, but there are some reports of successful percutaneous recanalization and stent implantation. Conversely, percutaneous angioplasty, with or without stent insertion, is the treatment of choice for infrarenal aortic stenosis (Fig. 26.22b,c,d). The procedure is technically successful in approximately 85 per cent of cases and the clinical patency rate is approximately 72 per cent at 5 years. Potential complications such as distal embolization or aortic rupture have been reported but are rare. The 5-year clinical patency rate is less than that for aortic surgery but the risk of early major complication is less.

AORTOENTERIC FISTULA

A direct communication between the aortic lumen and the gastrointestinal tract is a rare but potentially fatal *(a)*   *(b)*   *(c)*   *(d)*

Figure 26.22 *Stenosis of the abdominal aorta treated with angioplasty and an expandable metallic stent. (a) Initial angiogram showing a short, tight stenosis of the mid-abdominal aorta (arrow). Well-developed collaterals are present. (b) Following deployment of a metal stent (Wallstent, Boston Scientific). The stent shows a pronounced waist at the level of the stenosis (arrow). (c) Dilatation of the stent and stenosis with an angioplasty balloon. (d) Completion angiography.*

cause of gastrointestinal bleeding. The condition most commonly occurs in those patients who have previously had an abdominal aortic aneurysm repair, particularly if the graft has become infected. The fistula usually communicates between the proximal anastomotic suture line of the graft and the third part of the duodenum. Primary aortoenteric fistulae may also occur, usually in association with an aortic aneurysm. Despite the potential for severe, life-threatening haematemesis and melaena, there is often a history of small episodes of gastrointestinal bleeding, which should always raise the possibility of the diagnosis when there has been previous aortic surgery or if an aneurysm is palpable. Preoperative diagnosis can be difficult. Endoscopy should be the preliminary investigation but may fail to identify the fistula if the third part of the duodenum cannot be reached. Other potentially useful investigations are barium meal, CT or aortography with a lateral series to demonstrate the anterior aortic wall. False-negative imaging is not uncommon in aortoenteric fistula and the diagnosis may not be confirmed until laparotomy.

FURTHER READING

Audet, P., Therasse, E., Oliva, V.L. *et al.* 1998: Infra-renal aortic stenosis: long-term clinical and hemodynamic results of percutaneous transluminal angioplasty. *Radiology* **209**, 357–63.

Boxerman, J.L., Mosher, T.J., McVeigh, E.R., Atalar, E., Lima, J.A.C., Bluemke, D.A. 1988: Advanced MR imaging techniques for evaluation of the heart and great vessels. *Radiographics* **18**, 543–64.

Dailey, P.O., Trueblood, H.W., Stinson, E.B., Wuerflein, R.D., Shunway, N.E. 1970: Management of acute aortic dissection. *Annals of Thoracic Surgery* **10**, 2373–47.

DeBakey, M.E., Henly, W.S., Colley, D.A., Morris, G.C. Jr, Crawford, E. Beall, A.C. 1965: Surgical management of dissecting aneurysms of the thoracic aorta. *Journal of Thoracic & Cardiovascular Surgery* **49**, 130–49.

Kuhlman, J.E., Pozniak, M.A., Collins, J., Knisely, B. 1998: Radiographic and CT findings of blunt chest trauma: aortic injuries and looking beyond them. *Radiographics* **18**, 1085–106.

Mitchell, R.S., Miller, D.C., Dake, M.D., Semba, C.P., Moore, K.A., Sakai, T. 1999: Thoracic aortic aneurysm repair with an endovascular stent graft: the 'first generation'. *Annals of Thoracic Surgery* **67**, 1971–4.

Patel, N.H., Stephens, J.E. Jr, Mirvis, S.E., Shanmuganathan, K., Mann, F.A. 1998: Imaging of acute thoracic aortic injury due to blunt trauma: A review. *Radiology* **209**, 335–48.

Prince, M.R., Grist, T.M., Debatin, J.F. 1999: *3D contrast MR angiography*. New York, NY: Springer Verlag.

Slonim, S.M., Miller, D.C., Mitchell, R.S., Semba, C.P., Razavi,

M.K., Dake, M.D. 1999: Percutaneous balloon fenestration and stenting for life-threatening ischemic complications in patients with acute aortic dissection. *Journal of Thoracic & Cardiovascular Surgery* **117**, 1118–26.

Suarez de Lezo, J., Pan, M., Romero, M. *et al.* 1999: Immediate and follow-up findings after stent treatment for severe coarctation of aorta. *American Journal of Cardiology* **83**, 400–6.

27

Veins

SIMON C. WHITAKER

ANATOMY AND METHODS OF IMAGING

The venous system may be assessed by venography, ultrasound, computed tomography (CT) or magnetic resonance imaging (MRI). The presence of thrombus may also be imaged with isotope scintigraphy and MRI.

VENOGRAPHY

A venogram is a series of radiographs of one or more veins, taken as radiopaque contrast medium is injected into a tributary. The technique of the examination varies according to the part of the venous system being studied.

LOWER LIMB VENOGRAPHY

The examination is performed in a fluoroscopy room with a tilting table. A tourniquet is applied at the ankle and a cannula inserted into a suitable vein on the dorsum of the foot. Leaving the ankle tourniquet in place to occlude the superficial veins and encourage preferential filling of the deep system, 50 ml of non-ionic contrast agent are injected by hand with a head-up table tilt of about 45° to slow dissipation of the contrast agent. The process is observed with fluoroscopy and, when opacification is sufficient, frontal and oblique radiographs are taken of the calf together with frontal views of the knee and thigh (Fig. 27.1). Finally, a film of the pelvis is taken as the patient is returned to the horizontal position and the leg elevated, to show the iliac veins and lower inferior vena cava (IVC).

Modifications to this technique have been used for the investigation of chronic venous disease. **Descending venography**, used to demonstrate incompetence of the deep veins or of the long saphenous vein, requires cannulation of the common femoral vein, following which contrast agent is injected as the patient performs a Valsalva manoeuvre. **Varicography** involves injection of contrast agent directly into superficial varicose veins in order to identify individual perforating veins.

Normal appearances

In the normal subject there are three columns of veins in the calf, which are medial to lateral posterior tibial, peroneal and anterior tibial veins (Fig. 27.1). The veins are usually paired and run alongside their respective arteries. The popliteal and superficial femoral veins are usually single, but these may also be duplicated as variations in venous anatomy are common. The common femoral vein is formed a few centimetres below the inguinal ligament by the confluence of the deep and superficial femoral veins. In the pelvis, the external and internal iliac veins join to form the common iliac veins, which pass over their corresponding arteries to unite at the level of L5 forming the IVC. The long and short saphenous veins constitute the superficial venous system of the leg. The long saphenous passes medially in the calf and thigh to join with the

Figure 27.1 *Lower limb venogram. Normal study showing contrast within the calf veins and the popliteal vein. The valves in the calf veins are clearly seen.*

Figure 27.2 *Inferior vena cavogram. An angiographic catheter has been placed via the right common femoral vein with its tip at the confluence of the iliac veins. The arrow indicates the position of the left renal vein, shown by the stream of unopacified blood entering the IVC.*

common femoral vein via the saphenous opening in the deep fascia. The short saphenous vein passes posteriorly in the calf and usually joins the popliteal vein just above the level of the knee joint. The saphenous veins and their superficial tributaries communicate with the deep veins via a number of small perforating veins.

Both superficial and deep venous systems of the leg contain valves, which allow flow in a cranial direction only. Perforating veins also contain valves, which allow flow from superficial to deep veins.

Contraindications and complications

The risk of serious complication following venography with modern contrast agents is remote and consequently there are few contraindications to the procedure. However, the use of intravenous contrast does carry a small risk of adverse reaction to the agent. The development of deep vein thrombosis, as a consequence of lower limb venography, is a rare but recognized complication when ionic contrast agents are used. It has also been reported following non-ionic contrast but, even if a causal relationship does exist, the risk is very much smaller when non-ionic agents are used.

PELVIC VENOGRAPHY AND INFERIOR VENA CAVOGRAPHY

The pelvic veins and the lower IVC are normally shown in a good quality conventional lower limb venogram. To show these structures specifically, a short cannula is placed in the femoral vein using the Seldinger technique. Sequential radiographs of the pelvis are taken as contrast medium is injected by hand or by using a pump. Simultaneous injection into both common femoral veins may be made if both sides of the pelvis are to be examined. Where the IVC is the principal interest, contrast injection may be made using a pigtail catheter placed at the confluence of the common iliac veins (Fig. 27.2). Intravenous catheters should be used with caution in the pelvic veins and the IVC when proximal deep vein thrombosis is suspected, to avoid dislodgement of thrombus and subsequent pulmonary embolism.

The IVC receives lumbar veins, the right gonadal vein, two renal veins (the left renal vein receiving the left adrenal and gonadal veins), right adrenal vein, hepatic veins and phrenic veins, before passing through the caval opening in the diaphragm at the level of T8.

SUPERIOR VENA CAVOGRAPHY

In a similar manner to inferior vena cavography, the superior vena cava (SVC) can be demonstrated by contrast injection into one or both median antecubital veins, or by injection at its origin using a catheter inserted from either arm.

The SVC is quite short and is the final common pathway for venous drainage from the head, neck and upper limbs, being formed by the junction of the right and left brachiocephalic veins. Its single tributary is the azygos vein, which ascends alongside the lower thoracic vertebral bodies passing forwards in the right lateral aspect of the mediastinum, passing the origin of the right main bronchus and entering the SVC posteriorly.

UPPER LIMB VENOGRAPHY

To demonstrate the axillary and subclavian veins, a cannula is inserted into the ipsilateral median ante-cubital vein, and sequential images of the shoulder/upper chest are taken as contrast is injected with the patient supine. To show the forearm veins, the injection may be made into a vein on the dorsum of the hand with a tourniquet around the upper arm.

VISCERAL VENOGRAPHY

The **hepatic veins** are demonstrated by selective retrograde injection of contrast into one or more of the veins, using a catheter introduced from a femoral vein or from the right internal jugular vein (Fig. 27.3). Measurements of the hepatic venous pressure may be made at the same examination. Pressures recorded when the catheter tip is wedged in a small venous tributary provide an indirect measurement of the portal venous pressure.

The **renal veins** are also shown by selective contrast injection. It is usual to perform an inferior vena cavogram first, to demonstrate any thrombus protruding into the IVC lumen.

The **portal vein** may be demonstrated by indirect or direct transhepatic portography. **Indirect portography** is performed by selective contrast injection into the splenic artery. Images are taken during the venous phase as contrast passes from the spleen into the portal vein. **Direct portography** requires placement of a catheter into the portal vein itself either by a percutaneous transhepatic route or by a transjugular, intrahepatic route (see Figs 27.20 and 27.28). In both cases the portal vein must be patent, so direct portography cannot be used to demonstrate portal vein occlusion.

Figure 27.3 *Hepatic venogram. A catheter has been passed from the femoral vein in the groin, up the IVC and into the hepatic vein.*

Direct portography is technically more difficult than the indirect alternative, and percutaneous transhepatic access carriers a risk of haemorrhage.

Both indirect and direct portography are invasive procedures. They are usually reserved for specific purposes, such as portal vein localization during the TIPSS procedure or portal vein sampling. When the clinical requirement is to determine portal vein patency, ultrasound, CT or MRI offers better, non-invasive alternatives.

CROSS-SECTIONAL IMAGING

ULTRASOUND

Most veins are visible to ultrasound, the one notable exception being the superior vena cava. Doppler and, in particular, colour Doppler ultrasound (Plate 17, opposite p. 358), are important facilities for venous imaging which allow non-invasive demonstration of venous occlusion or venous incompetence. The IVC is normally visible but its orientation, at right angles to the ultrasound probe, makes Doppler assessment of blood flow difficult, except in thin patients. There are no contraindications to its use, but ultrasound may be difficult in obese patients or in the presence of marked oedema. The use of ultrasound is discussed in more detail below.

COMPUTED TOMOGRAPHY

Contrast-enhanced CT can be used to show veins and their neighbouring structures and is particularly useful

Figure 27.4 *Inferior vena cava shown on a CT of the abdomen. I = inferior vena cava; RV = renal vein; A = aorta; SMA = superior mesenteric artery; L = liver; K = right and left kidneys.*

for central venous strictures such as the superior and inferior vena cavae (Fig. 27.4) and the portal vein. Thrombus is identified as a filling defect within the vessel lumen and compression by an adjacent mass is readily demonstrated.

MAGNETIC RESONANCE VENOGRAPHY

Non-contrast-enhanced, time-of-flight and phase contrast MR angiographic techniques are both applicable to venous imaging (Fig. 27.5). Three-dimensional contrast-enhanced methods, either direct or indirect, are also effective. For direct contrast MR venography, heavily diluted contrast is injected into a tributary during image acquisition. Normal strength contrast injected into an antecubital vein is used for indirect venography. Image acquisition is timed to coincide with the venous phase of contrast enhancement, before significant equilibration with extracellular fluid occurs.

(a)

(b)

Figure 27.5 *MR angiography of pelvic veins. (a) Two-dimensional time-of-flight study, showing the pelvic veins and the IVC in a normal patient (EI = external iliac vein; CI = common iliac vein; IVC = inferior vena cava). (b) Three-dimensional contrast-enhanced MR angiography of the upper femoral and pelvic veins showing extensive left iliofemoral deep vein thrombosis. Tramlines of contrast are seen around the clot in the left femoral veins (curved arrows). The left iliac veins do not opacify and there is a filling defect in the lower IVC, which indicates protrusion of thrombus from the left iliac vein orifice (straight arrows). (By courtesy of Dr A. Moody, Department of Academic Radiology, University Hospital Nottingham.)*

IMAGING OF THROMBUS

Venous imaging is frequently directed towards the detection of thrombus as, for instance, in the diagnosis of deep vein thrombosis. Most modalities, such as venography, do so indirectly by focusing on non-thrombosed, normal blood. A new method, involving MRI, produces images of the thrombus itself. The technique relies on the shortening of T1 that occurs in freshly thrombosed blood to produce a high signal, which contrasts with adjacent normal blood and other tissues (Fig. 27.6). Any vein in the body is accessible to MRI in this way and the results in deep vein thrombosis and pulmonary embolism are promising. As the thrombus ages, so the T1 shortening and high signal intensity from the thrombus decline, allowing some measure of the age of the thrombus. This is of potential benefit for the assessment of recurrent symptoms in patients with a previous history of deep vein thrombosis.

VENOUS DISEASE

LOWER LIMB

DEEP VEIN THROMBOSIS

Conditions that predispose to the development of deep vein thrombosis include recent surgery (particularly orthopaedic procedures involving the lower limb), trauma, pregnancy, oral contraceptives, immobility, obesity and malignant disease. The clinical picture at presentation varies depending on the extent of thrombosis. Isolated calf vein thrombosis may present with pain and tenderness in the calf alone but, if the more proximal veins are involved, there will also be oedema of the leg. Very extensive thrombosis produces massive leg oedema and may limit blood flow through the limb to the extent that there is incipient venous infarction and gangrene, a serious condition known as **phlegmasia caerulea dolens**. The long-term consequences of deep vein thrombosis also depend on the extent of the original thrombus. The sequelae of isolated calf vein thrombosis are likely to be minor or non-existent, whereas there is a high incidence of chronic venous disease following involvement of the superficial femoral or more proximal veins. Confirmation of the diagnosis is necessary before commencing treatment with anticoagulants because the accuracy of clinical diagnosis on its own is poor. The usual imaging methods for deep vein thrombosis are venography and ultrasound.

Lower limb venography

Thrombus shows as a serpiginous filling defect within the vessel lumen on the venogram. As clot retraction

Figure 27.6 *Direct thrombus MRI, showing deep vein thrombosis in the left calf (arrows). The technique relies on the T1 shortening that occurs in relatively fresh thrombus. (By courtesy of Dr A. Moody, Department of Academic Radiology, University Hospital Nottingham.)*

occurs, the thrombus does not occupy the entire cross-section of the vein and is outlined by 'tramlines' of contrast between it and the vein wall (Fig. 27.7). When deep vein thrombosis is very extensive, obstruction of the deep veins may be complete, with the result that the venogram shows only a mesh of fine collateral veins with no filling of the main deep veins.

Ultrasound

Deep vein thrombosis may be detected with conventional ultrasound alone. Fresh thrombus is non-echogenic and difficult to distinguish from normal blood, but it quite rapidly becomes echogenic and visible (Fig. 27.8). Thrombus of any age within a vein prevents its collapse when it is subjected to manual compression using the ultrasound probe. This compression test can, with reasonable reliability, detect thrombus in the femoral and popliteal veins, with the exception of the segment within the adductor canal.

Colour Doppler ultrasound increases both the speed and reliability of detection of deep vein thrombosis by ultrasound. Thrombus is shown by an absence of flow, at rest or in response to gentle calf compression, or by flow that is only present in part of the lumen (Plate 18, opposite p. 358). The femoral and popliteal veins are

Figure 27.7 *Lower limb venogram showing thrombus (arrows).*

readily examined with colour Doppler and, in most subjects, the calf veins can also be assessed (Plate 19, opposite p. 358).

The pelvic veins are more difficult to examine with ultrasound because of overlying bowel. If, however, the common femoral vein is patent and shows normal variation in flow with the cardiac and respiratory cycles, it is likely that the iliac veins are patent as well. When there is

Figure 27.8 *Deep vein thrombosis. Ultrasound of the common femoral vein showing the echogenic column of thrombus in the vein lumen (arrows).*

doubt about the integrity of the pelvic veins, a conventional venogram should be performed to resolve the issue.

Doppler ultrasound or venography?

Venography provides excellent visualization of the deep veins and for many years has been the standard investigation for the detection of deep vein thrombosis. There are, however, some important disadvantages to venography:

- Ionizing radiation is used.
- Venepuncture is uncomfortable.
- There is a small risk of complications that may arise as a result of the procedure.
- Children tolerate venography poorly.
- Some causes of lower limb swelling, such as ruptured Baker's cyst (Fig. 27.9) or muscle haematoma, show indirectly nor not at all.

For these reasons venography is now being superseded by Doppler ultrasound.

Advantages of Doppler ultrasound include:

- It is painless and does not carry any risk for the patient.
- Ionizing radiation is not used.
- It is well tolerated, making it ideal for use in children and during pregnancy.
- It is capable of detecting deep venous thrombosis in the femoral and popliteal veins with an accuracy that is close to venography.
- Diagnoses of Baker's cyst, muscle haematoma and other soft-tissue abnormalities that are sometimes mistaken for deep vein thrombosis may be made and the distinction between cellulitis and deep vein thrombosis is usually apparent.

In common with other ultrasound examinations, the success of vascular ultrasound is related to the experience of the operator and the quality of equipment used. Ultrasound of the pelvic veins and the inferior vena cava may be difficult because of overlying bowel gas, and the superior vena cava cannot be seen at all.

Magnetic resonance imaging

MRI can be used to image the thrombus directly (see Fig. 27.6). This technique may be used when other methods are not appropriate, for instance when there is allergy to intravenous contrast material, pregnancy, or when the limb is encased in plaster.

Investigation of aetiology

When extensive deep vein thrombosis involving the iliac veins has occurred in the absence of an obvious

Figure 27.10 *Extrinsic iliac vein compression. Iliac venography via short catheter in the common femoral vein shows a prominent indentation in the lateral aspect of the common iliac vein (arrows) owing to neoplastic lymph node enlargement.*

Figure 27.9 *Baker's cyst. (a) Venography shows lateral deviation of the popliteal vein (arrows). (b) Ultrasound in the same patient confirms rupture of a Baker's cyst (C) with fluid tracking down into the calf. The posterior surface of the tibia has been drawn in.*

for this purpose. CT or MRI may also be helpful, depending on the clinical circumstances.

ASSESSMENT OF VARICOSE VEINS

Varicose veins of the lower limb may be either primary or secondary. The most common cause of secondary venous disease is **deep vein thrombosis**. Whether primary or secondary, superficial varicosities will be associated with one or more **incompetent communications** with the deep venous system, the identification of which is essential for successful treatment. Typical sites of incompetence are the saphenofemoral junction, the saphenopopliteal junction and perforating veins in the thigh (Hunter's veins) or calf. Clinical examination can detect simple saphenofemoral and saphenopopliteal incompetence and the larger perforating veins, but in complex cases (for instance recurrence of varicose veins after surgery) further information will be needed from Doppler ultrasound or venography.

Doppler ultrasound

The patient is first examined supine to show the femoral veins and the saphenofemoral junction. Deep venous or

predisposing cause, it may be appropriate to search for an underlying abnormality, such as an abdominal or pelvic mass compressing the proximal veins (Fig. 27.10). Abdominal ultrasound is a useful starting point

Figure 27.11 *Recurrent long saphenous incompetence following surgery. A tortuous collateral has developed (arrows) that connects the long saphenous vein (arrowheads) to the common femoral vein.*

Figure 27.12 *Incompetent perforating vein. Ultrasound of the calf showing a perforating vein (P) crossing the deep fascia (F and arrows). See also Plate 21 (opposite p. 358).*

saphenofemoral incompetence is shown by asking the patient to perform a Valsalva manoeuvre while the vein is observed with colour Doppler. In normal veins antegrade flow reduces or ceases when the intra-abdominal pressure rises, whereas incompetent veins show reversal of flow (Plate 20, opposite p. 358). Long saphenous incompetence may stem from the saphenofemoral junction or from a mid-thigh perforator. Patients who have had previous saphenofemoral ligation may develop recurrent long saphenous incompetence via new collateral vessels forming between the common femoral vein and the long saphenous vein remnant (Fig. 27.11).

The calf is examined for short saphenous incompetence and the presence of perforating veins with the patient sitting or standing. Perforators are visible as vessels that cross the plane of the deep fascia (Fig. 27.12; Plate 21, opposite p. 358). Those that are clinically significant communicate with subcutaneous varicose vessels and are usually dilated. Most will also show deep to superficial blood flow in response to calf compression, but the flow patterns in varicose veins can be complex, and some significant perforators will be missed if this criterion is used alone.

Venography

Modifications to the technique of lower limb venography have been used for the investigation of chronic venous disease. Tourniquets applied at different levels in the calf during venography may help to determine the level of incompetent perforators. Varicography, performed by injecting contrast material directly into the superficial varicosities, is also used to localize perforators. Descending venography involves the injection of contrast agent into the common femoral vein while the patient performs a Valsalva manoeuvre. The deep or long saphenous veins opacify if they are incompetent.

When used in the assessment of chronic venous disease, both ultrasound and venography require experienced operators but, carefully performed, they will give results that are comparable to each other.

UPPER LIMB

Axillary or subclavian vein thrombosis can occur because of indwelling catheters, extension of central venous thrombosis secondary to mediastinal disease, prothrombotic syndrome or vasculitis, but may also occur in otherwise fit patients. Either Doppler ultrasound or venography (Fig. 27.13). can be used to confirm the diagnosis. Thrombus within the axillary or subclavian veins has the same radiographic or colour Doppler sonographic appearance as it does in the lower limb. Compression ultrasound cannot be used for the axillary and subclavian veins since they are protected from compression by the clavicle.

CENTRAL VEINS

IVC OBSTRUCTION

This occurs as a result of thrombosis or of involvement by adjacent lesions. Thrombosis usually results from **extension of thrombus** from pelvic or lower-limb deep vein thrombosis (Fig. 27.14), but may also arise by extension of clot from other thrombosed tributaries, particularly the renal veins. **Renal tumours** are noted for their ability to spread along the lumen of the renal vein and into the IVC, an event that may also lead to secondary thrombosis. **Adjacent pathologies** may cause narrowing, displacement or obstruction of the IVC.

Figure 27.13 *Axillary vein thrombosis. The brachial vein is patent (arrow) but the axillary vein is occluded by thrombus. A mass of fine collateral veins around the axilla is shown instead.*

Figure 27.15 *Thrombus in a dilated IVC (V) shown on a contrast-enhanced CT. A thin rim of contrast is visible between the thrombus and vein wall.*

Examples include retroperitoneal disease such as lymphadenopathy or retroperitoneal fibrosis, neoplasia such as hepatic, adrenal, renal, duodenal or pancreatic tumours, and other masses such as aortic aneurysms.

Ultrasound and CT are usually the first investigations for the assessment of IVC occlusion. Thrombus can be seen at ultrasound as echogenic luminal material and at contrast-enhanced CT as a non-enhancing defect within the lumen (Fig. 27.15). CT is particularly useful when there is extrinsic involvement of the IVC (Fig. 27.16). In comparison, inferior cavography is invasive and does not give information about the nature and extent of pathology outside the IVC lumen. Inferior

Figure 27.14 *Thrombus within the IVC. Inferior vena cavogram showing thrombus arising out of the left common iliac vein orifice (arrows). The angiographic catheter (curved arrow) has been passed into the IVC from the right common femoral vein.*

Figure 27.16 *Contrast-enhanced CT scan of the abdomen of a child showing an enormous retroperitoneal and para-aortic tumour (T) (neuroblastoma) with anterior displacement of the IVC (V) and aorta (A). The liver (L) is pushed across to the left. The branches of the coeliac axis (arrows) are also displaced.*

cavography is generally performed as a preliminary study prior to the insertion of a vena cava filter (see below).

SUPERIOR VENA CAVAL SYNDROME

Stenosis or occlusion of the SVC leads to the distressing condition of superior vena caval syndrome, characterized by cyanosis and oedema of the head, neck and arms, together with orbital oedema and proptosis. Some patients complain of headache. SVC obstruction may be due to benign strictures (such as may occur in mediastinal fibrosis or in vasculitic syndromes), but in most cases obstruction is due to neoplastic lesions in the mediastinum. SVC stenosis may also occur as a result of long-term central venous catheters. Superior vena cavography, contrast-enhanced CT or MRI must be used as the first investigations, as the SVC cannot be assessed with ultrasound.

VISCERAL VEINS

HEPATIC VEINS

Thrombosis or occlusion of the main hepatic veins leads to the **Budd–Chiari syndrome**, which comprises abdominal pain, ascites and hepatomegaly. The condition can occur as a result of hypercoagulable states, such as polycythaemia rubra vera, tumours or trauma, but in many cases the cause is unknown. The caudate lobe of the liver is usually spared because it drains directly into the IVC by small veins that remain patent. As a consequence of the impaired function of the rest of the liver, caudate lobe hypertrophy often results. A similar clinical presentation to Budd–Chiari syndrome may result from membranous obstruction of the terminal portion of the IVC. The diagnosis of Budd–Chiari syndrome may be made by colour Doppler ultrasound, hepatic venography, contrast-enhanced CT, MRI or liver biopsy.

Colour Doppler ultrasound

The normal hepatic veins are clearly visible and flow within them is readily demonstrated using Doppler ultrasound. When the hepatic veins are occluded, they are difficult to visualize and no flow can be shown. Instead, many small collateral vessels are visible. In established cases of Budd–Chiari syndrome the caudate lobe may become markedly hypertrophied.

Hepatic venography

Until the advent of CT and MRI, the diagnosis of Budd–Chiari syndrome was made with hepatic venography or liver biopsy. When the main hepatic veins are occluded, it may be difficult or impossible to catheterize them. When selective cannulation is successful, contrast injection may show thrombus in the lumen or, in chronic cases, a mass of fine collaterals instead of the usual branching pattern of the normal veins (Fig. 27.17).

(a)

(b)

Figure 27.17 *Budd–Chiari syndrome. (a) Acute stage. Selective hepatic venography showing occlusive thrombus with the lumen of the main hepatic vein. (By courtesy of Dr R.H.S. Gregson, University Hospital Nottingham.) (b) Chronic stage. In this case, a hepatic venogram shows that, although the main vein is patent, the normal branching pattern of its tributaries is lost and a mesh of fine collaterals is visible instead. Compare with a normal hepatic venogram (Fig. 27.3). (By courtesy of Dr G. Steele, Derbyshire Royal Infirmary.)*

CT and MRI

The appearances at contrast-enhanced CT may be diagnostic. There is a characteristic mottling to the pattern of contrast enhancement of the hepatic parenchyma, and occluding material may also be visible in the IVC (Fig. 27.18). Features that may be detected on MRI include inhomogeneity of signal intensity and intrahepatic anastomoses. Both CT and MRI will detect general hepatic enlargement in the acute stage, and disproportionate caudate lobe enlargement in long-standing cases and ascites.

Figure 27.18 *Budd–Chiari syndrome. CT showing patchy contrast enhancement of the liver. The IVC also contains thrombus (arrow) and there is some ascites (arrowheads).*

Figure 27.19 *Portal vein thrombosis. CT showing recent portal vein thrombosis. Clot is visible as a filling defect within the vein (arrows). The scan also shows fatty change within most of the liver and a small amount of ascites (arrowheads). See also Plate 22, opposite p. 358. (By courtesy of Dr S. Amar, University Hospital Nottingham.)*

PORTAL VEIN

Portal vein thrombosis

In most cases, patency of the portal vein can be demonstrated with colour Doppler ultrasound (Plate 22, opposite p. 358). However, Doppler ultrasound is not a completely reliable test, since very slow flow may be undetectable. If the portal vein appears normal but blood flow cannot be shown, confirmatory evidence of portal vein occlusion such as the presence of collateral veins should be sought (Plate 23, opposite p. 358). If there is doubt about the ultrasound diagnosis of portal vein occlusion, further imaging with contrast-enhanced CT (Fig. 27.19) or MRI will be necessary.

Portal hypertension

Portal hypertension is usually due to hepatic disease. The hepatic abnormality may be presinusoidal (such as in schistosomiasis), sinusoidal (as in cirrhosis) or post-sinusoidal (as in Budd–Chiari syndrome or hepatic veno-occlusive disease). Portal hypertension may also be due to extrahepatic conditions such as portal vein occlusion. The commonest cause of portal hypertension in western countries is alcoholic cirrhosis.

The main adverse effect of portal hypertension is the development of varices, which are enlarged tortuous venous collaterals that form between the portal and systemic circulations (Fig. 27.20).

RENAL VEINS

Renal vein thrombosis can occur in a number of conditions such as dehydration, hypercoagulable states, renal tumours, renal parenchymal disease, renal trauma and caval thrombosis. It may be sudden and complete (leading to venous infarction of the kidney) or subacute, in which case perfusion of the kidney is maintained but the nephrotic syndrome occurs as a sequel. In complete renal vein thrombosis, the presence of thrombus within the vein may be visualized with ultrasound, CT, MRI or venography, and the intravenous urogram will show an enlarged, poorly or non-functioning kidney with a reduced or absent nephrogram. In subacute renal vein thrombosis, thrombus may be confined to tributaries of the main renal vein, requiring selective renal venography for its demonstration.

INTERVENTIONAL PROCEDURES

VENOUS THROMBOLYSIS

Catheter-directed thrombolysis, with the use of streptokinase, urokinase or recombinant tissue plasminogen

(a)

(b)

Figure 27.20 *Gastric varices. (a) Transjugular, transhepatic portogram, performed as part of the TIPS procedure (see also p. 299) showing large varices (V). (b) Completion portogram following construction of the shunt and embolization of the varices with Gianturco steel coils (arrows). S = Sengstaken tube.*

activator (rt-PA), is an established method of treatment for arterial occlusion. The technique has also been used in the management of selected patients with extensive, iliofemoral deep vein thrombosis. The thrombolytic agent is administered by infusion through a catheter placed directly into the occluding thrombus. There is an increased risk of thromboembolism because of fragmentation of the dissolving thrombus, so a temporary vena caval filter is deployed as the first stage of the procedure (Fig. 27.21). In about 50 per cent of cases, thrombolysis will reveal an underlying venous anomaly or abnormality, which can be treated by the insertion of a stent (see below). Successful recannalization leads to rapid resolution of the acute symptoms such as oedema. Whether successful thrombolysis reduces the risk of subsequent chronic venous disease in the postphlebitic limb is yet to be determined.

VENOUS STENTS

Expandable metallic stents are cylindrical in shape and constructed from stainless steel or nitinol in such a way that they can be collapsed into or onto a narrow diameter delivery device. Examples are the **Wallstent** and the **Gianturco stent** (Fig. 27.22). When deployed in strictures smaller than their maximum diameter, stents generate a constant radial dilating force within the lesion. As a result, significant expansion of the stent often occurs in the days following insertion, even in

lesions that have proved resistant to balloon dilatation. Pathological examination of stents that have been in place for weeks or months has shown that they often become incorporated into the vessel wall during this period.

Venous stents are used for the treatment of obstruction of major veins, such as the iliac veins and the IVC or the brachiocephalic veins and the SVC. Radiotherapy is used to treat malignant strictures but relief is not achieved immediately. Benign strictures may be treated by surgical bypass but these have a poor record of long-term patency.

Technique

The position and extent of the stricture are first delineated using venography (Fig. 27.23a). Thrombus may be present and this must be cleared before stent insertion by thrombolysis. With the lumen free of clot, the stricture is traversed using a guidewire and catheter advanced from an appropriate tributary such as the right internal jugular vein or the right common femoral vein. The stent delivery system is then introduced and the stent deployed under fluoroscopic guidance (Fig. 27.23b).

Results

The results are usually very gratifying. For instance, in the case of superior vena caval obstruction, there is immediate relief of headache with resolution of oedema

(a)

(c)

Figure 27.21 *Venous thrombolysis. (a) Initial venogram showing complete thrombosis of the left iliac veins. (b) Completion study following lysis and stent insertion. (c) The temporary vena caval filter inserted at the beginning of the procedure. Embolic thrombus (T) is visible within the filter, which cleared sufficiently with continuation of lysis for a further 12 hours.*

(b)

over the next 24 hours. The long-term patency of the SVC after stent insertion is good. Most patients with malignant strictures will die from the underlying condition without recurrence of the symptoms of SVC obstruction, but in a small number, signs of obstruction will return owing to overgrowth of tumour at the stent margins. Encouraging long-term patency has also been reported in benign disease.

Figure 27.22 *Self-expanding vascular stent: Wallstent (Boston Scientific).*

(a)   *(b)*

Figure 27.23 *Venous stent. (a) SVC stenosis (arrows) due to a mediastinal tumour, shown after simultaneous contrast injection into both antecubital veins. RBV = right brachiocephalic vein; LBV = left brachiocephalic vein; RA = right atrium. (b) Same patient 4 days after insertion of a linked pair of self-expanding Gianturco stents (S) within the stricture.*

INFERIOR VENA CAVAL FILTERS

The majority of patients with deep vein thrombosis or pulmonary embolism can be managed satisfactorily with anticoagulation alone. Difficulties arise when pulmonary embolism occurs despite effective anticoagulation, or when anticoagulant treatment is complicated or contraindicated. In these circumstances, an inferior vena caval filter is inserted to act as a trap for emboli originating in the pelvis and lower limbs.

There are a number of varieties of vena caval filters (Fig. 27.24). Most are permanent implants such as the Greenfield filter, Antheor filter and Bird's Nest filter.

The Greenfield and Antheor filters both present funnel-shaped cages to the venous flow from the pelvis. The funnel shape causes trapped emboli to be held in the central portion of the filter, away from the vein wall, to reduce the likelihood of IVC occlusion. The Bird's Nest filter consists of two V-shaped wire barbs, which fix to the IVC wall, connected by a fine wire mesh. The mesh fills the IVC lumen and traps embolic particles (Fig. 27.25). Temporary vena caval filters are available, which remain attached to an intravenous catheter, allowing their later removal. These devices are used to provide temporary protection from pulmonary embolism during periods of excessively high risk.

(a)   *(b)*   *(c)*

Figure 27.24 *Types of vena caval filters. (a) Greenfield filter (Boston Scientific), (b) Antheor filter (Boston Scientific) and (c) Bird's Nest filter (Cook Inc., Bloomington, USA).*

Figure 27.25 Bird's Nest vena caval filter (Cook Inc., Bloomington, USA.) Inferior vena cavogram performed immediately after insertion. The arrows point to the four anchoring feet of the filter (see also Fig. 27.24c). Thrombus (T) is present in the IVC below the filter, arising from the left iliac vein. R = renal veins.

Technique

The right femoral vein is usually used for access unless the lower IVC or right iliac veins are occluded, in which case the right internal jugular vein is used. Preliminary inferior vena cavography is essential to show the level of the renal veins, to demonstrate the presence and extent of any thrombus within the IVC itself and to measure the size of the IVC. With the exception of the Bird's Nest filter, which has no predefined shape and can be used in any size cava, vena caval filters should not be used if the diameter of the IVC is too large because this increases the risk of filter migration. The filter is normally deployed below the level of the renal veins so that, should IVC thrombosis occur, the renal veins will not be affected. In some circumstances infrarenal placement may not be possible, necessitating deployment in the suprarenal cava.

Complications

The main risks of IVC filters are IVC occlusion and migration of the filter. With modern filters, the risk of complication is low. Typically, the rate of recurrent pulmonary embolism is reduced to less than 5 per cent.

HICKMAN LINE INSERTION

A Hickman line is a central venous catheter inserted via a subclavian vein that is used for long-term venous access. Typical uses for Hickman lines are the administration of chemotherapy or parenteral nutrition. In order to reduce the chance of infection, the entry points at the skin and the subclavian vein wall are kept as far apart as practical by passing the catheter through a 10–15 cm long subcutaneous tunnel before it enters the vein. The tip of the catheter lies in the SVC where the flow rate and the lumen calibre are greatest.

Technique

A venogram is performed first via an antecubital vein. Using this venogram for guidance, the point where the subclavian vein crosses the undersurface of the clavicle is identified and punctured. A guidewire is passed into the subclavian vein and then into the SVC. Next, a 10–15 cm subcutaneous track is created from the venepuncture site to a point above and lateral to the nipple. The Hickman catheter is passed through this track and then advanced into the vein through a removable sheath until its tip is in the SVC. The catheter hub is fixed to the skin and the skin wounds are sutured.

Complications

The most important complication that may occur is catheter infection and septicaemia. If infection cannot be controlled the catheter will need to be removed. For this reason, insertion is always performed in a clean environment under antibiotic prophylaxis. Other complications that may occur are catheter malposition, catheter thrombosis and cutaneous inflammation at the catheter entry site.

REMOVAL OF INTRAVASCULAR FOREIGN BODY

The vascular system may play host to a variety of foreign bodies. Most are iatrogenic, such as catheter fragments and misplaced embolization coils. The site at which the foreign body locates depends on its size, shape and pliability. Venous foreign bodies will commonly pass to the central veins and from there to the right ventricle and pulmonary arteries. Arterial foreign bodies will be carried to distal sites such as the lower limb. Percutaneous removal with an appropriate retrieval device is the best method of managing such intravascular foreign material.

Figure 27.26 *Goose-Neck snare (Micro-Vena) used for retrieval of intravascular foreign bodies. The loop is manipulated around the object and tightened by withdrawing it into the catheter.*

Technique

A variety of retrieval devices exist. The simplest and perhaps the most elegant is the Goose-Neck snare (Fig. 27.26). The loop is manipulated around the foreign body and then tightened against the guiding catheter by traction on the external wire. Once grasped, the foreign body is withdrawn to the catheter entry site. If small enough it can be simply pulled out, but large objects may require a cut-down. Fortunately, percutaneous foreign body removal has a high rate of success. Complications are few but there is the potential for vascular injury. Catheter manipulation across the right heart may lead to arrhythmias, and care must be employed when objects are retrieved from the right ventricle, in order to avoid injury to the chordae tendinae.

VENOUS EMBOLIZATION

Venous embolization is employed in relatively few clinical settings. Examples include the treatment of varicocele, oesophageal varices (as part of the TIPSS procedure) and some venous malformations of the central nervous system.

Varicocele embolization

A varicocele is an abnormal dilatation of the pampiniform plexus of veins in the scrotum which occurs in

(a)

(b)

Figure 27.27 *Varicocele embolization following unsuccessful surgery. (a) Initial venography showing a dilated and very tortuous left gonadal vein. (b) Following embolization with Gianturco coils (Cook Inc., Bloomington, USA) confirming occlusion of the varicocele.*

Figure 27.28 *Direct percutaneous transhepatic portography and venous sampling in a patient with suspected insulinoma. After the catheter has been positioned, contrast injection is made into the splenic vein (SV). The main portal vein (PV) is also shown. The superior mesenteric vein is not shown, but non-opacified blood from it can be seen entering the portal vein (arrow). The numbers indicate the levels of insulin from samples taken at each site and show a step-up in concentration in the distal splenic vein. An insulinoma was subsequently removed from the tail of the pancreas.*

manoeuvre, is important to demonstrate the anatomy of the gonadal vein and its tributaries. From this study, the appropriate sites for venous occlusion, which will isolate the varicocele, can be determined (Fig. 27.27a). Embolization at these points is then performed, usually with coils (Fig. 27.27b).

VENOUS SAMPLING

Venous sampling is a technique for localization of small endocrine tumours. It is used when inappropriately high hormone levels are present but conventional imaging methods have failed to demonstrate the source. Veins draining the likely site of origin are selectively catheterized and a blood sample taken from each for hormone assay. The results are then plotted on an image of the venous anatomy (Fig. 27.28). Abnormally high hormone levels are found in the veins draining the location of the tumour. In some cases, sampling is performed following injection of the appropriate secretagogue to increase the sensitivity of the test. Venous sampling is applicable to many different hormone-secreting lesions, such as pituitary, parathyroid, thyroid, adrenal, pancreatic and carcinoid tumours. It is, however, an expensive examination to perform and there is scope for error because of the considerable variability in venous anatomy and patterns of drainage.

FURTHER READING

Armon, M.P., Whitaker, S.C., Tennant, W.G. 1997: Catheter-directed thrombolysis of iliofemoral deep vein thrombosis. A new approach via the posterior tibial vein. *European Journal of Vascular & Endovascular Surgery* **13**, 413–16.

Moody, A.R., Pollock, J.G., O'Connor, A.R., Bagnall, M. 1998: Lower-limb venous thrombosis: direct MR imaging of the thrombus. *Radiology* **209**, 349–55.

Prince, M.R., Gist, T.M., Debatin, J.F. 1999: *3D Contrast MR angiography.* New York, NY: Springer Verlag.

Verhaeghe, R., Stockx, L., Lacroix, H., Vermylen, J., Baert, A.L. 1997: Catheter-directed lysis of iliofemoral vein thrombosis with use of rt-PA. *European Radiology* **7**, 996–1001.

approximately 10–20 per cent of healthy males. Symptoms include reduced testicular growth in the adolescent and scrotal pain, swelling or infertility in the adult. The great majority of cases involve the left side of the scrotum, with a small number involving both sides. Rarely the right side is involved alone. A small number of varicoceles are found to be secondary to venous compression by an intra-abdominal or pelvic mass such as a lymphoma.

The appropriate gonadal vein is catheterized with an angiographic catheter introduced via either a common femoral vein or the right internal jugular vein. Pre-embolization venography, with hand injection of contrast agent while the patient performs a Valsalva

Index

Page numbers in *italic* indicate an illustration that appears on a different page from its text.